COVID-19 and Well-being

LIFE IN THE PANDEMIC

OECD

BETTER POLICIES FOR BETTER LIVES

Please cite this publication as:
OECD (2021), *COVID-19 and Well-being: Life in the Pandemic*, OECD Publishing, Paris, *https://doi.org/10.1787/1e1ecb53-en*.

ISBN 978-92-64-87183-0 (print)
ISBN 978-92-64-50537-7 (pdf)

Corrigenda to publications may be found on line at: *www.oecd.org/about/publishing/corrigenda.htm*.

Foreword

This report examines the emerging evidence on well-being outcomes for OECD countries in the first 15 months after COVID-19 was declared a pandemic by the World Health Organisation (i.e. March 2020 – June 2021). As part of the *How's Life?* series of reports, it follows the structure of the OECD Well-Being Framework, spanning current well-being, inclusion and sustainability. Thus, the report provides a holistic picture of how people's lives have been affected so far, how these impacts have differed across population groups, and what is happening to the stocks of resources (natural, economic, human and social capital) that help to sustain well-being over time. In addition, the report considers how a well-being lens can inform policy development and the design of pandemic recovery strategies, as well as to achieve stronger strategic alignment across public agencies and between public, private and civil society actors.

The report was prepared by the OECD WISE Centre. The authoring team consisted of: Margreet Frieling (Chapter 1); Gaia Bottura (Chapters 2 and 5); Jessica Mahoney (Chapters 3, 6 and 9); Lara Fleischer (Chapters 4, 7 and 10); Hae Ryun Kim (Chapter 8); and Carrie Exton (Chapter 11). Statistical support was provided by Mónica Quinza Armenta. Carrie Exton led the project and content editing, Marco Mira d'Ecole provided additional supervision and editing, and the report was published under the direction of Romina Boarini. Martine Zaida, Anne-Lise Faron, Julia Carro and Sonia Primot coordinated and assisted communications and publishing, and Gísli Gylfason designed the country profiles. Meral Gedik formatted and typeset the manuscript for publication. Patrick Hamm copy edited the work.

The report has benefitted from valuable comments provided by national delegates to the OECD Committee on Statistics and Statistical Policy and the Working Party on Social Policy under the OECD Employment, Labour and Social Affairs Committee. Their contributions and advice are very gratefully acknowledged.

We are also grateful to many colleagues in the OECD and beyond for their help, comments, insights and data, and edits either on draft text or in relation to specific queries. They include, but are not limited to:

- Andrea Bassanini, Sandrine Cazes, Michele Cecchini, Valerie Frey, Pauline Fron, Emily Hewlett, Alexander Hijzen, Chris James, Sebastian Könings, Gaetan Lafortune, Thomas Liebig, Pascal Marianna, David Morgan, Veronica Nilsson, Marissa Plouin, Christopher Prinz, Glenda Quintini, Angelica Salvi Del Pero, Shunta Takino and Chloé Touzet (OECD Employment, Labour and Social Affairs Directorate);
- Aimée Augilar Jaber, Katia Karousakis and Edward Perry (OECD Environment Directorate);
- Tracey Burns and Miyako Ikeda (OECD Education Directorate);
- Benoît Arnaud, Rachida Dkhissi, Annabelle Mourougane, Bettina Wistrom, Isabelle Ynesta, and Jorrit Zwijnenburg (OECD Statistics and Data Directorate);
- Boris Cournede and Federica De Pace (OECD Economics Department);
- Nadim Ahmad, Andrés Fuentes Hutfilter, Andrew Paterson, Lisanne Raderschall, and Paolo Veneri, (OECD Centre for Entrepreneurship, SMEs, Regions and Cities);
- Monica Brezzi, Marcos Díaz Ramírez, Santiago Gonzalez (OECD Public Governance Directorate);
- Janine Treves (OECD Public Affairs and Communications Directorate);
- Mario Barreto and Rachele Poggi (International Transport Forum);
- Musa Erdogan and Timothy Goodson (International Energy Agency);
- Jorge Castro, Mental Health Evidence & Research (World Health Organization);
- Susan Purcell, Market Strategy & Understanding (Ipsos);
- Hannes Kroeger and Laura Buchinger, (German Institute for Economic Research, DIW Berlin);
- Ezter Sandor, Sarah Farrell and Daphne Nathalie Ahrendt (Eurofound).

Table of contents

FIGURES

TABLES

Reader's guide

General methods and data considerations

As a starting point, this report draws on the same indicators and sources used in the *How's Life? 2020* report. This is feasible for some aspects of material well-being and economic capital in particular, as well as for data from the Gallup World Poll, used in the absence of harmonised official data sources for a limited number of indicators. However, for other outcomes, the report relies on a number of ad-hoc studies and new data collections that have emerged during the crisis. At the national level, these sources range from experimental time use studies (UK Office of National Statistics) to 'crowdsourced' mental health data (Statistics Canada), a Household Pulse Survey (United States Census Bureau), and the SOEP-Cov study in Germany. In other cases, existing data collections have been adapted – for example, Stats NZ introduced supplemental well-being questions in the Household Labour Force Survey in 2020, providing quarterly estimates of outcomes such as life satisfaction. At the international level, novel data collections include the Eurofound *Living, Working and COVID-19 Study;* the Imperial College London/YouGov *COVID-19 Public Monitor*, and the *REpresentations, PErceptions and ATtitudes on COVID-19* (REPEAT) survey from Sciences Po. Within the OECD, existing data collections such as the *Risks That Matter* survey have been adapted to address COVID-19 relevant concerns.

Several of the data sources used in the Evidence Scan build on existing survey vehicles and questionnaire items, but in some cases, the absence of comparable baseline data makes it difficult to provide an accurate account of pandemic *impacts*. The uneven and intersectional impacts of the pandemic across the population emphasise the need for large-sample representative studies that enable data to be disaggregated and cross tabulated with confidence – which is not always possible for smaller ad hoc studies. At the same time, the process of data collection has itself been heavily disrupted by the pandemic. For example, several data producers switched from face-to-face to other survey modes. The exceptional circumstances also mean that online-only methods and unconventional sampling strategies have occasionally been adopted (e.g. convenience sampling methods used for the Eurofound study). Post-hoc adjustments to survey weights are often applied to correct for the most easily addressed sources of bias, but these methods do not fully address the non-representativeness of the data when, for example, respondents are self-selecting.

Due to the constraints of the available data, some OECD countries have better coverage than others, direct country comparisons are not always feasible, and good 2019 baseline data are often lacking. It is also not possible to apply the more rigorous data quality standards adopted in *How's Life?* throughout this report. Instead, the chapters include brief boxes that describe key data sources, and results should be interpreted with these methodological details in mind.

Note on the timing of data collections, and particularly the Gallup World Poll 2020

Throughout the first 15 months of the pandemic covered by this report, well-being outcomes have been a moving target. It is rarely safe to generalise results beyond the months in which data were collected, as both disease risk and pandemic restrictions shifted – and often in different cycles among different OECD countries. All figures in this report therefore specify the month and year of data collection, as appropriate. A variety of online dynamic dashboards can be consulted to obtain information about the pandemic context in each OECD country at different points in time during 2020 and 2021. For example, the OECD Coronavirus web pages https://www.oecd.org/coronavirus/en/, and the Our World in Data COVID-19 data explorer https://ourworldindata.org/coronavirus.

For most comparative data, fieldwork dates are broadly harmonised across countries. However, as discussed in Chapter 3, Box 3.4, the fieldwork dates for the Gallup World Poll vary across OECD countries, from February-March 2020, to November-December 2020. Gallup World Poll data are used in this report to illustrate two aspects of subjective well-being (life satisfaction and affect balance), as well as social network support, feelings of safety, and trust in government. Table 1 describes some key pandemic context variables in each OECD country both during the time of the Gallup World Poll fieldwork, and during the year to date by the end of the fieldwork period in 2020. Sample sizes were approximately 1000 people in all OECD countries except Iceland, where it was 501. Prior to 2020, data in the majority of OECD countries was already collected entirely via telephone interviewing. However, in 14 OECD countries (Chile, Colombia, Costa Rica, the Czech Republic, Estonia, Greece, Hungary, Israel, Lithuania, Latvia, Mexico, Poland, the Slovak Republic and Turkey) interviews previously conducted face-to-face in 2019 were switched to telephone-based in 2020, which may result in some mode effects. In this publication, all countries with data collection method switches are marked with † in figures.

Table 1. Gallup World Poll fieldwork dates and COVID-19 context variables

Country Code	Fieldwork start date	Fieldwork end date	Rate of excess deaths during fieldwork (compared to 2015-19)	COVID-19 deaths during fieldwork period	Rate of excess deaths from start of 2020 to end of fieldwork	Total COVID-19 deaths from start of 2020 to end of fieldwork	Stringency Index, average during fieldwork
AUS	04-02-2020	22-03-2020	5%	7	5%	7	23
AUT	24-08-2020	19-09-2020	8%	29	3%	788	37
BEL	19-08-2020	19-09-2020	4%	137	10%	9 977	54
CAN	03-08-2020	21-09-2020	11%	327	11%	9 217	66
CHL	11-09-2020	16-11-2020	14%	3 227	17%	14 819	82
COL	21-08-2020	27-10-2020	48%	15 057	26%	30 154	74
CRI	15-09-2020	04-01-2021	..	..	..	..	58
CZE	09-10-2020	28-11-2020	69%	7 694	14%	8 467	65
DNK	14-09-2020	10-10-2020	2%	42	0%	669	49
EST	14-10-2020	20-11-2020	2%	20	1%	88	37
FIN	26-03-2020	13-05-2020	8%	288	1%	299	62
FRA	07-09-2020	02-10-2020	8%	1 624	7%	32 230	49
DEU	24-08-2020	10-09-2020	6%	154	2%	9 386	54
GRC	23-09-2020	24-10-2020	5%	236	4%	574	55
HUN	19-10-2020	17-11-2020	37%	2 222	2%	3 190	51
ISL	31-08-2020	12-10-2020	2%	0	1%	10	41
IRL	17-08-2020	12-09-2020	..	..	..	..	67
ISR	24-09-2020	19-10-2020	33%	953	10%	2 209	85
ITA	24-08-2020	16-09-2020	7%	311	10%	35 707	54
JPN	07-08-2020	08-10-2020	..	..	..	..	32
KOR	25-08-2020	07-10-2020	..	..	..	..	53
LTU	08-10-2020	26-11-2020	22%	412	3%	506	53
LVA	10-09-2020	31-10-2020	1%	39	-2%	74	37
MEX	08-09-2020	18-11-2020	54%	37 518	49%	101 676	72
NLD	11-03-2020	15-05-2020	34%	5 677	14%	5 680	74
NOR	24-03-2020	04-05-2020	4%	207	-1%	208	74
NZL	17-02-2020	23-03-2020	7%	0	5%	0	26
POL	25-09-2020	24-10-2020	28%	2 145	6%	4 438	34
PRT	20-03-2020	16-04-2020	18%	714	2%	714	82
SVK	09-09-2020	09-10-2020	7%	24	1%	61	37
SVN	13-03-2020	18-04-2020	3%	74	-1%	74	76
ESP	24-08-2020	17-09-2020	15%	2 017	18%	30 663	62

SWE	30-03-2020	29-04-2020	34%	3 051	7%	3 143	62
CHE	07-09-2020	09-10-2020	3%	69	3%	1 793	39
TUR	03-10-2020	23-10-2020	..	..	..	..	71
GBR	17-08-2020	12-09-2020	2%	599	14%	56 957	66
USA	16-03-2020	08-05-2020	28%	87 499	14%	87 560	68

Note: Luxembourg was not included in the 2020 Gallup World Poll. Data relating to excess mortality are sourced from (OECD, n.d.[1]); excess deaths are measured as the increase in the number of reported deaths from all causes during the time period, compared to the average number from 2015-19 for the same period. The Stringency Index is sourced from the COVID-19 Government Response Tracker (Hale et al., 2021[2]). It runs from 0 (least stringent) to 100 (most stringent), and combines data on school closures, workplace closures, cancellation of public events, restrictions on gatherings, closing of public transport, stay-at-home requirements, restrictions on internal movement, and international travel controls.

Source: OECD calculations based on the Gallup World Poll (2021[3]) (database), https://www.gallup.com/178667/gallup-world-poll-work.aspx; OECD (n.d.[1]), COVID-19 Health Indicators (database) https://stats.oecd.org/index.aspx?queryid=104676#; Hale et.al (2021[2]), "A global panel database of pandemic policies (Oxford COVID-19 Government Response Tracker)", Nature Human Behaviour, Vol. 5/4, pp. 529-538, http://dx.doi.org/10.1038/s41562-021-01079-8

Note on terminology for the inclusion chapters

Some of the inequalities addressed in the inclusion chapters (5, 6 and 7) pertain to aspects of diversity for which data collection was already sparse before 2020. Context and country matter for how terms such as "race", "ethnicity", "migrant status" and "Indigenous identity" are understood - and with the exception of migrant status (when defined as people born abroad), there are no internationally comparable definitions for describing these very different aspects of diversity. Measurement approaches and regulations that underpin the collection of what is often considered sensitive data differ across OECD governments, with practices clustered in three broad categories (Figure 1). All OECD countries collect information on diversity proxies such as country of birth.[1] A small majority (mostly Eastern European countries as well as the United Kingdom and Ireland) gather additional information on race and ethnicity. Finally, only a handful of countries in the Americas and Oceania collect data on Indigenous identity. By addressing these different aspects of diversity, this chapter does not imply that the situation, including the legal status, of different minority communities across the OECD is the same and that these can be directly compared. Rather, it aims to provide evidence on the well-being impacts such communities have faced during the pandemic and which can help devise locally appropriate policy solutions.

The norms around appropriate terminology are evolving even in countries that are advanced in diversity data collection. For instance, in the United Kingdom, the Commission on Race and Ethnic Disparities recommended in March 2021 that the government stop using the term "BAME" (Black, Asian and minority ethnic) because it emphasises certain ethnic groups (Asian and Black) and excludes others (Mixed, Other and white ethnic minority groups) (Commission on Race and Ethnic Disparities, 2021[4]). The government is currently considering its response to the Commission's recommendations. In Canada, the term "visible minority" is an official demographic category defined by the Canadian Employment Equity Act, and is used by Statistics Canada in their work. The Employment Equity Act defines visible minorities as "persons, other than Aboriginal peoples, who are non-Caucasian in race or non-white in colour". The visible minority population consists mainly of the following groups: South Asian, Chinese, Black, Filipino, Latin American, Arab, Southeast Asian, West Asian, Korean and Japanese (Statistics Canada, 2015[5]). However, the question of appropriate terminology is currently being reviewed in Canada, in the context of a task force on modernizing the Employment Equity Act (Department of Finance Canada, 2021[6]). This report has generally used the terminology adopted by data producers at the time of writing, while recognising that the racial and ethnic categories used are socially constructed and situational rather than static (Balestra and Fleischer, 2018[7]).[2]

Figure 1. Diversity collection practices across the OECD

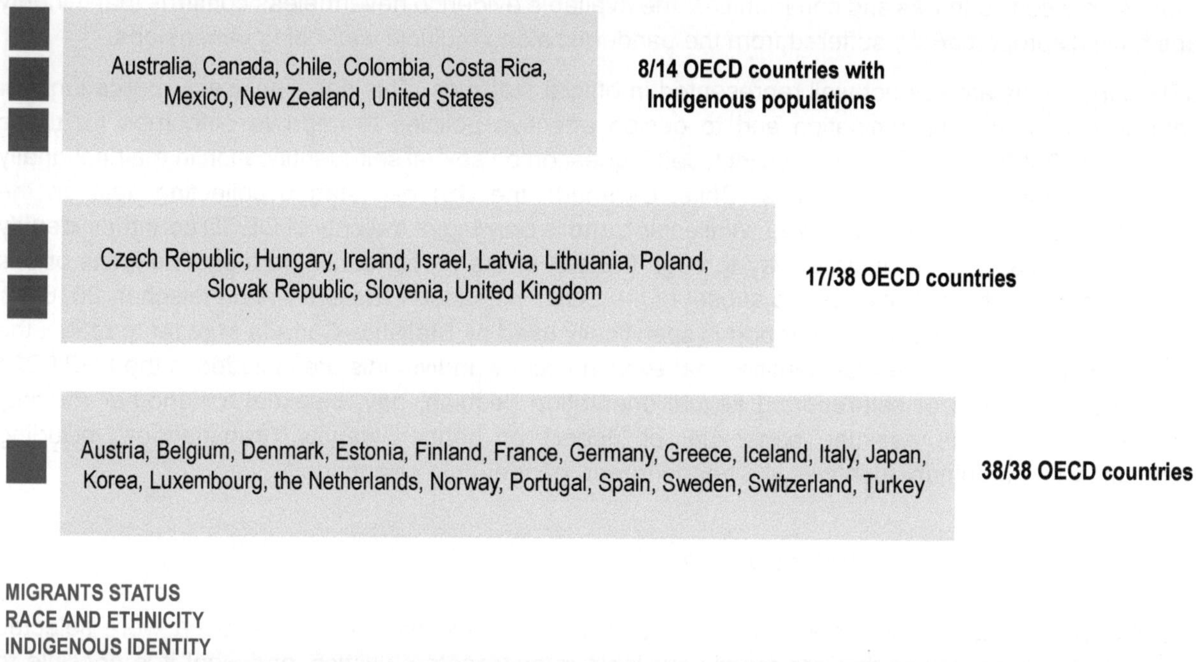

Note: A country is listed as collecting a type of diversity data if at least one source (e.g. census, sample survey, population registry) includes relevant information. As not all OECD countries have Indigenous populations, the denominator is set at 14 for this category.
Source: Balestra, C. and L. Fleischer (2018[7]), "Diversity statistics in the OECD: How do OECD countries collect data on ethnic, racial and indigenous identity?", *OECD Statistics Working Papers*, No. 2018/09, OECD Publishing, Paris, https://dx.doi.org/10.1787/89bae654-en.

Assessing the extent to which COVID-19 has affected different racial and ethnic communities is challenging. Basic statistics on the number and characteristics of COVID-19 cases are registered by national health systems, based on administrative sources such as testing and hospitalisations. Not all OECD countries consistently record diversity information (or other key socio-economic variables) in case numbers, hospital records or on death certificates, or do not always transmit these data for the compilation of national health and mortality statistics. For example, information on ethnicity or migrant status on death certificates is not transferred to the federal level in Germany; is incompletely recorded in Scotland; and not at all in England, Wales and Northern Ireland. This implies that data from census records, death registrations and hospital statistics in the latter countries have to be linked to provide information about the impact of COVID-19 by ethnicity (OECD, 2020[8]; ONS, 2020[9]). Many states in the United States have been slow to implement this practice: in May 2020, 51% of cases and 88% of deaths had an identified race (though states have been working to identify the race of deaths previously recorded without) and by September 2020, only 65% of new cases included an identified race/ethnicity code (The COVID Tracking Project, 2020[10]; NPR, 2020[11]). A year on, 39% of all cumulative cases recorded by April 2021 lacked this information (CDC, 2021[12]). American Indians and Alaska Natives in the United States and First Nations, Inuit and Métis communities in Canada, many of whom operate their own health systems, are also not officially required to report COVID-19 data. What is more, numbers of confirmed cases by ethnicity or origin are impacted by the ability of each country to reach the most vulnerable groups. For example, rates of testing among Veterans in the United States up to July 2020 have been found to be lower for Hispanic/Latino and Black communities compared to whites, for instance (Rentsch et al., 2020[13]). Hence, relative COVID-19 related risks among groups, especially those of younger ages less likely to show symptoms, are likely to be underestimated. Moreover, many population surveys, especially the non-official and experimental ones launched throughout 2020 to capture the pandemic's psychosocial impact in real-time, often either do not contain questions on identity, or have such small sample sizes that any statements would be misleading. With these caveats in mind, and recognising that the situation is constantly evolving and varies between countries and communities, the available evidence nevertheless confirms that minority groups have disproportionally suffered from the pandemic along multiple well-being dimensions.

LGBTI+ populations are still not well represented in official statistics. This has significant implications for our ability to measure discrimination and to design effective policies to improve outcomes for these populations. In 2019, 15 OECD countries included a question on sexual self-identification in their nationally representative surveys and 3 countries (Chile, Denmark, the US) had started collecting data on the transgender population (OECD, 2019[14]). While this trend is growing, a majority of OECD countries identify the LGBTI+ population in an indirect way through the sex of the respondent's partner. The limits of this approach are clear as it only captures a subset of the LGBT population (Balestra and Fleischer, 2018[7]).[3] The LGBTQ2+ acronym found in this report is specifically used by Statistics Canada in order to reflect the broad scope of gender and sexual identities that exist in society. Individuals are included in the LGBTQ2+ population on the basis of self-reported sexual orientation (lesbian, gay, bisexual, or another minority sexual identity such as asexual, pansexual or queer) or gender identity (transgender, including respondents with non-binary identities like genderqueer, gender fluid or agender).

Breakdowns considered in inclusion analyses

Age and education ranges considered in the inequalities sections throughout this report were selected according to the breakdowns that are readily available in aggregate statistics, and what it is possible to compile on an internationally comparable basis.

- Specific age ranges for each indicator are reported in the respective figure or figure note.
- The education ranges refer to the highest level of education completed, and correspond to ISCED levels 0-2 for "below upper secondary" level (i.e. less than primary, primary and lower secondary); 3-4 for "upper secondary" level (i.e. secondary and post-secondary non-tertiary education); and 5-8 for "tertiary" level. For individual country-level mappings to the ISCED 2011 classifications, please see http://uis.unesco.org/en/isced-mappings.
- Indicators sourced from the Gallup World Poll form an exception and correspond to completed elementary education or less (up to eight years of basic education), completed some secondary education up to three years tertiary education (nine to 15 years of education), and completed four years of education beyond "high school" and/or received a four-year college degree. These levels are described as "primary", "secondary" and "tertiary" in the report.
- In a small number of cases, data disaggregations lead to small effective sample sizes. Where this is the case, asterisks are used as described in the figure notes to signal small effective sample sizes. Data are not reported where fewer than 100 observations are available. ** denotes countries with between 100 and 300 observations per category; * denotes countries with between 301 and 500 observations per category. Where no asterisks are used, this indicates that more than 500 observations per category and per country are available.

Conventions for figures in the report

- In each figure, data labelled "OECD" are simple mean averages of the OECD countries displayed, unless otherwise indicated. Whenever data is available for less than all 38 OECD countries, the number of countries included in the calculation is specified in the figure (e.g. OECD 33).
- A weighted OECD average has been chosen in instances where the OECD convention is to provide this type of average. Where used, this is specified in the figure notes along with details of the weighting methodology. For example, when data are population-weighted this is done according to the size of the population in different countries, as a proportion of the total OECD population. Similarly, when OECD total sums instead of averages are used, this is indicated as "OECD Total".
- Where trend lines are shown in the figures, the OECD averages refer to only those countries with data available for every consecutive year, since the OECD average needs to consider the same sample of countries in each year. As only countries with a complete time series and no gaps can be included, this can sometimes lead to different OECD averages for trend lines versus the latest and earliest available time points.
- Each figure specifies the time period covered, and figure notes provide further details when data refer to different time periods for different countries. Countries are referred to by their ISO codes (Table 2).

Table 2. ISO codes for countries and word regions

AUS	Australia	**FIN**	Finland	**MEX**	Mexico
AUT	Austria	**FRA**	France	**NLD**	Netherlands
BEL	Belgium	**GBR**	United Kingdom	**NOR**	Norway
BRA	Brazil	**GRC**	Greece	**NZL**	New Zealand
CAN	Canada	**HUN**	Hungary	**OECD**	OECD average
CHE	Switzerland	**IRL**	Ireland	**POL**	Poland
CHL	Chile	**ISL**	Iceland	**PRT**	Portugal
COL	Colombia	**ISR**	Israel	**RUS**	Russian Federation
CRI	Costa Rica	**ITA**	Italy	**SVK**	Slovak Republic
CZE	Czech Republic	**JPN**	Japan	**SVN**	Slovenia
DEU	Germany	**KOR**	Korea	**SWE**	Sweden
DNK	Denmark	**LTU**	Lithuania	**TUR**	Turkey
ESP	Spain	**LUX**	Luxembourg	**USA**	United States
EST	Estonia	**LVA**	Latvia	**ZAF**	South Africa

References

Balestra, C. and L. Fleischer (2018), "Diversity statistics in the OECD: How do OECD countries collect data on ethnic, racial and indigenous identity?", *OECD Statistics Working Papers*, No. 2018/09, OECD Publishing, Paris, https://dx.doi.org/10.1787/89bae654-en. [7]

CDC (2021), *COVID-19 Hospitalization and Death by Race/Ethnicity*, https://www.cdc.gov/coronavirus/2019-ncov/covid-data/investigations-discovery/hospitalization-death-by-race-ethnicity.html#footnote01 (accessed on 11 February 2021). [12]

Commission on Race and Ethnic Disparities (2021), *Foreword, introduction, and full recommendations*, https://www.gov.uk/government/publications/the-report-of-the-commission-on-race-and-ethnic-disparities/foreword-introduction-and-full-recommendations#full-recommendations (accessed on 17 June 2021). [4]

Department of Finance Canada (2021), *Budget 2021: A Recovery Plan for Jobs, Growth, and Resilience, Annex 4: Gender, Diversity, and Quality of Life Statement*, https://www.budget.gc.ca/2021/report-rapport/anx4-en.html (accessed on 17 June 2021). [6]

Gallup (2021), *Gallup World Poll*, https://www.gallup.com/analytics/318875/global-research.aspx (accessed on 18 June 2021). [3]

Hale, T. et al. (2021), "A global panel database of pandemic policies (Oxford COVID-19 Government Response Tracker)", *Nature Human Behaviour*, Vol. 5/4, pp. 529-538, http://dx.doi.org/10.1038/s41562-021-01079-8. [2]

NPR (2020), *As Pandemic Deaths Add Up, Racial Disparities Persist — And In Some Cases Worsen*, https://www.npr.org/sections/health-shots/2020/09/23/914427907/as-pandemic-deaths-add-up-racial-disparities-persist-and-in-some-cases-worsen?t=1608509692531&t=1612899321921 (accessed on 9 February 2021). [11]

OECD (2020), "What is the impact of the COVID-19 pandemic on immigrants and their children?", *OECD Policy Responses to Coronavirus (COVID-19)*, OECD Publishing, Paris, https://dx.doi.org/10.1787/e7cbb7de-en. [8]

OECD (2019), *Society at a Glance 2019: OECD Social Indicators*, OECD Publishing, Paris, https://dx.doi.org/10.1787/soc_glance-2019-en. [14]

OECD (n.d.), *COVID-19 Health Indicators (database)*, https://stats.oecd.org/index.aspx?queryid=104676# (accessed on 19 September 2021). [1]

ONS (2020), *Updating ethnic contrasts in deaths involving the coronavirus (COVID-19), England and Wales: deaths occurring 2 March to 28 July 2020*, https://www.ons.gov.uk/peoplepopulationandcommunity/birthsdeathsandmarriages/deaths/articles/updatingethniccontrastsindeathsinvolvingthecoronaviruscovid19englandandwales/deathsoccurring2marchto28july2020#main-points (accessed on 11 February 2021). [9]

Rentsch, C. et al. (2020), "Patterns of COVID-19 testing and mortality by race and ethnicity among United States veterans: A nationwide cohort study", *PLOS Medicine*, Vol. 17/9, http://dx.doi.org/10.1371/journal.pmed.1003379. [13]

Statistics Canada (2015), *Visible minority of person*, https://www23.statcan.gc.ca/imdb/p3Var.pl?Function=DEC&Id=45152 (accessed on 17 June 2021). [5]

The COVID Tracking Project (2020), *The COVID Racial Data Tracker*, https://covidtracking.com/race (accessed on 9 February 2021). [10]

Notes

[1] In general, collecting migration-related information on the foreign-born population and their children is a crude method for capturing diversity. Although such data are relatively readily available and often considered as 'objective', their use as proxy for ethnicity or race is problematic. The country of birth of a person neither takes account of the diversity of the country of origin of the individual or the parents (e.g. 'white' people in the United Kingdom that were born in former British colonies) nor does it capture cultural affiliation, or the inherently self-perceived aspect of belonging to an ethnic group. This view is also reflected in the UN Principles and Recommendations for Population and Housing Censuses, which state that country of birth or citizenship as well as questions on religion and language should not be taken as providing proper ethnic data.

[2] People may change how they identify themselves over time or they may identify themselves differently in different environments, which can be important for the interpretation of data and the dynamics of race and ethnicity.

[3] People may change how they identify themselves over time or they may identify themselves differently in different environments, which can be important for the interpretation of data and the dynamics of race and ethnicity.

Abbreviations and acronyms

ABS	Australian Bureau of Statistics
AFP	Agence France-Presse
AIHW	Australian Institute of Health and Welfare
ANU	Australia National University
ATP	American Trends Panel
APA	American Psychological Association
BKA	Bundeskriminalamt (Federal Criminal Police Office Germany)
BLS	Bureau of Labor Statistics (the United States)
BMI	Body Mass Index
BMBF	Bundesministerium für Bildung und Forschung (German Federal Ministry of Education and Research)
CAMS	Copernicus Atmosphere Monitoring Service
CBC	Canadian Broadcasting Corporation (Canada)
CBS	Central Bureau of Statistics (Israel); Statistics Netherlands
CEPREMAP	Centre pour la recherche économique et ses applications (France)
CCHS	Canadian Community Health Survey
CDC	Centers for Disease Control and Prevention (United States)
COPD	Chronic Obstructive Pulmonary Disease
COVID-19	Coronavirus disease of 2019
CPS	Current Population Survey
CSO	Central Statistics Office (Ireland)
DALY	Disability-adjusted life-year
DANE	Departamento Administrativo Nacional de Estadística (National Administrative Department of Statistics) (Colombia)
DfE	Department for Education (England)
DIW	Deutsches Institut für Wirtschaftsforschung (German Institute for Economic Research)
DIY	Do it yourself craft and building activities
ECLAC	Economic Commission for Latin America
EHIS	European Health Interview Survey
EU	European Union
EU-SILC	European Union Statistics on Income and Living Conditions
EQLS	European Quality of Life Survey
EPA	Environmental Protection Agency (United States)
FBI	Federal Bureau of Investigation (United States)
GAD	Generalised Anxiety Disorder
GDP	Gross Domestic Product
GBP	Pound sterling
GFC	Global Financial Crisis (2008)
GFCF	Gross Fixed Capital Formation
GSS	General Social Survey (Canada, New Zealand)

HCSP	Haut Conseil de la Santé Publique (France)
HLFS	Household Labour Force Survey (New Zealand)
ICNL	The International Center for Not-for-Profit Law
IDEA	International Institute for Democracy and Electoral Assistance
IEA	International Energy Agency
IFRC	International Federation of Red Cross and Red Crescent Societies
ILO	International Labour Organisation
IMF	International Monetary Fund
INE	Instituto Nacional de Estadísticas (National Institute of Statistics) (Chile)
INSEE	Institut national de la statistique et des études économiques (National Institute of Statistics and Economic Studies) (France)
IPU	Inter-Parliamentary Union
LFPR	Labour Force Participation Rate
LFS	Labour Force Survey
LMS	Labour Market Survey
LGBTI+	Lesbian, gay, bisexual, transgender and intersex
LGBTQ+	Lesbian, gay, bisexual, transgender and queer
LGBTQI2S	Lesbian, gay, bisexual, transgender, queer (or questioning), intersex and two-spirit
MNS	Mental, neurological and substance abuse disorders
NCHS	National Center for Health Statistics (United States)
NEET	Young people not in education, employment or training
NHIS	National Health Interview Survey (United States)
NPR	National Public Radio (United States)
ONS	Office for National Statistics (United Kingdom)
OPN	Opinions and Lifestyle Survey (United Kingdom)
PHQ	Patient Health Questionnaire
PISA	Program for International Student Assessment
PYLL	Potential years of life lost
QALY	Quality-adjusted life-year
RIA	Regulatory impact assessment
SARS	Severe acute respiratory syndrome
SDSN	Sustainable Development Solutions Network
SOEP	Sozio-oekonomisches Panel (Socio-Economic Panel) (Germany)
SPS	Social Pulse Survey (Colombia)
UN	United Nations
UNDP	United Nations Development Programme
UNED	Universidad Estatal a Distancia (Costa Rica)
UNESCO	United Nations Educational, Scientific and Cultural Organization
UNODC	United Nations Office on Drugs and Crime
UN WOMEN	United Nations Entity for Gender Equality and the Empowerment of Women
USD	United States Dollar
VET	Vocational Education and Training
WHO	World Health Organisation

Executive summary

The pandemic has touched on every aspect of people's well-being

The COVID-19 pandemic is having far-reaching consequences for how we live, work and connect with one another, as well as for the economic, human, social and environmental systems that support well-being over time. Excess deaths in OECD countries averaged 16% between March 2020 and early May 2021, leading to a 7-month fall in OECD-average life expectancy in 2020 alone. Government support helped to sustain OECD average household income levels in 2020, and stemmed the tide of unemployment, even as average hours worked fell sharply, and nearly 1 in 3 people reported at least one financial difficulty. Data from 15 OECD countries suggest that over one-quarter of people were at risk of depression or anxiety in 2020. Confinement measures brought new challenges in terms of school closures, unpaid care work, and domestic violence. Some pressures on well-being eased in the earliest stages of the pandemic (e.g. carbon emissions fell, road deaths reduced, trust in government rallied, and gender-gaps in unpaid home and care work narrowed), but all now show strong signs of reverting back to business as usual. And as the pandemic has worn on, more people are feeling worn out. In early 2021, one-third of people reported feeling too tired after work to do necessary household chores, up from 22% in 2020. Feelings of loneliness, division and disconnection from society also grew between mid-2020 and the first half of 2021.

Experiences of the pandemic have varied widely depending on age, gender, race and ethnicity, as well as jobs, pay and skills

The crisis has hit people who were already struggling the hardest. Typically, disadvantage accumulates and intersects in ways not easy to see in the data we have, and this can understate how well-being challenges pile up for certain groups of people. In the case of age, older people have been much more likely to suffer severe outcomes or death due to COVID-19 infection, making reduced social contact an especially important precaution for them. At the same time, younger adults have experienced some of the largest declines in mental health, social connectedness and subjective well-being in 2020 and 2021, as well as facing job disruption and insecurity.

The relationship between well-being, race and ethnicity is complex – and a broader range of socio-economic factors, including living and working conditions as well as deep-seated forms of racism and discrimination, can help explain why different racial and ethnic communities have experienced divergent outcomes during COVID-19. In those OECD countries with data, COVID-19 mortality rates for some ethnic minority communities have been more than twice those of other groups, while ethnic minority workers have been more likely to lose their jobs during the pandemic. Mental health deteriorated for almost all population groups on average in 2020, but gaps in mental health by race and ethnicity are also visible.

Average well-being outcomes also differed by gender, as well as across different household types, during the pandemic. Excess deaths have been higher for men than for women, yet women are more likely to experience long COVID, saw larger falls in mental health, and felt lonelier. At the same time, women have often been on the frontline of pandemic care, whether in their jobs or doing unpaid care work at home. Housing conditions and how we live together took on a new significance for well-being in the pandemic. Life satisfaction fell particularly for couples living with children during 2020, while single parents and those living alone were almost twice as likely to feel lonely, compared to the population as a whole.

Whether and where people work has affected their exposure to both COVID-19 and the wider impacts of the crisis. Teleworking helped to protect people and their jobs, particularly for the well-paid and highly-skilled, but was not an option for the majority of workers. Data from 11 OECD countries showed workers in the bottom earnings quartile were twice as likely to stop working, and nearly half as likely to telework, compared to those in the top quartile. Losing work means losing more than your salary: unemployed people were more than twice as likely to feel lonely and to feel left out of society compared to the employed. At a time when 1 in 5 European OECD households are struggling to make ends meet, and 1 in 7 feel "likely" to lose their jobs within 3 months, new pressures on living costs are taking hold: OECD average house prices grew by almost 5% in 2020, and rental prices by nearly 2%, while energy costs are also on the rise.

Stocks of natural, human and social capital will need re-building after the crisis

In addition to the impacts of the pandemic on children and young people, damage to stocks of natural, economic, human and social capital have long-run consequences for societal well-being. Building back better must mean addressing the climate and biodiversity crises that threaten future well-being, as well as building up human and social infrastructure. Labour market underutilisation in OECD countries reached 17% in 2020, and 13% of people aged 15-29 were not in employment, education or training (NEET), erasing gains made since the 2007-8 crisis. Pandemic strains meant more people accumulated future health risks such as weight gain and increased alcohol consumption. Trust (in people and in institutions) has been an important resilience factor, with higher trust contributing to COVID-19 containment. Nevertheless, some of the early gains in trust enjoyed by several governments have since been eroded. By early 2021, 1 in 3 people felt left out of their societies (up from 1 in 5 in mid-2020), and the majority of adults in 12 OECD countries felt that their country was "more divided now than before the coronavirus outbreak". Youth and women continue to be under-represented in pandemic decision-making: by March 2021, women made up only 35% of COVID-19 task force members on average in 27 OECD countries.

Well-being outcomes are a moving target: frequent, timely data are essential

Throughout the first 15 months of the pandemic covered by this report, well-being outcomes have been a moving target, as both disease risk and restrictions shifted. The rush to meet new information needs, and the difficulty of data collection in a pandemic, posed new challenges for data quality. This has placed a premium on the high-quality, high-frequency, large-sample data collections that are typical of some economic indicators, but rare in the case of social, relational and environmental outcomes. Some national statistical offices in the OECD area responded with significant innovation, showcased throughout this report, ranging from high-frequency household 'pulse' surveys, to new internet-based surveys, and experimental time-use surveys. These innovations delivered important insights that could be further enhanced through improved international coordination and standardisation on methods.

Well-being evidence can help refocus, redesign, realign and reconnect policy

A return to business as usual would miss an important opportunity for governments to tackle several interconnected environmental, economic, social, and relational challenges which pre-date COVID-19. The wide-ranging effects of the crisis on well-being also call for a joined-up policy approach to recovery. Chapter 1 describes five illustrative policy channels that offer "triple wins", through coordinated cross-government action that will raise both current and future well-being while also promoting opportunities for all. These channels include: a focus on sustainable, inclusive, high-quality jobs; broadening uptake of lifelong learning; raising well-being for disadvantaged children and young people; strengthening mental and physical health promotion and prevention; and strengthening public sector capacity on both well-being analysis and citizen engagement. The chapter also sets out how well-being evidence can support policy makers in *refocusing* policies and recovery packages towards the outcomes that matter most to people, in *redesigning* policy content from a more multidimensional perspective, *realigning* policy practice across government silos, and in *reconnecting* people with the public institutions that serve them.

1 Building back better lives: Using a well-being lens to refocus, redesign, realign and reconnect

After an initial focus on the emergency response to COVID-19, governments are now developing recovery strategies that could lay the foundations for future well-being, shaping the long-term paths for economies and societies. This chapter looks at how a well-being lens can inform policy prioritisation and the design of recovery strategies, and can help achieve stronger strategic alignment across public agencies and between public, private and civil society organisations. Building on the evidence presented in the following chapters, it identifies common well-being priorities across OECD countries in the wake of the pandemic. The chapter then describes five strategic policy channels that can help address these well-being priorities in ways that simultaneously raise current and future well-being while promoting opportunities for all. Ultimately, achieving such well-being synergies requires new ways of working within the system of government and across the public and private sectors and civil society.

Introduction

The COVID-19 crisis has highlighted the strong interdependencies between social, economic and environmental outcomes. The pandemic rapidly cascaded from a public health crisis to a global economic and social crisis, impacting people's lives in a multitude of different ways, with both short- and potentially long-term consequences. The effects of the pandemic have been aggravated by pre-existing well-being challenges, ranging from air pollution (Cole, Ozgen and Strobl, 2020[1]; Wu et al., 2020[2]) to crowded households (Chen and Krieger, 2021[3]), and from job and financial insecurity (OECD, 2020[4]) to obesity (Alberca et al., 2020[5]; Dietz and Santos-Burgoa, 2020[6]) and cigarette smoking (Patanavanich and Glantz, 2020[7]; Reddy et al., 2021[8]). The pandemic has also brought increased attention to how threats to biodiversity, such as habitat destruction and wildlife exploitation, can increase the risk of infectious diseases being transferred across species (United Nations, 2020[9]; Gottdenker et al., 2014[10]). COVID-19 has been described as both a wake-up call and a dress rehearsal for other crises, including climate change (Guterres, 2020[11]).

After an initial focus on addressing the health emergency and the economic and jobs crises that accompanied it, governments' attention has now turned to stimulus measures to support the recovery. Across OECD countries, the fiscal stimulus in response to the COVID-19 crisis has been larger than that which followed the 2008 financial crisis, with additional spending or foregone revenues implemented or planned between January 2020 and mid-March 2021 amounting to around 16.4% of GDP on average (OECD, 2021[12]). COVID-19 recovery packages will have considerable implications for the long-term paths of societies (Buckle et al., 2020[13]). At the same time, governments face several interconnected economic, social and environmental challenges that predate the health crisis, implying that a return to business as usual would miss an important window to tackle these underlying vulnerabilities and risks (OECD, 2020[14]; OECD, 2020[15]; Hepburn et al., 2020[16]). Instead, well-designed recovery packages could serve dual purposes in building back better: on the one hand, repairing the damage caused by COVID-19, and on the other, setting countries on a stronger, greener, more inclusive and more resilient path, ready to tackle the upcoming crises of the future (OECD, 2020[14]; OECD, 2021[17]; Hepburn et al., 2020[16]).[1]

A well-being lens can be used to shape a more comprehensive and balanced approach to building forward, by helping to:

- **refocus** – firmly focusing government action on what matters most to the well-being of people and society, building on evidence about both current and future well-being outcomes, as well as inequality of opportunity across all dimensions of people's lives (Box 1.1)
- **redesign** – designing policy in a coherent and integrated way that systematically considers potential impacts across multiple well-being objectives, inclusion and sustainability, rather than focusing on a single (or very narrow range of) objective(s) "here and now" independently of others
- **realign** – aligning the system of government such that it is better able to collaboratively work towards societal priorities, by shifting the focus from narrower outputs of individual departments towards shared outcome-based objectives, and
- **reconnect** – strengthening the connections between government, the private sector and civil society based on a joint understanding of what well-being means and how it can be improved.

This chapter explores each of these four ways in which a well-being approach can help to build back better in more detail. Based on the well-being evidence analysed throughout the report, the first section of this chapter identifies common well-being priorities for recovery. These include the need to: increase the job and financial security of households, and particularly those most affected by the crisis; promote equality of opportunity and mitigate the scarring effects of the crisis on the most vulnerable individuals and workers, with a focus on youth, women and the low-skilled; lift the burden of poor physical and mental health; take strong action on climate change and environmental degradation; contain the increase of child poverty; and reinforce trust in others and in public institutions as the basis for greater social cohesion in the future.

The second section of this chapter illustrates how a well-being perspective can help inform the redesign of public policy by systematically considering well-being outcomes in policy development upstream rather than correcting for negative impacts ex post. To provide some concrete examples, five strategic policy channels are outlined that can simultaneously address multiple objectives (for current well-being, inclusion and sustainability) in the wake of the pandemic. These are: 1) supporting the creation of inclusive and high-quality jobs in the low-carbon economy; 2) broadening access to lifelong learning where it is needed the most; 3) using a whole-of-government approach to raise the well-being of disadvantaged children and young people; 4) strengthening mental and physical health promotion and prevention; and 5) reinforcing trust by enhancing public sector transparency and decision-making, establishing meaningful citizen participation on a more ongoing basis, and investing in local communities and social capital.

The third and fourth parts of this chapter look at the institutional mechanisms that are needed to support a well-being approach to public policy. More coherent and effective approaches to raising societal well-being require new ways of working within government as well as between the public sector, private sector and civil society. Recent decades have seen a growing number of governments using well-being frameworks and evidence to help inform government agenda-setting and budgeting, to help embed a longer-term focus within the system of government and to strengthen policy coherence (both between sectors and between different levels of government) in working towards well-being objectives. A well-being approach can also help create stronger connections between public, private and civil society actors in working towards well-being. Practical examples of this are presented in the last section of this chapter.

Box 1.1. Using the OECD Well-Being Framework to analyse the diverse impacts of the pandemic on people's lives

The OECD Well-being Framework guides the OECD's work on monitoring trends in current well-being outcomes, inclusion and the sustainability of well-being across member and partner countries. It underpins the *How's Life?* report series published on a bi- or triennial basis since 2011. The Framework (Figure 1.1) features two central pillars: current well-being (on top), which addresses living conditions here and now, as well as inequalities in their distribution; and resources for future well-being (on the bottom), which considers the stocks, flows and risk and resilience factors that shape well-being over time and for future generations (OECD, 2020[18]).

Current well-being comprises 11 dimensions. For the purposes of this report, the dimensions have been clustered into three broad groups:

- **Material conditions,** encompassing Income and Wealth, Housing, and Work and Job Quality
- **Quality-of-life,** spanning Health, Subjective Well-being, Knowledge and Skills, and Environmental Quality,
- **Community relations**, which covers Social Connections, Work-Life Balance, Safety and Civic Engagement.

National averages often mask large differences in how different population groups are doing. Moreover, inequalities in one well-being dimension (e.g. Health, Housing, or Safety) can produce inequalities of opportunity in other dimensions. Measuring the distribution of well-being is therefore a core aspect of the approach. The **inclusion** section of this report (Chapters 5, 6 and 7) addresses in particular how COVID-19 has affected population groups differently, as well as overall deprivation rates.

The final section of the evidence scan relates to **sustainability.** In the OECD Well-Being Framework, the systemic resources that underpin future well-being are expressed in terms of four types of capital, i.e. stocks that endure over time but are also affected by decisions taken (or not taken) today. Economic Capital includes both man-made (physical) and financial assets. Natural Capital encompasses natural assets (e.g. stocks of natural resources, land cover, species biodiversity), as well as ecosystems and their services (e.g. oceans, forests, soil and the atmosphere). Human Capital refers to the skills and future health of individuals. Finally, Social Capital refers to the social norms, shared values and institutional arrangements that foster co-operation.

Figure 1.1. The OECD Well-Being Framework

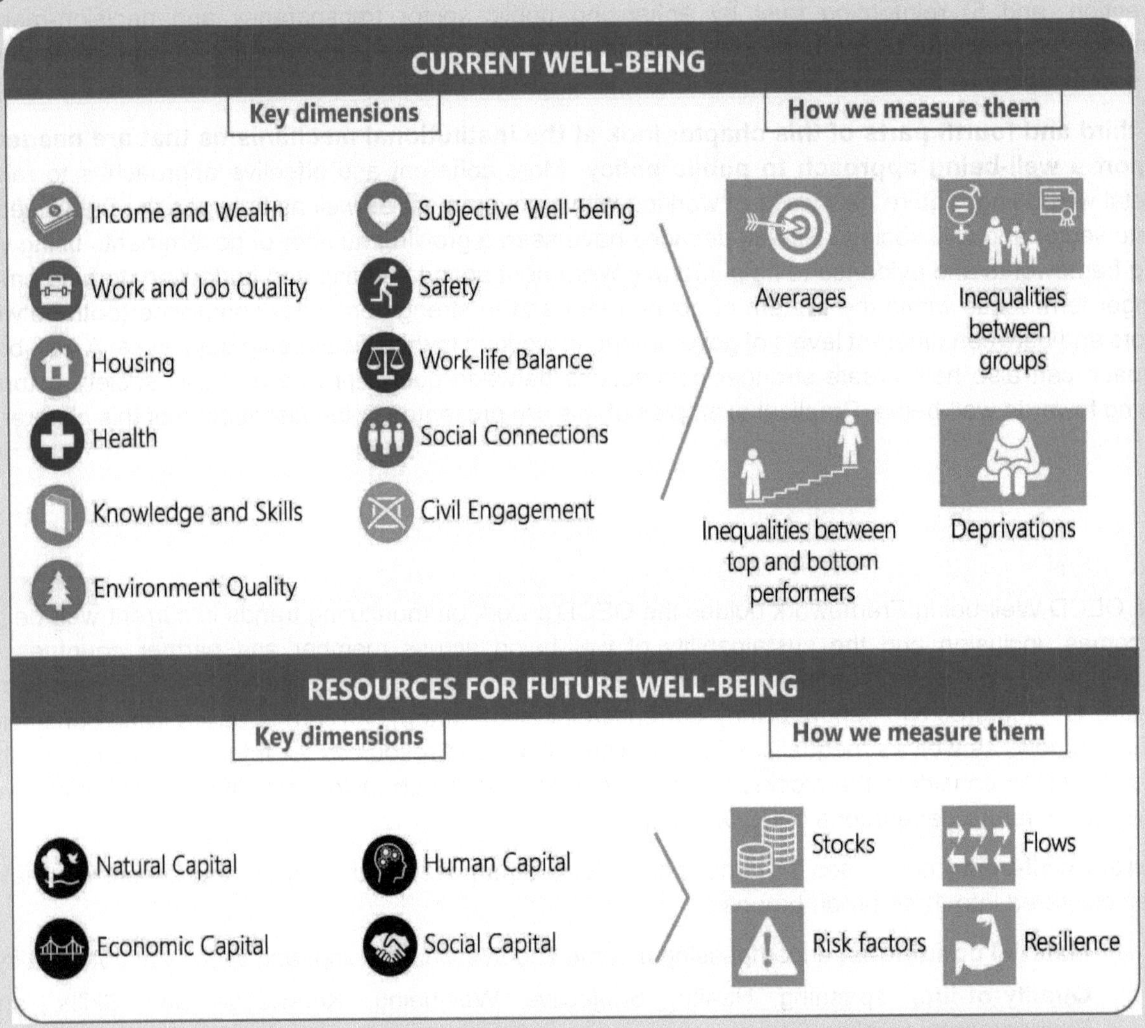

Source: OECD (2020[18]), *How's Life? 2020: Measuring Well-Being*, OECD Publishing, Paris, https://dx.doi.org/10.1787/9870c393-en.

Using a well-being approach to Refocus: Putting People and Planet First

The COVID-19 crisis has highlighted the unique and fundamental role of government in safeguarding people's well-being. From the timely and extensive interventions to manage the health and sanitary crisis, to the strong financial support provided to households, workers and small and medium companies, governments have demonstrated an unprecedented leadership in protecting people's lives and livelihoods. This focus ought to be maintained when designing recovery packages, whilst also integrating actions to address long-standing threats to well-being, such as biodiversity loss and climate change.

Directly targeting well-being outcomes, by explicitly building well-being considerations into policy upstream, is an efficient and cost-effective way to design policies that address social and environmental pressures of both a structural and cyclical nature. A well-being approach is about attending to the root causes of social and environmental vulnerabilities and imbalances and creating economic systems that do good for people and the planet by design (Nozal, Martin and Murtin, 2019[19]; Trebeck and Williams, 2019[20]). The post-pandemic recovery creates new opportunities to set in place the foundations for more resilient, equitable and sustainable societies and economies (OECD, 2021[21]). While a strong economic recovery is essential, ultimately it is the quality and form of the recovery that will determine its contribution to societal well-being.

Common well-being priorities for COVID-19 recovery strategies

What outcomes would COVID-19 recovery strategies prioritise if the well-being of current and future generations were front and centre? Determining policy priorities for a strong recovery is a challenging task for any government given the multiplicity of objectives to be simultaneously achieved. A well-being approach can give structure to this priority-setting process, by providing a framework for systematically scanning evidence on current well-being, distributional outcomes and resources for future well-being, to identify the areas of greatest need. This type of systematic evidence scanning is best done at the national and subnational level, since both pandemic experiences and economic, social and environmental contexts and policy settings vary substantially both across and within OECD countries. Nevertheless, building on the evidence presented in the following chapters, some concerns that are common to many OECD countries can be identified (Figure 1.2).

While OECD countries had markedly different patterns of performance across the dimensions of the OECD Well-Being Framework before the pandemic (OECD, 2020[18]), **this evidence scan highlights several common priorities that need to be central in country recovery strategies**. These include the need to:

- increase the job and financial security of individuals and households hit hardest by the pandemic
- promote opportunities for all and mitigate the scarring effects of the crisis on minorities, youth and women
- lift the increasing burden of poor physical and mental health
- take strong action on climate change, biodiversity loss and environmental degradation
- improve well-being outcomes for vulnerable children and young people, and
- reinforce trust in others and in public institutions.

Each of these priorities is discussed in more detail below.

The pandemic has raised the urgency of addressing existing well-being concerns

Increasing the job and financial security of individuals and households hit hardest by the pandemic

Increasing job and financial security is a key priority in response to one of the worst jobs crises since the Great Depression (OECD, 2020[22]). Job and household financial insecurity were already of concern prior to the pandemic and addressing these issues has become critically urgent now. Around 2016, more than a third (36%) of people in OECD countries were already financially insecure, meaning they would risk falling into poverty if they had to forgo three months of their income (OECD, 2020[18]). Similarly, the share of non-standard workers (i.e. part-time, temporary and self-employed workers) has been growing in recent decades,[2] with more than a third of workers in OECD countries being in non-standard employment (ILO, 2016[23]; OECD, 2019[24]).

Figure 1.2. Overview of common well-being concerns among most OECD countries in the wake of the pandemic

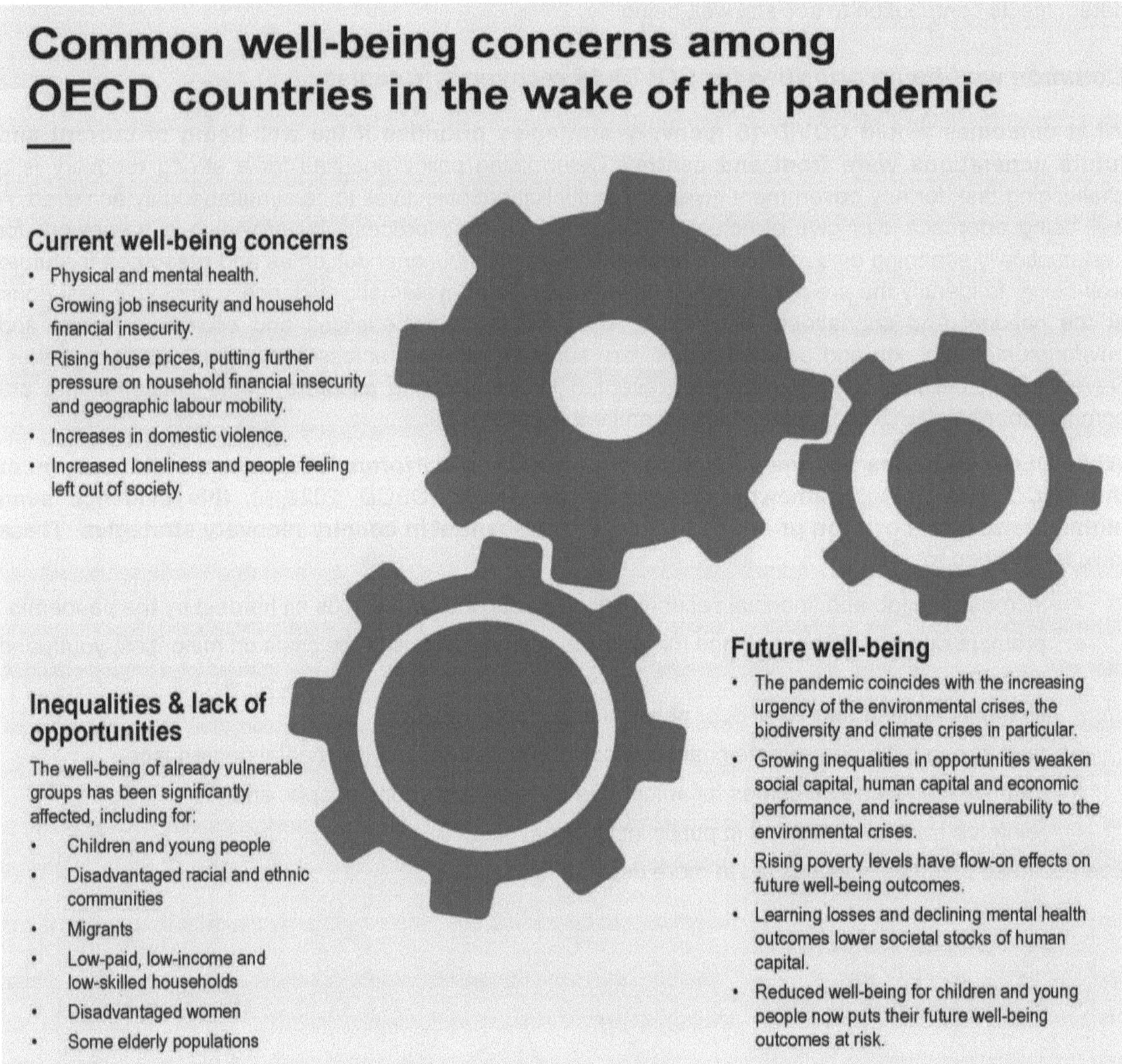

The pandemic's impact on employment and hours of work at the onset of the crisis was, on average, ten times bigger than that observed in the first months of the Global Financial Crisis in 2008 (OECD, 2020[22]). By October 2020, 37% of respondents in a representative sample of 25 000 adults from 25 OECD countries who participated in the 2020 OECD Risks that Matter survey indicated that their household had experienced at least one job-related disruption, such as a job loss, a reduction in work hours and/or a pay cut (OECD, 2021[25]). Among households that lost a job during the pandemic, 68% indicated having trouble paying bills (OECD, 2021[25]). In addition to non-standard workers, women, youth and low-income workers have been particularly exposed to the risk of job losses (see Chapter 5).

Housing cost overburden is putting further pressure on the financial security of low-income households (OECD, 2021[26]) (see Chapter 2). Real house prices as well as rental prices increased in most OECD countries between 2005 and 2019, constraining the ability of low-income households to spend on other essentials, such as food, health care and education (OECD, 2020[18]). Between 2019 and 2020, real house prices continued to grow significantly in most OECD countries, while rent prices remained stable or grew only slightly – likely due to caps on rent prices and other artificial rent suppression measures (OECD, 2021[26]). The economic fallout of COVID-19 has heightened housing insecurity for some households (OECD, 2021[27]). For example, in April-May 2020, 10% of people in 22 OECD European countries reported being behind in paying utility bills and 8% in making rent or mortgage payments (Eurofound, 2020[28]). An August 2020 study found that 25% of United States adults had trouble paying bills and 16% had problems paying their rent or mortgage; among lower-income adults, the same shares were 46% and 32% respectively, i.e. around twice as high (Parker, Minkin and Bennett, 2020[29]). The recent OECD report on *Building Better Housing Policies* provides an overview of what governments can do to design policies for more efficient, inclusive and sustainable housing (OECD, 2021[30]).

Promoting opportunities for all and mitigating the scarring effects of the crisis on minorities, youth and women

The unequal impacts of the pandemic are compounding both long-standing inequalities of opportunity across OECD countries and declining social mobility. Around 2016, the average income of the richest 10% of the OECD population was already about nine times that of the poorest 10%, up from seven times in the mid-1980s (OECD, 2019[31]). This report shows that people and groups who were already vulnerable before the COVID-19 pandemic have been particularly affected by it. Those with lower levels of education or income, women, young people and people with dependent children are more likely to have lost their jobs, to have experienced job-related disruption and to report financial difficulties (see Chapter 5). For example, on average across EU countries, the labour income loss following the pandemic was 4 times higher for workers in the bottom income quintile than for those in the top income quintile. The learning loss caused by school closures has particularly affected already disadvantaged children who have faced higher barriers and challenges to remote learning (see Chapter 6) (OECD, 2020[32]). In the Netherlands, which features an equitable system of school funding and one of the world's highest rates of broadband access, learning losses still proved to be up to 60% larger among students from less-educated homes compared to the general population (Engzell, Frey and Verhagen, 2021[33]).[3] Other reports have emphasised the increased risks of domestic violence that women and children have faced during the shutdown (OECD, 2020[32]; OECD, 2021[34]). While mental health deteriorated for everyone in 2020, certain groups – including women, those with lower education levels, the unemployed, young people, the elderly and frontline workers – have experienced especially large declines (see Chapter 6). The limited data that are available suggest that the well-being of migrants and certain racial and ethnic communities has also been hit particularly hard (see Chapters 5, 6 and 7). In addition, regional differences – both between and within countries – have further magnified, emphasising the importance of place-based recovery approaches (OECD, 2021[35]). Unless strong policy action is taken, these growing inequalities in well-being outcomes will not only undermine the well-being of those who are worse off, but also that of society at large, as inequality in society goes hand in hand with lower educational and population health outcomes

(Wilkinson and Pickett, 2007[36]; Pickett and Wilkinson, 2015[37]), lower levels of interpersonal trust (Uslaner, 2002[38]; Zak and Knack, 2001[39]) and lower economic performance (OECD, 2014[40]; McAdams, 2007[41]).

Lifting the burden of poor physical and mental health

Recovery strategies will also need to lift the burden of mental and physical ill-health that weighs heavily on individuals, societies and economies. Addressing the health emergency has been the top priority for policy makers following the pandemic outbreak. It will need to remain a long-term priority going forward, with a strong focus on both physical and mental health outcomes. Losses of loved ones, jobs and incomes, disruption of essential health services and deferred care, increased social isolation and loneliness, and heightened stress and anxiety all have long-term consequences for people's physical and mental health, over and above the direct impacts of the crisis on excess mortality (see Chapters 3 and 6). Across 15 OECD countries in the period between April and December 2020, over 70% of people on average avoided going to hospitals or health centres to seek treatment, due to fear of exposure to the virus, thus putting physical health outcomes at risk (Chapter 3). Evidence from eight OECD countries with comparable pre-pandemic data show that risk for anxiety and depression rose significantly in the onset of the pandemic, from April through December 2020, and these rates remained elevated in the early months of 2021 (Chapter 3) (OECD, 2021[42]). Since the outbreak started, many adults reported experiencing "stress, anxiety, or sadness that was difficult to cope with alone", including 33% of people in the United States, between 23% and 26% of people in Canada, Australia, New Zealand and France, and between 10% and 18% of people in Sweden, the Netherlands and Norway (The Commonwealth Fund, 2020[43]) (OECD, 2021[42]). At the same time, across OECD countries, many mental health services were completely or partially disrupted following the pandemic outbreak, with 57% of OECD countries reporting disruptions to services for older adults; 57% reporting disruptions in psychotherapy, counselling, and psychosocial interventions; 48% in work-related mental health programmes; and 52% in school mental health programmes (Chapter 3).

The COVID-19 health impacts are adding to existing concerns about worsening health outcomes across OECD countries. Across OECD countries, more than half of the population is now overweight (OECD, 2019[44]), and life expectancy already showed signs of plateauing or declining in some OECD countries prior to the pandemic (OECD, 2020[18]). In the EU, around 550 000 people of working-age die prematurely every year due to non-communicable diseases, amounting to 3.4 million life-years and EUR 115 billion in economic potential lost annually (Nozal, Martin and Murtin, 2019[19]). Mental health issues are one of the largest and fastest-growing categories of the burden of disease worldwide, with half of people across the OECD area experiencing a mental health issue in their lifetime (OECD, 2019[45]). At the same time, there is an enduring gap between the need for mental health treatment and people's access to it: around 2016, on average across OECD countries, 67% of working-age adults with mental distress reported that they wanted help but did not get it (OECD, 2021[46]). As the flow-on effects of ill-health on wider personal and societal outcomes are significant, affecting educational outcomes, employment outcomes, child well-being outcomes and subjective well-being, both physical and mental health are urgent priorities that should lie at the core of countries' recovery packages (United Nations, 2020[47]; Nozal, Martin and Murtin, 2019[19]).

Investment in ongoing critical well-being concerns needs to be accelerated to safeguard the sustainability of well-being going forward

Taking strong action on climate change and environmental degradation

As countries battle the COVID-19 crisis, they are also in a race against time to avoid an environmental catastrophe (OECD, 2021[48]) (see Chapter 11). Environmental challenges such as climate change, biodiversity loss and air pollution pose severe systemic risks to the well-being of current and future generations in ways that are highly unequally distributed (OECD, 2021[48]). A wide range of studies show how climate change and environmental degradation negatively affect physical health (Manisalidis et al., 2020[49]; Rossati, 2017[50]; Karbalaei et al., 2018[51]), mental health (Filipova et al., 2020[52]; Cunsolo and Ellis, 2018[53]; Hayes et al., 2018[54]; Obradovich et al., 2018[55]), livelihoods and poverty (Kabir and Serrao-Neumann, 2020[56]). Recent OECD analysis emphasised how the impacts of environmental degradation are concentrated among vulnerable groups and households, who are more likely to be exposed to their harmful effects, more susceptible to negative impacts, and more limited in their abilities to cope and recover from them. These groups include lower socio-economic households, as well as the young and the old (OECD, 2021[48]; Islam and Winkel, 2017[57]).

COVID-19 recovery efforts therefore need to be strongly integrated with concerted action on the environmental crises. While an early fall in greenhouse gas (GHG) emissions over the pandemic may have seemed like a positive effect, it is highly unlikely that these reductions will outlive the pandemic (OECD, 2021[48]; O'Callaghan and Murdock, 2021[58]) (see also Chapter 11). Initial short-term reductions in CO_2 emissions will not have a significant impact on future climate risks unless they are coupled with robust mitigation measures as part of the recovery packages (Buckle et al., 2020[13]). As the environmental crises could cause social and economic damages far greater than those caused by COVID-19, strong action on climate change and other environmental crises is critical for achieving a resilient recovery (OECD, 2021[48]). The OECD is supporting countries in this endeavour through policy analyses and recommendations to tackle the COVID-19 crisis in a holistic way that concurrently addresses environmental, social and economic well-being priorities (OECD, 2020[14]; OECD, 2020[59]; OECD, 2019[60]; OECD, 2020[15]; OECD, 2021[48]; Buckle et al., 2020[13]).

Timely action is needed now to mitigate greater risks in the future

Improving well-being outcomes for vulnerable children and youth

Putting vulnerable children and young people at the heart of the recovery is essential to ensure a resilient recovery. Children and young people have been less at-risk of developing severe physical health symptoms linked to COVID-19 than older age cohorts (WHO, 2020[61]). Nonetheless, the crisis has had significant impacts on their current well-being (especially in terms of employment, education, mental health and disposable income) as well as on their future opportunities and trajectories (particularly for students from disadvantaged backgrounds, those with learning disabilities, young people from racial and ethnic minority groups and those in temporary employment) (see Chapters 6 and 9) (OECD, 2020[32]; OECD, 2020[62]). School closures, social distancing and confinement have increased learning gaps and the risk of poor nutrition among children and young people. They have worsened their exposure to the impacts of poor housing quality, domestic violence and abuse, and raised their anxiety and stress, while at the same time reducing their access to vital family and care services (OECD, 2020[32]).

COVID-19's impact on children and young people could have long-term effects on their well-being outcomes. Early projections suggest that the pandemic could lead to significant rises in child poverty rates (OECD, 2021[63]). Children are over-represented amongst those living in poverty: in 2017-18, children made up 26% of those living in income poverty across OECD countries, despite representing only around 21% of the population (OECD, 2021[63]). The loss of relationships and learning opportunities that early care and education programs provide can exacerbate the large achievement gaps between children from low-income families and their peers (Office of the Assistant Secretary for Planning and Evaluation, 2021[64]; Barnett and Jung, 2021[65]). Learning losses due to school closures could also have long-term impacts. Estimates from the World Bank suggest that during the first phase of the crisis, students in primary and secondary school may have lost one-third of a school year of learning (see Chapter 3). These learning losses are likely to exacerbate pre-existing educational inequalities, as they are greater for already disadvantaged children who are less likely to live in good home-learning environments (OECD, 2020[66]; OECD, 2021[63]). The amount of learning loss is also likely to differ between countries, as countries with the lowest educational performance tended to fully close their schools for longer periods of time in 2020. This implies that education systems with poorer learning outcomes in 2018 were more likely to suffer from greater losses of in-person learning time in 2020 (OECD, 2021[67]).

Available evidence points to a rising prevalence of mental distress among young people (see Chapter 6) (OECD, 2021[68]). In most countries, mental health issues among young people have doubled or more following the pandemic outbreak (OECD, 2021[68]). Whereas prior to the pandemic, young people were less likely to report symptoms of anxiety or depression than the general population, post-pandemic most countries are seeing a higher share of young people experiencing such symptoms compared to the general population (OECD, 2021[68]). In the United States, more than one in four young people in a nationally representative survey of 13 to 19 year olds reported losing sleep because of worry, feeling unhappy or depressed, feeling constantly under strain, or experiencing a loss of confidence in themselves (Margolius et al., 2020[69]).Young people's life satisfaction has also fallen more than that of any other age cohort (Chapter 6) (OECD, 2020[62]). Levels of loneliness, a key risk factor for mental health, have been particularly high among young people (Varga et al., 2021[70]; Weissbourd et al., 2021[71]). Across 27 European countries, 18-34 year-olds were the most likely to report feeling lonely "more than half of the time", "most of the time" or "all of the time" in spring 2020 (32%) and summer 2020 (28%), well above the general population shares of 26% and 21% respectively (OECD, 2021[68]).

Young people have also suffered from a higher risk of job and income loss than other age cohorts (see Chapter 5). While the number of young people not in education, employment or training (NEET) has been declining over the past few years, the pandemic has led to a reversal of this trend (Chapter 9). In the second quarter of 2020, the OECD average unemployment rate for workers aged 15-24 was 18.5%, more than twice as high as that of workers aged 25 or over (7.4%) (OECD, 2021[72]). This was partly driven by the fact that young people are more likely to work in non-standard employment or jobs in customer-facing industries (OECD, 2020[22]). The earnings loss has also been higher for young workers (aged 16-34) compared to middle-aged workers (aged 35-65) (respectively 5.8% and 4.5%) (see Chapter 5). Faced with this loss of income, young people are more likely to fall into poverty, as they have fewer savings to fall back on. With fewer than 5 in 10 young people expressing trust in government across OECD countries, these heightened challenges can further deteriorate youth's relationship with public institutions and democratic processes, as already experienced in the aftermath of the 2007-2008 financial crisis (OECD, 2020[62]). Taken together, the well-being deprivations and inequalities that children and young people face not only compromise their well-being now, but are also likely to shape their health, educational, employment and civic participation outcomes later in life (Chapter 9) (OECD, 2020[32]; OECD, 2019[73]). A resilient recovery should therefore put children and young people at the centre so as to prevent the crisis from leaving long-lasting scars on their well-being going forward (OECD, 2021[74]).

Reinforcing trust in others and in public institutions

Reinforcing trust is fundamental to building back better. Social capital has played a vital role in determining the effectiveness of countries' emergency response to the COVID-19 crisis (Borgonovi and Andrieu, 2020[75]). Social capital refers to the social norms, shared values and institutional arrangements that foster co-operation within and between groups in society (see Chapter 10). It includes trust in public institutions and in others in society and a willingness to contribute to shared outcomes that have been pivotal in government strategies to combat the pandemic, such as through adherence to social distancing requirements, the use of contact tracing and the roll-out of vaccine programmes. Data from across OECD countries shows that both trust in institutions and interpersonal trust were key factors for successful pandemic management (Chapter 10). For instance, across European regions, trust in policy makers pre-outbreak was associated with higher decreases in mobility around the time of lockdown announcements in mid-March 2020 (Bargain and Aminjonov, 2020[76]). Data up until July 2020 from Europe and the United States, as well as a study including all OECD members, indicate that higher interpersonal trust has been associated with more hygienic practices, greater compliance with social distancing and, consequently, lower mortality rates (Bartscher et al., 2020[77]; Helliwell et al., 2021[78]; DIW, 2021[79]; Makridis and Wu, 2021[80])[4] (see Chapter 10).

Despite initial increases in trust following the pandemic outbreak, social capital cannot be taken for granted, and it is an essential area requiring more investment. While people's trust in institutions in 2020 was at its highest since records began in 2006, still only 50% of people in OECD countries reported confidence in national governments in 2020 (see Chapter 10). Many countries have experienced an increase in trust in government following the pandemic outbreak, and some have seen rises in trust in other people in the first half of 2020, pointing to a unifying or "rallying around the flag" effect in the face of a common threat (Chapter 10). However, it remains to be seen whether these increases in trust are long-lived. Previous pandemics and crises, such as the 1918–19 Spanish flu and the 2008 Global Financial Crisis, have had long-lasting negative effects on trust in others and in government. By early 2021, many countries were observing a turning point in their trust in government's capacities to handle the crisis and to implement coherent policies (OECD, 2021[12]). Data from the third round of the Eurofound *Living, Working, and COVID-19 survey* show that trust in government started to decline among the 22 OECD countries in the sample, from 5.2 on a scale of 1 to 10 in June-July 2020 to 4.2 in February-March 2021, with similar patterns observed in other OECD regions (Chapter 10). Trust in others, for which more limited data are available, continued to rise until early 2021 in Germany, but returned to 2018 baseline levels by September 2020 in New Zealand (Chapter 10). In addition, after being split in June-August 2020 on whether the pandemic has brought people together, by February-May 2021 the majority of adults in 12 OECD member countries found their country to be "more divided now than before the coronavirus outbreak" (Chapter 10).

The unequal impacts of the crisis, widespread disinformation and difficult recovery times ahead are likely to challenge levels of trust going forward. Increasing levels of inequality in societies are set to weaken trust in others and in public institutions (Uslaner, 2002[38]; Zak and Knack, 2001[39]). Despite the large expansion of social protection systems in OECD countries during the crisis, many people feel that governments should do more to ensure economic and social security and to address gaps in social protection (OECD, 2021[25]). Data from the third round of the Eurofound *Living, Working, and COVID-19 survey* show that only 14% of people across 22 European countries surveyed in spring 2021 felt that support measures were fair, down from 22% in summer 2020. Additional challenges are being posed by the wave of disinformation that has accompanied the spread of COVID-19 and has magnified distrust among certain groups (OECD, 2020[81]; OECD, 2021[12]). With difficult recovery times ahead, the value that social capital brings to societies should not be taken for granted, making investment in it an essential underpinning of effective recovery strategies (OECD, 2021[82]; OECD, 2021[12]; Brezzi, Gonzáles and Prats, 2020[83]; The British Academy, 2021[84]).

Using a well-being approach to Redesign

Given their interdependencies, well-being priorities for building back better cannot be achieved in isolation. This stands in stark contrast with the traditionally siloed approach to policy design within government ministries and departments, where policies on economic, environmental and social issues are often conceived, developed and implemented largely separately from each other. Siloed government systems in which each ministry works towards its own set of objectives, provide few incentives for departments to invest in outcomes that fall under the responsibility of other departments (APPG, 2014[85]). Policy designed this way is less likely to lead to a coherent and sustainable strategy and is more likely to miss opportunities for synergies than policy designed through a common framework and an agreed set of outcomes that transcend individual departments.

The post-pandemic pressures on public finances further raise the importance for recovery measures to consider key societal goals simultaneously rather than sequentially or in isolation

(Buckle et al., 2020[13]). It is more efficient to design coherent policies upstream than to have to correct for negative externalities after-the-fact. The increased pressures on government budgets make it all the more essential that governments deploy public spending in the most strategic and coherent way possible, focusing on the policies and programmes that will deliver the highest well-being returns on investment. This consideration asks for recovery pathways that focus on achieving multiple benefits in an integrated way, in order to cost-effectively generate both near-term and longer-term benefits for societal well-being across social, economic and environmental domains (Buckle et al., 2020[13]). Well-being frameworks can help identify opportunities for interventions by one policy agency to support the objectives of other policy agencies – as seen, for example, in integrated approaches to mental health, employment and skills policies (OECD, 2021[42]). At the same time, a well-being lens offers a structured approach to anticipate and mitigate risks in areas where well-intended actions in one policy area may trigger problems in others that would then require additional expenditure to address – as in the case of COVID-19 recovery strategies that could have harmful or mixed impacts on pressing environmental objectives (OECD, 2021[86])(see Chapter 11).

A well-being approach looks at government objectives as interconnected goals, focusing on the complementary roles that different policies play in improving them (APPG, 2019[87]). A well-being approach encourages governments to take a three-dimensional view of decision-making that simultaneously considers impacts on 1) current well-being; 2) inclusion; and 3) the sustainability of well-being over time. As such, well-being frameworks do not replace sectoral, inter-sectoral, regional or sub-population frameworks or analysis. They rather bring them together in an overarching, whole-of-government framework that enables policy makers to see the bigger picture and key interlinkages, like a "macroscope" for public policy (Winkler, 2009[88]; Karacaoglu, 2021[89]).

Assessing policies for their multidimensional well-being impact, ex ante rather than ex post, can lead to better strategic alignment and stronger cross-government collaboration in addressing societal priorities. In addition, multidimensional frameworks can draw attention to well-being issues that are commonly overlooked or left unaddressed in more traditional analysis, but which can nonetheless form barriers to progress in other areas. While considering externalities and spill-over effects has long been an important part of the work of policy analysts, there are often large inconsistencies between government agencies in how systematically this is done – and different parts of government have different definitions of what it means to improve people's well-being (Whitby, Seaford and Berry, 2014[90]). Putting a set of core societal objectives at the heart of all policies makes such assessments more systematic in three important ways: 1) each agency is asked to assess the impacts of its policies and practices on multidimensional outcomes; 2) the domains and dimensions of societal well-being considered by each agency are more comprehensive; and 3) the indicators used to measure and report on these domains and dimensions are more consistent.

Five illustrative examples of recovery channels that can simultaneously raise current, distributional and future well-being outcomes

The nature and scope of recovery pathways will vary across countries, reflecting national priorities and circumstances (Buckle et al., 2020[13]). Every country context is different, and no one-size-fits-all policy solutions to improve societal well-being exist. Nonetheless, this section provides illustrative examples of recovery channels that can simultaneously contribute to addressing current well-being concerns, promoting equal opportunities, and improving future well-being outcomes in the wake of the pandemic ("triple win channels"). Examples of such channels are:

- Supporting the creation of sustainable, inclusive and high-quality jobs
- Using lifelong learning to reduce inequalities of opportunity
- Strengthening mental and physical health promotion and prevention

- Using a whole-of-government approach to raise the well-being of disadvantaged children and young people
- Reinforcing trust by strengthening public sector competencies and values, and by encouraging meaningful citizen participation.

These "triple win" channels are not exhaustive, nor do they represent a comprehensive recovery agenda focused on well-being. They are rather meant as examples of how well-being frameworks can help identity strategic directions for recovery packages that can contribute to well-being across multiple dimensions, groups and time-periods (i.e. short and long-term) (see Table 1.1). They point to the value of embedding broader outcome-based frameworks across government that encourage more systematic consideration of the range of outcomes that shape societal well-being throughout policy development and implementation. The examples further illustrate how a well-being lens can help draw policy attention to important determinants of societal well-being that often remain unaddressed (e.g. the importance of social connectedness for mental and physical health outcomes). Applying a well-being lens also encourages broadening other policy tools and frameworks that determine what has value for public investment (e.g. cost-benefit analysis, the system of national accounts). Lastly, the examples illustrate how taking a wider well-being lens can support a more preventative approach to public policy by systematically considering well-being both today and tomorrow.

Supporting the creation of sustainable, inclusive and high-quality jobs

Work plays a central role in recovery strategies and is where many challenges of current well-being, lack of equal opportunities, and future well-being intersect (Sandbu, 2020[91]; OECD, 2020[15]; Hepburn et al., 2020[16]). In the matter of a few months, the COVID-19 pandemic turned from a public health crisis into a jobs crisis whose full extent is still unfolding (OECD, 2020[22]; OECD, 2021[72]). Job creation is therefore an essential component of any recovery strategy. Importantly, from a well-being perspective, the *quality* and *form* of job creation matters as much as its quantity. Two broad areas offer strong opportunities for making jobs work for raising current and future well-being and for promoting equal opportunities: 1) the green economy; and 2) the education, health and wider care sectors.

Supporting job creation while greening the economy

Greening the economy can create new opportunities to enhance current well-being, reduce inequalities and contribute to a more sustainable future. Policy choices made in the COVID-19 recovery will shape whether these opportunities are realised (OECD, 2020[15]; OECD, 2021[48]). Various sectors offer significant prospects for rapid green job creation, including in renewable energy, energy efficiency, green transport and ecosystem restoration (OECD, 2020[15]; Hepburn et al., 2020[16]; O'Callaghan and Murdock, 2021[58]). Investment in these sectors can create jobs quickly, and can contribute to more equitable and sustainable economic development (O'Callaghan and Murdock, 2021[58]):

- Investment in *housing and building energy efficiency* can reduce the cost of living and improve health outcomes (OECD, 2021[27]) (OECD, 2020[92]). This is particularly so for vulnerable groups, as the energy costs and the health burden of poorly insulated housing disproportionally falls on lower-income households, ethnic minorities, families with children, the elderly and households with disabilities (OECD, 2020[92]; González-Eguino, 2015[93]).
- Investment in *renewable energy* offers both short- and long-term employment opportunities. In addition, it can help improve electricity affordability (Dowling et al., 2020[94]) and create health benefits through reduced air pollution (Alvarez-Herranz et al., 2017[95]; Kampa and Castanas, 2008[96]).
- Investment in *green transport and infrastructure* helps to improve health outcomes, both by reducing air pollution (Buckle et al., 2020[13]; Buekers et al., 2014[97]) and by encouraging active transport (Pucher et al., 2010[98]).

- Investment in *natural ecosystem restoration and conservation* can create relatively low-skilled jobs quickly and in the longer-term helps support food security and poverty reduction (Adams, 2004[99]; Zhen et al., 2014[100]). In addition, increased access to green spaces can help promote mental and physical health (Chapter 3).

A strong focus on inclusiveness is needed to ensure that economic support for green job creation can indeed improve well-being for all (OECD, 2021[48]). Gains in green employment will come with job losses in other sectors, and those who will be able to pick up green jobs are not necessarily those who have lost or will lose their jobs. Inclusive policies are therefore pivotal to carefully navigate the differential impacts of the green transition on regions and people and to support a just transition. For example, while the sectors that are most negatively affected by the green transition are largely male-dominated, at the same time women remain under-represented in many green growth sectors, such as renewable energy, pointing to the need for gender-sensitive policies (OECD, 2021[48]; IRENA, 2019[101]). To date, green jobs also tend to score low on ethnic diversity. In the United Kingdom, for example, environmental jobs are the second-least ethnically diverse profession, after farming (Norrie, 2017[102]). Older workers – who make up a relatively large share of workers in carbon-intensive industries in some countries – are more vulnerable, since they often face above-average displacement challenges (OECD, 2021[48]). An integrated approach is therefore needed that accompanies investment in green growth with policies to facilitate labour reallocation, as well as ensuring well-targeted income support measures for those who initially stand to lose (OECD, 2021[48]). Measures to support the geographic mobility of workers at risk of losing their jobs in shrinking industries are also important (OECD, 2021[35]), as are reforms to improve access to affordable housing. In addition, strong place-based policies are needed – building on social dialogue – to ease the structural adjustment of local economies (OECD, 2021[48]).

Improving worker well-being means a focus on creating *good* jobs, not just *more* jobs. Attention needs to be given to earnings quality, labour market security and the quality of the working environment (OECD, 2015[103]). Although having a job promotes mental health and well-being, work of poor psycho-social quality (e.g. characterised by low levels of control, high job demands, high job insecurity and/or unfair pay) is not associated with any better mental health and sometimes even worse mental health than unemployment (OECD, 2015[104]; OECD, 2012[105]; Milner, Krnjacki and LaMontagne, 2017[106]; Butterworth et al., 2013[107]). High-quality jobs benefit firms' productivity as well as workers' well-being (Saint-Martin, Inanc and Prinz, 2018[108]). Longitudinal data from Australia further indicates that when parents hold poor-quality jobs their children show higher emotional and behavioural difficulties, after controlling for income, parent education, family structure and work hours (Strazdins et al., 2010[109]). Ensuring that job creation goes hand in hand with good job quality is therefore essential for workers and their families as well as for businesses and wider society.

Box 1.2. Synergies between climate goals and wider well-being in the COVID-19 recovery

A recent OECD working paper describes how focusing on wider well-being outcomes can accelerate progress in addressing the COVID-19 and environmental crises. The paper *Addressing the COVID-19 and climate crises* provides an analytical framework to assess recovery policy options in the light of potential synergies between climate goals and wider well-being goals, with a particular focus on recovery measures in the surface transport and residential sectors (Buckle et al., 2020[13]).

The paper distinguishes between three stylised pathways for the pandemic recovery in relation to climate goals: 1) a *Rebound* pathway, which prioritises a rapid re-establishment of economic growth and macroeconomic stability, without prioritising CO_2 emissions reductions and progress on wider social or environmental objectives; 2) a *Decoupling* pathway, which aims to restore economic growth and macroeconomic stability as well as achieving an absolute decoupling of CO_2 emissions (i.e. emissions would be flat or falling while GDP rises); and 3) a *Wider well-being* pathway, which integrates economic recovery, CO_2 emission reductions and wider well-being outcomes.

The paper lays out what the three pathways would mean in the case of the transport and residential sectors, using modelling data to contrast the three scenarios. In the case of transport, for instance, a Rebound scenario focuses on boosting economic growth, jobs and disposable incomes by fostering low-occupancy private vehicle ownership without introducing environmental conditionality. The policy rationale behind a Rebound approach is centred on physical movement (vehicles, passengers and ton-kilometres) and speed as central performance indicators for the sector. In a Decoupling pathway there would be strong incentives for low-carbon mobility, with associated well-being benefits from a reduction in environmental impacts (e.g. reduced air pollution and related improvements in health outcomes). However, a Decoupling pathway remains rooted in a "supporting mobility for economic growth" mindset and does not seek to transform transport systems. As a result, private, low-occupancy car use remains the dominant model, disfavouring shared and active transport modes. In contrast a Wider well-being recovery pathway shifts the focus towards cleaner vehicles and fuels, and redesigns the transport and urban system so that shared and active transport become central.

Urban transport scenarios mirroring such principles show that CO_2 emissions related to vehicle use would increase by 8% between 2015 and 2030 in a Rebound (business-as-usual) type scenario. In the Decoupling scenario – focused on automation and electrification with private vehicles remaining dominant – CO_2 emissions would fall by 7%. The biggest gains would be achieved in the Wider well-being scenario, which shifts the focus from mobility to accessibility by complementing accelerated automation and electrification with the transformation of the surface transport sector towards a higher use of shared and high-occupancy vehicles, as well as walking and cycling. The Wider Well-being scenario could reduce CO_2 emissions related to vehicle use by an estimated 30% as well as generating wider well-being benefits in terms of health, affordability of services, and safety and security.

A Wider well-being pathway could therefore considerably speed up emission reductions in addition to generating well-being benefits, by focusing on systemic change rather than incremental improvement of existing systems. While some investments in Wider well-being pathways may imply higher up-front costs, these pathways would have higher returns in terms of both climate and well-being outcomes. Moreover, some actions within this strategy (e.g. road-space redistribution) could both imply lower costs and result in rapid and significant improvements for both the environment and well-being.

Supporting job creation in the education, health and wider care sector

The education, health and wider care sector provides another important avenue to create sustainable jobs that contribute to the well-being of current and future generations and can help promote opportunities for all (NEF, 2020[110]). The pandemic has highlighted the importance of certain economic sectors, sometimes referred to as the "foundational economy", that are particularly important for meeting basic needs and making a "good life" possible by "keeping us safe, sound and civilised" (The Foundational Economy, n.d.[111]). Following the 2008 financial crisis, important parts of the foundational economy, including the health and wider care sector, have been a target for reduced spending, leading to a "care deficit" that has weakened many countries' resilience in the face of the COVID-19 crisis (De Henau and Himmelweit, 2020[112]; Van Gool and Pea, 2014[113]; Aponte et al., 2020[114]). Yet these activities play an important role in building the human and social capital that underpin both well-being and a healthy, sustainable economy, something that current national accounting practices are not well-equipped to incorporate (see Box 1.3).

Building social infrastructure can contribute to current well-being, reduce inequalities and deliver long-term benefits. Effective and well-targeted investment in social infrastructure, such as education, health and wider care services, can strengthen human capital by increasing educational and health outcomes, and address the inequalities within them, whilst also boosting employment and enabling sustainable economic growth (Nozal, Martin and Murtin, 2019[19]). Moreover, as a job creation strategy, the employment boost of investing in social infrastructure is often larger than that associated with investments in physical infrastructure (Richardson and Denniss, 2020[120]; Hill, 2020[121]; De Henau and Himmelweit, 2020[112]). Data for Australia, Denmark, Germany, Italy, Japan, the United Kingdom and the United States indicate that investment in the construction industry would generate half the number of new jobs that would be generated by a similar level of investment in the care industry (De Henau et al., 2016[119]).

Box 1.3. National accounts and public value

The overarching well-being goals of society are not equally considered in traditional national accounting (Canry, 2020[115]). The core national accounting frameworks are still largely structured around labour and physical capital as the two major production factors, accounting for the value of some forms of natural capital and human capital only in satellite accounts.[5] This means that, while public expenditure on the construction of schools, hospitals, care homes and nurseries, including the wages of building workers, is classified as capital expenditure (i.e. "investment"), expenditure to pay for the wages of teachers, doctors, nurses and care workers is classified as current expenditure in the central framework (i.e. "consumption") and is recognised as investment in human capital only in satellite accounts (Elson, 2016[116]). In addition, social capital is not accounted for in the system of national accounts (World Bank, 2005[117]). This has important consequences, as government rules and practices tend to be more tolerant of deficits incurred through making capital rather than current expenditure (Truger, 2016[118]). This partly explains the popularity of spending on physical (rather than social) infrastructure to reinvigorate the economy in recessionary times (De Henau et al., 2016[119]).

Economic support for the education, health and wider care sectors can also play an important role in helping to reverse the damaging impacts of COVID-19 on gender equality (Hill, 2020[121]). Whereas investment in the construction industry would increase the gender employment gap, social infrastructure investment decreases this gap (De Henau et al., 2016[119]). The gender impacts of recovery spending are important as women, despite having been on the frontline of the fight against COVID-19, are bearing a disproportionate share of its negative impacts. In many countries, women have been particularly badly affected by higher financial insecurity, the increased burden of unpaid care, worsening mental health, increased loneliness as well as higher domestic violence (OECD, 2020[122]; Aponte et al., 2020[114]) (see Chapters 5, 6 and 7). Support measures for the education, health and wider care sectors can help counteract some of these negative impacts in two important ways. First, investment in good-quality early childcare enables more women to take up employment. Second, as women make up 70% of the global health and social care workforce (Aponte et al., 2020[114]), investment in social infrastructure can help balance fiscal support for industries that remain male-dominated, including many green growth sectors.[6]

Promoting opportunities for all through lifelong learning

Lifelong learning is another area of possible multiple benefits and is vital for effective re-employment strategies following the pandemic (OECD, 2021[48]; Ramos et al., 2020[123]; Hepburn et al., 2020[16]). Lifelong learning is a central component of promoting a just transition to greener economies, which many countries are aiming to accelerate in the wake of the pandemic, both by facilitating labour reallocation and by addressing existing skills gaps and shortages in a number of green sectors, such as renewable energy and energy and resource efficiency (OECD, 2020[15]; OECD, 2021[48]; OECD, 2021[124]). Moreover, the growing focus on digitalisation alongside existing trends of automation, globalisation, population ageing and increased migration flows means that a pro-active approach to lifelong learning is gaining further importance (OECD, 2021[124]; OECD, 2019[125]) (Box 1.4). Lifelong learning also has important benefits for subjective well-being and physical and mental health (Dolan, Fujiwara and Metcalfe, 2012[126]; Manninen et al., 2014[127]). Participation in learning strengthens adults' psycho-social resources, which promotes their self-esteem, identity, purpose and social integration and helps them cope with change and adversity (Hammond, 2004[128]; Manninen et al., 2014[127]). These benefits of participation in adult learning are particularly strong for vulnerable groups, including people with lower levels of education and the elderly (Manninen et al., 2014[127]; Narushima, Liu and Diestelkamp, 2018[129]).

Currently, disadvantaged adults receive little training in most OECD countries (OECD, 2019[130]; OECD, 2021[124]). While lifelong learning has a unique potential to raise current and future well-being outcomes and to help address inequalities, the adults who need further training and learning the most are the least likely to benefit from it. Evidence from the Programme for the International Assessment of Adult Competencies (PIAAC) shows that most adult learning is job-related (Desjardins, 2020[131]). Adults who have low educational qualifications, earn little and are unemployed and/or older have the lowest chances of participating in job-related formal and non-formal training (Figure 1.3). In contrast, highly skilled adults make ample use of the broader range of opportunities that are available to them to upskill or reskill, thereby further increasing the gap between the high- and low-skilled (OECD, 2019[125]). Where lifelong learning has been specifically targeted towards vulnerable groups, early school leavers and migrants appear to be the main target groups, leaving the learning needs of many other vulnerable groups unaddressed (Tuparevska, Santibáñez and Solabarrieta, 2020[132]).

Figure 1.3. Disadvantaged adults receive little training in most OECD countries

Share of adults participating in job-related formal or non-formal training, OECD 30

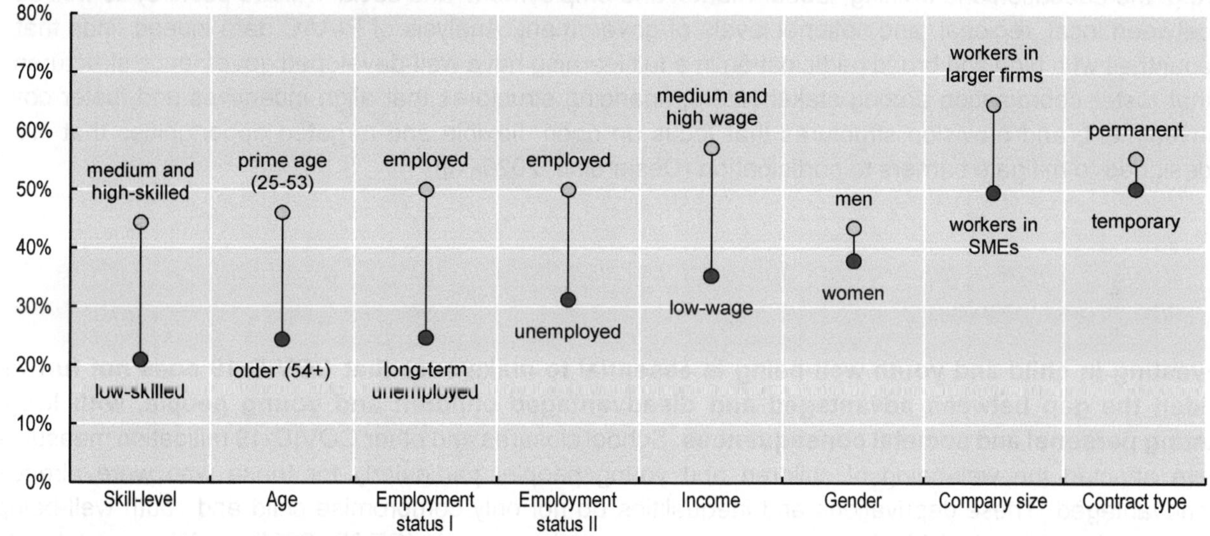

Note: Average of 30 OECD countries participating in PIAAC 2012-2015. This average excludes Colombia, Costa Rica, Iceland, Latvia, Luxembourg, Mexico, Portugal and Switzerland.

Source: *Survey of Adult Skills* (PIAAC) 2012, 2015, as reported in Chart 2, OECD (2019[130]), *Policy brief. Future-ready adult learning systems*, OECD Publishing, Paris, http://www.oecd.org/employment/skills-and-work/adult-learning/Policy-Brief-Future-ready-adult-learning-2019-EN.pdf.

StatLink https://stat.link/h3dlxz

Ensuring inclusive approaches to lifelong learning is even more relevant given the growing importance of digital skills in the wake of the pandemic (OECD, 2021[124]). The COVID-19 pandemic has highlighted the value of digital skills and solutions in times of crisis, and is accelerating the rise of the digital economy. Digitalisation holds great potential for lifelong learning, and online course offerings are growing rapidly. However, while online courses can make access to training easier for many adults by addressing barriers of time, scheduling and location, the pre-requisite to have basic digital skills and devices risks further limiting access to learning opportunities for those with lower levels of digital proficiency or limited access to digital infrastructure (OECD, 2020[133]). Data from PIAAC (2012, 2015, 2018) show that, on average across OECD countries, 43% of adults score at the lowest levels of digital proficiency (Level 1 or below, on a scale ranging from Level 1 to Level 3[7]) (OECD, 2019[134]). Addressing this digital divide has become increasingly important to make sure that lifelong learning can benefit all (OECD, 2021[124]).

Box 1.4. Future-ready adult learning systems

A comprehensive policy agenda is needed to increase the future readiness of countries' adult learning systems (OECD, 2019[135]). The OECD report *Getting Skills Right: Future-Ready Adult Learning Systems* includes an online dashboard on priorities for online learning, comparing countries in terms of: the urgency of updates to the adult learning system; the learning system's coverage and inclusiveness; the flexibility of learning opportunities and the availability of guidance; alignment with labour market needs; perceived impact; and financing (OECD, 2019[136]). To improve learning system's coverage and inclusiveness, the report includes best practice examples of ways to: 1) reach out and provide information and guidance on opportunities for education and training; 2) remove common barriers to participation by vulnerable groups; 3) offer targeted support to those most in need of up- and re-skilling, but least likely to participate; and 4) further engage employers in the provision of adult learning. The report stresses the importance of strong and ongoing collaboration across the many stakeholders in the adult learning system. This includes stronger alignment both between different ministries and sectors (e.g. the education and training, labour market and employment, and social welfare sectors) as well as between local, regional, and national levels of government. Analysis of PIAAC data indeed finds that countries with high and broad participation in adult learning have well-developed governance structures that foster coordination among stakeholders; financing structures that align incentives and foster co-investment; and provision structures that focus on open, flexible and targeted opportunities that are designed to mitigate barriers to participation (Desjardins, 2020[131]).

Using a whole-of-government approach to raise the well-being of disadvantaged children and young people

Investing in child and youth well-being is essential to make sure that COVID-19 does not further widen the gap between advantaged and disadvantaged children and young people, with long-lasting personal and societal consequences. School closures and other COVID-19 mitigation measures have affected the well-being of children and young people, particularly for those who were already disadvantaged. These deprivations and inequalities do not only compromise child and youth well-being now, but also shape individual and societal outcomes going forward (OECD, 2020[32]). The societal well-being returns from investing in children and young people are very high: for instance, a longitudinal study following children through to the age of 35, shows that each dollar invested in high-quality birth-to-five programs for disadvantaged children generated a benefit of over 7 dollars by the age of 35, taking into account the children and their parents' subsequent life outcomes, including their health, educational outcomes, employment outcomes, and participation in crime (García et al., 2016[137]; Reynolds et al., 2011[138]; OECD, 2016[139]). Not all intervention programmes for children show the same cost-benefit ratio, but there is wide evidence that the benefits outweigh the costs for many of them (Hendren and Sprung-Keyser, 2020[140]; Rea and Burton, 2020[141]; Rosholm et al., 2021[142])

The multifaceted challenges in raising child and youth well-being calls on governments to develop comprehensive child and youth well-being strategies that can guide inter-agency collaboration (OECD, 2019[73]; OECD, 2020[143]). Vulnerable children and young people need coherent and coordinated support throughout child and young adulthood and in their transition to an autonomous life. As of April 2020, while 76% of OECD countries had an operational national or federal multi-year youth strategy in place, only 20% of them are fully participatory, budgeted, monitored and evaluated according to the OECD Assessment Framework of National Youth Strategies (OECD, 2020[143]). In most OECD countries, child and youth policies are developed in silos without sufficient consideration of how the range of factors shaping child and youth well-being interact (OECD, 2019[73]). Individual agency approaches that focus on single aspects of child and youth well-being, such as learning difficulties, early school leaving or childhood obesity, are unlikely to be effective if they do not address other barriers to healthy child and youth development, such as family circumstances, housing security, domestic violence, or mental health problems (OECD, 2015[144]).

Comprehensive child and youth well-being strategies can help overcome siloed approaches by identifying overarching child and youth well-being objectives against which policies can be assessed, efforts can be aligned, and accountability can be enhanced. A lack of institutional mechanisms for horizontal coordination across ministries represents a significant barrier to effective whole-of-government approaches, as indicated by 45% of government entities who are in charge of youth affairs across OECD countries (OECD, 2020[143]). At the strategic level, whole-of-government approaches to child and youth policies require clear allocation of mandates and responsibilities across ministerial portfolios and different levels of government (OECD, 2020[143]). Ideally, one ministry or a dedicated agency should take responsibility for coordinating the strategy and ensuring overall accountability (OECD, 2019[73]). At the implementation level, a joined-up strategy forms the basis for more integrated, person-centred service provision, for example through co-location or case management, which is associated with better programme outcomes for vulnerable groups (OECD, 2015[144]). OECD work identifies six priority policy areas around which comprehensive child well-being strategies could be organised, building on best-practice examples from a wide range of countries (Box 1.5), and forthcoming work will describe how various OECD governments are tackling a more strategic approach to child well-being (OECD, 2021[145]).

Box 1.5. Six priority areas for comprehensive child well-being strategies

The OECD report *Changing the odds for vulnerable children* outlines six priority areas around which child well-being strategies should be organised:

1. **Policies empowering vulnerable families**, focused on early intervention and prevention. For example, providing opportunities for parents to gain parenting skills, knowledge, and resources; working together with families to reduce specific risks to child well-being; and investing in whole-of-community approaches to support vulnerable children.
2. **Policies strengthening children's emotional and social skills**. For example, enhancing the role of schools in promoting good emotional and social well-being; providing timely and accessible early intervention for children with mental health difficulties; ensuring smooth transitions of young people onto adult mental health services; providing opportunities for vulnerable children to build relationships with supportive adults and role models, as well as access to extra-circular activities; and empowering children online and building digital resilience.
3. **Policies strengthening child protection**. For example, making child protection services more child-centred and accessible, and investing in improving outcomes for children in out-of-home care.
4. **Policies improving educational outcomes**. For example, increasing participation of vulnerable children in early childhood education and care; improving the quality of early childhood education and care that vulnerable children receive; adopting measures to reduce inequity in education; preventing early school leaving and providing early action for school leavers; and supporting the integration of migrant children in schools.

5. **Policies improving health outcomes**. For example, improving the quality and accessibility of pre-natal care for key groups; improving access to parental leave for low-income families and those with children with additional needs; ensuring access to health care for children from low-income families and with additional health needs; and ensuring access to adequate nutrition for low-income children and pregnant women.
6. **Policies reducing income poverty**. For example, creating better quality jobs for working parents and removing barriers to taking up employment; and ensuring social benefits reach the poorest families and those with children with additional needs.

Source: (OECD, 2019[73]) *Changing the odds for vulnerable children.* Paris: OECD Publishing.

Strengthening mental and physical health promotion and prevention

The pandemic has made the incorporation of health in all policies a reality, albeit not in the way it was intended (Van den Broucke, 2020[146]). Improving mental and physical health was already an important policy priority before the pandemic hit and has become even more urgent now, given the possible long-term implications for physical and mental health outcomes. Investing in physical and mental health has strong benefits for both current and future well-being as well as reducing inequalities. Health is one of the strongest factors associated with people's satisfaction with life (Boarini et al., 2012[147]; Dolan, Peasgood and White, 2008[148]). Poor health weighs heavily on individuals as well as society as a whole by limiting people's opportunities to lead fulfilled, productive lives (OECD, 2021[149]; OECD, 2021[46]; OECD, 2019[44]; OECD, 2019[45]). For example, poor mental health contributes to worse educational outcomes, higher unemployment, and poorer physical health (OECD, 2019[150]; Hewlett and Moran, 2014[151]). Similarly, harmful alcohol consumption and obesity increase the risk of chronic disease, reduce life expectancy, and are related to worse mental health outcomes as well as higher risk of unemployment (OECD, 2021[149]; OECD, 2021[46]; OECD, 2019[44]).

Improving health outcomes is key to addressing inequalities and raising the well-being of future generations. People who are disadvantaged tend to have worse health outcomes than the better-off or better educated (OECD, 2019[152]). A two-way causal relationship, often referred to as the "health-poverty trap", means that disadvantaged people can get trapped in a negative feedback loop between poor health and poverty (Ridley et al., 2020[153]). For example, poor mental health makes it harder to do well in school and work, which can lead to greater risk of poverty, which is itself a risk factor for poor mental health. Improving parental mental health outcomes is also an important part of supporting child and youth well-being. Parental mental health problems can have intergenerational well-being effects through their impact on children's cognitive, emotional, social, and behavioural development as well as their physical health (Harvard University Centre on the Developing Child, 2009[154]; Jarde et al., 2016[155]; Manning and Gregoire, 2006[156]).

With health systems already under pressure, a more preventative health approach is urgently needed (OECD, 2019[44]; OECD, 2015[157]; Patel et al., 2018[158]). Policies targeting the root causes of ill-health are increasingly important given the mounting pressures on the health system due to the pandemic, ongoing population ageing, and the growing prevalence of people with multiple chronic conditions (OECD, 2019[44]). Currently, on average, OECD countries allocate less than 3% of their health spending to prevention activities, with most of it spent on monitoring programmes, such as check-ups and dental examinations (Gmeinder, Morgan and Mueller, 2017[159]; European Commission, 2017[160]). While the cost-effectiveness of preventative health measures depends on a wide range of factors, including the successfulness of policy targeting, there are many preventative health measures that are highly cost-effective (OECD, 2021[149]; OECD, 2021[46]; OECD, 2019[44]; Masters et al., 2017[161]). For example, interventions in the areas of mental health promotion, promoting healthy behaviours, housing interventions, screening, vaccination, and healthy employment programmes have been shown to have early returns on investment within the first 5 years, with additional benefits in the longer-term (WHO, 2014[162]). Careful analysis of the costs and benefits of specific interventions, rather than broad generalisations, nonetheless remains critical. In doing so, it is important to account for the wider well-being benefits of preventative health care spending, including impacts on educational, employment, and child development outcomes, rather than limiting cost-benefit analysis to the health care sector alone.

A well-being approach can help support a more preventative approach to improving health outcomes. Firstly, well-being analysis helps to clarify the interconnections between health and other well-being outcomes. This enables more comprehensive and pro-active interventions to enhance health outcomes that recognise the drivers of good health as well as those of illness (Patel et al., 2018[158]) (Box 1.6). Secondly, a well-being approach makes health promotion a shared objective across government rather than leaving it up to one ministry or part of government. This is fundamental because progress on the health agenda necessitates a whole-of-government approach (OECD, 2015[157]; OECD, 2019[44]; OECD, 2019[45]), where health is seen as a vehicle to enable people to do what they have reason to value rather than merely a destination, like a hospital or a care home (Button, 2021[163]). Thirdly, a well-being approach helps to embed a stronger future-focus in the system of government, encouraging greater appreciation of the long-term value of investments made in health today. Forthcoming OECD work illustrates these points in relation to population mental health, by describing the interrelationships between mental health and wider well-being (including social connections, safety, housing, jobs, income and more), and discussing evidence on the benefits of more integrated policy approaches (OECD, 2021[164]; OECD, 2021[165]).

Box 1.6. Links between social connectedness and health

A preventative approach to public health needs to consider the importance of social connectedness for physical and mental health outcomes. Chapters 4 and 7 describe how the need for social distancing following the pandemic outbreak has disrupted people's sense of connectedness. For example, data from several countries shows that feelings of loneliness doubled to nearly tripled during lockdown and extended beyond lockdown periods.

Social relationships can "get under our skin"

A lack of social connectedness predicts early death as much as major health risk behaviours like smoking (Berkman et al., 2000[166]; Cacioppo and Cacioppo, 2018[167]). Supportive relationships can help buffer the adverse effects of life's stressors on health outcomes and can strengthen the immune system (Uchino, 2006[168]). For example, in studies of patients with HIV, those who had less emotional support in the baseline year were found to have fewer helper T-cells[1] in subsequent years to combat the disease (Theorell et al., 1995[169]). Social connectedness also leads to more functional and adaptive coping styles and better self-regulation (Cohen and Wills, 1985[170]). Experiments show that participants who are exposed to social exclusion are less likely to engage in healthy behaviour, quit sooner on a frustrating task, and are less able to focus their attention (Baumeister et al., 2005[171]). In addition, social connections influence health behaviours through processes of social influence, giving rise to growing interest in social network approaches for health behaviour changes (Hunter et al., 2017[172]).

Social connectedness has persistent and cumulative effects on mental health

Social connectedness also plays an important role in protecting against poor mental health. Loneliness is a unique predictor of depression and anxiety (Cacioppo et al., 2006[173]). For children, loneliness and social isolation have persistent and cumulative effects on later mental health outcomes (Caspi et al., 2006[174]; Qualter et al., 2010[175]). For young adults, family and school connectedness are powerful determinants of their levels of anxiety and psychological distress (Bond et al., 2007[176]). Social relationships also play an important role in protecting older people against depression (Cruwys et al., 2013[177]) and cognitive decline (Bennett et al., 2006[178]; Haslam, Haslam and Jetten, 2014[179]). The size of these effects is considerable: studies have shown that memory loss among older people who were least socially connected worsened at twice the rate of those who were most connected over a six-year period (Ertel, Glymour and Berkman, 2008[180]).

Social prescribing as part of a "whole-person" and preventative approach to health care

Several countries are starting to apply a more preventative and holistic approach to health care that more explicitly considers the importance of the social determinants of ill-health. For instance, in the United Kingdom, "social prescribing" enables GPs, nurses, hospital discharge teams, police, and other primary care professionals to refer patients and clients to trained "link workers". Link workers support people in developing and achieving a personalised set of health and social goals by engaging with local, non-clinical services and initiatives. These can range from debt management workshops and career coaching to gym classes and walking groups. Social prescribing can particularly benefit people with long-term conditions, those who need support with their mental health, who are lonely or isolated, and/or have complex social needs which affect their well-being (NHS, n.d.[181]).

Note: 1. T-cells play a central role in the body's immune response system.
Source: (Frieling, Krassoi Peach and Cording, 2018[182])

Reinforcing trust by strengthening public sector competencies and values, encouraging meaningful citizen participation

COVID-19 has demonstrated the important role of social capital in determining societal well-being outcomes. Social capital has influenced the effectiveness of countries' responses to the COVID-19 crisis. In addition, earlier research has shown how shared pro-social norms and institutional arrangements that foster cooperation between groups are associated with better democratic performance (LaPorta et al., 1997[183]; Putnam, 2000[184]; Algan and Cahuc, 2013[185]; Berning and Ziller, 2017[186]), increased economic growth (Zak and Knack, 2001[39]; Knack and Keefer, 1997[187]), higher overall educational performance (Putnam, 2000[184]; Knack and Keefer, 1997[187]), greater safety in society (Wilkinson, Kawachi and Kennedy, 1998[188]; Sampson, Raudenbush and Earls, 1997[189]), and higher overall experienced well-being (Algan and Cahuc, 2013[185]; OECD, 2017[190]).

Recovery strategies should focus on ensuring high public sector competencies and values as well as ensuring meaningful citizen participation (OECD, 2017[191]). Despite the likely temporary boost to institutional trust in 2020, still only 51% of people trust their government, which weakens governments' ability to raise support for ambitious recovery plans. Widespread mis- and disinformation further undermines trust, amplifies fears, and sometimes leads to harmful behaviours (OECD, 2020[81]). Low trust is associated with resistance, even to things that seem to be in a person's overall best interest (OECD, 2017[191]). For example, hesitancy about Covid-19 vaccination has been evident in many countries and governments' actions to garner trust are essential to the successfulness of vaccination campaigns (OECD, 2021[82]). This means that strong public sector competencies (responsiveness and reliability) and values (integrity, openness/ inclusiveness, and fairness) are even more important now as key drivers of institutional trust (OECD, 2017[191]; OECD, 2020[192]; Murtin, Fleischer and Siegerink, 2018[193]; OECD, 2021[12]). In turn, trust in public institutions forms the basis for strong collective action in building forward (OECD, 2017[191]).

Open government reforms can foster a culture of governance based on the principles of transparency, integrity, accountability, and stakeholder participation (OECD, 2016[194]). As the last section of this chapter will discuss in more detail (see *Using a well-being lens to Reconnect*), transparent and timely public communication, as well as ongoing and inclusive citizen participation in the design of recovery strategies, are essential to better understand and address public concerns and to strengthen public confidence in the effectiveness of recovery pathways (OECD, 2020[81]; OECD, 2021[82]). The OECD *Toolkit* *and Case Navigator for Open Government* offers practical guidance for building an open government programme, from concept development through to implementation and monitoring and evaluation (OECD, 2021[195]). In addition, the *OECD Serving Citizens Framework* helps to assess country performance in terms of access, responsiveness, and quality of services (OECD, 2019[196]; OECD, 2021[12]).

The pandemic has highlighted the important role that social protection plays in times of crisis – as well as the gaps in coverage that weaken its effectiveness. The COVID-19 crisis has exposed weaknesses in OECD countries' social protection systems (OECD, 2020[197]; OECD, 2021[72]). Even in countries with the most advanced systems of social protection, certain groups of workers and their families have missed out on adequate social protection: workers with non-standard jobs – including the self-employed, temporary and informal workers, and those who work very short hours – are often not covered by insurance-based unemployment and sickness benefit schemes. Others, who were already out of work before the crisis, have faced prolonged hardship (OECD, 2020[197]). The situation is worse in countries with large informal sectors and weak social protection systems, where many people have lost or will lose work without any access to income support (OECD, 2020[197]). Surveys highlight that despite the large expansion of social protection systems in OECD countries during the crisis, demands for greater government support are common, regardless of experienced job security during the pandemic; on average, 68% of all participants to the OECD Risks That Matter survey felt that their government should be doing more to ensure citizens' social and economic security, ranging from 41% in Denmark to 93% in Chile (OECD, 2021[25]).

Ex ante screening of policy impacts on specific population groups can identify where policy risks creating or exacerbating inequalities of opportunity. For example, the Canadian government uses its Gender-based Analysis Plus (GBA+) to mainstream assessments of the potential impacts of government actions on diverse groups of people, based on gender, as well as other factors such as age, ethnicity, indigenous heritage, geographic location, socio-economic status, family status and disability status. In response to the COVID-19 crisis, Canada has used its GBA+ system to understand how emergency response and recovery spending was likely to impact on existing inequalities and experiences of diverse peoples (Government of Canada, 2020[198]). While half of OECD countries have now introduced gender budgeting, very few countries undertake ex ante assessments of budgetary decisions on income inequality and poverty (OECD, 2019[199]). Similarly, the use of ex-ante regulatory impact assessments to assess implications of regulatory and policy decisions for different groups in society remains limited. Nonetheless, several countries, including Austria, France, Germany, and New Zealand, have developed "youth checks" to incorporate youth considerations more systematically into policymaking and legislation (OECD, 2020[143]).

Table 1.1 **provides an overview of the expected well-being gains of the five recovery channels described in this chapter, in terms of current, distributional, and future well-being outcomes.** As mentioned above, these channels are not exhaustive, nor do they represent a comprehensive well-being focused recovery agenda. Ultimately, the most suitable channels to raise societal well-being depend on countries' unique contexts. Nonetheless, the five channels provide examples of strategies that can deliver benefits in terms of improving current well-being outcomes, promoting opportunities for all and strengthening future well- being. Identifying such synergies is essential to be able to address the current impacts of the COVID-19 pandemic in an equitable and sustainable way. Importantly, the discussion of the five channels has highlighted that achieving these synergies goes beyond prioritising and allocating funding alone. It depends on strong policy design and implementation that builds in well-being considerations up front rather than trying to correct for them after the fact (OECD, 2018[200]). Regardless of their potential, even well-allocated recovery spending can have unintended consequences if impacts on other well-being outcomes are left unconsidered or unaddressed throughout the policy design or implementation process (Hepburn et al., 2020[16]; Agrawala, Dussaux and Monti, 2020[201]). The following section therefore looks at the required processes and mechanisms in the system of government to underpin an effective well-being approach.

Table 1.1. Overview of the five illustrative recovery channels and their expected well-being gains

Recovery channel	Related well-being priorities	Expected current well-being gains	Reduction in inequalities	Expected future well-being gains
Supporting the creation of inclusive and high-quality jobs, with a focus on job creation in: 1) the green sector; and sustainable, 2) the education, health, and wider care sector	Increase the job and financial security of individuals and households hit hardest by the pandemic. Curb the tide on growing well-being inequalities. Take strong action on climate change, biodiversity loss and environmental degradation.	Direct gains Increased job and financial security. However, creating good quality jobs is as important as creating more jobs as low quality jobs are associated with worse health outcomes. Indirect gains Investment in the green sector can help reduce the cost of living, improve health outcomes, and can support energy and food security. Investing in the education, health, and wider care sector can help improve educational and health outcomes.	Direct gains Green jobs can help reduce regional disparities in employment. However, a strong inclusive approach in relation to gender, age, race and ethnicity, and geographic location is needed to ensure that economic support for green job creation reduces rather than reproduces existing inequalities. Investment in the health, education and wider care sector can help reverse the particularly damaging impacts of the pandemic on women's job and financial security. Indirect gains Investment in the energy efficiency sector can help reduce the cost of living for vulnerable groups. Investing in the education, health, and wider care sector can help address health and educational inequalities. Investing in good quality early childcare enables more women to take up employment.	Green job creation contributes to improved environmental outcomes and more sustainable economic development. Investing in the education, health, and wider care sector strengthens human capital.
Using lifelong learning to reduce inequalities	Increase the job and financial security of individuals and households hit hardest by the pandemic. Promote opportunities for all and mitigate the scarring effects of the crisis on minorities, youth and women. Take strong action on climate change, biodiversity loss and environmental degradation.	Adult learning is associated with higher subjective well-being and better physical and mental health.	The health and subjective well-being benefits of participation in adult learning are particularly strong for vulnerable groups, including people with lower levels of education and the elderly. However, existing data shows that adults who need further training and learning the most are the least likely to benefit from existing adult education.	Lifelong learning increases human capital and supports a just transition to greener economies.
Using a whole-of-government approach to raise the well-being of disadvantaged children and young people	Improve well-being outcomes for vulnerable children and young people. Promote opportunities for all and mitigate the scarring effects of the crisis on minorities, youth and women.	Improved overall well-being outcomes for vulnerable children and young people.	Reduced inequalities in well-being outcomes between advantaged and disadvantaged children and young people as well as across generations.	Child and youth well-being deprivations and inequalities to a large extent shape individual and societal outcomes going forward.

Strengthening mental and physical health promotion and prevention	Lift the increasing burden of poor physical and mental health. Promote opportunities for all and mitigate the scarring effects of the crisis on minorities, youth and women. Increase the job and financial security of individuals and households hit hardest by the pandemic. Improve well-being outcomes for vulnerable children and young people.	Poor mental and/or physical health limits people's opportunities to lead fulfilled, productive lives and impacts on a wide range of well-being outcomes, including life satisfaction, educational outcomes, employment outcomes, and life expectancy.	A stronger focus on mental and physical health promotion and prevention can help address the "health-poverty trap", through which disadvantaged people can get stuck in a negative feedback loop between poverty and negative health outcomes.	Improving health outcomes strengthens human capital as well as well-being for future generations, as health disadvantages for parents can have long-term, intergenerational effects on child development.
Reinforcing trust by strengthening public sector competencies and values, and by encouraging meaningful citizen participation	Reinforce trust in others and in public institutions. Promote opportunities for all and mitigate the scarring effects of the crisis on minorities, youth and women.	High levels of trust and pro-social norms are associated with greater safety in society, stronger civic engagement, and higher overall experienced well-being.	Strengthening government responsiveness and values of fairness and integrity, and providing inclusive opportunities for citizen participation to help create more equal opportunities for people to thrive.	High levels of trust and pro-social norms can improve democratic performance, strengthen economic growth, and is associated with higher overall educational performance, thereby strengthening human capital.

Using a well-being approach to Realign

Using a more integrated and coherent approach to building forward and raising well-being asks for a more unified governance system. The COVID-19 pandemic has highlighted the unique and fundamental role of government in safeguarding people's well-being. The crisis has also shown that large shifts in both behaviours and policies are possible once the scale of an emergency is clear and sufficient political and public support is present, even when current pain is needed for long-term gain (Sandbu, 2020[91]; Hepburn et al., 2020[16]). Then, if the core objective of good governance is to safeguard the well-being of current and future generations, how can governance systems be better attuned to reach these goals? While the most effective approaches, models and tools will need to be tailored to local circumstances, there are at least five institutional building blocks that underpin a well-being approach to addressing the post-pandemic priorities:

- **Multidimensional well-being monitoring** - using a multidimensional well-being lens to monitor societal progress and measure policy outcomes, including current and distributional well-being outcomes as well as resources for future well-being
- **Evidence-based priorities** - prioritising policy objectives based on multidimensional well-being evidence
- **Long-term focus** - embedding a long-term focus in governance systems and prioritising prevention
- **Integration and collaboration** - strengthening horizontal and vertical policy coherence to enable an integrated and collaborative approach to addressing multiple well-being priorities
- **Actively connecting** to private and civil society stakeholders in defining well-being issues and identifying and implementing ways to address them.

Over the last decade, components of this governance infrastructure have been implemented in various countries around the world, but not yet in a fully integrated way (Karacaoglu, 2021[89]). This section will focus on the first four of these institutional building blocks. The last section of this chapter *(Using a well-*

being lens to Reconnect) will then look at the importance of actively connecting to civil society and the private sector to jointly drive a strong, inclusive, and sustainable recovery based on a collective sense of purpose.

Multidimensional well-being monitoring

The COVID-19 crisis calls on governments to apply a multidimensional lens to societal progress. To help inform better decision-making, a growing number of governments have broadened their measurement and monitoring frameworks to go "beyond GDP" and "measure what counts" for the well-being of people today and in the future (Stiglitz, Fitoussi and Durand, 2019[202]) (Figure 1.4). Although any well-being framework needs to be anchored within a local context, at a minimum a well-being approach requires measurement of current well-being, of inequalities across well-being outcomes, and of resources for future well-being. In addition, measures of transboundary effects help assess country impacts on well-being elsewhere, for example in terms of carbon footprints, foreign aid, or export of waste (OECD, 2020[203]; Stats NZ, 2018[204]; CBS, 2020[205]).

Establishing well-being frameworks through an inclusive and transparent participatory process is fundamental to ensure legitimacy and public support for the framework used to assess societal progress. In the development of local well-being frameworks, many governments have engaged in wide public consultation processes to develop a shared vision of what matters most to societal well-being (Exton and Shinwell, 2018[207]). For example, in 2015 the federal government of Germany initiated a 6-month long national dialogue with 200 events around the country, reaching out to a large diversity of citizens, to get a better understanding of citizens' perspectives on well-being as the basis for the development of the *Gut Leben in Deutschland* (Good Living in Germany) framework. Some countries, including France, Italy, and New Zealand, as well as Scotland, have built well-being reporting requirements into legislation, with mandated opportunities for public consultation and input. For example, Scottish Ministers have a duty to consult on, develop and publish a new set of National Outcomes for Scotland at least every five years (Durand and Exton, 2019[208]). This helps ensure that public accountability for well-being outcomes extends beyond electoral cycles (Durand and Exton, 2019[209]; Ormston, Pennycook and Wallace, 2021[210]). However, a well-being-oriented recovery needs to go beyond reporting requirements alone.

Well-being evidence-based priorities

Going beyond reporting requirements is essential to truly integrate well-being data in the way that recovery strategies and policies are prioritised and designed. Using comprehensive well-being evidence as the basis for COVID-19 recovery agenda setting is essential to ensure that they target the societal well-being areas that are most in need. In recent years, the government budget process, which gives form to the government's priorities, has been used to more strongly link well-being evidence to government agenda setting and policy prioritisation (Ormston, Pennycook and Wallace, 2021[210]; Durand and Exton, 2019[208]; OECD, 2019[211]). For example, in 2019 New Zealand released its first Wellbeing Budget (Box 1.7). Following on from its GBA+ budget analysis (see above), the Government of Canada is also working to better incorporate well-being measures into its budget decision-making (Government of Canada, 2021[212]); to that end, it released a new "Quality of Life Framework"[8] along with its 2021 Budget to articulate a vision of what it means to have a good quality of life in Canada. This framework serves as a tool to better identify investment priorities. Investments in federal datasets (including to improve levels of disaggregation) will help to advance Canada's existing GBA+ practice within the context of the new Quality of Life Framework. Other countries and regions have similarly expressed an interest in more closely integrating well-being frameworks into their budgetary processes, including Ireland (Government of Ireland, 2021[213]), Iceland (Jakobsdóttir, 2020[214]), and Wales (Future Generations Commissioner for Wales, 2019[215]).

Figure 1.4. National well-being frameworks across the OECD, selected countries

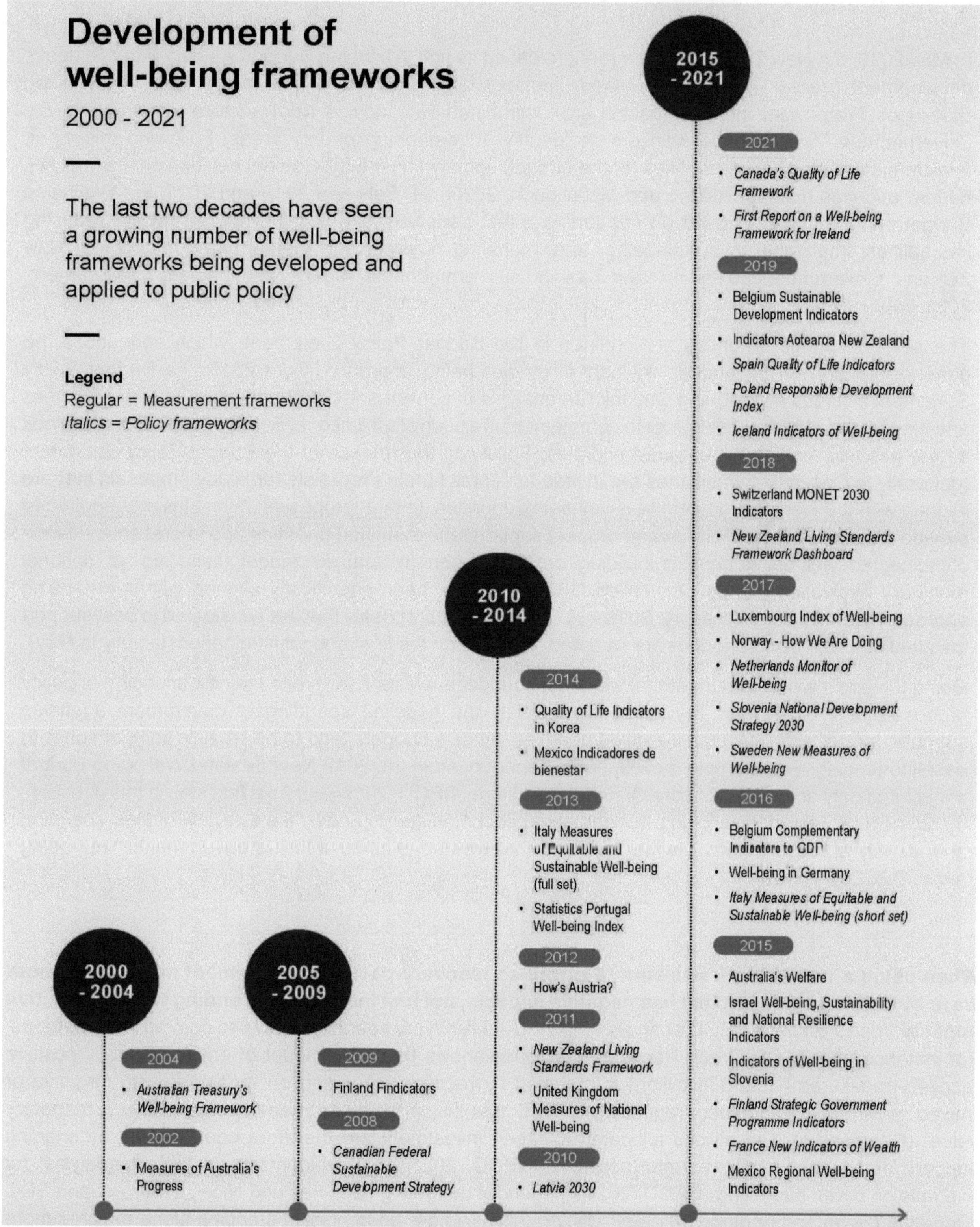

Note: Launch time refers to the actual release of a framework, rather than the commissioning of its development. Number of indicators refers to the dashboards as of Q3 2019 unless specified otherwise. Measures of Australia's Progress was discontinued in 2013, and the Australian Treasury's Well-being Framework in 2016. Australia's Welfare reports have been published since 1993.
Source: Exton and Fleischer (forthcoming[206]).

Box 1.7. The New Zealand Wellbeing Budget

In May 2019, the New Zealand Government released its first Wellbeing Budget. As part of the Budget's development process, the New Zealand Treasury used analysis of well-being data in its Living Standards Framework indicator dashboard[1], combined with advice from sectoral experts and the Government's Chief Science Advisors, to identify 12 well-being priority areas. Following this input, ministers shortlisted seven priorities for the budget, upon which the full Cabinet decided on the final five budget priorities (Huang, Renzio and Mccullough, 2020[216]). Between 2019 and 2021, the Wellbeing Budget priorities have focused on supporting a just transition, shaping the future of work, reducing inequalities, improving child well-being, and improving physical and mental health outcomes (New Zealand Government, 2018[217]; New Zealand Government, 2019[218]; New Zealand Government, 2021[219]).

The selected budget priorities are outlined in the Budget Policy Statement, which announces the general direction of the budget. As part of its well-being approach, from 2019, the Budget Policy Statement includes a Wellbeing Outlook (an analysis of current and distributional well-being outcomes and resources for future well-being) to complement the budget's traditional Economic and Fiscal outlook as the basis for setting government priorities. Following the release of the Budget Policy Statement (generally in December), ministries are invited to submit funding requests for policy proposals that are aligned with the identified government well-being priorities. In their proposals, ministries are required to provide evidence of how their funding request supports the identified priorities and to present evidence on expected well-being impacts building on a cost-benefit analysis model (including an optional monetary evaluation component, called CBAx) that has been specifically aligned with a well-being approach (New Zealand Treasury, 2018[220]). Those policy proposals that are considered to best support the identified well-being priorities are selected, upon which the final budget is released (usually in May).

Going forward it will be important that well-being budget analysis is not limited to new spending or policy proposals only but to also review how effectively the baseline spending of government agencies supports (or detracts from) the identified priorities, as new budgets tend to be small in comparison with baseline funding. For example, new spending announced in the 2019 New Zealand Wellbeing Budget constituted only around 4% of core Crown expenditure (OECD, 2019[221]). As a first step in this direction, the 2019 New Zealand Wellbeing Budget asked each Minister to undertake a review of their spending and identify at least 1% of baseline spending that was not aligned with the government's well-being aims (OECD, 2019[221]).

Note: 1. https://lsfdashboard.treasury.govt.nz

When using a well-being framework to prioritise recovery packages, alignment needs to go both ways by curbing spending that has negative impacts, not just increasing spending that has positive impacts. In this respect, OECD analysis of COVID-19 recovery spending points to contradictory patterns. For instance, the OECD Green Recovery Database shows that the amount of environmentally positive recovery measures (USD 336 billion) is matched by recovery spending on measures with negative or "mixed" environmental impacts (equalling to USD 334 billion for those measures that have a monetary value) (Chapter 11). The billions allocated to green investment are therefore counteracted by ongoing support for environmentally harmful activities (OECD, 2021[86]). Developments in budget analysis, for example on green budgeting (OECD, 2021[86]), gender budgeting (Downes and Nicol, 2020[222]), and SDG budgeting (Hege and Brimont, 2018[223]; UNDP, 2020[224]) are an important stepping stone towards more comprehensive and coherent well-being budget approaches. France's new methodology for green budgeting, for instance, identifies environmentally friendly as well as environmentally damaging expenditures (Fetet and Postic, 2020[225]). As most recovery funds will be spent via public procurement, the strategic use of public procurement is also an important instrument for governments to operationalise gender, green, and SGD budgeting and to ensure that recovery spending will contribute to the identified well-being priorities (OECD, 2019[226]). For example, in a recent review of the German federal public procurement system, the OECD assessed how the country's public procurement system affects well-being in Germany, building on the OECD Framework for Measuring Well-Being and Progress (OECD, 2019[227]).

Long-term focus

Misalignment between COVID-19 recovery measures and long-term societal goals may lower well-being over time (Buckle et al., 2020[13]). Well-being frameworks can support more future-focused and anticipatory policies (Box 1.5). They can help to underpin long-term development strategies, by clarifying tensions as well as possible synergies between current and future well-being outcomes (OECD, 2019[211]). To help deal with such tensions and synergies in practice, some countries have enshrined the rights of future generations in their Constitution or have established dedicated accountability and oversight institutions, such as Finland's Committee for the Future, to strengthen consideration of long-term well-being outcomes (OECD, 2020[143]; Durand and Exton, 2019[208]). Others, like New Zealand and Germany are looking at the impact of public procurement strategies on resources for future well-being (New Zealand Government Procurement, 2018[228]; OECD, 2019[227]). Wales created a Future Generations Commissioner, as well as establishing a legal obligation for public bodies to better incorporate long-term well-being considerations into policy making to strengthen accountability for sustainable development (Box 1.8).

Box 1.8. Embedding a long view: The Welsh Well-being of Future Generations Act

The Well-being of Future Generations (Wales) Act 2015 requires all public bodies to place seven well-being goals - informed by a large-scale public consultation process - at the centre of their decision-making. These seven goals are: a prosperous Wales, a resilient Wales, a more equal Wales, a healthier Wales, a Wales of cohesive communities, a Wales of vibrant culture and thriving Welsh language, and a globally responsible Wales. The Act makes it clear that each of these goals is as important as the others and that, as much as possible, public bodies must work towards all of them rather than focusing on one or two in isolation. In addition, the Act sets out five ways of working by public bodies to achieve the seven well-being goals:

- **Thinking long-term**: Meeting the needs of the present without compromising the ability of future generations to meet their own needs.
- **Integration**: Considering how the public body's objectives may impact upon each of the seven well-being goals or on the objectives of other public bodies
- **Involvement**: Involving people with an interest in achieving the well-being goals and ensuring that those people reflect the diversity of the area which the body serves
- **Collaboration**: Acting in collaboration with any other person (or different parts of the body itself) that could help the body meet its well-being objectives
- **Prevention**: Acting to prevent problems occurring or getting worse to help public bodies meet their objectives

Transparency and accountability are an important part of the Act. The Future Generations Commissioner is the guardian for the interests of future generations in Wales and supports the public bodies listed in the Act to work towards achieving the well-being goals. When the Future Generations Commissioner for Wales makes recommendations to a public body, this body must publish a response. If the public body does not follow a recommendation, it must explain why, and what alternative action it will take. In addition, Audit Wales is responsible for assessing the extent to which the 44 public bodies that are subject to the duties of the Act are operating in accordance with the sustainable development principle (including the "five ways of working" mentioned above) when setting their well-being objectives and taking steps to meet them. The Auditor General must provide a report on his examinations to the National Assembly for Wales at least a year before each Assembly election (Audit Wales, 2020[229]).

Source: www.futuregenerations.wales/about-us/future-generations-act/

Integration and collaboration

The pandemic has highlighted the need for strong alignment across government to be able to deliver the most effective policy responses. The COVID-19 crisis has emphasised the need to strengthen the strategic role played by Centres of Government, beyond crisis response coordination, in establishing more anticipatory and integrated governance (OECD, 2020[203]; OECD, 2021[12]). A study of 26 OECD countries indicates that during the pandemic, 77% of Centres of Government supported more cross-ministerial co-ordination activities and 73% involved more stakeholders in co-ordination meetings. However, only around one-quarter of these centres benefitted from an increase in their financial resources, and roughly the same share experienced an increase in staffing levels (OECD, 2021[12]). More broadly, a lack of integration and coordination of strategies, policies and implementation has long been recognised as one of the main impediments to sustainable development (OECD, 2019[211]). Inconsistent policies and fragmented programmes entail a higher risk of duplication, inefficient spending, a lower quality of service, and difficulty in meeting goals. Ultimately, such shortcomings lead to a reduced capacity to deliver and to unsustainable choices and pathways that stand in the way of a resilient recovery (OECD, 2019[211]; De Coning, 2007[230]). The associated costs – both in terms of reduced well-being and resilience and of higher financial spending – are significant. In the United States, for example, the US Government Accountability Office has estimated that actions from Congress and executive branch agencies to reduce fragmentation, overlap and duplication in government programmes from 2011 to 2018 have generated about USD 262 billion in reported financial benefits (GAO, 2019[231]).

Only a unified public service can ensure the cross-agency leadership and commitment that is necessary to drive a strong, inclusive, and sustainable recovery (OECD, 2020[203]; Buckle et al., 2020[13]; OECD, 2019[211]). A well-being approach encourages this by requiring policy agencies to work together towards shared well-being objectives, aligning their own sectoral goals with overarching priorities to enhance current, distributional and future well-being outcomes. As mentioned above, even though considering policy externalities has for long been part of the work of many policy analysts and executives, there are often large differences between government agencies in terms of how this is done. For example, in the first iteration of its Wellbeing Budget process, the New Zealand Treasury found that some agencies were more accustomed to providing rigorous analysis across well-being dimensions and domains than others (Huang, Renzio and Mccullough, 2020[216]). A well-being approach can help make multidimensional assessments more systematic by defining a core set of well-being priorities against which all policy decisions need to be evaluated. This helps to ensure that all government agencies are engaged in multidimensional well-being analysis, that there is consistency in the domains and dimensions considered, and that they build on the same set of core indicators for each of these domains and dimensions.

Several institutional mechanisms can be used to support more integrated policy analysis and decision-making (OECD, 2019[211]). At a strategic level, national well-being and sustainability strategies can help align the unique roles that different agencies and bodies play in raising well-being. For example, Finland's national sustainability strategy (*The Finland we want by 2050*) brings together existing sector-based long-term strategies within one overarching framework with a common timeline up to 2050. Collaboration requirements for budget proposals can also help encourage alignment of ministerial strategies towards post-crisis well-being priorities. For instance, in New Zealand, once well-being budget priorities have been defined, government ministries are required to work together to put forward budget bids that target the overarching well-being priorities. Budget bids from ministries need to demonstrate cross-agency and cross-portfolio collaboration in the development of the initiative. Ministers are appointed to coordinate the budget bids to help drive policy integration. As a result, the 2019 New Zealand budget saw as many as 10 agencies come together to jointly put in a budget bid to help address issues of family and sexual violence (Huang, Renzio and Mccullough, 2020[216]). Alongside these changes to its budget process, New Zealand has amended its Public Service Act to enable government agencies to more easily work together on cross-cutting priorities through new joint venture structures (Box 1.9).

Box 1.9. Joint ventures: Sharing resources to work on cross-cutting well-being priorities

The New Zealand Public Service Act 2020 (New Zealand Public Service Commission, 2020[232]) aims to support a more adaptive, agile and collaborative public service. It enables public sector chief executives to come together in a joint venture to promote an integrated, whole-of-government approach. Joint ventures cut through existing organisational boundaries by giving public service providers the tools and options to swiftly organise themselves around specific issues, without the cost, complexity and slowness of having to create a new, separate department.

Joint ventures create collective responsibility for achieving an agreed set of outcomes, while making it easier to join up people and resources from across the public service to work on common issues. Budget appropriations go directly to the joint venture itself, and a group of chief executives, rather than one of them, shares accountability for the budget spending, collectively reporting to one Minister. Joint ventures have their own staff, funding and assets, which make it easier to work on cross-cutting topics with suppliers and partners as they can be contracted by the joint venture itself rather than by individual agencies.

Source: www.publicservice.govt.nz

In addition to stronger horizontal alignment between ministries, an effective and efficient recovery asks for stronger alignment between the different levels of government (OECD, 2021[233]; OECD, 2019[211]). Stronger alignment and coordination between national and sub-national levels of government is needed to optimise the potential of each level of government in contributing to post-crisis priorities. Sub-national governments play a vital role in achieving well-being objectives. They carry important responsibilities for many well-being areas, such as education, social protection, health, housing and community amenities. A unique strength of local governments is that they are in more direct contact with their communities, including the most vulnerable groups, for example, through social workers and frontline staff (OECD, 2018[200]). Across OECD countries, sub-national governments are responsible for around 63% of public staff spending, 49% of public procurement, 59% of public investment and 40% of total government expenditures (OECD, 2018[200]). Increasing decentralisation across OECD countries further emphasises the importance of sound multi-level governance arrangements (OECD, 2019[234]; OECD, 2017[235]). Strong vertical alignment and coordination also provides unique opportunities for peer learning and upscaling of successful approaches by sub-national governments, who are in many ways leading the application of well-being metrics and concepts in public policy (Whitby, Seaford and Berry, 2014[90]) (Box 1.10).

Box 1.10. Local governments leading the way: The Amsterdam City Doughnut

Using the Amsterdam City Doughnut to refocus, redesign, realign, and reconnect

In April 2020, the City of Amsterdam released its first Amsterdam City Doughnut.[9] The City Doughnut is a localised version of Raworth's Doughnut Economics model, in which the inner ring sets out the minimum outcomes that are needed to lead a good life while the outer ring represents the ceiling of social and planetary boundaries beyond which future well-being is put at severe risk (Raworth, 2018[236]). By assessing where Amsterdam city is currently "undershooting" and "overshooting" its boundaries, the city has been able to define a set of objectives for Amsterdam to be thriving within its ecological and social boundaries.

The City Doughnut was developped based on a participative approach, including seven workshops in diverse neighbourhoods across Amsterdam, to reflect the lived experience of Amsterdam's residents. The resulting Doughnut vision and strategy is used to bring together a network of city actors in the Amsterdam Doughnut Coalition, involving citizens' networks, alongside government, businesses and knowledge institutions. Together, these actors work towards city-wide initiatives and co-creation for well-being, underpinned by the Doughnut framework.

New perspectives for policy development: Early examples of the Doughnut in action

The City Doughnut is used by policymakers, the wider Amsterdam Doughnut Coalition, and their stakeholders as a guide for thinking about opportunities and challenges, synergies and tensions, and alternative policy options. For example, the City Doughnut has been influential in the development of Amsterdam's construction project, Strandeiland (Beach Island). Beach Island was reclaimed from the waters with sand carried by boats run on low-emission fuel and its foundations were laid using processes that do not hurt local wildlife. Beach Island's future neighbourhood is designed to produce zero emissions and to prioritise social housing and access to nature. The City of Amsterdam has introduced new standards for sustainability and circular use of materials for contractors in all city-owned buildings. This means that anyone wanting to build on Beach Island needs to provide a "materials passport" for their buildings, so that whenever the buildings are taken down, the city can reuse the parts.

The City Doughnut has also influenced the city's responses to the COVID-19 crisis. For instance, when the Netherlands went into lockdown in March 2020, the City of Amsterdam realised that thousands of residents did not have access to computers, which were becoming increasingly important to be able to take part in society. Rather than buying new devices - which would have been expensive and generate e-waste - the city arranged a collection of old and broken laptops from residents who could spare them, hired a firm to refurbish them, and distributed 3 500 refurbished laptops to those in need.

Source: www.amsterdam.nl, (Van Doorninck and Schouten, 2020[237]) and (Nugent, 2021[238]).

To date, very few countries have put a joint well-being framework at the heart of their multi-level governance approach, but the Welsh Well-being of Future Generations Act provides an example of how this could work (OECD, 2020[239]) (Box 1.11). Using a well-being framework across different levels of government can help streamline multi-level approaches in building back better. The Welsh example also highlights the importance of harmonised measurement of core well-being outcomes at national, regional, and local levels to support vertical alignment for raising well-being. While many countries have taken steps over the last two decades to harmonise well-being measurement at the national level (Figure 1.4), the ability to disaggregate national well-being data to regional and local levels remains a challenge in many countries (OECD, 2014[240]). Collaboration and harmonisation in data collection can bring value to both national and subnational analysis and interpretation. Lessons needs to be drawn from the well-being monitoring response to the COVID-19 crisis, which saw many public agencies from different sectors and geographic levels collect well-being data, each using their own set of instruments and survey questions. Even within central government, a lack of common frameworks for data collection and data sharing remains an important obstacle for effective cross-agency collaboration (OECD, 2021[12]).

Box 1.11. Vertical alignment through the Well-being of Future Generations (Wales) Act

The Welsh Well-being of Future Generations Act is unique in that it requires public bodies *at all levels* to work together towards the achievement of the 7 identified well-being priorities, based on the "5 ways of working" (Box 1.8). In total, 44 public bodies are currently subject to the duties of the Act, ranging from the Welsh Government to local health boards, fire and rescue authorities, the national parks authority, and several national bodies (such as the Arts Council, Higher Education Funding Council, and Sport Wales). As the Act applies to Welsh Minsters and national councils as well as local authorities, it forms an important mechanism to encourage both horizontal and vertical coherence across government towards shared well-being objectives.

The Act established Public Services Boards (PSBs) for each local authority area in Wales. These are required to consult on and publish: 1) a regular assessment of the state of economic, social, environmental, and cultural well-being in its area; 2) a local well-being plan, setting out local objectives and strategies to contribute, within the local area, to achieving the overarching well-being goals; and 3) an annual progress report, specifying the steps taken to meet the PSB well-being objectives. These local well-being assessments, plans and progress reports need to be shared with the Welsh Ministers, the Commissioner for Future Generations, the Auditor General for Wales, as well as the local authority's overview and scrutiny committee.

The requirements of the Act thus place a well-being duty on all public bodies and support multi-level alignment in their well-being strategies. Importantly, it does so in a way that allows flexibility for context-appropriate goals and strategies at the local level.

Source: www.futuregenerations.wales/about-us/future-generations-act/

An ongoing challenge for strengthening policy integration and coherence is the need for better understandings of the interconnectedness of well-being outcomes and ways to reflect this in policy design and implementation. Civil servants responsible for policy development in specific domains may have little knowledge of the concepts of well-being, well-being metrics, or their application to public policy (Durand and Exton, 2019[208]). The need for multi-dimensional assessments can quickly push analysts beyond their areas of expertise and place considerable demands on time and capacities. Several of the well-being initiatives led by national governments have begun to include components of civil service capacity-building. For example, the United Arab Emirates' Wellbeing Academy[10] offers (virtual) programmes to federal and local government entities on how to integrate the principles of well-being into their programmes, policies, and services. In the United Kingdom, the Treasury's Green Book provides non-technical guidance on how to appraise and evaluate policies, projects and programmes for their impact on well-being (HM Treasury, 2018[241]; Durand and Exton, 2019[208]). Multi-disciplinary teams or commissions can also play an important role in bringing together the wide array of specialist knowledge that is needed to identify integrated pathways towards greater societal well-being. Multidisciplinary capability is particularly important for central government agencies but there is also value in further considering how the knowledge base that underpins each of the post-crisis well-being priorities can be made more readily accessible across the system of government. For example, establishing advisory roles for selected well-being priorities within each government agency can help create "knowledge linking pins". The practical reality is that being able to consult with someone internally is much more likely to happen than finding and reaching out to someone externally to provide advice, even if the internal person is only a first port of call.

Strengthening evidence on *what worked* can help accelerate progress on raising well-being in the post-pandemic recovery (Karacaoglu, 2021[89]). Gathering better evidence on the extent to which policies and programmes have raised well-being, and their associated costs, is essential to help inform better policies for better lives. This is even more important because most existing studies on the drivers of well-being tend to focus on average effects, whereas most policy interventions focus on very specific groups or areas of interest (Smith, 2021[242]). In a recent effort to distill lessons learned from green stimulus measures following the Global Financial Crisis that could inform recovery measures in response to the COVID-19 pandemic, the OECD has noted a remarkable scarcity of ex post evaluations (Agrawala, Dussaux and Monti, 2020[201]). This scarcity of evidence on "what worked" limits the knowledge that can be gained from past experiences to inform responses to upcoming issues. Where ex post evaluations were undertaken, distributional consequences were often overlooked (Agrawala, Dussaux and Monti, 2020[201]). This points to the importance of applying more comprehensive frameworks , encompassing current and distributional outcomes and resources for future well-being, when evaluating the success of specific government programmes. Some countries have established dedicated institutes, such as the *What Works* Centre for Wellbeing in the United Kingdom, to help bring together academic expertise and knowledge on "what works", as valuable input into ongoing policy development to improve well-being (Box 1.12).

Box 1.12. The United Kingdom What Works Centre for Well-being

In the United Kingdom, the *What Works* Centre for Well-being aims to develop and share evidence that governments, businesses, and civil society can use to improve well-being across the country. Rather than focusing on a specific sector, the What Works Centre for Well-being provides advice to all government agencies on the drivers and measurement of well-being outcomes as well as on how to integrate well-being evidence into public policy. It forms part of a network of seven *What Works* Centres in the United Kingdom addressing different policy issues or geographic regions. These centres help ensure that high quality, independently assessed evidence shapes decision-making at every level by:

- collating existing evidence on the effectiveness of policy programmes and practices
- producing synthesis reports and systematic reviews in areas where they do not currently exist
- encouraging policy-makers to use these findings to inform their decisions by sharing findings in an accessible way, including through regular newsletters, courses, and learning events.

Source: https://whatworkswellbeing.org

Using a well-being lens to Reconnect

The recovery challenges ahead urge governments to more actively reach out to different stakeholders to set shared priorities, align actions and mobilise resources (OECD, 2019[211]). Diverse stakeholders – including public agencies, businesses and industry, civil society and academics – all have pivotal roles to play in alleviating the impacts of the COVID-19 crisis and in building back better (OECD, 2020[203]). A key strength of a well-being approach is that it helps connect government goals with what is most important for the well-being of current and future generations, particularly as country well-being frameworks are often based on large-scale consultations. The resulting frameworks offer a structure for dialogue between governments, citizens and other actors on how to build back better, using a language that resonates with citizens from diverse backgrounds. Well-being frameworks can help citizens better understand the current state of their society, allow them to see where they can add value, and provide them with data to hold their government to account.

Citizens' and external stakeholder participation in public policy development and decision-making weakened during the pandemic, as did the usual system of checks and balances to a certain degree. Already before the pandemic in 2018, only 40% of people in 26 European OECD countries on average believed the political system in their country allows people like them to have a say in what the government does, with the less educated, less wealthy, unemployed, and older people feeling the least empowered to influence their institutions (OECD, 2021[12]; Murtin, Fleischer and Siegerink, 2018[193]). In autumn 2020, on average across 25 OECD countries, 49% of OECD Risks that Matter survey respondents reported that they did not think their government considered the views of people like them (OECD, 2021[25]). Indeed, the speed and scale at which governments had to implement their response to COVID-19 have posed risks for transparency and openness as governments were fast-tracking emergency regulations, policies and procurement (Chapter 10) (OECD, 2021[12]).[11] Although these changes in government processes were often made in light of the extraordinary public health threat they faced, it is important to avoid risks of "mission creep", restore a proper system of checks and balances, and strengthen citizen participation efforts as soon as possible (OECD, 2020[192]).

Effective public communication and ongoing dialogue between governments and citizens are key success factors for joining up forces to building forward (OECD, 2020[81]; OECD, 2020[243]). COVID-19 has put the spotlight on the fundamental role of timely and transparent public communication to strengthen and maintain trust in government and to mobilise collective action (OECD, 2020[81]). Among other things, it has highlighted the importance of making communication more inclusive by focusing on getting to hard-to-reach groups that are necessary for a whole-of-society response (OECD, 2021[244]). In addition, strengthening representative deliberative processes can play an important role in building a shared understanding of post-crisis priorities and to improve trust between citizens and government. Representative deliberative processes refer to a randomly selected group of people - who are broadly representative of their community - spending significant time learning and collaborating through facilitated deliberation to reach collective recommendations for policy makers (OECD, 2020[243]). Throughout such processes, governments can learn more about citizens' perspectives, issues and concerns in response to the crisis, particularly of those who are most vulnerable. At the same time, citizens can gain deeper understandings of the - often complex - interplay between the well-being outcomes at stake and can play a more direct role in public agenda setting and decision-making.

Governments are increasingly carrying out open government reforms and are using representative deliberative processes to help deliver better policies, strengthen democracy and build trust (Figure 1.5). The range of policy issues that are being addressed through representative deliberative processes – such as citizens' assemblies, juries and panels - has been wide and increasing (OECD, 2020[243]).[12] In response to the pandemic, several OECD countries have held online public forums to consult with citizens on their experiences of, and opinions on, recovery responses. For example, the Finnish Ministry of Finance, in partnership with the Dialogue Academy and Timeout Foundation, has organised a series of Lockdown Dialogues on how the crisis has affected citizens' lives and is reshaping their country (OECD, 2021[245]). The French parliament has hosted a virtual public forum to gather citizens' opinions on the direction of France's policy priorities post-COVID-19 (Open Government Partnership, 2020[246]). Some governments, including Norway and New Zealand, have also held special press conferences for children to answer their questions about the pandemic (The Guardian, 2020[247]; Financial Times, 2020[248]).

Reaching out to those who face higher barriers or are less used to or willing to "get involved" is essential to make recovery strategies more responsive to people who are under-served or less-heard. This includes youth, whose well-being has been deeply affected by the crisis but whose political weight has decreased across OECD countries due to population ageing (OECD, 2020[143]). While young people's trust in government edged up following the pandemic outbreak - as it has for all age groups

(Chapter 10) - going forward this trust may be challenged by governments' abilities to adequately support young people's well-being needs in the post-crisis period. The circulation of COVID-19 misinformation on social media, which is a key source of news for many young people, could also pose threats to young people's trust in government (Brennen et al., 2020[249]). At the same time, child and youth demonstrations around the world prior to the pandemic clearly show young people's motivation to address global challenges (OECD, 2020[143]). During the pandemic, young people and their organisations have also provided crucial help in mitigating the impact of the COVID-19 crisis on the most vulnerable in society, including the elderly (OECD, 2020[62]) (see also Chapter 10). Strengthening the relationships between youth and public institutions, by engaging them throughout the policy cycle and promoting their participation and representation in policymaking, is therefore important to further align their actions. The forthcoming OECD *Youth Action Plan* will set out a toolkit of measures that countries and stakeholders can use to empower young people and promote better outcomes in terms of their employment, education, and participation in public life (OECD, n.d.[250]). National Youth Strategies are also being adopted in an increasing number of OECD countries: in 2020, 25 OECD countries had a National Youth Strategy in place; 80% of these strategies aim to improve the access to and responsiveness of public services to young people; and 84% seek to integrate youths' own views and concerns in public policies (OECD, 2021[12]).

Figure 1.5. A deliberative wave has been building over time

Number of representative deliberative processes per year in 18 OECD countries plus the European Union, 1986 – October 2019

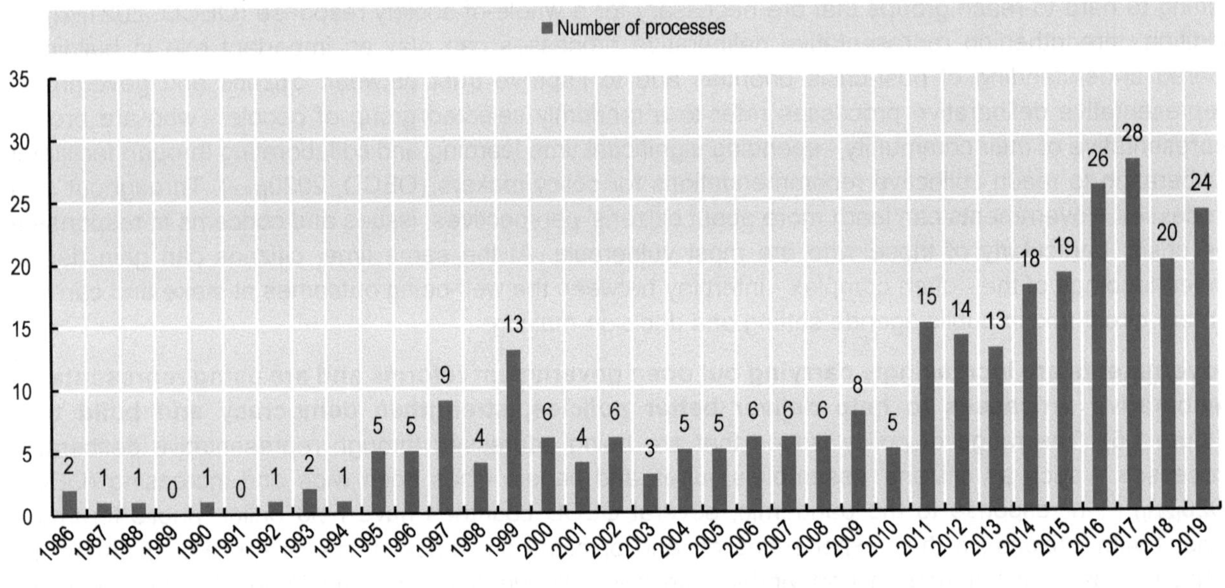

Note: n = 282; data is based on 18 OECD countries that were members in 2019, plus the European Union. Processes that spanned over multiple years are noted by the year of their completion (except for permanent ongoing processes).
Source: OECD (2020[243]), *Catching the deliberative wave*, Highlights 2020, Figure 5, OECD Publishing, Paris, http://www.oecd.org/gov/open-government/innovative-citizen-participation-new-democratic-institutions-catching-the-deliberative-wave-highlights.pdf.

StatLink https://stat.link/p4ub93

Creating permanent or ongoing deliberative structures can support continuous collaboration between governments and citizens in the process of building forward. Despite positive developments in the use of deliberative processes, citizen engagement has yet to become part of the day-to-day work of policy makers. While in 92% of OECD countries, policy makers consult early on draft regulations with selected groups, open consultations tend to be more common only at a late stage of policy development (OECD,

2018[200]; OECD, 2021[12]). Moreover, to date, most representative deliberative processes for public decision-making have been one-off, with topics being defined top-down by public decision makers (OECD, 2020[243]). Further institutionalising the role of citizens in developing strategies for building back better is important to mobilise collective support and action for the chosen direction of travel. For example, in 2019, a permanent Citizens' Council was established in Ostbelgien (the German-speaking part of Belgium) to constitute its third fundamental democratic institution alongside the Parliament and the Executive. The main objectives of the Citizens' Council are to give citizens a permanent voice in the process of decision-making, to establish a systematic monitoring system to ensure that they are heard, and to increase accountability and reinvigorate the agenda-setting power of common citizens (OECD, 2020[243]).

A well-being approach can also help inform stronger strategic alignment between the public and private sector in building back better. The involvement of businesses is important: first, because of the direct role they play in improving employee well-being; and second, because of the way their products and services affect societal well-being outcomes. A shared (outcome based) framework can help counteract the idea that the public and private sectors have opposing interests and can help further align their efforts in working towards societal well-being priorities (Wade, 2021[251]). Better measurement of and reporting on the wider well-being impacts of businesses can also improve their financial performance. Business sustainability ranking and standards have been shown to significantly impact shareholder value (Lyon and Shimshack, 2015[252]), stock-market valuation (Clark, Feiner and Viehs, 2015[253]), and companies' financial performance (Eccles, Ioannou and Serafeim, 2014[254]; BCG, 2017[255]). More conscious consumers and investors further drive the need for businesses to better measure and report on their impacts and contributions to societal well-being (Shinwell and Shamir, 2018[256]). Using a comprehensive well-being framework adds particular value in doing so as businesses, just like many government agencies, tend to focus on certain elements of societal well-being and can easily lose sight of the bigger well-being picture.

Despite the global rise in Corporate Social Responsibility (CSR) reporting, significant data and measurement challenges persist in both official statistics and in business efforts to measure non-financial business performance. National statistical offices and the wider statistical and research communities could play an important role to help align national and business efforts to measure well-being outcomes (Shinwell and Shamir, 2018[256]; OECD, forthcoming[257]). To that end, (OECD, forthcoming[257]) uses the OECD Well-being Framework as a starting point for measuring the broad societal and environmental impacts of businesses on different groups of stakeholders – including employees, consumers, suppliers, society at large and future generations.

Social dialogue can help translate the core dimensions of well-being frameworks into business models that increase well-being for all while protecting the planet. In response to the COVID-19 pandemic, social dialogue between governments, employers and workers has played a crucial role in reaching agreements to strengthen labour market resilience, improve worker protection against the spread of the virus, and to develop flexible but balanced working-time arrangements (Global Deal, OECD and ILO, 2020[258]). Going forward, social dialogue will be fundamental to enable an inclusive and sustainable recovery. The importance of social dialogue is the driver of the Global Deal,[13] a multi-stakeholder partnership that aims to encourage governments, businesses, unions and other organisations to make commitments to enhance social dialogue. In addition, Business for Inclusive Growth – a public-private partnership between the OECD and 35 major global companies – supports work to strengthen more inclusive business models (Box 1.13).

During the COVID-19 crisis the social economy has also demonstrated its unique capacity to help address market and government failures in inclusive and sustainable ways (Box 1.14). Social entrepreneurs are a natural partner for governments seeking to improve societal well-being. In line with the principles of a well-being economy (Nozal, Martin and Murtin, 2019[19]), social entrepreneurship is about "doing business for societal and environmental good". Its main goal is to address societal challenges in an innovative way by targeting social impact primarily rather than profit maximisation. By linking economic and social value creation, social enterprises play an important role in helping to reshape the post-crisis economy by promoting more inclusive and sustainable economic models (OECD, 2020[259]). They can create new jobs, be a vehicle for better service delivery, boost citizens' participation in their local communities, and turn innovative ideas into action for the benefit of the common good, all while generating tax revenues (European Union and OECD, 2016[260]).

Box 1.13. Business for Inclusive Growth Coalition

Business for Inclusive Growth (B4IG) is a strategic partnership between the OECD and 35 major global companies that works to fight against inequalities of opportunities. Launched in 2019 at the G7 Leaders' Summit, B4IG leverages relevant OECD data, analysis and standards to help companies move towards more inclusive business models.

Each Chairperson or CEO of B4IG member companies has signed the Pledge to Fight against Inequalities, which covers three main areas of inclusive growth:

- advancing human rights in direct operations and supply chains
- building inclusive workplaces
- strengthening inclusion in companies' value chains and ecosystems.

The B4IG coalition is developing a measurement framework and methodology that can be used to assess their progress in implementing the Pledge, drawing on the OECD Well-being Framework and impact measurement work stream. B4IG organises its work via three main actions: Working Groups, an Incubator, and an Inclusive Growth Financing Forum. By sharing best practices, developing new solutions, launching pilot programs, and developing metrics to better evaluate inclusive growth efforts, B4IG shows how businesses can contribute to a sustainable and inclusive future for all.

Government recovery strategies should provide a clear role for the social economy and identify actions to support their impact and scale (OECD, 2020[259]; OECD/European Union, 2017[261]). Social entrepreneurs' values-based approach to economic activities can help transform society and the economy by:

- successfully demonstrating alternative ways of conducting economic activities, inspiring other economic actors to follow and mainstream these practices;
- unlocking new economic sectors such as textile recycling, which has been pioneered by social economy organisations since the 1960s and has since experienced an increase in the number of economic actors entering this field; and
- revitalising local economies and providing services in remote areas. A distinctive strength of the social economy is that their economic activities typically build on local roots, mobilising and empowering local actors, including those who are vulnerable. They are therefore particularly well-suited to help respond to local well-being issues in the wake of the pandemic (OECD, 2020[259]).

Box 1.14. Masques-Coronavirus.Brussels: Social economy collaboration towards well-being

Masques-Coronavirus.Brussels is a government-supported social economy initiative that worked to improve well-being by addressing market and state failures during the COVID-19 crisis. In response to shortages in personnel protective equipment, two social enterprises from Brussels, EcoRes and Travie, joined forces to meet the urgent demand for masks for frontline health care personnel.

EcoRes is a sustainable innovation lab specialised in the circular economy, while Travie is a work integration social enterprise that employs people with disabilities. With the support of the Brussels-Capital Region, a collaborative and decentralised production line of masks was established. Students from a fashion design school designed the mask pattern and conducted a tutorial on the design. Mask kits were then pre-cut and prepared by Travie and delivered by the social enterprise Urbike to a network of volunteering citizens who sewed the masks according to quality standards. More than 2 000 people were involved and produced 240 000 reusable masks for frontline caregivers in 1.5 months.

This project demonstrates the capacity of the social economy to:

- address urgent well-being needs and improve quality of life for people and their communities
- react with agility and foster solidarity in extreme situations
- rally local actors and mobilise different resources (funding, volunteering, knowledge) from a range of actors (government, citizens, social economy organisations, professionals)
- design, experiment with and consolidate innovative approaches to economic activities and new ways of working together between individuals, organisations and local governments.

Source: Adapted from OECD (2020[259]), Social economy and the COVID-19 crisis, Box 2

Conclusion

This chapter has considered the ways in which a well-being approach can guide the process of building back better in the wake of the COVID-19 pandemic by helping governments *refocus*, *redesign*, *realign* and *reconnect*. Using a multidimensional framework to assess key elements of current and future well-being enables governments to focus their recovery efforts on the well-being areas of greatest need - including pre-pandemic vulnerabilities that have been exacerbated by the crisis. This includes the need to increase job and financial security and to improve opportunities for all - including among children and young people as well as across generations. To build forward more resiliently, strong action on the environmental crises needs to be a central part of all recovery efforts but a pro-active approach is also needed to help reinforce trust and social capital. In addition, addressing the personal and societal burden of poor mental and physical health is critical to strengthen people's quality of life and to enable families, communities, businesses, economies and societies to thrive.

Different pathways can enable governments to simultaneously improve current and future well-being while reducing inequalities. This chapter has identified five such pathways: 1) supporting the creation of sustainable, inclusive, and high-quality jobs, including in the green economy and the health, education and wider care sectors; 2) using lifelong learning to reduce inequalities; 3) using a whole-of-government approach to raise the well-being of disadvantaged children and young people; 4) strengthening mental and physical health promotion and prevention; and 5) reinforcing trust by strengthening public sector competencies and values and encouraging meaningful citizen participation on a more ongoing basis. These "triple win" channels constitute examples of policy directions that build on synergies between *current*, *distributional* and *future* well-being outcomes, rather than a comprehensive well-being policy agenda. The most suitable and effective well-being approaches will ultimately depend on country's unique local contexts and well-being priorities. Nonetheless, the discussion of these five channels has illustrated how well-being frameworks can help to identity strategic directions for recovery that can contribute to well-being across multiple dimensions, groups and time-periods; how potential synergies between well-being objectives often remain unrealised; and how a well-being lens can help broaden policy thinking about what has value for public investment and what the best ways are to address societal concerns.

Building back better lives in a more integrated way asks for new ways of working within government and with private and civil society actors. Improving governments' awareness of the impact of their recovery measures on the multiple dimensions of current well-being, inequalities and future well-being is fundamental to be able to build back more coherently, efficiently, and effectively. It requires all government agencies to focus on a system of interconnected goals, rather than on individual targets that can be met by individual agencies. Recent decades have seen important initiatives in this direction from governments around the world. These initiatives go beyond measuring and reporting on well-being, to actively using well-being frameworks and data to inform policy priorities and budget decisions, to encourage more holistic, coherent and forward-looking policy initiatives, and to align actions between public, private, and civil society stakeholders based on a shared sense of purpose.

The wide-ranging impacts of the pandemic on well-being highlight the need for a whole-of-government response and a joined-up, forward-looking recovery. The COVID-19 pandemic has highlighted the radical uncertainty and complexity of the world in which policy makers are acting. In these uncertain and complex environments there are no silver bullets and no single organisation holds the range of knowledge or information required to arrive at desired outcomes (Karacaoglu, 2021[89]). What is needed is a shift in the focus of public policy from looking for optimal solutions to narrowly defined problems to building resilience by investing in environmental, social, human, and economic capital (Karacaoglu, 2021[89]). Doing so builds on the core elements of collaboration, integration, and anticipation that characterise a well-being approach to public policy.

References

Adams, W. (2004), "Biodiversity conservation and the eradication of poverty", *Science*, Vol. 306/5699, pp. 1146-1149, http://dx.doi.org/10.1126/science.1097920. [99]

Agrawala, S., D. Dussaux and N. Monti (2020), "What policies for greening the crisis response and economic recovery?: Lessons learned from past green stimulus measures and implications for the COVID-19 crisis", *OECD Environment Working Papers*, No. 164, OECD Publishing, Paris, https://dx.doi.org/10.1787/c50f186f-en. [201]

Alberca, R. et al. (2020), "Obesity as a risk factor for COVID-19: an overview", *Critical Reviews in Food Science and Nutrition*, http://dx.doi.org/10.1080/10408398.2020.1775546. [5]

Algan, Y. and P. Cahuc (2013), *Trust, Growth and Well-being: New Evidence and Policy Implications*, IZA, Bonn, http://repec.iza.org/dp7464.pdf (accessed on 13 March 2021). [185]

Alvarez-Herranz, A. et al. (2017), "Energy innovation and renewable energy consumption in the correction of air pollution levels", *Energy Policy*, Vol. 105, pp. 386-397, http://dx.doi.org/10.1016/j.enpol.2017.03.009. [95]

Aponte, M. et al. (2020), *From insights to action. Gender equality in the wake of COVID-19*, UN Women, New York, http://www.unwomen.org (accessed on 25 March 2021). [114]

APPG (2019), *A spending review to increase wellbeing*, The All Party Parliamentary Group on Wellbeing Economics, London, https://wellbeingeconomics.co.uk (accessed on 25 March 2021). [87]

APPG (2014), *Wellbeing in four policy areas*, All Party Parliamentary Group on Wellbeing Economics, London, https://b.3cdn.net/nefoundation/ccdf9782b6d8700f7c_lcm6i2ed7.pdf (accessed on 7 April 2021). [85]

Audit Wales (2020), “So what’s different? Findings from the Auditor General’s sustainable development principle examinations”, https://www.wao.gov.uk/sites/default/files/Well-being-of-Future-Generations-report-eng_11.pdf (accessed on 5 June 2021). [229]

Bargain, O. and U. Aminjonov (2020), “Trust and Compliance to Public Health Policies in Times of COVID-19”, http://bordeauxeconomicswp.u-bordeaux.fr/2020/2020-06.pdf (accessed on 21 June 2021). [76]

Barnett, W. and K. Jung (2021), *Seven Impacts of the Pandemic on Young Children and their Parents: Initial Findings from NIEER’s December 2020 Preschool Learning Activities Survey*, National Institute for Early Education Research, New Brunswick, New Jersey, https://nieer.org/research-report/seven-impacts-of-the-pandemic-on-young-children-and-their-parents-initial-findings-from-nieers-december-2020-preschool-learning-activities-survey. [65]

Bartscher, A. et al. (2020), “Social Capital and the Spread of Covid-19: Insights from European Countries”, *SSRN Electronic Journal*, http://dx.doi.org/10.2139/ssrn.3616714. [77]

Baumeister, R. et al. (2005), “Social exclusion impairs self-regulation”, *Journal of Personality and Social Psychology*, Vol. 88/4, pp. 589-604, http://dx.doi.org/10.1037/0022-3514.88.4.589. [171]

BCG (2017), *Total societal impact: A new lens for strategy*, Boston Consulting Group, Boston, http://www.bcg.com/publications/2017/total-societal-impact-new-lens-strategy (accessed on 11 April 2021). [255]

Bennett, D. et al. (2006), “The effect of social networks on the relation between Alzheimer’s disease pathology and level of cognitive function in old people: a longitudinal cohort study”, *Lancet Neurology*, Vol. 5/5, pp. 406-412, http://dx.doi.org/10.1016/S1474-4422(06)70417-3. [178]

Berkman, L. et al. (2000), “From social integration to health: Durkheim in the new millennium”, *Social Science and Medicine*, Vol. 51/6, pp. 843-857, http://dx.doi.org/10.1016/S0277-9536(00)00065-4. [166]

Berning, C. and C. Ziller (2017), “Social trust and radical right-wing populist party preferences”, *Acta Politica*, Vol. 52/2, pp. 198-217, http://dx.doi.org/10.1057/ap.2015.28. [186]

Boarini, R. et al. (2012), *What makes for a better life?: The determinants of subjective well-Being in OECD countries – Evidence from the Gallup World Poll*, OECD Publishing, Paris, https://doi.org/10.1787/5k9b9ltjm937-en (accessed on 7 April 2021). [147]

Bond, L. et al. (2007), “Social and school connectedness in early secondary school as predictors of late teenage substance use, mental health, and academic outcomes”, *Journal of Adolescent Health*, Vol. 40/4, pp. 357.e9-357.e18, http://dx.doi.org/10.1016/j.jadohealth.2006.10.013. [176]

Borgonovi, F. and E. Andrieu (2020), “Bowling together by bowling alone: Social capital and COVID-19”, *Social Science and Medicine*, Vol. 265, p. 113501, http://dx.doi.org/10.1016/j.socscimed.2020.113501. [75]

Brennen, J. et al. (2020), *Types, sources, and claims of COVID-19 misinformation*, Reuters Institute for the Study of Journalism, https://reutersinstitute.politics.ox.ac.uk/types-sources-and-claims-covid-19-misinformation (accessed on 23 March 2021). [249]

Brezzi, M., S. Gonzáles and M. Prats (2020), "All you need is trust. Informing the role of government in the COVID-19 context", *The OECD Statistics Newsletter* 73, http://dx.doi.org/10.2307/j. [83]

Buckle, S. et al. (2020), *Addressing the COVID-19 and climate crises: Potential economic recovery pathways and their implications for climate change mitigation, NDCs and broader socio-economic goals*, OECD and IEA, Paris, http://www.oecd.org/environment/cc/ccxg.htm (accessed on 3 June 2021). [13]

Buekers, J. et al. (2014), "Health and environmental benefits related to electric vehicle introduction in EU countries", *Transportation Research Part D: Transport and Environment*, Vol. 33, pp. 26-38, http://dx.doi.org/10.1016/j.trd.2014.09.002. [97]

Butterworth, P. et al. (2013), "Common mental disorders, unemployment and psychosocial job quality: is a poor job better than no job at all?", *Psychological medicine*, Vol. 43/8, pp. 1763-1772, http://dx.doi.org/10.1017/S0033291712002577. [107]

Button, D. (2021), *Social care reform: ambition vs reality*, New Economics Foundation, http://www.neweconomics.com (accessed on 11 April 2021). [163]

Cacioppo, J. and S. Cacioppo (2018), *The growing problem of loneliness*, Lancet Publishing Group, http://dx.doi.org/10.1016/S0140-6736(18)30142-9. [167]

Cacioppo, J. et al. (2006), "Loneliness as a specific risk factor for depressive symptoms: Cross-sectional and longitudinal analyses", *Psychology and Aging*, Vol. 21/1, pp. 140-151, http://dx.doi.org/10.1037/0882-7974.21.1.140. [173]

Canry, N. (2020), "Why and how should human capital be measured in National Accounts?", *Economie et Statistique* 517-518-519, pp. 61-79, http://dx.doi.org/10.24187/ecostat.2020.517t.2023. [115]

Caspi, A. et al. (2006), "Socially isolated children 20 years later: Risk of cardiovascular disease", *Archives of Pediatrics and Adolescent Medicine*, Vol. 160/8, pp. 805-811, http://dx.doi.org/10.1001/archpedi.160.8.805. [174]

CBS (2020), *Monitor Brede Welvaart & de Sustainable Development Goals 2020 [Monitor of Broad Prosperity and the Sustainable Development Goals 2020]*, Centraal Bureau Statistiek , The Hague, http://www.cbs.nl/nl-nl/publicatie/2020/21/monitor-brede-welvaart-de-sustainable-development-goals-2020 (accessed on 3 June 2021). [205]

Chen, J. and N. Krieger (2021), "Revealing the unequal burden of COVID-19 by income, race/ethnicity, and household crowding: US county versus zip code analyses.", *Journal of public health management and practice : JPHMP*, Vol. 27 Suppl 1, pp. S43-S56, http://dx.doi.org/10.1097/PHH.0000000000001263. [3]

Clark, G., A. Feiner and M. Viehs (2015), *From the stockholder to the stakeholder: How sustainability can drive financial outperformance*, University of Oxford and Arabesque Partners, London, https://arabesque.com/research/From_the_stockholder_to_the_stakeholder_web.pdf (accessed on 11 April 2021). [253]

Cohen, S. and T. Wills (1985), "Stress, social support, and the buffering hypothesis", *Psychological Bulletin*, Vol. 98/2, pp. 310-357. [170]

Cohn, A. et al. (2019), "Civic honesty around the globe", *Science*, Vol. 365/6448, pp. 70-73, http://dx.doi.org/10.1126/science.aau8712. [264]

Cole, M., C. Ozgen and E. Strobl (2020), "Air pollution exposure and COVID-19. Discussion Paper Series. IZA DP No. 13367." 13367, p. 31. [1]

Cruwys, T. et al. (2013), "Social group memberships protect against future depression, alleviate depression symptoms and prevent depression relapse", *Social science & medicine (1982)*, Vol. 98, http://dx.doi.org/10.1016/J.SOCSCIMED.2013.09.013. [177]

Cunsolo, A. and N. Ellis (2018), "Ecological grief as a mental health response to climate change-related loss", *Nature Climate Change*, Vol. 8/4, pp. 275-281, http://dx.doi.org/10.1038/s41558-018-0092-2. [53]

De Coning, C. (2007), *Coherence and coordination in United Nations Peacebuilding and Integrated Missions - A Norwegian perspective. NUPI Report*, Norwegian Institute of International Affairs, Oslo, https://gsdrc.org/document-library/coherence-and-coordination-in-united-nations-peacebuilding-and-integrated-missions-a-norwegian-perspective/ (accessed on 11 March 2021). [230]

De Henau, J. and S. Himmelweit (2020), *The gendered employment gains of investing in social vs. physical infrastructure: evidence from simulations across seven OECD countries*, The Open University, Innovation Knowledge and Development Director, http://www.open.ac.uk/ikd/publications/working-papers (accessed on 25 March 2021). [112]

De Henau, J. et al. (2016), *Investing in the care economy: A gender analysis of employment stimulus in seven OECD countries*, UK Women's Budget Group, London. [119]

Desjardins, R. (2020), *PIAAC Thematic report on adult learning. OECD Education Working Paper 223*, OECD Publishing, Paris, http://www.oecd.org/edu/workingpapers (accessed on 11 March 2021). [131]

Dietz, W. and C. Santos-Burgoa (2020), "Obesity and its implications for COVID-19 mortality", *Obesity*, Vol. 28/6, p. 1005, https://doi.org/10.1002/oby.22818. [6]

DIW (2021), *Corona-Pandemie: Vertrauensvolle Menschen sind eher zur Impfung bereit und halten sich eher an AHA-Regeln*, https://www.diw.de/de/diw_01.c.820366.de/publikationen/diw_aktuell/2021_0066/corona-pandemie__vertrauensvolle_menschen_sind_eher_zur_impfung_bereit_und_halten_sich_eher_an_aha-regeln.html (accessed on 24 June 2021). [79]

Dolan, P., D. Fujiwara and R. Metcalfe (2012), *Review and update of research into the wider benefits of adult learning*, Department for Business, Innovation and Skills, http://www.simetrica.co.uk/wp-content/uploads/2020/03/Review-and-Update-of-Adult-Learning.pdf (accessed on 10 March 2021). [126]

Dolan, P., T. Peasgood and M. White (2008), "Do we really know what makes us happy? A review of the economic literature on the factors associated with subjective well-being", *Journal of Economic Psychology*, Vol. 29/1, pp. 94-122, http://dx.doi.org/10.1016/j.joep.2007.09.001. [148]

Dowling, J. et al. (2020), "Role of long-duration energy storage in variable renewable electricity systems", *Joule*, Vol. 4/9, pp. 1907-1928, http://dx.doi.org/10.1016/j.joule.2020.07.007. [94]

Downes, R. and S. Nicol (2020), "Designing and implementing gender budgeting – a path to action", *OECD Journal on Budgeting*, https://dx.doi.org/10.1787/689198fa-en. [222]

Durand, M. and C. Exton (2019), "Adopting a well-being approach in central government: Policy mechanisms and practical tools", in *Global Happiness Policy Report 2019*, Sustainable Development Solutions Network, New York, http://www.happinesscouncil.org. [208]

Durand, M. and C. Exton (2019), "Adopting a Well-Being Approach in Central Government: Policy Mechanisms and Practical Tools", in *Global Happiness Policy Report 2019*, Sustainable Development Solutions Network, New York, http://www.happinesscouncil.org/. [209]

Eccles, R., I. Ioannou and G. Serafeim (2014), "The impact of corporate sustainability on organizational processes and performance", *Management Science*, Vol. 60/11, pp. 2835-2857, http://dx.doi.org/10.1287/mnsc.2014.1984. [254]

Economist Intelligence Unit (2020), *Democracy Index 2020: In sickness and in health?*, https://www.eiu.com/n/campaigns/democracy-index-2020/ (accessed on 21 June 2021). [271]

Elson, D. (2016), "A gender-equitable macroeconomic framework for Europe", in Himmelweit, S., G. Cozzi and H. Bargawi (eds.), *Economics and austerity in Europe: Gendered impacts and sustainable alternatives*, Routledge, Milton Park. [116]

Engzell, P., A. Frey and M. Verhagen (2021), "Learning loss due to school closures during the COVID-19 pandemic", *Proceedings of the National Academy of Sciences of the United States of America*, Vol. 118/17, http://dx.doi.org/10.1073/PNAS.2022376118. [33]

Ertel, K., M. Glymour and L. Berkman (2008), "Effects of social integration on preserving memory function in a nationally representative US elderly population", *American Journal of Public Health*, Vol. 98/7, pp. 1215-1220, http://dx.doi.org/10.2105/AJPH.2007.113654. [180]

Eurofound (2020), *Living, working and COVID-19*, Publications Office of the European Union, Luxembourg. [28]

European Commission (2017), *State of Health in the EU. Companion report 2017*, Publications Office of the European Union, Luxembourg, http://dx.doi.org/10.2875/870704. [160]

European Union and OECD (2016), *Policy brief on scaling the impact of social enterprises: Policies for social entrepreneurship*, http://dx.doi.org/10.2767/45737. [260]

Eurostat, OECD and UNECE (2020), *Webinar on well-being and sustainability: A broader framework for wellbeing and sustainability in the system of national accounts. Working paper 2.6*, https://unece.org/fileadmin/DAM/stats/documents/ece/ces/ge.20/2020/mtg1/2.6_Broader_Framework_for_Wellbeing.pdf (accessed on 3 June 2021). [270]

Exton, C. and L. Fleischer (forthcoming), "The Future of the OECD Well-being Dashboard", *OECD Statistics Working Papers*, No. forthcoming, OECD Publishing, Paris. [206]

Exton, C. and M. Shinwell (2018), "Policy use of well-being metrics: Describing countries' experiences", *OECD Statistics Working Papers*, No. 2018/07, OECD Publishing, Paris, https://dx.doi.org/10.1787/d98eb8ed-en. [207]

Fetet, M. and S. Postic (2020), *France's green budget: What's next?*, https://www.i4ce.org/france-green-budget-climate/ (accessed on 2 April 2021). [225]

Filipova, T. et al. (2020), *Mental health and the environment. How European policies can better reflect the impact of environmental degradation on people's mental health and well-being*, Institute for European Environmental Policy (IEEP) and the Barcelona Institute for Global Health (ISGlobal), Brussels. [52]

Financial Times (2020), *Norway's PM moves to allay children's coronavirus fears | Financial Times*, http://www.ft.com/content/38357156-6786-11ea-800d-da70cff6e4d3 (accessed on 8 June 2021). [248]

Frieling, M., E. Krassoi Peach and J. Cording (2018), *Social connectedness and wellbeing*, Ministry of Social Development, Wellington. [182]

Future Generations Commissioner for Wales (2019), *How the Welsh Government draft budget is taking account of the Well-being of Future Generations Act. A Briefing for Assembly Members*, Future Generations Commissioner for Wales, Cardiff. [215]

GAO (2019), *US Government Accountability Office 2019 Annual Report*, US Government Accountability Office, Washington, https://www.gao.gov/products/gao-19-285sp (accessed on 11 March 2021). [231]

García, J. et al. (2016), *There is more to gain by taking a comprehensive approach to early childhood development*, http://www.heckmanequation.org (accessed on 18 May 2021). [137]

Global Deal, OECD and ILO (2020), *Social dialogue, skills and COVID-19*, http://www.theglobaldeal.com/resources/2020%20Global%20Deal%20Flagship%20Report.pdf (accessed on 17 June 2021). [258]

Gmeinder, M., D. Morgan and M. Mueller (2017), "How much do OECD countries spend on prevention?", *OECD Health Working Papers*, No. 101, OECD Publishing, Paris, https://dx.doi.org/10.1787/f19e803c-en. [159]

González-Eguino, M. (2015), "Energy poverty: An overview", *Renewable and Sustainable Energy Reviews*, Vol. 47, pp. 377-385, http://dx.doi.org/10.1016/j.rser.2015.03.013. [93]

Gottdenker, N. et al. (2014), "Anthropogenic Land Use Change and Infectious Diseases: A Review of the Evidence", http://dx.doi.org/10.1007/s10393-014-0941-z. [10]

Government of Canada (2021), *Budget 2021*, http://www.budget.gc.ca/2021/report-rapport/toc-tdm-en.html (accessed on 1 June 2021). [212]

Government of Canada (2020), *Economic and Fiscal Snapshot 2020*, Government of Canada, Ottawa, https://www.canada.ca/content/dam/fin/publications/efs-peb/homepage/EFS2020-eng.pdf (accessed on 18 March 2021). [198]

Government of Canada (n.d.), *Gender-based Analysis Plus (GBA+)*, https://women-gender-equality.canada.ca/en/gender-based-analysis-plus.html (accessed on 8 April 2021). [262]

Government of Ireland (2021), *Budget 2021 Wellbeing and the Measurement of Broader Living Standards in Ireland*, Department of Finance. [213]

Guterres, A. (2020), *Opening remarks at the UN General Assembly, 22 September 2020*, http://www.un.org/sg/en/content/sg/speeches/2020-09-22/address-the-opening-of-the-general-debate-of-the-75th-session-of-the-general-assembly (accessed on 25 March 2021). [11]

Hammond, C. (2004), "Impacts of lifelong learning upon emotional resilience, psychological and mental health: Fieldwork evidence", *Oxford Review of Education*, Vol. 30/4, pp. 551-568, http://dx.doi.org/10.1080/0305498042000303008. [128]

Harvard University Centre on the Developing Child (2009), *Maternal depression can undermine the development of young children. Working paper no. 8*, Harvard University , Cambridge, MA, http://www.developingchild.harvard.edu (accessed on 2 April 2021). [154]

Haslam, C., S. Haslam and J. Jetten (2014), "Social determinants of cognitive change: Identity processes as the source of both enhancement and decline", in Reynolds, K. and N. Branscombe (eds.), *The psychology of change: Life contexts, experiences, and identities*, Psychology Press, New York, https://espace.library.uq.edu.au/view/UQ:354812 (accessed on 19 March 2021). [179]

Hayes, K. et al. (2018), "Climate change and mental health: Risks, impacts and priority actions", *International Journal of Mental Health Systems*, Vol. 12/1, http://dx.doi.org/10.1186/s13033-018-0210-6. [54]

Hege, E. and L. Brimont (2018), *Integrating SDGs into national budgetary processes*, IDDRI, Paris, http://www.iddri.org (accessed on 18 March 2021). [223]

Helliwell, J. et al. (2021), "Happiness, trust, and deaths under COVID-19", in *The World Happiness Report 2021*, https://worldhappiness.report/ed/2021/happiness-trust-and-deaths-under-covid-19/#fn17 (accessed on 10 June 2021). [78]

Hendren, N. and B. Sprung-Keyser (2020), *A Unified Welfare Analysis of Government Policies*, Oxford University Press, http://dx.doi.org/10.1093/qje/qjaa006. [140]

Hepburn, C. et al. (2020), "Will COVID-19 fiscal recovery packages accelerate or retard progress on climate change?", *Oxford Review of Economic Policy*, Vol. 36, pp. S359-S381, http://dx.doi.org/10.1093/oxrep/graa015. [16]

Hewlett, E. and V. Moran (2014), *Making Mental Health Count: The Social and Economic Costs of Neglecting Mental Health Care*, OECD Health Policy Studies, OECD Publishing, Paris, https://dx.doi.org/10.1787/9789264208445-en. [151]

Hill, E. (2020), *Reducing gender inequality and boosting the economy: fiscal policy after COVID-19*, Committee for Economic Development of Australia, Sydney, http://www.ceda.com.au/ResearchAndPolicies/Research/Workforce-Skills/Labour-market-policy-after-COVID-19 (accessed on 25 March 2021). [121]

HM Treasury (2018), *The Green Book. Central government guidance on appraisal and evaluation*, HM Treasury, London, https://assets.publishing.service.gov.uk/government/uploads/system/uploads/attachment_data/file/938046/The_Green_Book_2020.pdf (accessed on 27 March 2021). [241]

Huang, C., P. Renzio and D. Mccullough (2020), *New Zealand's "WellBeing Budget": A new model for managing public finances?*, International Budget Partnership, Washington. [216]

Hunter, R. et al. (2017), "Social network interventions for health behaviour change: a systematic review", *The Lancet*, Vol. 390, p. S47, http://dx.doi.org/10.1016/s0140-6736(17)32982-3. [172]

ILO (2016), *Non-standard employment around the world. Understanding challenges, shaping prospects*, International Labour Office, Geneva. [23]

IRENA (2019), *Renewable energy: A gender perspective*, International Renewable Energy Agency, Abu Dhabi, http://www.irena.org/publications/2019/Jan/Renewable-Energy-A-Gender-Perspective (accessed on 19 March 2021). [101]

Islam, S. and J. Winkel (2017), *Climate change and social inequality*, United Nations Department of Economic and Social Affairs, New York, https://www.un.org/esa/desa/papers/2017/wp152_2017.pdf (accessed on 11 March 2021). [57]

Jakobsdóttir, K. (2020), "In Iceland, well-being is the measure of our success", *London Evening Standard*, https://www.standard.co.uk/comment/comment/iceland-wellbeing-measure-success-katrin-jakobsdottir-a4324791.html (accessed on 18 March 2021). [214]

Jarde, A. et al. (2016), "Neonatal outcomes in women with untreated antenatal depression compared with women without depression: A systematic review and meta-analysis", *JAMA Psychiatry*, Vol. 73/8, pp. 826-837, http://dx.doi.org/10.1001/jamapsychiatry.2016.0934. [155]

Kabir, M. and S. Serrao-Neumann (2020), "Climate change effects on people's livelihood", in Leal Filho W. et al. (eds.), *Climate Action. Encyclopedia of the UN Sustainable Development Goals*, Springer, Cham, http://dx.doi.org/10.1007/978-3-319-95885-9_7. [56]

Kampa, M. and E. Castanas (2008), "Human health effects of air pollution", *Environmental Pollution*, Vol. 151/2, pp. 362-367, http://dx.doi.org/10.1016/j.envpol.2007.06.012. [96]

Karacaoglu, G. (2021), *Love you: Public policy for intergenerational wellbeing*, Tuwhiri, Wellington. [89]

Karbalaei, S. et al. (2018), *Occurrence, sources, human health impacts and mitigation of microplastic pollution*, Springer Verlag, http://dx.doi.org/10.1007/s11356-018-3508-7. [51]

Knack, S. and P. Keefer (1997), "Does social capital have an economic payoff? A cross-country Investigation", *The Quarterly Journal of Economics*, Vol. 112/4, pp. 1251-1288, http://dx.doi.org/10.1162/003355300555475. [187]

LaPorta, R. et al. (1997), "Trust in large organizations", *American Economic Review Papers and Proceedings*, Vol. 87/2. [183]

Lyon, T. and J. Shimshack (2015), "Environmental Disclosure: Evidence From Newsweek's Green Companies Rankings", *Business & Society*, Vol. 54/5, pp. 632-675, http://dx.doi.org/10.1177/0007650312439701. [252]

Makridis, C. and C. Wu (2021), "How social capital helps communities weather the COVID-19 pandemic", *PLOS ONE*, Vol. 16/1, http://dx.doi.org/10.1371/journal.pone.0245135. [80]

Manisalidis, I. et al. (2020), *Environmental and health impacts of air pollution: A review*, Frontiers Media S.A., http://dx.doi.org/10.3389/fpubh.2020.00014. [49]

Manninen, J. et al. (2014), *Benefits of lifelong learning in Europe: Main results of the BeLL-Project research report*, European Union, Bonn, http://www.bell-project.eu (accessed on 11 March 2021). [127]

Manning, C. and A. Gregoire (2006), "Effects of parental mental illness on children", *Psychiatry*, Vol. 5/1, pp. 10-12, http://dx.doi.org/10.1383/psyt.2006.5.1.10. [156]

Margolius, M. et al. (2020), *The State of Young People during COVID-19: Findings from a Nationally Representative Survey of High School Youth*, America's Promise Alliance, Washington, D.C., https://www.americaspromise.org/resource/state-young-people-during-covid-19. [69]

Masters, R. et al. (2017), *Return on investment of public health interventions: A systematic review*, BMJ Publishing Group, http://dx.doi.org/10.1136/jech-2016-208141. [161]

McAdams, R. (2007), *The economic costs of inequality*, University of Chicago Law School , Chicago, https://chicagounbound.uchicago.edu/law_and_economics (accessed on 26 April 2021). [41]

Milner, A., L. Krnjacki and A. LaMontagne (2017), "Psychosocial job quality and mental health among young workers: A fixed-effects regression analysis using 13 waves of annual data", *Scandinavian Journal of Work, Environment and Health*, Vol. 43/1, pp. 50-58, http://dx.doi.org/10.5271/sjweh.3608. [106]

Murtin, F., L. Fleischer and V. Siegerink (2018), *Trust and its determinants: Evidence from the Trustlab experiment. Working Paper No. 89*, OECD Publishing , Paris, http://www.oecd.org/sdd/publicationsdocuments/workingpapers/ (accessed on 5 April 2021). [193]

Narushima, M., J. Liu and N. Diestelkamp (2018), "Lifelong learning in active ageing discourse: Its conserving effect on wellbeing, health and vulnerability", *Ageing and Society*, Vol. 38/4, pp. 651-675, http://dx.doi.org/10.1017/S0144686X16001136. [129]

NEF (2020), *Building a green stimulus for COVID-19. A recovery plan for a greener, fairer future*, New Economics Foundation, London, https://neweconomics.org/uploads/files/green-stimulus-covid.pdf (accessed on 22 March 2021). [110]

New Zealand Government (2021), *Budget Policy Statement 2021*, New Zealand Government, Wellington. [219]

New Zealand Government (2019), *Budget Policy Statement 2020*, New Zealand Government, Wellington. [218]

New Zealand Government (2018), *Budget Policy Statement 2018*, New Zealand Government, Wellington. [217]

New Zealand Government Procurement (2018), *Broader outcomes*, https://www.procurement.govt.nz/broader-outcomes/ (accessed on 14 April 2019). [228]

New Zealand Public Service Commission (2020), *Public service reforms*, New Zealand Public Service Commission | Te Kawa Mataaho, https://www.publicservice.govt.nz/our-work/reforms/ (accessed on 12 March 2021). [232]

New Zealand Treasury (2018), *Budget 2019: Guidance for agencies*, New Zealand Treasury , Wellington, http://www.treasury.govt.nz/publications/guide/budget-2019-guidance-agencies (accessed on 21 June 2021). [220]

NHS (n.d.), *Social prescribing*, https://www.england.nhs.uk/personalisedcare/social-prescribing/ (accessed on 19 March 2021). [181]

Norrie, R. (2017), *The two sides of diversity. Which are the most ethnically diverse occupations?*, The Policy Exchange, London, https://policyexchange.org.uk/wp-content/uploads/2017/03/The-two-sides-of-diversity-2.pdf (accessed on 19 March 2021). [102]

Nozal, A., N. Martin and F. Murtin (2019), *The economy of well-being: Creating opportunities for people's well-being and economic growth. SDD Working Paper No. 102*, OECD Publishing , Paris, http://www.oecd.org/sdd/publicationsdocuments/workingpapers/ (accessed on 5 April 2021). [19]

Nugent, C. (2021), "Could Amsterdam's new economic theory replace capitalism?", *Time*, https://time.com/5930093/amsterdam-doughnut-economics/ (accessed on 23 March 2021). [238]

Obradovich, N. et al. (2018), "Empirical evidence of mental health risks posed by climate change", *Proceedings of the National Academy of Sciences of the United States of America*, Vol. 115/43, pp. 10953-10958, http://dx.doi.org/10.1073/pnas.1801528115. [55]

O'Callaghan, B. and E. Murdock (2021), *Are we building back better? Evidence from 2020 and pathways to inclusive green recovery spending*, United Nations Environment Programme, Nairobi, https://wedocs.unep.org/bitstream/handle/20.500.11822/35281/AWBBB.pdf (accessed on 11 March 2021). [58]

OECD (2021), *A New Benchmark for Mental Health Systems: Tackling the Social and Economic Costs of Mental Ill-Health*, OECD Health Policy Studies, OECD Publishing, Paris, https://dx.doi.org/10.1787/4ed890f6-en. [46]

OECD (2021), *Brick by Brick: Building Better Housing Policies*, OECD Publishing, Paris, https://dx.doi.org/10.1787/b453b043-en. [30]

OECD (2021), *Building for a better tomorrow: Policies to make housing more affordable. Employment, Labour and Social Affairs Policy Briefs*, OECD Publising , Paris, http://oe.cd/affordable-housing-2021 (accessed on 15 June 2021). [27]

OECD (2021), *Drivers of Trust in Public Institutions in Finland*, OECD Publishing, Paris, https://dx.doi.org/10.1787/52600c9e-en. [245]

OECD (2021), *Economic Policy Reforms 2021: Going for Growth: Shaping a Vibrant Recovery*, OECD Publishing, Paris, https://dx.doi.org/10.1787/3c796721-en. [21]

OECD (2021), *Enhancing public trust in COVID-19 vaccination: The role of governments*, OECD Publishing , Paris, http://www.oecd.org/coronavirus/policy-responses/enhancing-public-trust-in-covid-19-vaccination-the-role-of-governments-eae0ec5a/ (accessed on 22 June 2021). [82]

OECD (2021), *Government at a Glance 2021*, OECD Publishing, Paris, https://dx.doi.org/10.1787/1c258f55-en. [12]

OECD (2021), *Meeting of the OECD Council at Ministerial Level 31 May - 1 June 2021: Key Issues Paper*, OECD Publishing, Paris, https://www.oecd.org/mcm/MCM_2021_C-MIN(2021)1.en.pdf. [17]

OECD (2021), *OECD Affordable Housing Database*, OECD, Paris, http://www.oecd.org/housing/data/affordable-housing-database/ (accessed on 15 June 2021). [26]

OECD (2021), *OECD Child Well-Being Data Portal*, https://www.oecd.org/social/family/child-well-being/data/education/. [145]

OECD (2021), *OECD Employment Outlook 2021: Navigating the COVID-19 Crisis and Recovery*, OECD Publishing, Paris, https://dx.doi.org/10.1787/5a700c4b-en. [72]

OECD (2021), *OECD Regional Outlook 2021: Addressing COVID-19 and Moving to Net Zero Greenhouse Gas Emissions*, OECD Publishing, Paris, https://dx.doi.org/10.1787/17017efe-en. [35]

OECD (2021), *OECD Skills Outlook 2021: Learning for Life*, OECD Publishing, Paris, https://doi.org/10.1787/0ae365b4-en. [124]

OECD (2021), *Preventing Harmful Alcohol Use*, OECD Health Policy Studies, OECD Publishing, Paris, https://dx.doi.org/10.1787/6e4b4ffb-en. [149]

OECD (2021), *Public communication: The global context and the way forward (forthcoming report)*, https://www.oecd.org/gov/open-government/oecd-international-report-on-public-communication.htm (accessed on 18 August 2021). [244]

OECD (2021), "Risks that matter 2020: The long reach of COVID-19", *OECD Policy Responses to Coronavirus (COVID-19)*, OECD Publishing, Paris, https://dx.doi.org/10.1787/44932654-en. [25]

OECD (2021), "Securing the recovery, ambition, and resilience for the well-being of children in the post-COVID-19 decade", *OECD Policy Responses to Coronavirus (COVID-19)*, OECD Publishing, Paris, https://dx.doi.org/10.1787/0f02237a-en. [63]

OECD (2021), "Supporting jobs and companies: A bridge to the recovery phase", *OECD Policy Responses to Coronavirus (COVID-19)*, OECD Publishing, Paris, https://dx.doi.org/10.1787/08962553-en. [74]

OECD (2021), "Supporting young people's mental health through the COVID-19 crisis", *OECD Policy Responses to Coronavirus (COVID-19)*, OECD Publishing, Paris, https://doi.org/10.1787/84e143e5-en. [68]

OECD (2021), "Tackling the mental health impact of the COVID-19 crisis: An integrated, whole-of-society response", *OECD Policy Responses to Coronavirus (COVID-19)*, OECD Publishing , Paris, https://doi.org/10.1787/0ccafa0b-en. [42]

OECD (2021), "The inequalities-environment nexus: Towards a people-centred green transition", *OECD Green Growth Papers*, No. 2021/01, OECD Publishing, Paris, https://dx.doi.org/10.1787/ca9d8479-en. [48]

OECD (2021), "The OECD Green Recovery Database: Examining the environmental implications of COVID-19 recovery policies", *OECD Policy Responses to Coronavirus (COVID-19)*, OECD Publishing, Paris, https://doi.org/10.1787/47ae0f0d-en. [86]

OECD (2021), *The State of School Education: One Year into the COVID Pandemic*, OECD Publishing, Paris, https://doi.org/10.1787/201dde84-en (accessed on 10 June 2021). [67]

OECD (2021), "The territorial impact of COVID-19: Managing the crisis and recovery across levels of government", *OECD Policy Responses to Coronavirus (COVID-19)*, OECD Publishing, Paris, https://doi.org/10.1787/a2c6abaf-en. [233]

OECD (2021), *The Toolkit and Case Navigator for Open Government*, OECD, Paris, http://www.oecd.org/gov/open-government/open-government-toolkit-navigator.htm (accessed on 30 April 2021). [195]

OECD (2021), "Towards gender-inclusive recovery", *OECD Policy Responses to Coronavirus (COVID-19)*, OECD Publishing, Paris, https://doi.org/10.1787/ab597807-en. [34]

OECD (2021), *Well-being and mental health – an integrated policy approach.* [164]

OECD (2021), *Well-Being and Mental Health project webpage*, http://www.oecd.org/wise/well-being-and-mental-health.htm. [165]

OECD (2020), *Building a coherent response for a sustainable post-COVID-19 recovery*, OECD Publishing, Paris, https://doi.org/10.1787/5b0fd8cd-en (accessed on 5 April 2021). [203]

OECD (ed.) (2020), *Building back better: A sustainable, resilient recovery after Covid-19*, OECD Publishing, Paris, https://read.oecd-ilibrary.org/view/?ref=133_133639-s08q2ridhf&title=Building-back-better-_A-sustainable-resilient-recovery-after-Covid-19 (accessed on 7 March 2021). [14]

OECD (2020), *Catching the Deliberative Wave: Innovative Citizen Participation and New Democratic Institutions*, OECD, Paris, http://www.oecd.org/gov/open-government/innovative-citizen-participation-new-democratic-institutions-catching-the-deliberative-wave-highlights.pdf (accessed on 23 March 2021). [243]

OECD (2020), "Combatting COVID-19's effect on children", *OECD Policy Responses to Coronavirus (COVID-19)*, OECD Publishing, Paris, https://doi.org/10.1787/2e1f3b2f-en. [32]

OECD (2020), "COVID-19 and the low-carbon transition: Impacts and possible policy responses", *OECD Policy Responses to Coronavirus (COVID-19)*, OECD Publishing, Paris, https://doi.org/10.1787/749738fc-en. [59]

OECD (2020), "COVID-19: Protecting people and societies", *OECD Policy Responses to Coronavirus (COVID-19)*, OECD Publishing, Paris, https://doi.org/10.1787/e5c9de1a-en. [4]

OECD (2020), *Education at a Glance 2020: OECD Indicators*, OECD Publishing, Paris, https://dx.doi.org/10.1787/69096873-en. [66]

OECD (2020), *Governance for Youth, Trust and Intergenerational Justice: Fit for All Generations?*, OECD Public Governance Reviews, OECD Publishing, Paris, https://dx.doi.org/10.1787/c3e5cb8a-en. [143]

OECD (2020), *Housing and Inclusive Growth*, OECD Publishing, Paris, https://dx.doi.org/10.1787/6ef36f4b-en. [92]

OECD (2020), *How's Life? 2020: Measuring Well-being*, OECD Publishing, Paris, https://dx.doi.org/10.1787/9870c393-en. [18]

OECD (2020), "Making the green recovery work for jobs, income and growth", *OECD Policy Responses to Coronavirus (COVID-19)*, OECD Publishing, Paris, https://doi.org/10.1787/a505f3e7-en (accessed on 5 April 2021). [15]

OECD (2020), *OECD Employment Outlook 2020: Worker Security and the COVID-19 Crisis*, OECD Publishing, Paris, https://dx.doi.org/10.1787/1686c758-en. [22]

OECD (2020), "Social economy and the COVID-19 crisis: current and future roles", *OECD Policy Responses to Coronavirus (COVID-19)*, OECD Publishing, Paris, https://dx.doi.org/10.1787/f904b89f-en. [259]

OECD (2020), "Supporting livelihoods during the COVID-19 crisis: Closing the gaps in safety nets", *OECD Policy Responses to Coronavirus (COVID-19)*, OECD Publishing, Paris, https://dx.doi.org/10.1787/17cbb92d-en. [197]

OECD (2020), "The Covid-19 crisis: A catalyst for government transformation?", *OECD Policy Responses to Coronavirus (COVID-19)*, OECD Publishing, Paris, https://doi.org/10.1787/1d0c0788-en (accessed on 19 May 2021). [192]

OECD (2020), *The Future of Regional Development and Public Investment in Wales, United Kingdom*, OECD Multi-level Governance Studies, OECD Publishing, Paris, https://dx.doi.org/10.1787/e6f5201d-en. [239]

OECD (2020), "The potential of online learning for adults: Early lessons from the COVID-19 crisis", *OECD Policy Responses to Coronavirus (COVID-19)*, OECD Publishing, Paris, https://dx.doi.org/10.1787/ee040002-en. [133]

OECD (2020), "Transparency, communication and trust: The role of public communication in responding to the wave of disinformation about the new Coronavirus", *OECD Policy Responses to Coronavirus (COVID-19)*, OECD Publishing, Paris, https://doi.org/10.1787/bef7ad6e-en (accessed on 27 April 2021). [81]

OECD (2020), "Women at the core of the fight against COVID-19 crisis", *OECD Policy Responses to Coronavirus (COVID-19)*, OECD Publishing, Paris, https://dx.doi.org/10.1787/553a8269-en. [122]

OECD (2020), "Youth and COVID-19: Response, recovery and resilience", *OECD Policy Responses to Coronavirus (COVID-19)*, OECD Publishing, Paris, https://dx.doi.org/10.1787/c40e61c6-en. [62]

OECD (2019), *Accelerating Climate Action: Refocusing Policies through a Well-being Lens*, OECD Publishing, Paris, https://dx.doi.org/10.1787/2f4c8c9a-en. [60]

OECD (2019), *Budgeting and Public Expenditures in OECD Countries 2019*, OECD Publishing, Paris, https://dx.doi.org/10.1787/9789264307957-en. [199]

OECD (2019), *Changing the Odds for Vulnerable Children: Building Opportunities and Resilience*, OECD Publishing, Paris, https://dx.doi.org/10.1787/a2e8796c-en. [73]

OECD (2019), *Dashboard on priorities for adult learning*, http://www.oecd.org/els/emp/skills-and-work/adult-learning/dashboard.htm (accessed on 15 June 2021). [136]

OECD (2019), *Getting Skills Right: Future-Ready Adult Learning Systems*, Getting Skills Right, OECD Publishing, Paris, https://dx.doi.org/10.1787/9789264311756-en. [135]

OECD (2019), *Government at a Glance 2019*, OECD Publishing, Paris, https://dx.doi.org/10.1787/8ccf5c38-en. [196]

OECD (2019), *Health at a Glance 2019: OECD Indicators*, OECD Publishing, Paris, https://dx.doi.org/10.1787/4dd50c09-en. [150]

OECD (2019), *Health for Everyone?: Social Inequalities in Health and Health Systems*, OECD Health Policy Studies, OECD Publishing, Paris, https://dx.doi.org/10.1787/3c8385d0-en. [152]

OECD (2019), *Making Decentralisation Work: A Handbook for Policy-Makers*, OECD Multi-level Governance Studies, OECD Publishing, Paris, https://dx.doi.org/10.1787/g2g9faa7-en. [234]

OECD (2019), *OECD Economic Surveys: New Zealand 2019*, OECD Publishing, Paris, https://dx.doi.org/10.1787/b0b94dbd-en. [221]

OECD (2019), *OECD Employment Outlook 2019: The Future of Work*, OECD Publishing, Paris, https://dx.doi.org/10.1787/9ee00155-en. [24]

OECD (2019), *OECD Mental health performance framework*, OECD Publishing, Paris, http://www.oecd.org/health/OECD-Mental-Health-Performance-Framework-2019.pdf (accessed on 18 March 2021). [45]

OECD (2019), *OECD Skills Strategy 2019: Skills to Shape a Better Future*, OECD Publishing, Paris, https://dx.doi.org/10.1787/9789264313835-en. [125]

OECD (2019), *Policy brief. Future-ready adult learning systems*, OECD Publishing, Paris, http://www.oecd.org/employment/skills-and-work/adult-learning/Policy-Brief-Future-ready-adult-learning-2019-EN.pdf (accessed on 1 April 2021). [130]

OECD (2019), *Public Procurement in Germany: Strategic Dimensions for Well-being and Growth*, OECD Public Governance Reviews, OECD Publishing, Paris, https://dx.doi.org/10.1787/1db30826-en. [227]

OECD (2019), *Recommendation of the Council on Policy Coherence for Sustainable Development*, OECD/LEGAL/0381, OECD, Paris, http://www.oecd.org/gov/pcsd/recommendation-on-policy-coherence-for-sustainable-development-eng.pdf (accessed on 14 May 2021). [211]

OECD (2019), *Reforming Public Procurement: Progress in Implementing the 2015 OECD Recommendation*, OECD Public Governance Reviews, OECD Publishing, Paris, https://dx.doi.org/10.1787/1de41738-en. [226]

OECD (2019), *Skills Matter: Additional Results from the Survey of Adult Skills*, OECD Skills Studies, OECD Publishing, Paris, https://dx.doi.org/10.1787/1f029d8f-en. [134]

OECD (2019), *Society at a Glance 2019: OECD Social Indicators*, OECD Publishing, Paris, https://dx.doi.org/10.1787/soc_glance-2019-en. [31]

OECD (2019), *The Heavy Burden of Obesity: The Economics of Prevention*, OECD Health Policy Studies, OECD Publishing, Paris, https://dx.doi.org/10.1787/67450d67-en. [44]

OECD (2018), *Opportunities for All: A Framework for Policy Action on Inclusive Growth*, OECD Publishing, Paris, https://dx.doi.org/10.1787/9789264301665-en. [200]

OECD (2017), *Multi-level Governance Reforms: Overview of OECD Country Experiences*, OECD Multi-level Governance Studies, OECD Publishing, Paris, https://dx.doi.org/10.1787/9789264272866-en. [235]

OECD (2017), *OECD Guidelines on Measuring Trust*, OECD Publishing, Paris, https://dx.doi.org/10.1787/9789264278219-en. [190]

OECD (2017), *Trust and Public Policy: How Better Governance Can Help Rebuild Public Trust*, OECD Public Governance Reviews, OECD Publishing, Paris, https://dx.doi.org/10.1787/9789264268920-en. [191]

OECD (2016), *2015 OECD Recommendation of the Council on Gender Equality in Public Life*, OECD Publishing, Paris, https://dx.doi.org/10.1787/9789264252820-en. [263]

OECD (2016), *Enhancing child well-being to promote inclusive growth*, OECD Publishing , Paris, http://www.oecd.org/officialdocuments/publicdisplaydocumentpdf/?cote=DELSA/ELSA(2016)7/REV1&doclanguage=en (accessed on 13 May 2021). [139]

OECD (2016), *Open Government: The Global Context and the Way Forward*, OECD Publishing, Paris, https://dx.doi.org/10.1787/9789264268104-en. [194]

OECD (2015), *Fit Mind, Fit Job: From Evidence to Practice in Mental Health and Work*, Mental Health and Work, OECD Publishing, Paris, https://dx.doi.org/10.1787/9789264228283-en. [104]

OECD (2015), *Integrating Social Services for Vulnerable Groups: Bridging Sectors for Better Service Delivery*, OECD Publishing, Paris, https://dx.doi.org/10.1787/9789264233775-en. [144]

OECD (2015), *Recommendation of the Council on Integrated Mental Health, Skills and Work Policy*, OECD/LEGAL/0420, OECD, Paris, https://legalinstruments.oecd.org/en/instruments/334 (accessed on 18 March 2021). [157]

OECD (2015), "The quality of working lives: Earnings mobility, labour market risk and long-term inequality", in *OECD Employment Outlook 2015*, OECD Publishing, Paris, https://dx.doi.org/10.1787/empl_outlook-2015-8-en. [103]

OECD (2014), *Focus on inequality and growth*, OECD, Paris, http://www.oecd.org/social/Focus-Inequality-and-Growth-2014.pdf (accessed on 10 April 2021). [40]

OECD (2014), *How's Life in Your Region?: Measuring Regional and Local Well-being for Policy Making*, OECD Publishing, Paris, https://dx.doi.org/10.1787/9789264217416-en. [240]

OECD (2012), *Sick on the Job?: Myths and Realities about Mental Health and Work*, Mental Health and Work, OECD Publishing, Paris, https://dx.doi.org/10.1787/9789264124523-en. [105]

OECD (forthcoming), "Measuring non-financial business performance through the lens of the OECD Well-being Framework", OECD Publishing, Paris. [257]

OECD (n.d.), *OECD Youthwise*, http://www.oecd.org/about/civil-society/youth/youthwise/ (accessed on 19 May 2021). [250]

OECD/European Union (2017), *Boosting Social Enterprise Development: Good Practice Compendium*, OECD Publishing, Paris, https://dx.doi.org/10.1787/9789264268500-en. [261]

OECD/Eurostat/WHO (2017), *A System of Health Accounts 2011: Revised edition*, OECD Publishing, Paris, https://dx.doi.org/10.1787/9789264270985-en. [267]

Office of the Assistant Secretary for Planning and Evaluation (2021), *COVID-19 and economic opportunity: Unequal effects on economic need and program response*, United States Department of Health and Human Services, https://aspe.hhs.gov/reports/covid-19-economic-opportunity-unequal-effects-economic-need-program-response. [64]

Open Government Partnership (2020), *A guide to Open Government and the Coronavirus: Protecting participation and deliberation*, http://www.opengovpartnership.org/documents/a-guide-to-open-government-and-the-coronavirus-protecting-participation-and-deliberation/ (accessed on 1 May 2021). [246]

Ormston, H., L. Pennycook and J. Wallace (2021), *Embedding a wellbeing framework in Northern Ireland. A contribution from Carnegie UK Trust to inform discussions around the Programme for Government consultation*, Carnegie UK Trust, Fife. [210]

Parker, K., R. Minkin and J. Bennett (2020), *Economic fallout from COVID-19 continues to hit lower-income Americans the hardest*, PEW Research Center, https://www.pewresearch.org/social-trends/2020/09/24/economic-fallout-from-covid-19-continues-to-hit-lower-income-americans-the-hardest/ (accessed on 4 October 2021). [29]

Patanavanich, R. and S. Glantz (2020), "Smoking is associated with COVID-19 progression: A meta-analysis", *Nicotine & Tobacco Research*, Vol. 22/9, pp. 1653-1656, http://dx.doi.org/10.1093/ntr/ntaa082. [7]

Patel, V. et al. (2018), "The Lancet Commission on global mental health and sustainable development", *The Lancet*, Vol. 392, pp. 1553-1598, http://dx.doi.org/10.1016/S0140-6736(18)31612-X. [158]

Pickett, K. and R. Wilkinson (2015), *Income inequality and health: A causal review*, Elsevier Ltd, http://dx.doi.org/10.1016/j.socscimed.2014.12.031. [37]

Pucher, J. et al. (2010), "Walking and cycling to health: A comparative analysis of city, state, and international data", *American Journal of Public Health*, Vol. 100/10, pp. 1986-1992, http://dx.doi.org/10.2105/AJPH.2009.189324. [98]

Putnam, R. (2000), *Bowling alone: The collapse and revival of American community*, Simon & Schuster, New York, http://bowlingalone.com/ (accessed on 13 March 2021). [184]

Qualter, P. et al. (2010), "Childhood loneliness as a predictor of adolescent depressive symptoms: An 8-year longitudinal study", *European Child and Adolescent Psychiatry*, Vol. 19/6, pp. 493-501, http://dx.doi.org/10.1007/s00787-009-0059-y. [175]

Ramos, G. et al. (2020), *Systemic thinking for policy making. The potential of systems analysis for addressing global policy challenges in the 21st century*, OECD Publishing, Paris. [123]

Raworth, K. (2018), *Doughnut economics: Seven ways to think like a 21st-century economist*, Cornerstone, London. [236]

Rea, D. and T. Burton (2020), "NEW EVIDENCE ON THE HECKMAN CURVE", *Journal of Economic Surveys*, Vol. 34/2, pp. 241-262, http://dx.doi.org/10.1111/joes.12353. [141]

Reddy, R. et al. (2021), "The effect of smoking on COVID-19 severity: A systematic review and meta-analysis", *Journal of Medical Virology*, Vol. 93/2, pp. 1045-1056, http://dx.doi.org/10.1002/jmv.26389. [8]

Reynolds, A. et al. (2011), "Age 26 Cost-Benefit Analysis of the Child-Parent Center early education program", *Child Development*, Vol. 82/1, pp. 379-404, http://dx.doi.org/10.1111/j.1467-8624.2010.01563.x. [138]

Richardson, D. and R. Denniss (2020), *Women lose from COVID-19, men to gain from stimulus*, The Australian Institute, Manuka. [120]

Ridley, M. et al. (2020), "Poverty, depression, and anxiety: Causal evidence and mechanisms", *Science*, Vol. 370/6522, http://dx.doi.org/10.1126/science.aay0214. [153]

Rosholm, M. et al. (2021), "Are Impacts of Early Interventions in the Scandinavian Welfare State Consistent with a Heckman Curve? A Meta-Analysis", *Journal of Economic Surveys*, p. joes.12400, http://dx.doi.org/10.1111/joes.12400. [142]

Rossati, A. (2017), *Global warming and its health impact*, NIOC Health Organization, http://dx.doi.org/10.15171/ijoem.2017.963. [50]

Saint-Martin, A., H. Inanc and C. Prinz (2018), "Job Quality, Health and Productivity: An evidence-based framework for analysis", *OECD Social, Employment and Migration Working Papers*, No. 221, OECD Publishing, Paris, https://dx.doi.org/10.1787/a8c84d91-en. [108]

Sampson, R., S. Raudenbush and F. Earls (1997), "Neighborhoods and violent crime: A multilevel study of collective efficacy", *Science*, Vol. 277/5328, pp. 918-924, http://dx.doi.org/10.1126/science.277.5328.918. [189]

Sandbu, M. (2020), *The post-pandemic brave new world*, pp. 4-9, http://www.imf.org/external/pubs/ft/fandd/2020/12/post-pandemic-brave-new-world-sandbu.htm (accessed on 11 March 2021). [91]

Shinwell, M. and E. Shamir (2018), *Measuring the impact of businesses on people's well-being and sustainability: Taking stock of existing frameworks and initiatives*, OECD Publishing, Paris, http://www.oecd-ilibrary.org/docserver/51837366-en.pdf?expires=1618132150&id=id&accname=guest&checksum=2E3FFA65A56741828C74196CB3025E5C (accessed on 11 April 2021). [256]

Smith, C. (2021), ""Policy Pitch" presentation at the 2021 McGill IHSP/ Canadian Policies for Better Lives conference", https://wellbeing.research.mcgill.ca/BetterLives2021/policyvideos/ (accessed on 1 June 2021). [242]

Stats NZ (2018), *Indicators Aotearoa New Zealand*, Stats NZ, Wellington, http://www.stats.govt.nz/assets/Consultations/indicators-aotearoa-new-zealand-nga-tutohu-aotearoa-consultation/indicators-aotearoa-new-zealand-measuring-our-well-being.pdf (accessed on 3 June 2021). [204]

Stiglitz, J., J. Fitoussi and M. Durand (2019), *For good measure: An agenda for moving beyond GDP*, The New Press, New York and London, http://dx.doi.org/10.1017/s004727942000063x. [202]

Strazdins, L. et al. (2010), "Job quality and inequality: Parents' jobs and children's emotional and behavioural difficulties", http://dx.doi.org/10.1016/j.socscimed.2010.02.041. [109]

The British Academy (2021), *Shaping the Covid decade. Addressing the long-term societal impacts of COVID-19*, The British Academy , London, http://www.thebritishacademy.ac.uk/documents/3239/Shaping-COVID-decade-addressing-long-term-societal-impacts-COVID-19.pdf (accessed on 11 April 2021). [84]

The Commonwealth Fund (2020), *Do Americans face greater mental health and economic consequences from COVID-19? Comparing the U.S. with other high-income countries*, http://www.commonwealthfund.org/publications/issue-briefs/2020/aug/americans-mental-health-and-economic-consequences-COVID19 (accessed on 20 May 2021). [43]

The Foundational Economy (n.d.), *What is the foundational economy?*, https://foundationaleconomy.com/introduction/ (accessed on 20 May 2021). [111]

The Guardian (2020), *Jacinda Ardern holds special coronavirus press conference for children | Coronavirus | The Guardian*, http://www.theguardian.com/world/2020/mar/19/jacinda-ardern-holds-special-coronavirus-press-conference-for-children (accessed on 8 June 2021). [247]

Theorell, T. et al. (1995), "Social support and the development of immune function in human immunodeficiency virus infection", *Psychosomatic Medicine*, Vol. 57/1, pp. 32-36, http://dx.doi.org/10.1097/00006842-199501000-00005. [169]

Trebeck, K. and J. Williams (2019), *The economics of arrival. Ideas for a grown-up economy*, Policy Press, Bristol. [20]

Truger, A. (2016), "Reviving fiscal policy in Europe: Towards an implementation of the golden rule of public investment", *European Journal of Economics and Economic Policies: Intervention*, Vol. 13/1, pp. 57-71, https://EconPapers.repec.org/RePEc:elg:ejeepi:v:13:y:2016:i:1:p57-71 (accessed on 5 April 2021). [118]

Tuparevska, E., R. Santibáñez and J. Solabarrieta (2020), "Equity and social exclusion measures in EU lifelong learning policies", *International Journal of Lifelong Education*, Vol. 39/1, pp. 5-17, http://dx.doi.org/10.1080/02601370.2019.1689435. [132]

Uchino, B. (2006), *Social support and health: A review of physiological processes potentially underlying links to disease outcomes*, http://dx.doi.org/10.1007/s10865-006-9056-5. [168]

UN (2020), *Satellite account for education and training: Compilation guide*, United Nations Economic Commission for Europe, New York and Geneva, https://unece.org/DAM/stats/publications/2020/ECECESSTAT20201.pdf (accessed on 3 June 2021). [266]

UN (2016), *Guide on measuring human capital*, United Nations Economic Commission for Europe, New York and Geneva. [265]

UN (n.d.), *System of Environmental Economic Accounting*, https://seea.un.org/ (accessed on 3 June 2021). [268]

UN (n.d.), *The SEEA Ecosystem Accounting*, https://seea.un.org/ecosystem-accounting (accessed on 3 June 2021). [269]

UNDP (2020), *Budgeting for the Sustainable Development Goals: Aligning domestic budgets with the SDGs. Guidebook 2020*, United Nations Development Programme, New York. [224]

United Nations (2020), *COVID-19 and the need for action on mental health. United Nations Policy Brief*, https://unsdg.un.org/sites/default/files/2020-05/UN-Policy-Brief-COVID-19-and-mental-health.pdf (accessed on 7 April 2021). [47]

United Nations (2020), *The Sustainable Development Goals Report*, https://unstats.un.org/sdgs/report/2020/The-Sustainable-Development-Goals-Report-2020.pdf (accessed on 31 July 2020). [9]

Uslaner, E. (2002), *The moral foundations of trust*, Cambridge University Press, Cambridge, http://dx.doi.org/10.1017/cbo9780511614934. [38]

Van den Broucke, S. (2020), "Why health promotion matters to the COVID-19 pandemic, and vice versa", *Health Promotion International*, Vol. 35/2, pp. 181-186, http://dx.doi.org/10.1093/HEAPRO/DAAA042. [146]

Van Doorninck, M. and S. Schouten (2020), "The Doughnut model for a fairer, greener Amsterdam", *Green European Journal*, http://www.greeneuropeanjournal.eu (accessed on 31 March 2021). [237]

Van Gool, K. and M. Pea (2014), *Health, austerity and economic crisis: Assessing the short-term impact in OECD countries. OECD Health Working Paper No. 76*, OECD Publishing , Paris, https://www.oecd-ilibrary.org/docserver/5jxx71lt1zg6-en.pdf?expires=1616408564&id=id&accname=guest&checksum=2BFCC9B56B8054CE0A0C773B9DE7A7C8 (accessed on 22 March 2021). [113]

Varga, T. et al. (2021), "Loneliness, worries, anxiety, and precautionary behaviours in response to the COVID-19 pandemic: a longitudinal analysis of 200,000 Western and Northern Europeans", *The Lancet Regional Health - Europe*, Vol. 2, p. 100020, http://dx.doi.org/10.1016/j.lanepe.2020.100020. [70]

Wade, R. (2021), "The opening of minds towards wellbeing", in Karacaoglu, G. (ed.), *Love you. Public policy for intergenerational wellbeing*, The Tuwhiri Project, Wellington. [251]

Weissbourd, R. et al. (2021), *Loneliness in America: How the pandemic has deepened an epidemic of loneliness and what we can do about it*, Harvard University , Cambridge, http://www.makingcaringcommon.org (accessed on 20 March 2021). [71]

Whitby, A., C. Seaford and C. Berry (2014), *The BRAINPOoL Project Final Report. Beyond GDP - From measurement to politics and policy*, World Future Council , Hamburg, http://www.brainpoolproject.eu (accessed on 12 March 2021). [90]

WHO (2020), *Statement – Older people are at highest risk from COVID-19, but all must act to prevent community spread*, http://www.euro.who.int/en/health-topics/health-emergencies/coronavirus-covid-19/statements/statement-older-people-are-at-highest-risk-from-covid-19,-but-all-must-act-to-prevent-community-spread (accessed on 29 March 2021). [61]

WHO (2014), *The case for investing in public health.*, World Health Organization Europe, Copenhagen. [162]

Wilkinson, R., I. Kawachi and B. Kennedy (1998), "Mortality, the social environment, crime and violence", *Sociology of Health & Illness*, Vol. 20/5, pp. 578-597, http://dx.doi.org/10.1111/1467-9566.00120. [188]

Wilkinson, R. and K. Pickett (2007), "The problems of relative deprivation: Why some societies do better than others", *Social Science and Medicine*, Vol. 65/9, pp. 1965-1978, http://dx.doi.org/10.1016/j.socscimed.2007.05.041. [36]

Winkler, O. (2009), *Interpreting economic and social data: A foundation of descriptive statistics*, Springer, Berlin, http://dx.doi.org/10.1007/978-3-540-68721-4. [88]

World Bank (2005), *Where Is the Wealth of Nations? Measuring Capital for the 21st Century*, World Bank, Washington, DC, http://dx.doi.org/10.1596/978-0-8213-6354-6. [117]

Wu, X. et al. (2020), *Exposure to air pollution and COVID-19 mortality in the United States: A nationwide cross-sectional study*, medRxiv, http://dx.doi.org/10.1101/2020.04.05.20054502. [2]

Zak, P. and S. Knack (2001), "Trust and growth", *Economic Journal*, Vol. 111/470, pp. 295-321, http://dx.doi.org/10.1111/1468-0297.00609. [39]

Zhen, N. et al. (2014), "Poverty reduction, environmental protection and ecosystem services: A prospective theory for sustainable development", *Chinese Geographical Science*, Vol. 24/1, pp. 83-92, http://dx.doi.org/10.1007/s11769-014-0658-5. [100]

Notes

[1] This report complements work currently underway at the OECD to develop a dashboard of indicators to monitor the COVID-19 recovery, as discussed at the 2020 and 2021 OECD Ministerial Council Meetings. While the present report focuses on describing well-being impacts in the first year of the pandemic, the recovery dashboard is a forward-looking exercise that aims to monitor OECD countries' progress towards a strong, green, inclusive and resilient recovery, based on a more limited set of indicators. The OECD Well-Being Framework has informed and shaped both of these activities.

[2] The increase in non-standard workers has mainly been driven by an increase in part-time workers.

[3] Findings are based on biannual test scores in core subjects for students aged 8 to 11 in a dataset covering 15% of Dutch primary schools from 2017 to 2020 (Engzell, Frey and Verhagen, 2021[33]).

[4] Control variables in the study included: the median age of the population; whether the country is an island; an exposure index measuring how close a country was to infections in other countries in the early stages of the pandemic (in March 31); measures of the extent to which a country was able to remember and apply the epidemic control strategies learned during the SARS epidemic of 2003; and whether the country has a female head of government (Helliwell et al., 2021[78]). In terms of the validity of the "wallet return" question, evidence from an experiment involving large numbers of wallets being dropped in 40 countries (some containing money and some not) suggests that there is a strong positive relation (r = 0.64) between expected and actual wallet return (Cohn et al., 2019[264]).

[5] While some types of natural resources such as *land, mineral and energy reserves*, and *non-cultivated biological resources, water resources and other natural resources* are recognised in the central national accounting framework, other types of natural resources as well as human and social capital are currently not recognised in the central framework of national accounts. A lot of relevant information is currently captured in the form of satellite accounts in several countries, for example, focusing on human capital (UN, 2016[265]), education and training (UN, 2020[266]), health care spending (OECD/Eurostat/WHO, 2017[267]), environmental-economic accounts (UN, n.d.[268]), and ecosystem accounting (UN, n.d.[269]). Work in relation to better capturing well-being and sustainability in the system of national accounts is ongoing as part of the System of National Accounts Research Agenda, aiming to bring more of these assets into the central framework (Eurostat, OECD and UNECE, 2020[270]).

[6] Ultimately, a gender-responsive approach to addressing the socio-economic impacts of the pandemic on men and women from diverse backgrounds relies on a dual approach (OECD, 2021[34]). Firstly, pro-active and targeted policies are needed to close identified gender gaps and level the playing field for men and women. This includes targeted measures to tackle specific challenges faced by women, such as gender-based violence. Secondly, in line with the OECD Recommendation on Gender Equality in Public Life, it is essential to mainstream gender-inclusive considerations throughout the policy cycle, to ensure that government action does not inadvertently reinforce existing gender stereotypes and inequalities (OECD, 2016[263]). For example, the Canadian government has mandated that its Gender-based Analysis Plus (GBA+) must be undertaken on all policies and proposals, including in response to the COVID-19 crisis. GBA+ is an analytical tool that policy makers use to examine the potential impacts (both intended and unintended) of a policy, plan, programme, or other initiative on diverse groups of people. It considers gender as well as other identity factors such as age, ethnicity, indigenous heritage, geographic location, socio-economic status, family status, and mental or physical disability status (Government of Canada, n.d.[262]).

[7] At Level 1, tasks typically require the use of widely available and familiar technology applications, such as e-mail software or a web browser. There is little or no navigation required to access the information or commands required to solve the problem. The problem may be solved regardless of the respondent's awareness and use of specific tools and functions (e.g. a "sort" function). The tasks involve few steps and a minimal number of operators (OECD, 2019[134]).

[8] Canada's Quality of Life Framework, "https://www.canada.ca/en/department-finance/services/publications/measuring-what-matters-toward-quality-life-strategy-canada.html

[9] Home to 55% of the world's population, cities have a unique responsibility and opportunity to shape intergenerational well-being outcomes. The Thriving Cities Initiative (TCI), a collaboration between C40 Cities, the Doughnut Economics Action Lab, and Circle Economy, is working with the cities of Amsterdam, Philadelphia, and Portland to pilot new ways of thinking, governance, and collaboration for a green and just future.

[10] https://wellbeingacademy.hw.gov.ae

[11] For example, although 20 of 26 governments (77%) consulted stakeholders on their COVID-19 response strategies, only 9 (35%) actively involved them in policy design (OECD, 2021[12]). In taking a risk-based approach in prioritising the most time-critical processes, stakeholder engagement practices used shorter consultation periods and more focused consultation activities, and in some cases, economic regulators put consultations on hold, recognising the limited ability of stakeholders to take part (OECD, 2021[12]). Moreover, with few exceptions, there were rarely formal channels created for the public to voice an opinion on or shape the evolution of the decided measures (Economist Intelligence Unit, 2020[271]). Among government initiatives in OECD countries to publish data on COVID-19 and responses in 2020, 77% were primarily for situational awareness, and there is limited evidence that open government data initiatives drove concrete action beyond public communication efforts (OECD, 2021[12])(see Chapter 10). In some countries, access to information requests by citizens were either delayed or their general timeline for completion officially extended or suspended (see Chapter 10).

[12] *Government at a Glance 2021* reports that the use of virtual consultations in regulatory policy-making has increased since 2017; from 35% to 62% of OECD countries for early-stage consultations, and from 41% to 57% of countries for late-stage consultations. In 92% of OECD countries, policy makers consult early on draft regulations with selected groups; open consultations are more common only at a late stage (OECD, 2021[12]).

[13] Initiated by Sweden in collaboration with the ILO and the OECD in 2016, the Global Deal brings together over 100 partners representing governments, business, trade unions, and civil society. https://www.theglobaldeal.com

2 Material conditions in the first year of COVID-19

COVID-19's impact on households' material conditions has been significant. Although government support ensured that average household income did not decrease as markedly as GDP in 2020, many households did nevertheless face financial difficulties. The pandemic led to the closure, both permanently and temporarily, of activities and businesses, and for many jobs teleworking is simply not an option. Despite unprecedented government action to support workers and employers, labour underutilisation rates nearly doubled, and there has been a steep reduction in hours worked. Overcrowded and poor-quality housing conditions increase vulnerability to COVID-19, while the lack of Internet access still prevents some people from working, studying or accessing services remotely. Housing cost overburden and sharp rises in rents and house prices have added to the difficulties faced by poorer households. These impacts have tended to hit vulnerable people and places the hardest, threatening to widen pre-existing inequalities.

2.1. Income and Wealth

While the COVID-19 pandemic has put large numbers of households in financial difficulty, the impact has been mixed within and across countries. Across OECD countries, government measures are being implemented with the aim of supporting households facing a considerable loss of labour income. As a result, real household income per capita did not decrease as markedly as GDP per capita, on average, in the OECD area in 2020. Nevertheless, many households are struggling financially.

Crisis measures taken by governments helped to cushion the impact on incomes…

Government measures shielded average household per capita income from the direct economic impacts of COVID-19 across the OECD area. As a result, while OECD real GDP per capita decreased by 5.1% cumulatively between 2019 and 2020, average real household disposable income per capita (i.e. after direct taxes and transfers) increased by 2.9% cumulatively (Figure 2.1 and Figure 2.2 Panel A).

GDP and household disposable income per capita followed divergent trends in 2020. Average household disposable income per capita reached its peak in Q2 2020 (with a 3.9% increase over the previous quarter) and progressively declined until Q4 2020. By contrast, after reaching its trough in Q2 2020 (with a 10.5% decline over the previous quarter), average GDP per capita increased up to Q4 2020 (Figure 2.1 and Figure 2.2 Panel B). Canada and the United States experienced a particularly marked increase in household disposable income per capita between 2019 and 2020, of 7.9% and 6.1% respectively, in both countries peaking in Q2 2020.

Government transfers to the household sector in response to the pandemic played a significant buffering role. Net cash transfers to households increased in most OECD countries between 2019 and 2020 (Figure 2.3, Panel A). In Canada, government net cash transfers to households increased by 20.7% between Q1 and Q2 2020, which explains why Canada experienced a larger increase in household disposable income per capita compared to other countries (Figure 2.3, Panel B). Over 8.9 million Canadians received income assistance from the Canada Emergency Response Benefit or enhanced Employment Insurance between 16 March and 26 September 2020, which helped many families to avoid low income. According to Statistics Canada's experimental estimates of weekly household income, the proportion of individuals living in families that had earnings below the Low-Income Measure – the Canadian poverty line – in April 2020 was 16 percentage points lower when pandemic benefits were taken into account than otherwise (22% versus 38%) (Government of Canada, 2021[1]; Beck et al., 2020[2]). Similarly, in the United States, government support through the April 2020 CARES Act contributed to the significant increase in household disposable income during the first two quarters of 2020 (OECD, 2020[3]).

The decrease in real household disposable income per capita between Q2 and Q4 2020 reflected the reduction of government transfers to households after the unprecedented support provided at the beginning of the pandemic (Figure 2.3, Panel B). Nevertheless, the United States enacted additional fiscal stimulus throughout the Coronavirus Response and Relief Supplemental Appropriations Act of 2021 and the American Rescue Plan Act of 2021, which is reflected in the large increase in household disposable income in Q1 2021. Local and regional actors have also played an increasingly important role in providing support to vulnerable businesses and households. They often implemented emergency support policies on behalf of national governments, complementing them with local actions to fill gaps for specific sectors or populations and helping local workers and firms navigate the sometimes-complex patchwork of schemes (OECD, 2021[4]).

Figure 2.1. In 2020, GDP decreased by 5.1% across the OECD area

GDP per capita, index

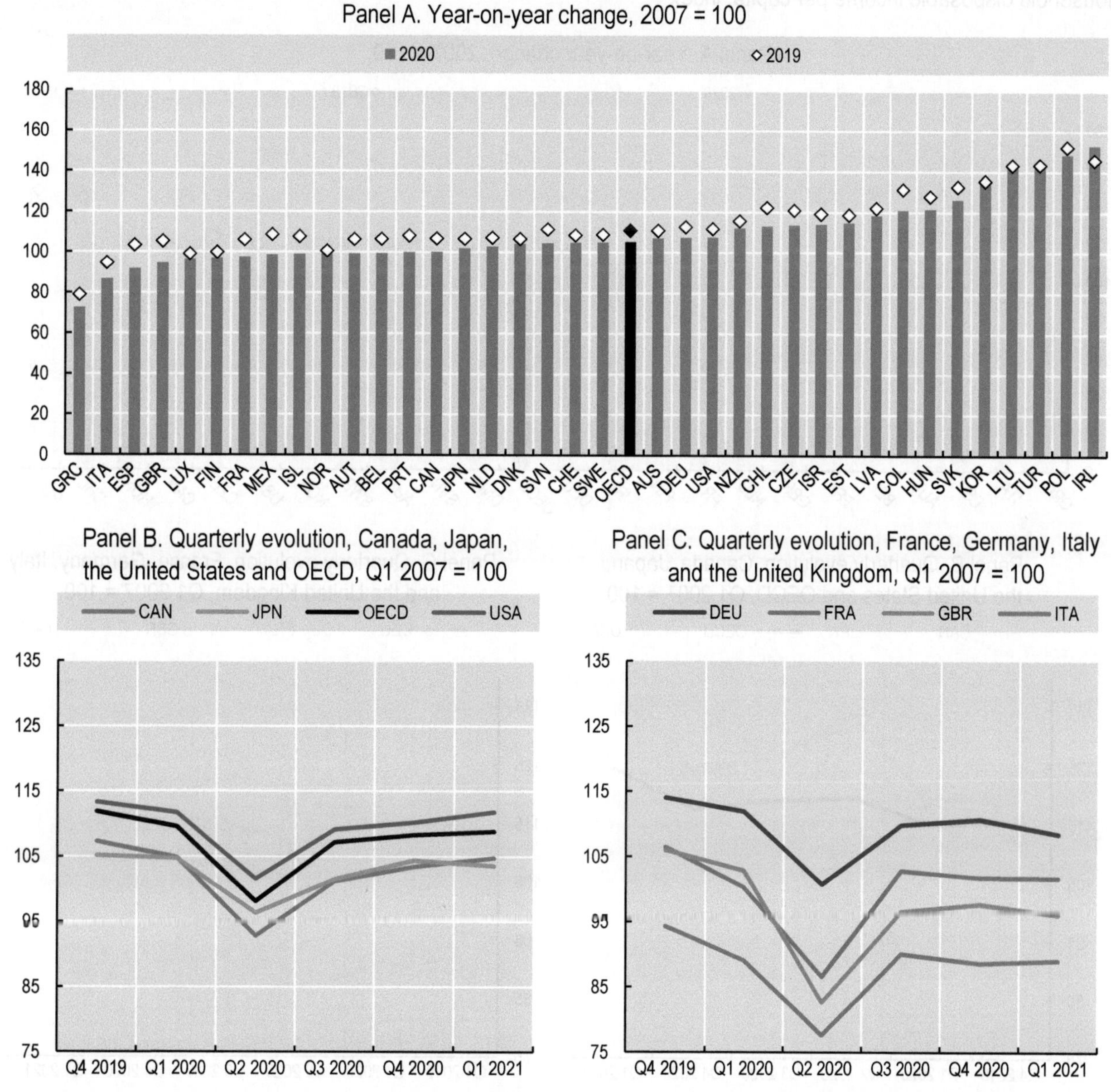

Note: The OECD average is calculated considering all the OECD countries as a single entity, and the final aggregate is divided by the total population.
Source: OECD (n.d.[5]), *Household Dashboard* (database), www.oecd.org/sdd/na/household-dashboard.htm.

StatLink https://stat.link/qtecnv

Figure 2.2. Government support measures shielded household disposable income during the pandemic

Household disposable income per capita, index

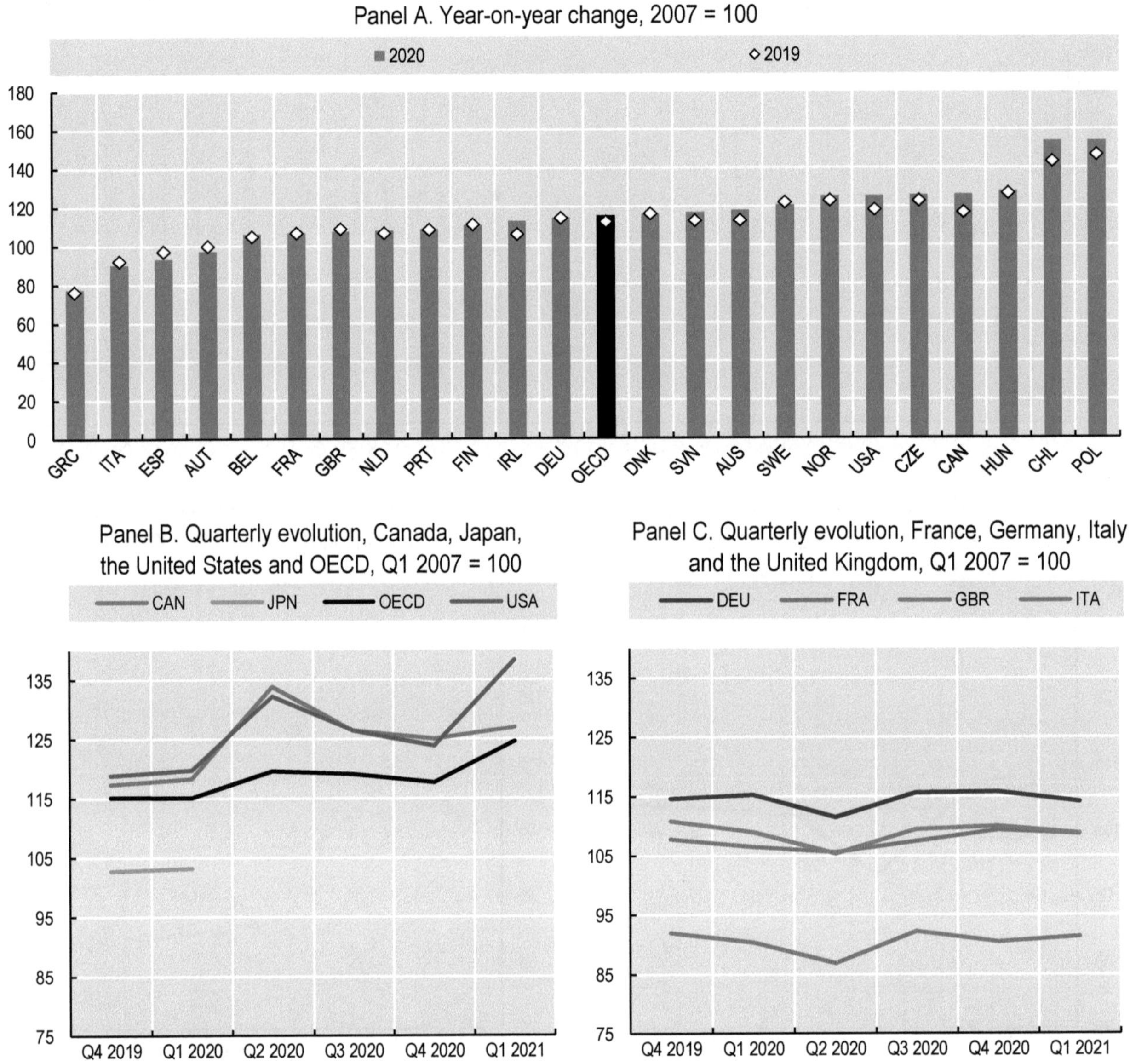

Note: The OECD average is calculated considering all the OECD countries as a single entity, and the final aggregate is divided by the total population. Data are available only in Q4 2019 and Q1 2020 for Japan.
Source: OECD (n.d.[5]), *Household Dashboard* (database), www.oecd.org/sdd/na/household-dashboard.htm.

StatLink https://stat.link/4nsgya

Figure 2.3. Net cash transfers to households increased in most OECD countries in 2020

Net cash transfers to households, index

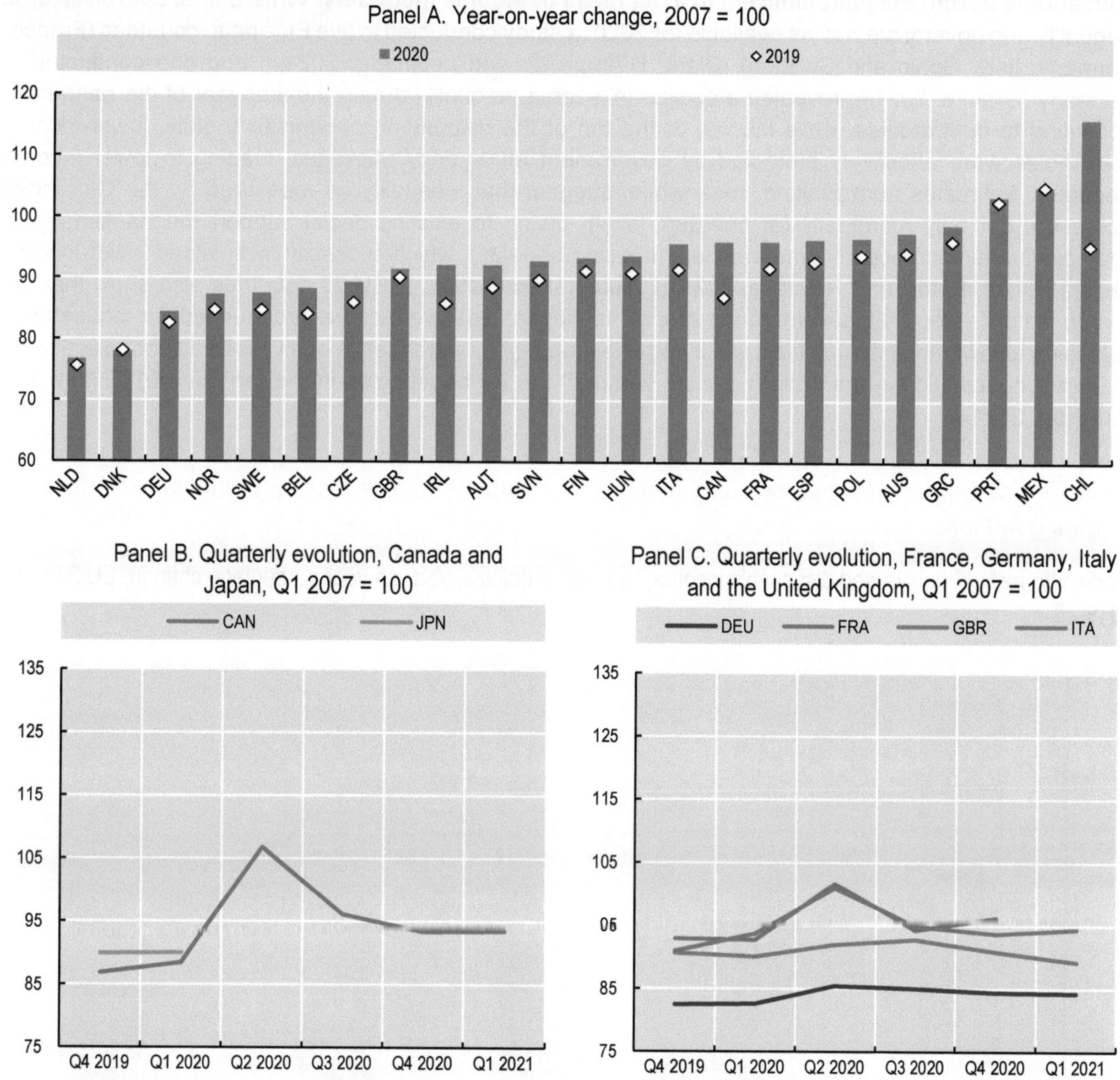

Note: Data are available only in Q4 2019 and Q1 2020 for Japan, and Q1 2021 data are missing for France.
Source: OECD (n.d.[5]), *Household Dashboard* (database), www.oecd.org/sdd/na/household-dashboard.htm.

StatLink https://stat.link/fb280h

… but the most vulnerable households have been facing financial difficulties

There is preliminary evidence for a small number of countries that government support to households during the pandemic led to a decrease in income inequality. While official data on income inequality and poverty are not yet available for 2020, a study conducted in five European countries (France, Germany, Italy, Spain and Sweden) (Clark, D'Ambrosio and Lepinteur, 2021[6]) and one conducted in Germany (Grabka, 2021[7]) revealed a decline in income inequality during the first year of the pandemic. According to both studies, while income at the top of the distribution decreased slightly, lower-income households were effectively protected by government emergency packages, leading to lower income inequality. Estimates from Finland, meanwhile, suggest that inequality as measured by the Gini index increased, but only marginally (at one-digit level), owing to existing social support mechanisms (e.g. unemployment insurance, income transfers, housing benefits), which successfully shielded lower-income deciles (Kyyrä, Pirttilä and Ravaska, 2021[8]). Eurostat estimates for EU 27 countries also show that the compensatory effects of government support[1] to households were more pronounced for households belonging to lower income quintiles, which experienced higher increases in equivalised disposable income (1.9% for households in the bottom quintile versus 0.5% for households in the top quintile) (Figure 2.4) (Eurostat, 2021[9]).

Figure 2.4. Government schemes compensated employment income losses, particularly for lower income quintiles

Median household equivalised disposable income, by income quintile, year-on-year percentage change, EU 27, 2019-20

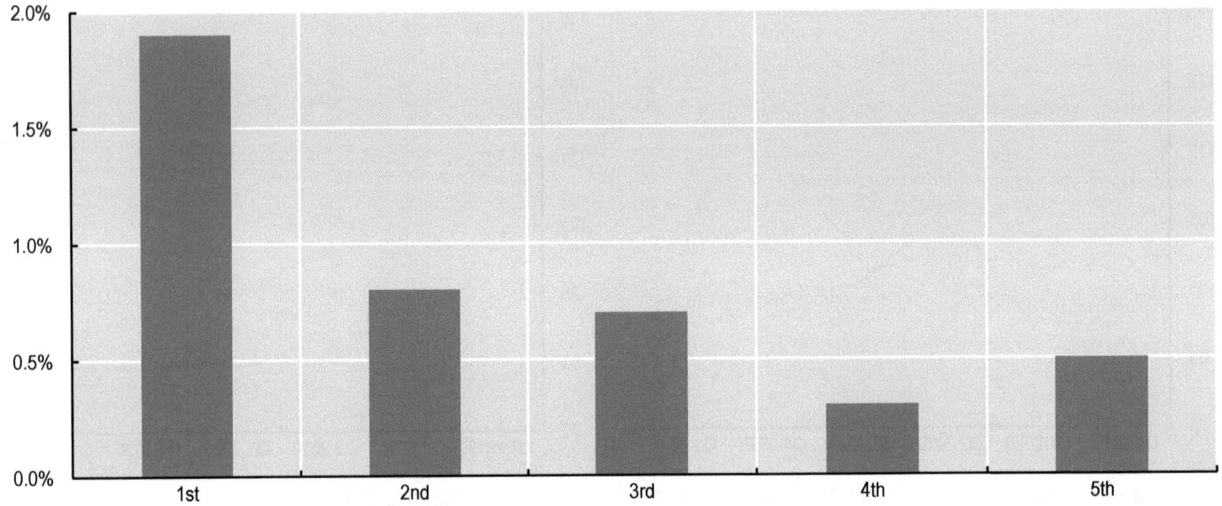

Note: EU 27 includes all member states of the European Union, including also Bulgaria, Croatia, Cyprus, Malta and Romania. All figures provided are part of the experimental statistics produced by Eurostat in the context of advanced estimates on income inequality and poverty indicators. The results refer to the yearly change 2019-2020. Uncertainty of the early estimates is particularly high in the current context, and a number of caveats and model assumptions should be considered.
Source: Eurostat (2021[9]), *Early estimates of income inequalities during the 2020 pandemic*, https://ec.europa.eu/eurostat/statistics-explained/index.php?title=Early_estimates_of_income_inequalities_during_the_2020_pandemic.

StatLink https://stat.link/s9bf0h

Despite strong government support, lower-income households are struggling financially. High rates of financial insecurity before the pandemic left many households vulnerable as they entered the crisis. On average across 28 OECD countries, OECD wealth distribution data indicate that 36% of people who were not income poor in 2016 were nevertheless at risk of falling into poverty within three months in the event of a sudden loss of income (OECD, 2020[10]).[2] When the pandemic hit, higher-income households were, on average, able to accumulate wealth by cutting discretionary spending on activities that were restricted during the lockdowns (e.g. restaurants, culture, travel) while lower income households – whose spending is largely not discretionary – were not able to reduce their spending to the same extent (refer to Chapter 5 for more information about financial difficulties across the income distribution). Data collected in September-October 2020 in 25 OECD countries as part of the OECD Risks That Matter Survey indicate that close to one third (31%) of respondents reported that they or their household experienced at least one form of financial difficulty since the pandemic began (Figure 2.5 – the figure note provides the full list of financial difficulties included). Countries with higher GDP per capita and with higher spending on social programmes show lower levels of financial difficulties in September-October 2020 (OECD, 2021[11]).

Figure 2.5. An average of 31% of respondents in 25 OECD countries have been struggling financially since the outbreak of COVID-19

Share of people reporting at least one financial difficulty since the start of the COVID-19 pandemic, Sept-Oct 2020

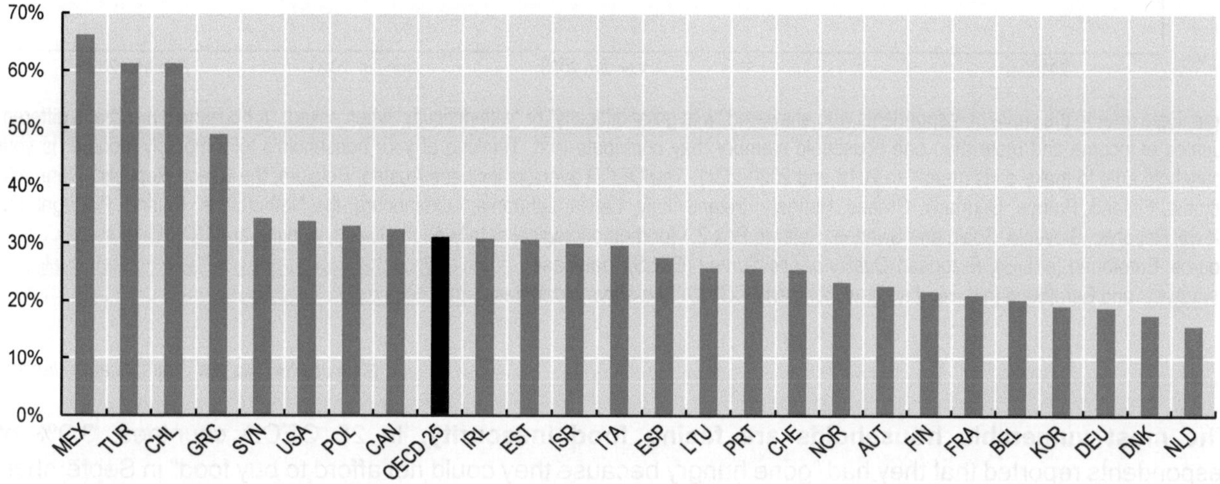

Note: Respondents were asked whether, at any time since the start of the COVID-19 pandemic, they (or their household) had experienced one or more of a range of specific finance-related events: failed to pay a usual expense; took money out of savings or sold assets to pay for a usual expense; took money from family or friends to pay for a usual expense; took on additional debt or used credit to pay for a usual expense; asked a charity or non-profit organisation for assistance because they could not afford to pay; went hungry because they could not afford to pay for food; lost their home because they could not afford the mortgage or rent; or declared bankruptcy or asked a credit provider for help. Respondents could select all the options that applied. The OECD average includes only those 25 countries shown.
Source: OECD (n.d.[12]), *Risks That Matter Survey*, http://oe.cd/RTM.

StatLink https://stat.link/0pxylg

Across 22 European OECD countries the share of households reporting difficulties to make ends meet increased in 2020. Questions on financial difficulty and savings have been included in the Eurofound Living, working and COVID-19 e-survey (see Box 2.1, below). These data indicate that in April-June 2020, just over one-fifth (21%) of people in 22 European OECD countries reported difficulty or great difficulty in making ends meet – a level that was broadly sustained in a second and third round of data collection in June-July 2020 and February-March 2021. These 2020-21 averages are well above the 14.5% level observed by the European Quality of Life Survey in 2016 (Figure 2.6).

Figure 2.6. Across European countries, financial struggles increased as a result of the pandemic

Share of people stating they have difficulty or great difficulty to make ends meet, European Quality of Life Survey (2016) and Living, working and COVID-19 e-survey (2020-21), OECD 22

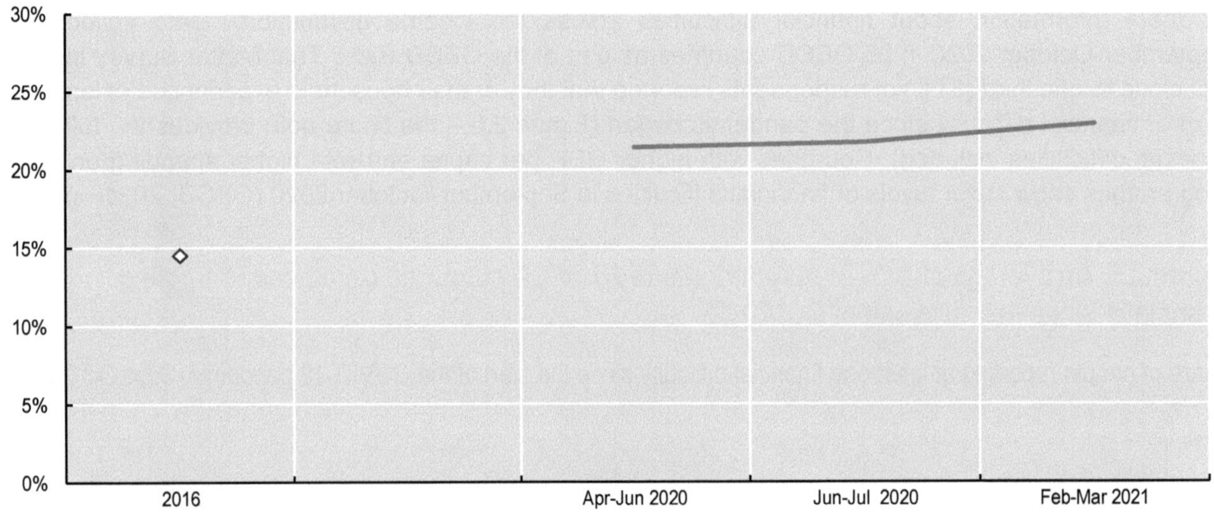

Note: Data refer to the share of respondents who answered "with great difficulty" or "with difficulty" when asked: "A household may have different sources of income and more than one household member may contribute to it. Thinking of your household's total monthly income: is your household able to make ends meet?" in 2016 and 2020-2021. The OECD average includes Austria, Belgium, the Czech Republic, Denmark, Estonia, Finland, France, Germany, Greece, Hungary, Ireland, Italy, Latvia, Lithuania, Luxembourg, the Netherlands, Poland, Portugal, the Slovak Republic, Slovenia, Spain and Sweden. Refer to Box 2.1 for methodological details on the Living, working and COVID-19 survey.
Source: Eurofound (n.d.[13]), *European Quality of Life Survey (EQLS)* (database), https://www.eurofound.europa.eu/data/european-quality-of-life-survey; and Eurofound (n.d.[14]), *Living, working and COVID-19 e-survey* (database), http://eurofound.link/covid19data.

StatLink https://stat.link/enikdy

The most vulnerable households are facing food insecurity. In 25 OECD countries, 3.9% of respondents reported that they had "gone hungry because they could not afford to buy food" in September-October 2020 (OECD, 2021[11]). Data collected in 22 European OECD countries in April-June 2020 indicate a much higher level of food insecurity: 13.6% of respondents reported that they went without fruit and vegetables, and 28.5% that they bought cheaper cuts of meat or bought less than wanted in the previous two weeks because money was needed for other essentials (Eurofound, n.d.[14]). Separate national studies also show worrying figures. A study from the United Kingdom revealed that between August 2020 and January 2021, 4.7 million adults experienced food insecurity (i.e. 9% of all households, compared to 7.6% in 2019). This includes 1.6 million adults who reported having had to go a whole day without eating due to not being able to afford or access food (Goudie and McIntyre, 2021[15]).[3] In Chile, 19.4% of households suffered from moderate/severe food insecurity in July 2020, and 11.5% in November 2020 (Ministerio Desarrollo Social y Familia, n.d.[16]) (Box 5.3).[4] In the United States, 20% of households indicated that they often or sometimes ran out of food before having enough money to buy more between 1 and 8 June 2020, slightly improving from April (23%) and May (22%) (Wozniak et al., 2020[17]) (Box 3.1). In Canada, between 4 and 10 May 2020 one in seven (14.6%) people reported that they lived in a household experiencing some form of food insecurity – ranging from food not lasting before there was money to buy more, to going hungry because there was not enough money for food – in the previous thirty days (Statistics Canada, 2020[18]).[5]

Box 2.1. Methods: The Eurofound Living, working and COVID-19 e-survey

The Eurofound Living, working and COVID-19 e-survey was launched in April 2020. It aims to investigate well-being, work, telework and people's financial situations across the European Union during the crisis.

Fieldwork and sampling

As of June 2021, three rounds of survey fieldwork had been completed: Round 1 from 9 April to 11 June 2020; Round 2 from 22 June 2020 for panel respondents and 25 June 2020 for public respondents, closing for both on 27 July 2020; and Round 3 from 15 February 2021 to 29 March 2021.

The survey was conducted online via the SoSciSurvey platform. It was open to respondents from all countries, but only promoted in the 27 European Union countries. In both Round 1 and Round 2 the recruitment of respondents was carried out via uncontrolled convenience sampling, by publishing the link to the survey on social media and distributing it among Eurofound's contacts and stakeholders, complemented by social media advertising targeting hard-to-reach groups. In Round 2 an additional panel element was introduced: Round 1 collected email addresses from respondents interested in participation in further survey rounds, who then received an invitation to complete Round 2 a few days before the questionnaire was launched to the public.

Cleaning and weighting, effective sample size

The final sample size after cleaning was of 53 918 for Round 1, 19 987 for Round 2 and 38 708 for Round 3. The weighting methodology was the same in all rounds. To produce country level and EU 27 averages, all individual responses were re-weighted to be representative of the demographic of each respondent's country. Data were weighted by age crossed with gender (in 12 age-gender combinations), urbanisation level (2 categories) and education level (2 categories). Weighting targets for each country included 2019 population estimates from Eurostat by age and gender, self-defined urbanisation levels by age and gender as measured in the 4th European Quality of Life Survey, and education levels by age and gender from the 2018 Labour Force Survey.

Source: Eurofound (n.d.[14]), *Living, working and COVID-19 e-survey* (database), http://eurofound.link/covid19data

2.2. Work and Job Quality

The COVID-19 crisis had an impact on both the quantity and quality of jobs. Early government measures aimed at containing the spread of the virus led to the closure of many activities and businesses. The relatively small increase in the unemployment rate in most OECD countries does not fully reflect the extent of the job crisis. As a large number of workers went on job retention schemes or were temporarily laid off, and as people who were out of work stopped actively looking for jobs (meaning that they are no longer counted in official unemployment rates),[6] overall labour underutilisation rates rose sharply across the OECD area. Teleworking reduced the immediate job consequences of physical-distancing measures in some sectors, but in practice it remains restricted to jobs that can be performed remotely – around 25% of all jobs in the EU 28 (Fana, Pérez and al., 2020[19]).

The pandemic's impact on unemployment varied across countries

The pandemic's impact on OECD labour markets has been significant. Between 2019 and 2020, OECD average unemployment rose by 1.7 percentage points (Figure 2.7, Panel A). In particular, following the onset of the crisis, the OECD unemployment rate rose from 5.4% in Q1 2020 to 8.6% in Q2 2020. This surge was largely driven by substantial increases in countries such as the United States and Canada (of 9.3 and 6.7 percentage points respectively), where large numbers of workers on temporary layoff increased unemployment figures (OECD, 2021[20]). Costa Rica, Colombia and Chile also experienced very large increases in unemployment between 2019 and 2020 (respectively of 7.9, 5.6 and 3.6 percentage points). By contrast, elsewhere in the OECD area – particularly in European countries, which made large use of job retention schemes – unemployment rates were relatively steady or even fell slightly in the first months of the pandemic (Figure 2.7, Panel B). The Q2 2020 falls in some European countries such as France and Italy do not generally indicate that labour market conditions improved, but rather that some jobless individuals stopped actively seeking work and therefore no longer met the international definition of unemployment.[7] This is borne out by the very substantial rises in the labour underutilisation rate in the second quarter of 2020 (Figure 2.8). The divergent patterns between the United States, Canada and other G7 countries continued as the pandemic progressed: while in Q3 and Q4 of 2020, unemployment rates were falling in North America, they were rising in Japan, Italy, the United Kingdom and France.

Differences in unemployment rates partly reflect differences in policy responses. Most OECD countries, and particularly those in Europe, relied on job retention schemes, which allow companies to reduce or entirely halt employees' work while keeping them employed with (part of) their salaries covered from government funds (OECD, 2021[20]). By contrast, the United States relied on temporary layoffs and unemployment insurance benefits: many companies released their workers when the crisis hit, often with the intention of hiring them back once economic activity resumed.[8] Although unemployment insurance benefits replaced a portion of earnings for many workers on temporary layoff, many lost their salary and sometimes their health insurance. These factors explain why the unemployment rate rose so much more in the United States and Canada compared to other OECD countries, as well as why it decreased substantially by Q3 2020, as businesses started to reopen and many workers on temporary layoff went back to work (OECD, 2021[20]). There are also differences in how national statistical offices classify people on "temporary layoff" – differences which normally have little impact on the comparability of unemployment statistics, but in times when layoffs affect larger numbers of people, the impact can be larger (OECD, 2021[20]; OECD, 2020[21]).

Job losses due to COVID-19 disproportionally affected vulnerable population groups. Indeed, younger, lower-income, less-educated individuals, as well as women, and people belonging to racial/ ethnic minorities and LGBTQ+ communities, who are over-represented in the industries most exposed to government closures and containment measures (e.g. leisure and hospitality, tourism, retail), were less often able to telework and were most likely to lose their jobs (see Chapter 5 for more information on how COVID-19 impacted labour market outcomes for different population groups).

These impacts also varied strongly across regions and types of employment. The regions most affected by the pandemic were those with a strong focus on tourism, leisure or cultural services, as well as those with many independent, temporary or informal workers, who are also the least likely to be covered by safety nets (OECD, 2021[4]). In particular, self-employed workers registered a 19% decrease in total hours worked between Q2 2019 and Q2 2020, a fall that was 12 percentage points larger than among dependent employees (OECD, 2021[20]). Small-and-medium enterprises (SMEs) are also over-represented in the sectors that have been more impacted by COVID-19. On average across OECD countries, SMEs are estimated to account for 75% of employment in the most affected sectors (see also Box 5.4) (OECD, 2021[4]).

Figure 2.7. The impact of COVID-19 on unemployment has varied across OECD countries

Share of the total labour force who are unemployed

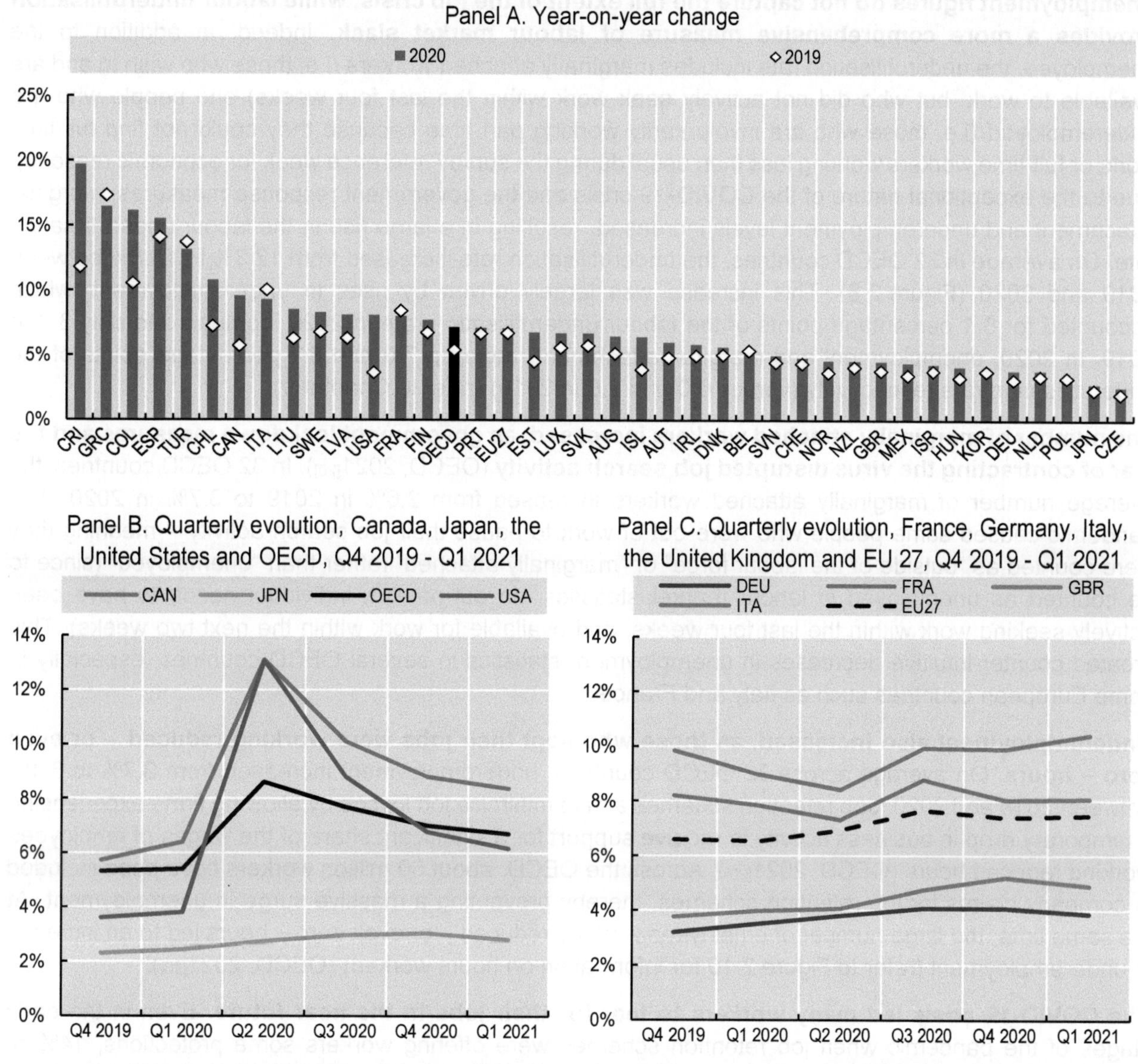

Note: The OECD area unemployment rate is calculated as the total number of unemployed people in all OECD countries as a percentage of the total labour force (i.e. the unemployed plus those in employment); this is equivalent to an average of unemployment rates of all OECD countries weighted by the labour force of each country. Data for Germany in 2020 are provisional and might be subject to low reliability due to technical issues with the introduction of the new German system of integrated household surveys.

Source: OECD (n.d.[5]), *Household Dashboard* (database), www.oecd.org/sdd/na/household-dashboard.htm.

StatLink https://stat.link/ea502y

Unemployment does not fully reflect the extent of the job crisis: labour underutilisation rates increased substantially, and job insecurity levels are high

Unemployment figures do not capture the full extent of the job crisis, while labour underutilisation provides a more comprehensive measure of labour market slack. Indeed, in addition to the unemployed, the underutilisation rate includes marginally attached workers (i.e. those who wish to and are available to work, but who did not actively seek work within the last four weeks) and people who are underemployed (i.e. those who are involuntarily working part-time because they could not find full-time work, or full-time workers working less than usual during the survey reference week for economic reasons). Due to the exceptional nature of the COVID-19 crisis and the government response measures, marginal attachment and underemployment levels increased, resulting in a large rise in the labour underutilisation rate. On average in 32 OECD countries, the underutilisation rate increased from 12.3% to 16.8% between 2019 and 2020 (Figure 2.8). This increase was largely driven by rises in underemployment, which accounted for 6.1 percentage points of the labour underutilisation rate in 2020, compared to only 3.7 in 2019. In 2020, unemployment and marginal attachment made up 7.0 and 3.7 percentage points of the underutilisation rate respectively (versus 6.0 and 2.6 in 2019) (refer to Chapter 9).

The number of marginally attached workers increased, as government lockdown measures and the fear of contracting the virus disrupted job search activity (OECD, 2021[20]). In 32 OECD countries, the average number of marginally attached workers increased from 2.6% in 2019 to 3.7% in 2020. The pandemic caused some people who were out of work to pause their job search activity – meaning they were counted as "outside of the labour force" or "marginally attached" rather than "unemployed" (since to be counted as unemployed in labour market statistics, an out-of-work individual needs to have been actively seeking work within the last four weeks, and available for work within the next two weeks). This created counter-intuitive decreases in unemployment statistics in several OECD countries, especially in some European countries such as Italy and France.

Underemployment also increased, as those who kept their jobs were working reduced – or even zero – hours. On average across 32 OECD countries, underemployment increased from 3.7% to 6.1% between 2019 and 2020. Job retention schemes aim to minimise job losses by allowing firms experiencing a temporary drop in business activity to receive support for a significant share of the wages of employees working reduced hours (OECD, 2021[20]). Across the OECD, about 60 million workers have been included in company claims for job retention schemes, thereby preventing a massive surge in unemployment. At the same time, the large number of employees working reduced – or even zero – hours led to an increase in underemployment (refer to Figure 2.10 for information on hours worked) (OECD, 2021[20]).

The COVID-19 crisis led many workers to fear for their jobs in the near future. Even in the early stages of the pandemic when job retention schemes were offering workers some protections, 14% of employees in 19 European OECD countries felt it was "likely" they would lose their job within three months (Figure 2.9). Feelings of job insecurity may be heightened among those with only temporary employment contracts, a group that represented 10.1% of all employed people of working age (15–64) in the second quarter of 2020 across the same European OECD countries (Eurostat, n.d.[22]). On average, feelings of job insecurity in these European countries improved slightly as the pandemic progressed, falling to 10% by June-July 2020 and to 9% by February-March 2021 (Figure 2.9).

Figure 2.8. Labour underutilisation in the OECD area almost doubled across the first two quarters of 2020

Labour underutilisation rate, as a share of the total labour force

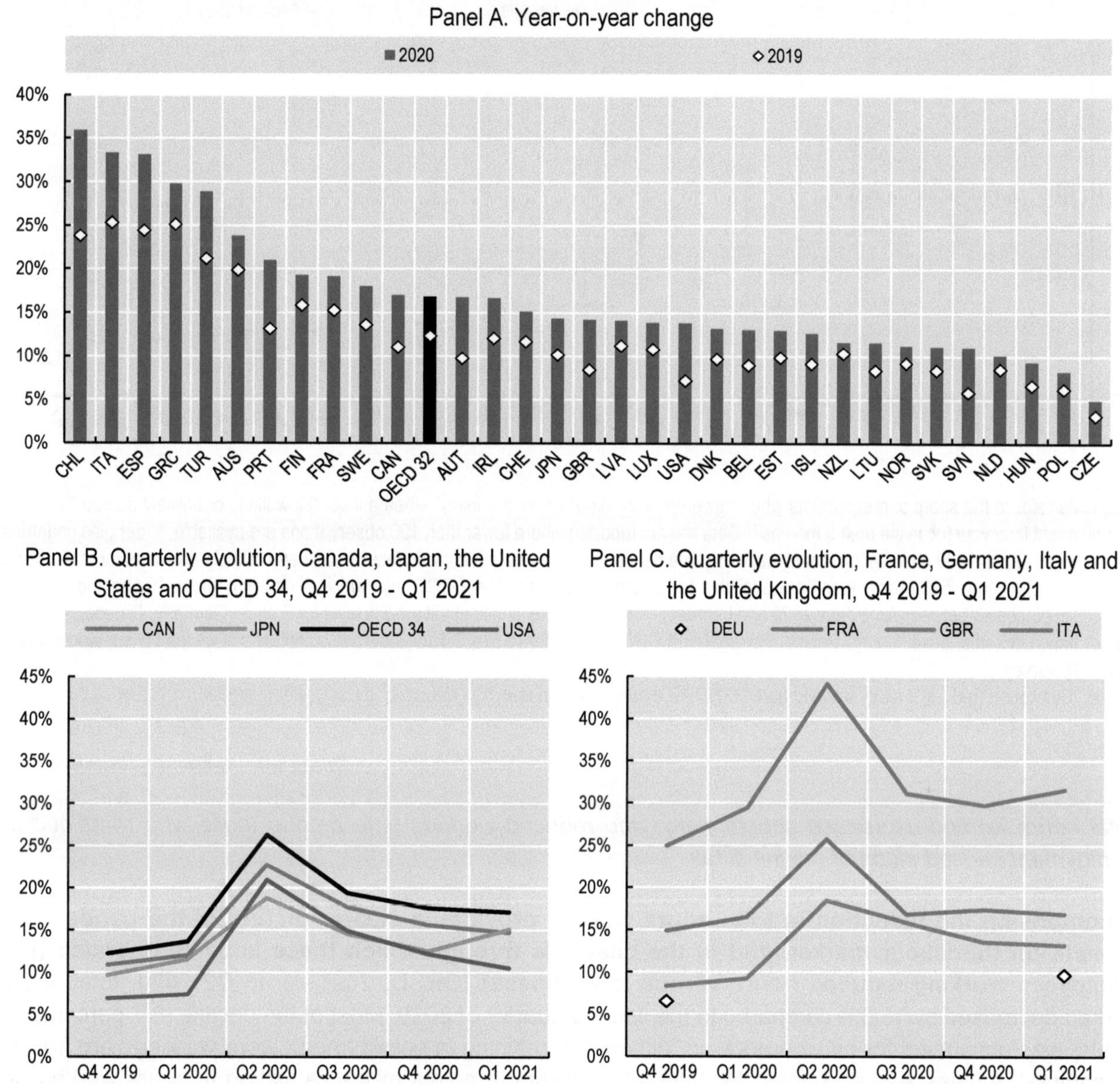

Note: The labour underutilisation rate includes the unemployed, marginally attached workers and the underemployed, expressed as a share of the total labour force. In Panel A, the OECD average excludes Colombia, Costa Rica, Germany, Israel, Korea and Mexico. Data for Germany in 2020 are not available due to the introduction of the new system of integrated household surveys since the beginning of 2020; those for Mexico in 2020 are not shown because of changes in survey collection during the year. In Panel B, the OECD average excludes Colombia, Costa Rica, Israel and Korea. Data for Germany are available only for Q4 2019 and Q1 2021.

Source: OECD (n.d.[5]), *Household Dashboard* (database), www.oecd.org/sdd/na/household-dashboard.htm.

StatLink https://stat.link/4yx5lu

Figure 2.9. In 19 European countries, nearly 1 in 7 workers feared for their jobs in April-June 2020

Share of people who felt "likely" to lose their jobs within three months, Apr-Jun 2020, Jun-Jul 2020, Feb-Mar 2021

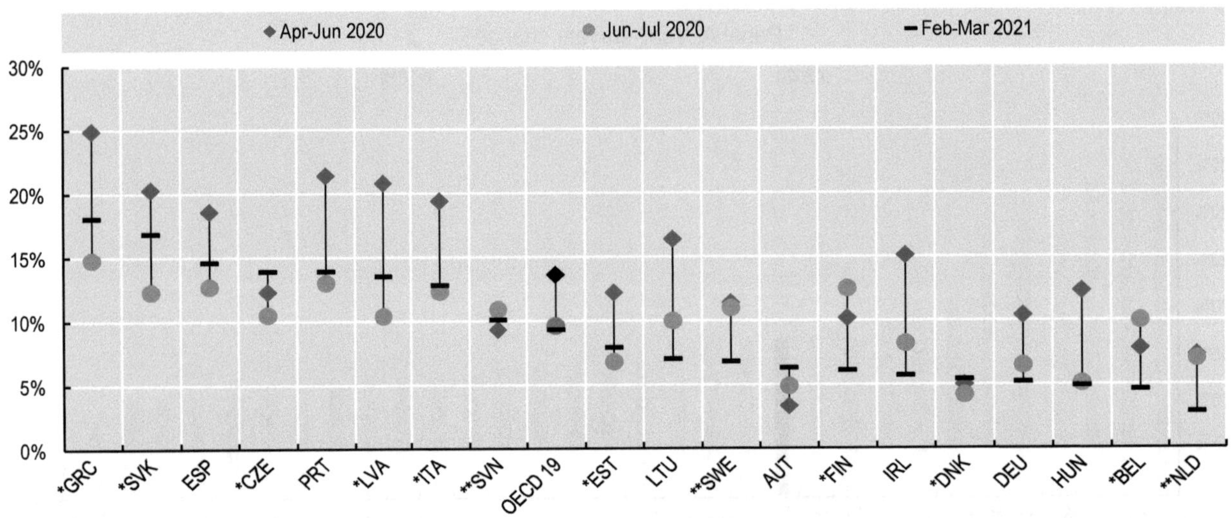

Note: Data refer to the share of respondents who answered "very likely" or "rather likely" when asked: "How likely or unlikely do you think it is that you might lose your job in the next 3 months?" Data are not reported where fewer than 100 observations are available. ** denotes countries with between 100 and 300 observations for at least one time period. * denotes countries with between 301 and 500 observations for at least one time period. More than 500 observations are available for all other countries. The OECD average includes only those 19 countries shown. Changes in outcomes between April-June 2020 and February-March 2021 are significant at the 5% level for France, Germany, Greece, Hungary, Ireland, Italy, Lithuania, Luxembourg, Poland, Portugal and OECD 19. Refer to Box 2.1 for methodological details on the Living, working and COVID-19 survey.
Source: Eurofound (n.d.[14]), *Living, working and COVID-19 e-survey* (database), http://eurofound.link/covid19data.

StatLink https://stat.link/15joi2

Total hours worked decreased substantially, and reduced working time among those who remained in employment caused much of the initial fall

Decomposing the reduction in total hours worked provides a clearer picture of the pandemic's impacts on the labour market, and of the channels through which these impacts operated (i.e. employees working reduced hours versus joblessness) (OECD, 2021[20]). In Q2 2020, total hours worked decreased by 15.3% compared to the second quarter of 2019. Most of the decline (8.7 percentage points) was accounted for by workers who, although remaining in employment, were working zero hours. By contrast, joblessness accounted for only 4.2 percentage points of the reduction in hours worked on average (OECD, 2021[20]). This was largely driven by European countries making extensive use of job retention schemes. In the United States, where many workers were laid off, the majority of unworked hours was channelled through joblessness (Figure 2.10) (OECD, 2021[20]). In the third quarter of 2020, as many employees went back to work after the first lockdown, total hours worked recovered in most OECD countries (just 4.3% below the third quarter of 2019), with joblessness accounting for the majority of the decrease. Nevertheless, in the fourth quarter of 2020, as a new wave of the virus brought further closures, working hours dropped again across the OECD (a 5.6% decrease compared to Q4 2019), with reduced working time once again accounting for the biggest share of this reduction (OECD, 2021[20]).

Figure 2.10. Across the OECD, total hours worked decreased by 15.3% in Q2 2020 year-on-year

Total hours worked, year-on-year percentage change, Q2 2019 - Q2 2020

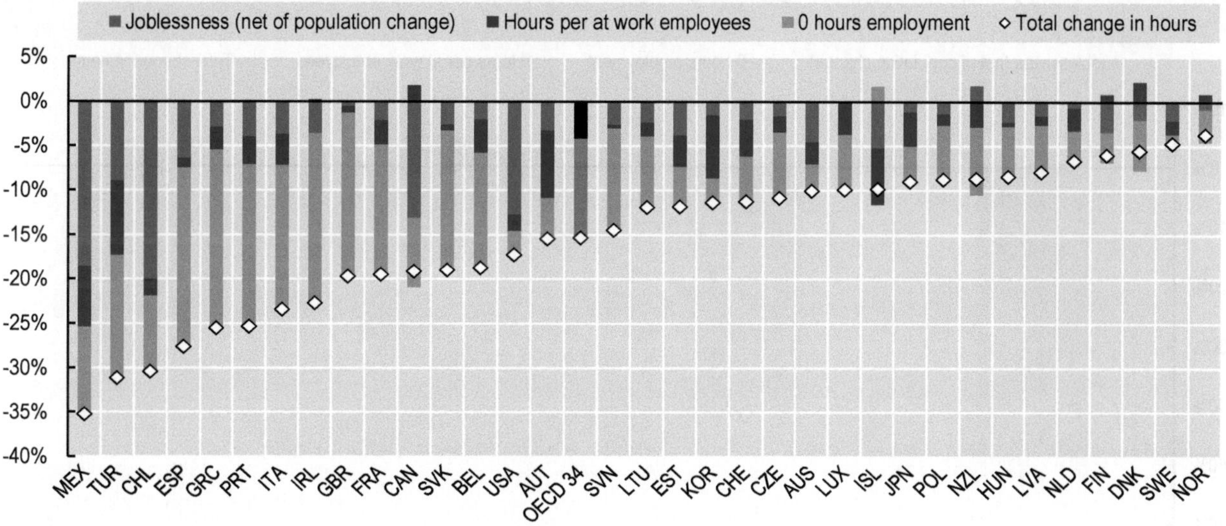

Note: The figure shows the contribution of each category to the change in total hours. The change in hours is decomposed into (a) the change in the average hours worked for at-work employees, (b) the net change in the level of 0-hour employees and (c) the net change in the level of jobless individuals (inactive and unemployed). Positive values for "joblessness" indicate net employment creation. See Annex 1.A in OECD (2021[20]) for details on the decomposition. Time series comparisons for Mexico require caution: in Q2 2020, the National Survey of Occupation and Employment (ENOE) was suspended and replaced with telephone interviews (ETOE) due to the domestic epidemic-related restrictions that were in place at that time in the country. The OECD average excludes Colombia, Costa Rica, Germany and Israel.

Source: OECD (2021[20]), *Employment Outlook 2021: Navigating the COVID-19 Crisis and Recovery,* OECD Publishing, Paris, https://doi.org/10.1787/5a700c4b-en.

StatLink https://stat.link/nbwhcv

Hours decreased the most in sectors such as hospitality, tourism, arts and leisure. For instance, in accommodation and food services, total hours worked more than halved in Q2 2020 compared to a year earlier on average across the OECD. In the arts sector, total hours worked fell by over 42% in Q2 2020 year-on-year (OECD, 2021[20]). By contrast, the financial and insurance activities and the information and communication sectors experienced an increase in hours worked in Q2 2020 compared to the previous year, probably due to the larger number of jobs that can be performed remotely in these sectors (Figure 2.11; see also (OECD, 2021[20]) for further detail).

Meanwhile, there is also evidence that those who could telework are working longer hours, on average. While the available data suggest that people whose work can be performed remotely were less likely to lose their jobs (Box 2.2), they have been working longer hours, on average, in many countries across Europe and North America (DeFilippis et al., 2020[23]). In June-July 2020, employees working exclusively from home in the EU 27 were most likely to report that their number of hours worked had increased, or increased a lot (Eurofound, 2020[24]). Similarly, in the United States in October 2020, 33% of those working entirely from home said they worked longer hours than before the pandemic, compared to 21% of those whose work cannot be done from home (Parker, Menasce Horowitz and Minkin, 2020[25]).

Figure 2.11. Working hours decreased the most in the accommodation and food services and arts sectors

Total hours worked, year-on-year percentage change, OECD 29, Q2 2019 - Q2 2020

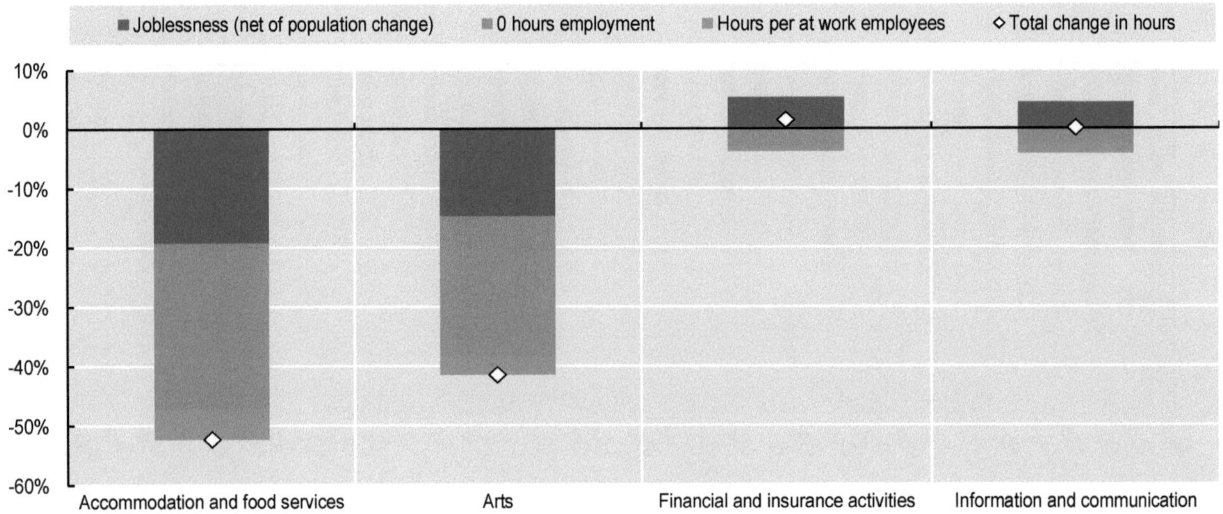

Note: The figure shows the contribution of each category to the change in total hours. The change in hours is decomposed into (a) the change in the average hours worked for at-work employees, (b) the net change in the level of 0-hour employees and (c) the net change in the level of jobless individuals (inactive and unemployed). Positive values for "joblessness" indicate net employment creation. See Annex 1.A in OECD (2021[20]) for further details on the decomposition. The OECD average excludes Australia, Canada, Colombia, Costa Rica, Germany, Iceland, Israel, Korea and New Zealand.
Source: OECD (2021[20]), *Employment Outlook 2021: Navigating the COVID-19 Crisis and Recovery,* OECD Publishing, Paris, https://doi.org/10.1787/5a700c4b-en.

StatLink https://stat.link/6wvkc0

Box 2.2. The relationship between teleworking opportunities and change in employment in the United States

A study from the US Bureau of Labor Statistics relied on employment estimates from the Current Population Survey (CPS, see Box 2.3) to assess how the possibility to telework acted as a protective factor for employment during the pandemic. Overall, from February to April 2020 employment in the United States decreased by 15.6%. In all industries, the drop in employment in occupations in which telework is not feasible (21.2%) was considerably larger than in occupations where telework is feasible (7.9%). Over the same time period, unemployment increased by 14.3 percentage points in occupations in which telework is not feasible, but only by 6.2 percentage points in occupations in which telework is feasible (with overall unemployment rising by 10.8 percentage points). This points to a strong relationship between employment loss and teleworking possibilities: in every industry except agriculture, workers in occupations in which telework is feasible experienced a smaller percentage decline in employment. The difference is particularly large in the information sector and the services industry, where employment fell by 37.3% and 35.9%, respectively, in occupations in which telework is not feasible, but by only 2.1% and 8.4% in occupations in which telework is feasible (Table 2.1).

Table 2.1. In the United States occupations where teleworking is possible registered a smaller decrease in employment

Difference in employment between occupations able to telework and those not able to telework, by employment sector, Feb-Apr 2020

Industry	Percentage of employed able to telework (Apr 2020)	Labour market outcomes		Percentage change in employment rate (Feb-Apr 2020)			Percentage point change in unemployment rate (Feb-Apr 2020)		
		Percentage change in employment rate (Feb-Apr 2020)	Percentage point change in unemployment rate (Feb-Apr 2020)	Able to telework	Not able to telework	Difference	Able to telework	Not able to telework	Difference
Financial activities	81.1	-6.1	3.7	-5.8	-7.2	1.4	2.8	7.2	-4.4
Information	80.4	-11.8	9.3	-2.1	-37.3	35.2	5.8	21.1	-15.3
Professional and business services	71.6	-9.6	5.5	-6.4	-16.8	10.4	3.5	10.0	-6.5
Public administration	57.0	-3.8	3.4	-1.5	-6.7	5.1	3.2	3.8	-0.6
Education and health services	47.9	-13.9	9.4	-12.5	-15.2	2.8	8.8	9.9	-1.1
Manufacturing	41.0	-13.7	9.2	-3.9	-19.5	15.5	4.3	12.3	-8.0
Mining, quarrying, and oil and gas extraction	40.3	-14.9	4.2	5.5	-24.8	30.3	4.2	5.1	-0.8
Other services	39.9	-27.2	19.4	-8.4	-35.9	27.5	10.6	24.3	-13.6
Transportation and utilities	32.7	-10.9	8.7	4.7	-16.9	21.6	4.9	10.4	-5.5
Wholesale and retail trade	26.5	-16.4	12.6	-9.4	-18.6	9.2	7.6	14.2	-6.6
Construction	20.7	-16.6	10.2	-11.9	-17.8	5.8	5.1	11.3	-6.2
Leisure and Hospitality	20.3	-42.0	32.1	-25.5	-45.1	19.6	22.9	34.1	-11.2
Agriculture, forestry, fishing and hunting	8.1	-1.2	-1.7	-4.3	-1.0	-3.3	-5.9	-1.3	-4.5
Total	45.8	-15.6	10.8	-7.9	-21.2	13.3	6.2	14.3	-8.1

Note: Calculations based on Feb-Apr 2020 Current Population Survey (CPS) data and O*NET job-content data.
Source: Dey et al. (2020[26]), *Ability to work from home: Evidence from two surveys and implications for the labor market in the COVID-19 pandemic*, US Bureau of Labor Statistics, https://www.bls.gov/opub/mlr/2020/article/ability-to-work-from-home.htm.

On average, earnings increased slightly in 2020, with large cross-country differences

Across the OECD area, average annual wages increased by 0.5% between 2019 and 2020. The pandemic's impact on wages varied however across countries, ranging from a 7.1% increase in Lithuania to a 9.6% decline in Chile (Figure 2.12). One reason for higher average wages is the change in the composition of employment. Indeed, during the COVID-19 crisis, low-paid workers were more likely to become unemployed (refer to Chapter 5), so average wages reflect the wages of higher-paid workers who experienced fewer job losses (ILO, 2020[27]). This composition effect was most powerful in countries with a high number of temporary layoffs, such as the United States. By contrast, in other countries, including European countries, where unemployment did not increase as much owing to job retention schemes, average wages remained relatively steady or declined, as working time was reduced or the nominal wages of workers were frozen or reduced (ILO, 2020[27]). Eurostat estimates show that, in EU 27 countries, losses in employment income were almost halved by government compensation schemes (Eurostat, 2020[28]).

It is estimated that, in the EU 27, the loss in labour income between 2019 and 2020 was particularly strong for some sectors and vulnerable population groups, such as low-income and young workers. The food and accommodation sector was hit the hardest, registering losses of almost 20% in labour income (Eurostat, 2020[28]). Meanwhile, labour income losses for workers in the bottom income quintile were estimated to be four times higher than those for earners in the top income quintile in the EU 27 (see Chapter 5) (Eurostat, 2021[9]).

Figure 2.12. Average annual wages increased marginally in 2020, but trends diverged strongly across OECD countries

Average annual wages, USD at 2020 PPPs, year-on-year percentage change, 2019-20

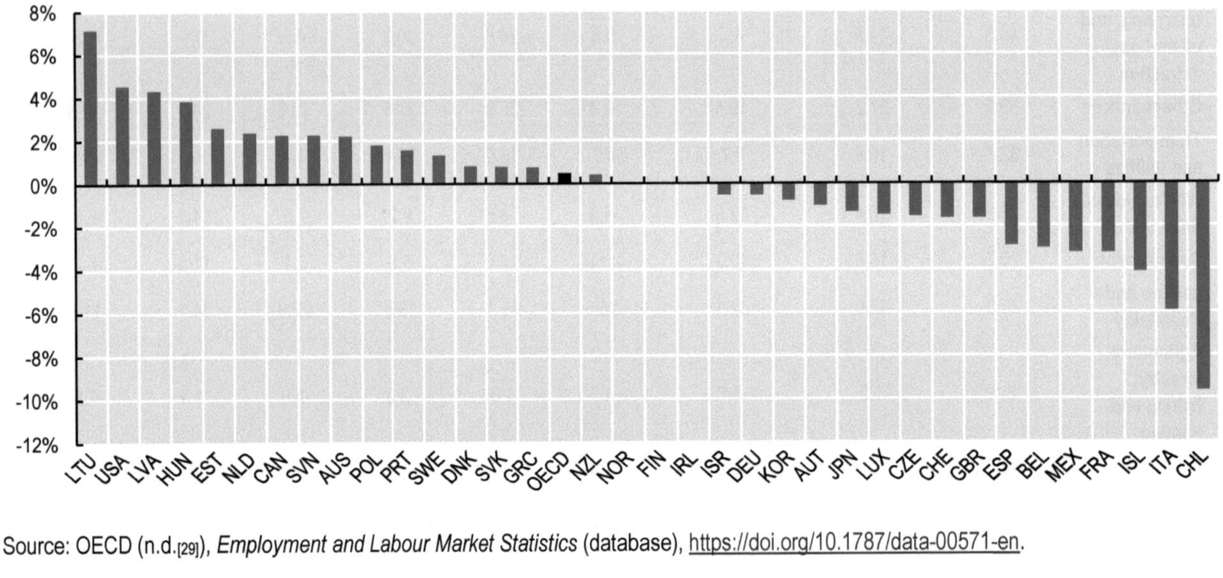

Source: OECD (n.d.[29]), *Employment and Labour Market Statistics* (database), https://doi.org/10.1787/data-00571-en.

StatLink https://stat.link/maurxf

Teleworking has become the normal way of working for around one-third of all employees, but not all jobs can be done remotely

With the closure of many workplaces as the pandemic hit, many companies and employees transitioned to working from home. In April-June 2020, survey data suggest that 39% of employees in 21 European OECD countries started teleworking as a result of COVID-19 (Figure 2.13) (Eurofound, n.d.[14]). In four countries (Finland, Luxembourg, Belgium and the Netherlands) the share was above 50%. Separate data from the United Kingdom Office for National Statistics indicate that 47% of people did some work from home in April-May 2020, 86% of whom did so as a result of the pandemic (see Box 2.3) (ONS, 2020[30]). In the United States, according to the Bureau of Labor Statistics, 35% of employees worked from home in May, and 31% in June (see also Box 2.3) (BLS, n.d.[31]).

A sizeable portion of employees also worked from home in June-July 2020 and February-March 2021. A second Eurofound survey wave conducted in June-July 2020 asked where respondents worked during the pandemic, with 46% saying that they worked from home across 22 European OECD countries. In February-March 2021, the share of respondents reporting this decreased to 41% (Eurofound, n.d.[14]).[9] Reflecting the changing nature of government restrictions, the share of people working exclusively from home decreased in the United Kingdom from a peak of 38% in June to 24% in July 2020 but then rebounded to 47% in early February 2021 (ONS, 2020[32]; Shine, 2021[33]). In the United States, the share of people working from home fell to 26% in July 2020, and continued decreasing to 23% in February and 17% in May 2021 (BLS, n.d.[31]). In Canada, a study by Statistics Canada indicates that, at the beginning of 2021, 32% of employees aged 15 to 69 worked most of their hours from home, compared to only 4% in 2016 (Mehdi and Morissette, 2021[34]). The figures presented above could, however, overestimate the share of people who teleworked during the pandemic. Data from the 2020 European Union Labour Force Survey indicate that, on average across five European OECD countries, 18.9% of employees worked from home (OECD, 2021[20]).[10]

Figure 2.13. Over a third of workers in 21 European OECD countries began working from home due to COVID-19

Share of respondents who started to work from home as a result of the COVID-19 crisis, Apr-Jun 2020

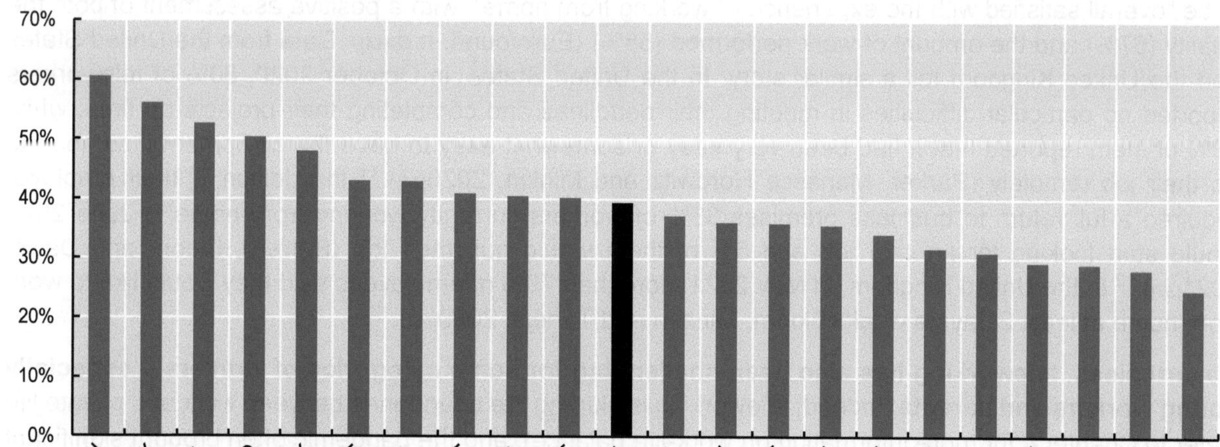

Note: Data refer to people who answered "yes" when asked: "Have you started to work from home as a result of the COVID-19 situation?" Data are not reported where fewer than 100 observations are available. * denotes countries with between 301 and 500 observations. More than 500 observations are available for all other countries. The OECD average includes only those 21 countries shown. Refer to Box 2.1 for methodological details on the Living, working and COVID-19 survey.

Source: Eurofound (n.d.[14]), *Living, working and COVID-19 e-survey* (database), http://eurofound.link/covid19data.

StatLink https://stat.link/ex5s1q

The shift to teleworking was not equally possible within and across countries. Indeed, teleworking has been restricted to employees working in jobs that could be performed remotely, mainly in sectors such as education, most of public administration, finance, insurance and telecommunications (Fana, Pérez and al., 2020[19]). It is estimated that, in the EU 28, only 25% of jobs are "teleworkable" (refer to Chapter 5 for more information on teleworking opportunities for different population groups) (Fana, Pérez and al., 2020[19]). In addition, the propo rtion of jobs with tasks amenable to remote working appears to be much higher in cities and capital regions than elsewhere. Compared to rural areas, the share of jobs amenable to remote working in cities is 13 percentage points higher (OECD, 2020[35]).

At the national level, several factors explain the different take-up of telework. For instance, prior teleworking experience supported the transition to working from home in countries such as the Netherlands, Sweden and Finland, where over 30% of employees worked from home at least sometimes in 2019 – well above the 10% share observed in over half of EU member states. Other explanatory factors include differences in countries' industrial structures (e.g. in 2019 and during the pandemic, telework was more common in countries with more employees in knowledge- and ICT-intensive services, such as Denmark, Sweden and Finland); the distribution of employment by firm size (e.g. in Sweden and Finland, firms with more than 50 employees account for a larger share of total employment in knowledge-intensive business services, where the prevalence of teleworking before the pandemic was more common); and workers' digital skills (e.g. workers with low or no digital skills number just 10% in the Netherlands, compared to an average of 20% in the EU 27) (JRC, 2020[36]). Access to teleworking is also affected by countries' regulations and firms' management cultures. Prior to the COVID-19 crisis, teleworking was higher in countries where workers had an enforceable right to request teleworking (e.g. the Netherlands, the United Kingdom), and highest in countries where this right was granted through collective bargaining (e.g. Denmark, Sweden) (see Chapter 5 in (OECD, 2021[20])).

A large share of employees wish to continue working from home. Between June 2020 and March 2021, almost half of all employed people in 22 European OECD countries (46%) would like to work from home at least several times a week after COVID-19 subsides; 15% of them would like to do so daily (Eurofound, n.d.[14]). In June-July 2020, most workers (60%) across 22 European OECD countries reported to be "overall satisfied with the experience of working from home", with a positive assessment of both the quality (67%) and the amount of work performed (55%) (Eurofound, n.d.[14]). Data from the United States and the United Kingdom tell a similar story. In the United States, in October 2020, 80% of teleworkers reported no particular difficulties in meeting their deadlines and completing their projects on time, while 86% of them reported that it had been very easy or somewhat easy to have the equipment they need to do their job remotely (Parker, Menasce Horowitz and Minkin, 2020[25]).[11] In addition, if their employer required a full return to business premises 36% of workers currently working from home in June 2021 would start looking for another job and 6% of them would quit their job (Barrero, Bloom and Davis, 2021[37]).[12] In the United Kingdom, in May 2021 more than 70% of employees said they would like to work from home at least 2 days a week (Bloom, Minzen and Taneja, 2020[38]).[13]

Nevertheless, teleworking has also been challenging for some categories of workers – especially young workers and parents. Indeed, teleworking is blurring the boundaries between work and private life (refer to Chapter 4 for more information on work-life balance), and the pandemic often brought significant new burdens for those with caring responsibilities (e.g. due to school or nursery closures, or the need to provide additional support to people who were shielding from the virus), which had to be juggled alongside teleworking duties. In addition, some workers, including teleworkers, have been feeling unmotivated and unsatisfied, as well as isolated and stressed (see Box 5.5 for more information on COVID-19 and teleworking).

Box 2.3. Innovation: Adapting data collections to capture labour market outcomes during the crisis

United Kingdom: Office for National Statistics' Online Labour Market Survey

As part of a wider response to the COVID-19 pandemic, the Office for National Statistics (ONS) has explored new ways to measure changes in the labour market, including through more rapid access to government data sources and the introduction of new online surveys. At the end of March 2020, the ONS launched the Online Labour Market Survey (LMS). The LMS has a mixed-mode design, online and face-to-face (but online by default). The current LMS design is still a prototype in development. The survey includes around 18 000 households per quarter. Respondents are asked questions on employment, unemployment and economic inactivity relating to a reference week one to two weeks prior to the interview. In addition, respondents are also asked if they did any work at home, and if their main reason for doing this was the COVID-19 pandemic. The LMS is based on random sample of households (addresses) drawn from the Postcode Address File. The geographical ordering of the frame implicitly stratifies the sample, ensuring a geographic spread of addresses. The quarterly sample is computed across 13 weeks, with each week containing a representative proportion of addresses, for each nation within the United Kingdom, as well as for large English regions.

According to the LMS, in April 2020, 47% of people in employment did some work at home, 86% of whom did so as a result of the COVID-19 pandemic. Working from home resulted in a reduction of hours worked for 34% of respondents, while 30% of them reported working more hours than usual. Women were slightly more likely than men to do some work at home (48% and 46% respectively), and young people (aged 16 to 24) were less likely to telework than older age groups. Homeworking was more frequent among occupations requiring higher educational attainment (such as managers, directors, senior officials) and more professional experience, relative to elementary or manual occupations (such as sales and customer service occupations). Lastly, white and ethnic minority groups had around the same proportion of people doing some work from home.

United States: Bureau of Labor Statistics Current Population Survey

The Bureau of Labor Statistics (BLS) added questions to the Current Population Survey (CPS) to help gauge the effects of the COVID-19 pandemic on the labour market. These questions were launched in May 2020 and will remain in the CPS until further notice. The CPS is a monthly sample survey of 60 000 eligible households conducted using a combination of live telephone and in-person interviews with household respondents. The newly added questions ask whether people teleworked or worked from home because of the pandemic; whether people were unable to work because their employers closed or lost business due to the pandemic; whether they were paid for that missed work; and whether the pandemic prevented job-seeking activities. All of these supplemental questions refer to activities preformed at any time during the "last 4 weeks" and follow the monthly labour force questions.

In June 2020, 31% of workers teleworked due to COVID-19, down from 35% in May. Women, workers over 25, full-time workers, and workers with higher educational attainment were more likely to have teleworked due to the COVID-19 pandemic. Workers in educational services, finance and insurance, or professional and technical services were more likely to work from home than workers employed in the accommodation and food services or in agriculture.

In addition, in June 2020, 16% of the civilian non-institutional population said that they had been unable to work at some point in the previous 4 weeks because their employer closed or lost business due to COVID-19 – that is, they did not work at all or worked fewer hours. Part-time workers were twice as likely as full-time workers to report not being able to work at some point in the previous 4 weeks due to the pandemic. Among those unable to work at some point in the last 4 weeks because of pandemic-related closures or lost business, 15% received at least some pay from their employer for the hours not worked. Those who usually work part-time were about half as likely as full-time workers to report being paid by their employer for the hours they did not work. People employed in personal care and service occupations were the least likely to be paid by their employer for the hours they missed (9% in June). Those employed in education, training or library occupations were the most likely to be paid (54%) by their employer.

Sources: ONS (2020[30]), *Coronavirus and homeworking in the UK: April 2020*, Office for National Statistics, https://www.ons.gov.uk/employmentandlabourmarket/peopleinwork/employmentandemployeetypes/bulletins/coronavirusandhomeworkingintheuk/latest and BLS (n.d.[31]), *Supplemental data measuring the effects of the coronavirus (COVID-19) pandemic on the labor market*, US Bureau of Labor Statistics, https://www.bls.gov/cps/effects-of-the-coronavirus-covid-19-pandemic.htm

2.3. Housing

Housing conditions play an important role in people's experience of COVID-19. While only limited data are available on housing conditions in 2020, pre-pandemic data highlight a number of risks and challenges in this area. Overcrowding and poor access to sanitation make it harder for vulnerable households to stay safe and contain the spread of the virus. A lack of electronic devices and/or home Internet access exclude people from teleworking and homeschooling as well as from receiving essential services and supports virtually (i.e. mental health services, services for students with disabilities, etc.). Poorer households are also more likely to be overburdened by increasing housing costs. Over the course of the pandemic, governments across the OECD enacted a number of housing measures to support households at risk (see, for example (OECD, n.d.[39]; OECD, 2021[40]).

Poor housing conditions put people's well-being at greater risk…

People living in poor housing conditions are more vulnerable to the physical and mental health effects of COVID-19. Pre-pandemic data indicate that 10.6% of households, on average, live in crowded conditions in OECD countries with this share exceeding 30% in Latvia and Mexico (Figure 2.14) (OECD, n.d.[39]). People living in overcrowded housing are at greater risk of infection, since it is harder to isolate symptomatic individuals and the same basic facilities are being shared by a large number of people. During lockdown periods, both people in overcrowded housing and people living alone face elevated risks to mental health. In addition, lack of access to basic sanitation (i.e. an indoor flushing toilet for the sole use of the household) – which is still an issue for 6.2% of poor households across OECD countries – makes it harder to contain the spread of COVID-19 between households living in close proximity (OECD, n.d.[39]).

Homeless people face huge difficulties in protecting themselves from the virus. They have no means of self-isolating, and where they do have shelter available it is typically in hostels with limited means of isolation or protection for at-risk individuals (such as those with existing health conditions). For example, data from the Australian Bureau of Statistics indicate that 44% of those considered "homeless" were living in severely crowded dwellings in 2016 (ABS, 2018[41]).[14] While country comparisons are challenging due to different definitions and methods of data collection, it is estimated that around 2.1 million people are homeless across OECD countries for which data are available (OECD, n.d.[39]).

Lack of Internet access or electronic devices is a challenge for the most vulnerable households. COVID-19 has accelerated the digital transition, making connectivity (both in terms of quantity and quality) even more critical. Individuals who do not have a sufficient number of computers or access to high-speed Internet at home could not telework, home-school, video-call friends and relatives, or reach remote services such as medical consultations or community support (e.g. delivery of groceries and medicines).

Across 33 OECD countries, 87.4% of households had access to the Internet at home in 2019, but this share is less than 60% in Colombia and Mexico (OECD, n.d.[42]). Even where Internet access is available, variable connection quality can still pose challenges to efficient and effective teleworking, remote schooling, etc. (refer to Chapter 5 for more information on digital divides).

Figure 2.14. Over one third of households in Mexico and Latvia live in overcrowded conditions

Share of households living in overcrowded conditions, 2019 or latest available year

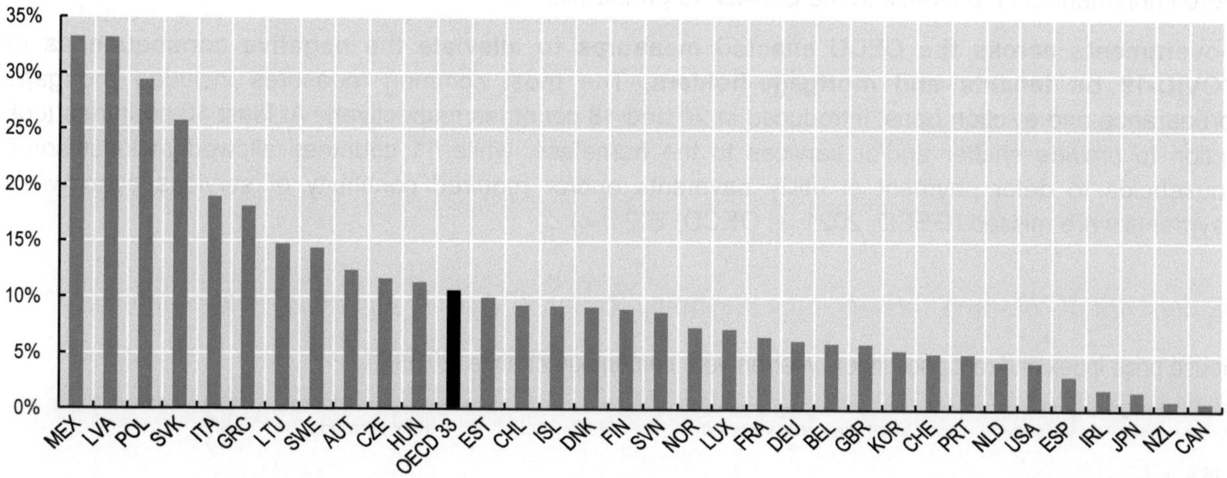

Note: A household is considered overcrowded if it does not have at its disposal a minimum number of rooms equal to: one room for the household; one room per adult couple in the household; one room for each single person aged 18 or over; one room per pair of single persons of the same sex between 12 and 17 years of age; one room for each single person between 12 and 17 years of age and not included in the previous category; and one room per pair of children under 12 years of age. The OECD average excludes Australia, Colombia, Costa Rica, Israel and Turkey, due to a lack of data. The latest available year is 2018 for Iceland, Ireland, Italy, Japan, Mexico, New Zealand and the United Kingdom, 2016 for Canada, 2014 for Germany and 2013 for Chile.
Source: OECD (n.d.[39]), *Affordable Housing* (database), https://www.oecd.org/housing/data/affordable-housing-database/; Statistics Korea, who provided data for Korea; and Statistics New Zealand, who provided data for New Zealand.

StatLink https://stat.link/cv6ug4

… and rising house and rent prices may threaten vulnerable households' finances

Reduced earnings and working hours threaten people's ability to meet housing costs. Workers who have lost their jobs, are temporarily laid off, or are working reduced hours for reduced pay may struggle to cover their monthly rent, mortgage or utilities payments. This is especially true for those households that are already overburdened by housing costs (OECD, 2021[40]). On average across OECD countries, 27.2% of the population in the bottom income quintile spent more than 40% of their disposable income on housing (i.e. rent and mortgage costs) before the COVID-19 crisis.

During the pandemic, many struggled to pay housing expenses. In April-June 2020, 10% of people in 22 European OECD countries reported being in arrears for their utility bills, a share that rose to 12% in February-March 2021 (Eurofound, n.d.[14]). In the same countries, 8% of people were in arrears for their rent/mortgage payments in both April-June 2020 and in February-March 2021 (Eurofound, n.d.[14]). In the United States, as of 16-21 July 2020, 12.5% of respondents were experiencing housing distress – i.e. they were late on their rent or mortgage payments, or their payments were deferred. Housing hardship in the United States was most common among families that identify as Black or Hispanic/Latino; those who lack a four-year college degree and renters (US Census Bureau, n.d.[43]).

A general rise in house and rent prices is worsening housing affordability, especially for poorer households. In 2018, housing costs accounted for around 20% of household disposable income in 34 OECD countries (OECD, 2020[10]). In a vast majority of OECD countries, house prices have been growing faster than general inflation since 2012, and data show that this continued to be the case in 2020 during the pandemic. On average, house prices rose by 4.7% from 2019 to 2020 across the OECD area. Prior to the COVID-19 crisis, rent prices had been systematically increasing in all but two OECD countries. Between 2019 and 2020, rental prices grew to a lesser extent than house prices, but still increased by 1.8% (Figure 2.15). This may reflect caps on rent prices and other artificial rent suppression measures that were implemented in response to the COVID-19 pandemic.

Governments across the OECD enacted measures to alleviate the negative consequences of COVID-19 on tenants and mortgage-holders. The most common measures included mortgage forbearance and eviction bans, introduced in 20 and 18 countries respectively. At least 10 countries took action to provide shelter and/or services to the homeless, while 11 countries allowed at least some households to defer payment of utility payments and/or required continuity of services even when payments were missed (OECD, 2021[40]; OECD, 2021[44]).

Figure 2.15. COVID-19 is threatening households' financial stability and housing affordability

House price index and rent price index, year-on-year percentage change, 2019-20

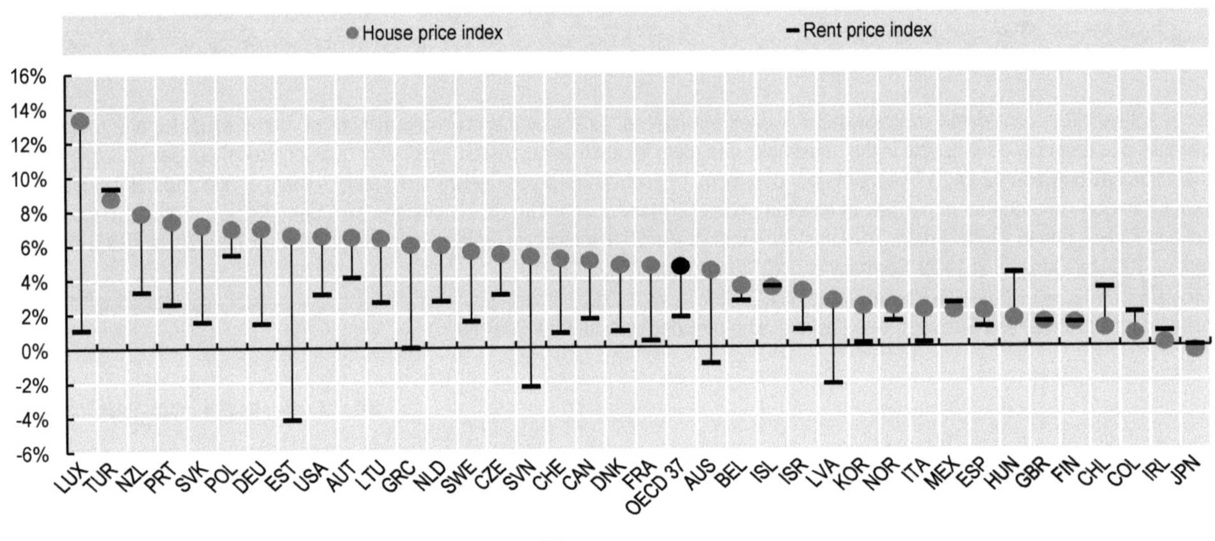

Note: The OECD average excludes Costa Rica, due to a lack of data.
Source: OECD (n.d.[45]), *Main Economic Indicators* (database), https://doi.org/10.1787/cbcc2905-en.

StatLink https://stat.link/i5elu6

Box 2.4. Further reading

- OECD (2020), *OECD Economic Outlook,* Volume 2020 Issue 2, OECD Publishing, Paris, https://dx.doi.org/10.1787/39a88ab1-en
- OECD (2020), *OECD Employment Outlook 2020: Worker Security and the COVID-19 Crisis*, OECD Publishing, Paris, https://doi.org/10.1787/1686c758-en
- OECD (2020), *Housing Amid Covid-19: Policy Responses and Challenges*, OECD Publishing, Paris, https://doi.org/10.1787/cfdc08a8-en
- OECD (2021), *Building for a better tomorrow: Policies to make housing more affordable*, *Employment, Labour and Social Affairs Policy Briefs*, OECD Publishing, Paris, http://oe.cd/affordable-housing-2021
- OECD (2021), *Brick by Brick: Building Better Housing Policies,* OECD Publishing, Paris, https://doi.org/10.1787/b453b043-en
- OECD (no date), *Affordable Housing database*, www.oecd.org/social/affordable-housing-database.htm
- OECD (2021), *OECD Employment Outlook 2021: Navigating the COVID-19 crisis and recovery,* OECD Publishing, Paris, https://doi.org/10.1787/5a700c4b-en

References

ABS (2018), *Census of Population and Housing: Estimating homelessness*, Australian Bureau of Statistics, https://www.abs.gov.au/statistics/people/housing/census-population-and-housing-estimating-homelessness. [41]

Barrero, J., N. Bloom and S. Davis (2021), *Let me work from home, or I will find another job*, VOX.org CEPR Policy Portal, https://voxeu.org/article/let-me-work-home-or-i-will-find-another-job. [37]

Beck, K. et al. (2020), *Experimental estimates of family weekly income for January to September 2020*, Statistics Canada, https://www150.statcan.gc.ca/n1/pub/75f0002m/75f0002m2020004-eng.htm. [2]

Bloom, N., P. Minzen and S. Taneja (2020), *Returning to the office will be hard*, VOX.org CEPR Policy Portal, https://voxeu.org/article/returning-office-will-be-hard. [38]

BLS (n.d.), *Supplemental data measuring the effects of the coronavirus (COVID-19) pandemic on the labor market*, US Bureau of Labor Statistics, https://www.bls.gov/cps/effects-of-the-coronavirus-covid-19-pandemic.htm (accessed on 10 May 2021). [31]

Clark, A., C. D'Ambrosio and A. Lepinteur (2021), *The fall in income inequality during COVID-19 in five European countries*, Society for the Study of Economic Inequality, http://www.ecineq.org/milano/WP/ECINEQ2020-565.pdf. [6]

DeFilippis, E. et al. (2020), *Collaborating during Coronavirus: The impact of COVID-19 on the nature of work*, National Bureau of Economic Research, https://www.nber.org/system/files/working_papers/w27612/w27612.pdf. [23]

Dey, M. et al. (2020), *Ability to work from home: Evidence from two surveys and implications for the labor market in the COVID-19 pandemic*, US Bureau of Labor Statistics, https://www.bls.gov/opub/mlr/2020/article/ability-to-work-from-home.htm (accessed on 23 May 2021). [26]

Eurofound (2020), *Living, working, and COVID-19*, COVID-19 series, Publications Office of the European Union, Luxembourg, https://www.eurofound.europa.eu/sites/default/files/ef_publication/field_ef_document/ef20059en.pdf. [24]

Eurofound (n.d.), *European Quality of Life Survey (EQLS) 2016*, https://www.eurofound.europa.eu/publications/report/2017/fourth-european-quality-of-life-survey-overview-report (accessed on 31 January 2021). [13]

Eurofound (n.d.), *Living, working and COVID-19 database*, https://www.eurofound.europa.eu/data/covid-19 (accessed on 13 August 2021). [14]

Eurostat (2021), *Early estimates of income inequalities during the 2020 pandemic*, https://ec.europa.eu/eurostat/statistics-explained/index.php?title=Early_estimates_of_income_inequalities_during_the_2020_pandemic (accessed on 13 August 2021). [9]

Eurostat (2020), *Impact of COVID-19 on employment income - advanced estimates*, https://ec.europa.eu/eurostat/statistics-explained/index.php?title=Impact_of_COVID-19_on_employment_income_-_advanced_estimates#A_sharp_decrease_in_the_median_employment_income. [28]

Eurostat (n.d.), *Temporary employees as a percentage of the total number of employees, by sex and age*, https://ec.europa.eu/eurostat/databrowser/view/LFSQ_ETPGA$DEFAULTVIEW/default/table (accessed on 15 February 2020). [22]

Fana, M., T. Pérez and E. al. (2020), *The COVID confinement measures and EU labour markets*, Joint Research Center (European Commission), Publications Office of the European Union, Luxembourg, https://publications.jrc.ec.europa.eu/repository/handle/JRC120578. [19]

Goudie, S. and Z. McIntyre (2021), *A crisis within a crisis: The impact of COVID-19 on household food security*, Food Foundation, https://foodfoundation.org.uk/wp-content/uploads/2021/03/FF_Impact-of-Covid_FINAL.pdf. [15]

Government of Canada (2021), *Canada Emergency Response Benefit and EI statistics*, https://www.canada.ca/en/services/benefits/ei/claims-report.html (accessed on 15 June 2021). [1]

Grabka, M. (2021), *Income inequality in Germany stagnating over the long term, but decreasing slightly during the coronavirus pandemic*, DIW, Berlin, https://www.diw.de/documents/publikationen/73/diw_01.c.817498.de/dwr-21-17.pdf. [7]

ILO (2020), *Global Wage Report 2020/2021: Wages and minimum wages in the time of COVID-19*, International Labour Organisation, https://www.ilo.org/wcmsp5/groups/public/---dgreports/---dcomm/---publ/documents/publication/wcms_762534.pdf. [27]

JRC (2020), *Telework in the EU before and after the COVID-19: Where we were, where we head to*, Joint Research Center (European Commission), https://ec.europa.eu/jrc/sites/default/files/jrc120945_policy_brief_-_covid_and_telework_final.pdf. [36]

Kyyrä, T., J. Pirttilä and T. Ravaska (2021), *The Corona crisis and household income: The case of a generous welfare state*, VATT Institute for Economic Research, Helsinki, https://www.doria.fi/bitstream/handle/10024/180378/vatt-mimeo-61-the-corona-crisis-and-household-income-the-case-of-a-generous-welfare-state.pdf?sequence=1&isAllowed=y. [8]

Mehdi, T. and R. Morissette (2021), *Working from home: Productivity and preferences*, Statistics Canada, https://www150.statcan.gc.ca/n1/pub/45-28-0001/2021001/article/00012-eng.htm. [34]

Ministerio Desarrollo Social y Familia (n.d.), *Encuesta Social COVID-19 (COVID-19 Social Survey) database*, http://observatorio.ministeriodesarrollosocial.gob.cl/encuesta-social-covid19 (accessed on 20 May 2021). [16]

OECD (2021), *Brick by Brick: Building Better Housing Policies*, OECD Publishing, Paris, https://dx.doi.org/10.1787/b453b043-en. [44]

OECD (2021), *Building for a better tomorrow: Policies to make housing more affordable. Employment, Labour and Social Affairs Policy Briefs*, OECD Publising, Paris, http://oe.cd/affordable-housing-2021. [40]

OECD (2021), *OECD Employment Outlook 2021: Navigating the COVID-19 Crisis and Recovery*, OECD Publishing, Paris, https://dx.doi.org/10.1787/5a700c4b-en. [20]

OECD (2021), *OECD Regional Outlook 2021: Addressing COVID-19 and Moving to Net Zero Greenhouse Gas Emissions*, OECD Publishing, Paris, https://dx.doi.org/10.1787/17017efe-en. [4]

OECD (2021), *Risks that Matter 2020: The long reach of COVID-19*, OECD Policy Responses to Coronavirus (COVID-19), OECD Publishing, Paris, https://doi.org/10.1787/44932654-en. [11]

OECD (2020), *Growth and economic well-being: Government support measures continue to shield household income from economic impact of COVID-19 in second quarter of 2020*, https://www.oecd.org/sdd/na/Growth-and-economic-well-being-oecd-11-2020.pdf. [3]

OECD (2020), *How's Life? 2020: Measuring Well-being*, OECD Publishing, Paris, https://dx.doi.org/10.1787/9870c393-en. [10]

OECD (2020), *OECD employment and unemployment statistics during the COVID-19 crisis*, https://www.oecd.org/sdd/labour-stats/OECD-employment-and-unemployment-%0A%0Astatistics-during-the-COVID-19-crisis.pdf. [21]

OECD (2020), *Regions and Cities at a Glance*, OECD Publishing, Paris, https://doi.org/10.1787/959d5ba0-en. [35]

OECD (n.d.), *Employment and Labour Market Statistics database*, https://doi.org/10.1787/data-00571-en (accessed on 13 August 2021). [29]

OECD (n.d.), *Household Dashboard database*, http://www.oecd.org/sdd/na/household-dashboard.htm (accessed on 13 August 2021). [5]

OECD (n.d.), *Main Economic Indicators database*, https://doi.org/10.1787/cbcc2905-en (accessed on 13 August 2021). [45]

OECD (n.d.), *OECD Affordable Housing database*, http://www.oecd.org/housing/data/affordable-housing-database/ (accessed on 15 June 2021). [39]

OECD (n.d.), *Risks That Matter Survey*, http://oe.cd/RTM (accessed on 15 May 2021). [12]

OECD (n.d.), *Telecommunications and Internet Statistics database*, https://doi.org/10.1787/tel_int-data-en (accessed on 11 September 2021). [42]

ONS (2020), *Coronavirus and homeworking in the UK: April 2020*, Office for National Statistics, https://www.ons.gov.uk/employmentandlabourmarket/peopleinwork/employmentandemployeetypes/bulletins/coronavirusandhomeworkingintheuk/latest#hours-worked (accessed on 23 May 2021). [30]

ONS (2020), *Coronavirus and the latest indicators for the UK economy and society: 1 October 2020*, Office for National Statistics, https://www.ons.gov.uk/peoplepopulationandcommunity/healthandsocialcare/conditionsanddiseases/bulletins/coronavirustheukeconomyandsocietyfasterindicators/1october2020. [32]

Parker, K., J. Menasce Horowitz and R. Minkin (2020), *How the Coronavirus outbreak has – and hasn't – changed the way americans work*, Pew Research Center, https://www.pewresearch.org/social-trends/2020/12/09/how-the-coronavirus-outbreak-has-and-hasnt-changed-the-way-americans-work/. [25]

Shine, C. (2021), *Working from home: Comparing the data*, Office for National Statistics, https://blog.ons.gov.uk/2021/05/17/working-from-home-comparing-the-data/. [33]

Statistics Canada (2020), *Food insecurity during the COVID-19 pandemic, May 2020*, https://www150.statcan.gc.ca/n1/en/pub/45-28-0001/2020001/article/00039-eng.pdf?st=glSvorSX. [18]

US Census Bureau (n.d.), *Measuring household experiences during the coronavirus pandemic*, https://www.census.gov/data/experimental-data-products/household-pulse-survey.html (accessed on 13 September 2021). [43]

Wozniak, A. et al. (2020), *COVID Impact Survey*, National Opinion Research Center, https://www.covid-impact.org/ (accessed on 9 August 2021). [17]

Notes

[1] Temporary policies enacted by governments as a response to COVID-19 have been simulated via the microsimulation model Euromod, and include actions such as wage compensation schemes, transfers from government to firms and households, lump-sum benefits, and reductions or exemptions on taxes.

[2] Namely, equivalised liquid financial assets below 25% of the national median income poverty line.

[3] Since the beginning of the pandemic, the Food Foundation has conducted seven nationally representative surveys on food insecurity in the United Kingdom through YouGov. Each survey included three questions on food insecurity sourced from the US Department of Agriculture's (USDA) Adult Food Security Survey Module 20: 1): Did (you/you or other adults in your household) ever cut the size of your meals or skip meals because there wasn't enough money for food? 2) Were you ever hungry but didn't eat because there wasn't enough money for food? 3) Did (you/the other adults in your household) ever not eat for a whole day because there wasn't enough money for food? YouGov survey respondents are drawn from a large pool of potential respondents. Active Sampling ensures that the right people are invited in the right proportions. In combination with statistical weighting, this ensures that results are representative of the country as a whole. Samples of at least 2 000 respondents (aged 18 or over) are weighted to match the adult UK population by age, gender and region, social class and highest education level.

[4] People who face uncertainties in their abilities to acquire food or who are forced to buy less/lower-quality food than usual are said to face moderate food insecurity, and people who often run out of food or that go one or more day without eating are said to face severe food insecurity.

[5] Between May 4 and 10, Statistics Canada collected the second wave of its new web panel survey, the Canadian Perspectives Survey Series (CPSS). 4 600 respondents from all 10 provinces participated in the CPSS during that time period. Food insecurity is based on a scale of six food experiences: food didn't last and no money to get more, sometimes or often; couldn't afford balanced meals, sometimes or often; adults in household skipped or cut size of meals; adults in household skipped or cut size of meals, 3 days or more; personally ate less because not enough money to buy food; and personally was hungry but didn't eat because couldn't afford food.

[6] The standard ILO classification of unemployment (followed by the OECD) defines unemployed persons as those who did not perform any paid work in the survey reference week, actively searched for work within the last 4 weeks, and would be available to start work within the next 2 weeks. In the context of the pandemic, some jobless individuals who want to work would nevertheless not meet this definition, either due to halting their job search (e.g. if in sectors closed by government restrictions) or due to caring responsibilities that span more than 2 weeks (e.g. home-schooling).

[7] See endnote 6 (above).

[8] The term temporary layoff refers to a worker whose employment contract is terminated (temporarily or permanently, severing employer obligations), but where there is an expectation that the employee may be recalled back to the same job in future. The term job-retention scheme covers a worker whose employment contract is maintained, but where his/her work is reduced or entirely halted, and (part of) his/her salary is covered from government funds.

[9] Although these data are higher than in April-June 2020, this could be due to the change in how the question was formulated – since data from the later two survey rounds also include respondents who worked from home routinely, even prior to the pandemic.

[10] The average includes the following five European countries: Austria (24.6%), France (26.1%), Germany (18.5%), Italy (12.1%) and Poland (13.3%).

[11] Data collected as part of a larger survey conducted between 13 and 19 October 2020. Everyone who took part in this survey is a member of the Center's American Trends Panel (ATP), an online survey panel that is recruited through national, random sampling of residential addresses. The survey is weighted to be representative of the United States adult population by gender, race, ethnicity, partisan affiliation, education and other categories. It included 5 858 respondents.

[12] Data are from the June 2021 Survey of Working Arrangements and Attitudes. 2 232 people who were currently working from home at least one day a week were asked the following question: How would you respond if your employer announced that all employees must return to the worksite 5+ days a week starting on 1 August 2021? (1) I would comply and return to the worksite; (2) I would start looking for a job that lets me work from home at least one or two days a week, but return to the worksite if I don't find one by 1 August. (3) I would quit my job on or before 1 August, regardless of whether I got another job. Responses were population-weighted to match population shares in the 2010 to 2019 Current Population Survey.

[13] Data is from a survey of 2 500 working-age employees conducted in May 2021 in the United Kingdom. The sample was re-weighted to match the Labour Force Survey figures by age, gender and education.

[14] In the context of the elements developed for the Australian Bureau of Statistics definition of homelessness, people living in "severely" crowded dwellings are considered to be homeless because they do not have control of, or access to, space for social relations.

3 Quality of life in the first year of COVID-19

As people contend with rising COVID cases and deaths, and cope with lockdowns, confinements and the economic fallout of the pandemic, their quality of life has been greatly altered. Both physical and mental health outcomes have declined. Preliminary evidence suggests that the resulting disruptions to schooling may be associated with serious long-term risks to children's life chances. Average life satisfaction has fallen slightly in most countries, but early evidence in some cases also suggests a surprising level of resilience. Like many other outcomes, subjective measures of well-being are sensitive to the timing of data collection within 2020, reflecting evolving changes in COVID risks, lockdown measures and the overall government response. This underscores the need to strengthen rapid data collection systems in order to monitor and react to individuals' changing circumstances in real time.

Quality of life has been dramatically impacted throughout the OECD by the COVID-19 pandemic. 30% of respondents from 15 OECD countries reported that their lives were greatly affected by the virus from June to December 2020; this percentage rose to 35% for the period January to June 2021 (Figure 3.1). Changes in material conditions (documented in Chapter 2) coupled with social distancing protocols and fears of the health impacts of the virus have meant that almost no aspect of everyday life has been untouched.

Figure 3.1. Over one-third of respondents report that COVID has greatly affected their lives

Share of respondents reporting that COVID-19 has greatly affected their lives, Jun 2020 - Jun 2021

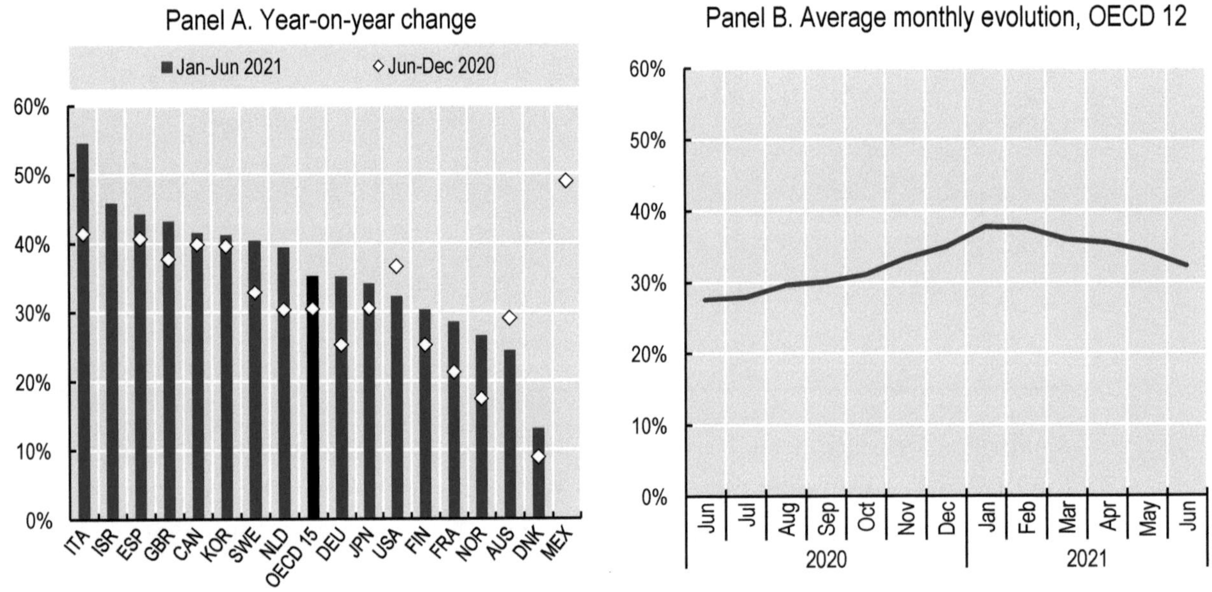

Note: Respondents answer the extent to which they agree with the statement, "My life has been greatly affected by coronavirus (COVID-19)" on a scale from 1 (not at all) to 7 (greatly affected). This figure refers to the share of respondents who answer either 6 or 7. Panel A depicts pooled averages from 2020 and 2021. 2020 pooled averages run from June through December, except for Mexico and the United States, which report pooled averages from June through September 2020. There are no 2020 data for Israel. The 2021 data are pooled averages from January through June, aside from the United States (February through June), the Netherlands (January through February), and Finland (January only). There are no 2021 data for Mexico. The OECD average includes the countries shown, except Israel and Mexico. Changes in outcomes between 2020 and 2021 are significant at the 5% level for all countries, including OECD 15, aside from Korea. In Panel B, the OECD average excludes Finland, the Netherlands and the United States, in addition to those excluded in Panel A, due to an incomplete time series.

Source: OECD calculations based on Imperial College London YouGov (2020[11]), *Covid 19 Behaviour Tracker Data Hub* (database), https://github.com/YouGov-Data/covid-19-tracker.

StatLink https://stat.link/v85ebg

3.1. Physical and mental health

3.1.1. Excess mortality and life expectancy

Excess mortality data – rather than COVID-19 fatality rates – provide a more accurate picture of the direct and indirect impacts of the pandemic on the mortality of OECD residents

COVID has impacted longevity both directly – through increased mortality, especially of the elderly population – but also indirectly, as both the supply and demand of routine health services have been curtailed due to the virus. The surge of COVID-19 cases across the OECD meant that hospitals were forced to reallocate resources to treat victims of the pandemic, yet in many cases they still found themselves understaffed and underequipped to handle the influx of patients: both those suffering from COVID-19 complications, and those seeking treatment for other health problems. Half of European countries recruited retired or inactive healthcare workers, and many also hired students who were in their final years of medical studies. In Italy, at the height of the first wave of the pandemic, 80% of pre-crisis beds in intensive care units (ICU) were estimated to be housing COVID-19 patients: in Ireland, France and Belgium, the figure was closer to 65%. To address these problems, countries transformed other wards to ICUs, created field hospitals, transferred patients to different regions with more capacity and partnered with private hospitals (OECD/European Union, 2020[2]).

The abrupt shift to treating COVID-19 patients resulted in disruptions to other health services. A report from the World Health Organization found that in Europe, the five health services most disrupted during pandemic peaks were rehabilitation services (91% of countries surveyed reported disruptions), dental services (91%), non-communicable disease treatment and diagnosis (76%), family planning (74%) and outreach for immunisations (63%) (European Observatory on Health Systems and Policies & WHO, 2020[3]).

Limited capacity, coupled with the population's fear of contracting the virus, resulted in fewer visits to health centres and hospitals. Across 15 OECD countries in the period April to December 2020, over 74% of people on average avoided going to hospitals or health centres to seek treatment; this share rose to 77% for the period January through June 2021 (Figure 3.2, Panel A). Monthly data for the OECD-12 average (Figure 3.2, Panel B) indicate that this fear dissipated somewhat from June to August 2020 but began rising steadily in September through the end of 2020. (The reasons for reduced visits to health centres are many. In addition to reductions in service provision and increased fear of contracting the virus, declines in visits may also be due to changes in activities and situations in which one might need to visit a health centre. For example, the observed reduction in traffic accidents and fatalities (Figure 4.7) and in seasonal flu cases (Jones, 2020[4]) both entail fewer visits to hospitals and/or health centres.)

Figure 3.2. On average in 2020, over 70% of people in 15 OECD countries avoided hospitals or health centres during the pandemic, with further increases in the early months of 2021

Share of the population who avoided health centres and hospitals over the past 7 days, Apr 2020 - Jun 2021

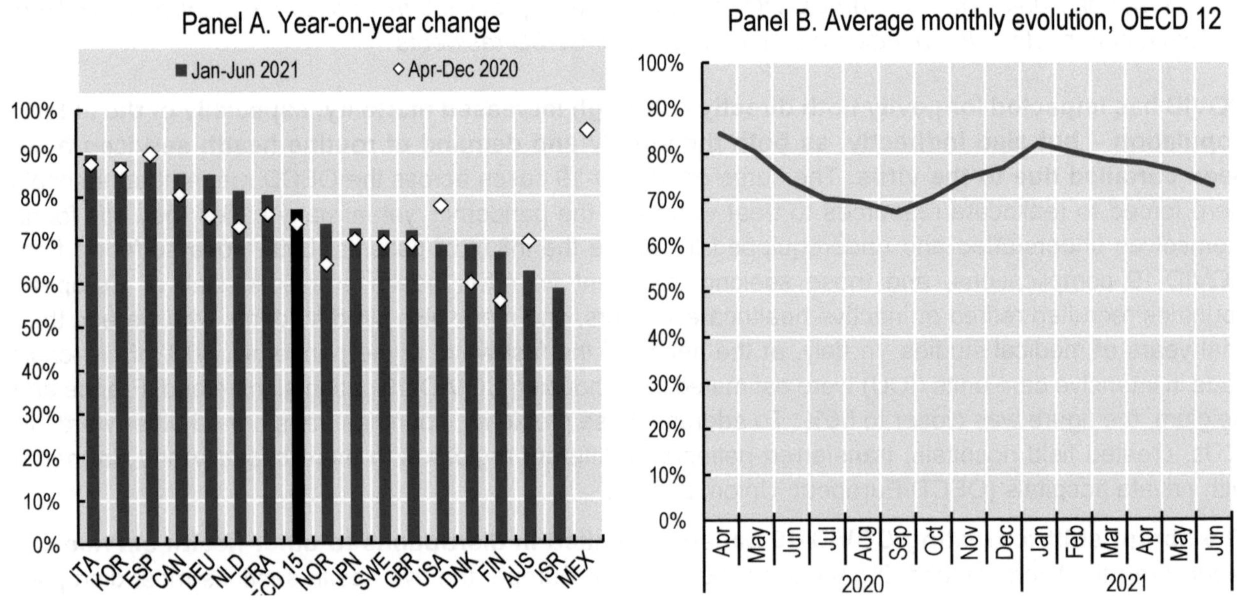

Note: Both figures depict the share of respondents who answered the question, "How often did you avoid going to hospital or other health-care settings over the past week?" with "always", "frequently" or "sometimes". The question does not identify the reason for individuals avoiding centres: i.e. whether based on fears of infection, or because health services were no longer available. Panel A depicts pooled averages from 2020 and 2021. 2020 pooled averages run from April through December, except for Mexico and the United States, which report pooled averages from April through September 2020. There are no 2020 data for Israel. The 2021 data are pooled averages from January through June, aside from the United States (February through June), the Netherlands (January through February) and Finland (January only). There are no 2021 data for Mexico. The OECD average includes the countries shown, except Israel and Mexico. Changes in outcomes between 2020 and 2021 are significant at the 5% level for all countries, including OECD 15. In Panel B, the OECD average excludes Finland, the Netherlands and the United States, in addition to those excluded in Panel A, due to an incomplete time series.

Source: OECD calculations based on Imperial College London YouGov (2020[1]), *Covid 19 Behaviour Tracker Data Hub* (database), https://github.com/YouGov-Data/covid-19-tracker.

StatLink https://stat.link/t52yku

Excess mortality statistics are better able to capture the overall effects of the pandemic on mortality than data on deaths attributed to COVID-19. Depending on the way in which death certificates are filled out in different countries, combined with variable COVID-19 testing availability and practices, certain fatalities may be coded as COVID-related in some jurisdictions but not in others. Furthermore, the pandemic has led to disruptions to preventative care and continuity of care; the pandemic is clearly contributing to any resulting negative health impacts, even though the official cause of death is not recorded as COVID-19. For this reason, excess mortality statistics provide a more accurate picture of the ways in which the pandemic has affected mortality rates (Morgan et al., 2020[5]). The excess mortality statistics used in this report are defined as the increase in all-cause mortality over the expected mortality based on historical trends (here, compared to average values from 2015-19). As can be seen in Figure 3.3, the total number of deaths in 33 OECD countries with data increased by 16%, on average, over the first year of the pandemic: from 11 March 2020 – when the World Health Organization first declared COVID-19 a global pandemic – to early May 2021, compared to the 2015-19 average.[1]

The OECD countries with the highest rates of excess mortality between March 2020 and early May 2021 include Mexico, Colombia, Chile, the Czech Republic, Poland, the Slovak Republic and the United States, where deaths were more than 20% higher than the 2015-19 average for this period. Conversely, a handful of countries – including Norway, Iceland and New Zealand – experienced about the same or *fewer* deaths in 2020-21 as compared to the baseline period. This decline reflects the success of early confinement measures in ensuring relatively low exposure to the virus (aided by geographic isolation and/or low population density). In addition, with the population staying home, there were fewer fatalities from non-COVID causes of death, such as road traffic accidents (see Figure 4.7) and other communicable illnesses, such as the seasonal flu (Jones, 2020[4]). It is also important to keep in mind the dynamic nature of the data:[2] different countries experience waves of the virus at different times. Panels B and C of Figure 3.3 depict excess death trends for G7 countries for which data are available. The virus peaked in Italy and France first, in early- to late-March 2020, whereas the first wave did not peak in the United Kingdom until mid-April. Some OECD countries had relatively low excess death rates in 2020 but saw an uptick in 2021 (OECD, forthcoming[6]). Early evidence suggests that excess mortality has, on average, been lower in the first half of 2021 (see Figure 3.3, Panels B and C) (Eurostat, 2021[7]), which may in part be due to the introduction of COVID-19 vaccines. However vaccination rates vary widely, both within and across OECD countries (OECD, 2021[8]).

There are large spatial inequalities of excess mortality within OECD countries: in many instances, within-country differences are larger than between-country disparities. On average, the hardest hit regions had excess mortality rates 17 percentage points higher than the least affected regions (Diaz Ramirez, Veneri and Lembcke, 2021[9]). More specifically, excess mortality in the worst affected regions of Mexico in 2020 was 60 percentage points higher than in the least affected areas of Mexico; the sub-national differences in Colombia were 90 percentage points. During the same time period, the gap between the most and least affected OECD countries was only 47 percentage points (Diaz Ramirez, Veneri and Lembcke, 2021[9]). In most OECD countries, metropolitan regions were hardest hit during the early months of the pandemic; however, the gap in excess mortality rates between metropolitan and remote regions diminished throughout 2020 and into 2021. While the virus was initially introduced to many countries through air travel in large metropolitan areas, as the pandemic has worn on it has spread to all areas within countries (Diaz Ramirez, Veneri and Lembcke, 2021[9]; OECD, 2020[10]).

Though it is too soon to say whether the pandemic has caused significant declines in life expectancy in OECD countries, preliminary evidence suggests that this is the case. As the pandemic lingers, and disproportionately affects certain groups more than others, the impact on life expectancy is gradually becoming apparent. Provisional estimates from 29 OECD countries show that life expectancy at birth has fallen by 0.6 years on average from 2019 to 2020 (Figure 3.4) (OECD, forthcoming[6]), declining in all but five countries.[3] A report published by the US National Center for Health Statistics (NCHS) in early 2021 found that life expectancy in the United States fell on average by one year, from 78.8 in 2019 to 77.8 in 2020 (Arias, Tejada-Vera and Ahmad, 2021[11]), the largest year-on-year decline since World War II. In addition to the immediate excess mortality associated with the pandemic, a longstanding literature identifies higher GDP growth and lower unemployment as two determinants of life expectancy gains over time (OECD, 2017[12]). While the relationship is indirect, a prolonged economic recession may have negative impacts on life expectancy in the long term.

Figure 3.3. In the first year of the pandemic, deaths increased by 16% on average across the OECD

Excess mortality, percentage change in total number of deaths from week 11 2020 to week 18 2021, compared to 2015-19 average

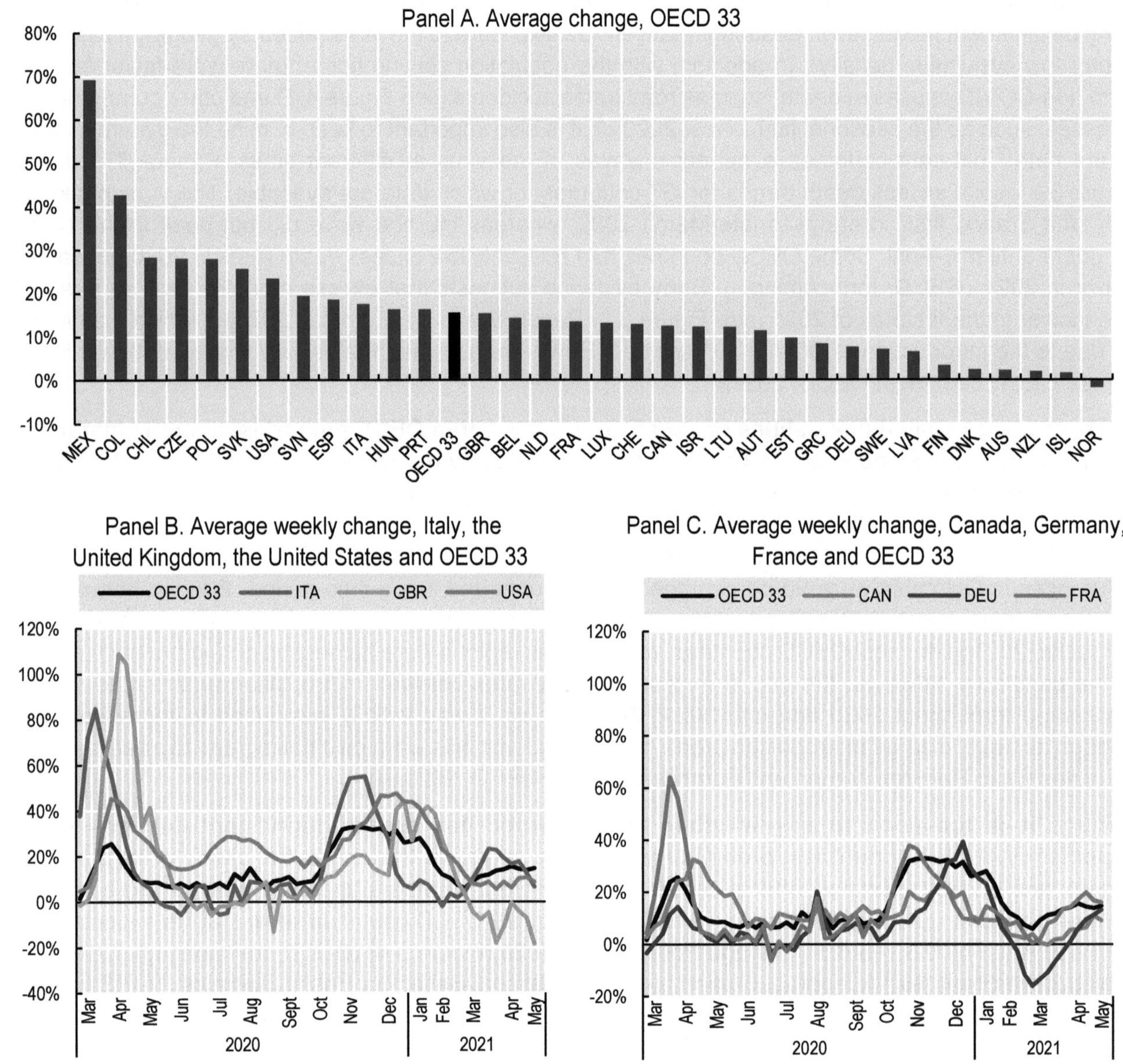

Note: Data refer to the increase in the number of reported deaths from all causes for the period March 2020 (week 11) to early May 2021 (week 18), compared to the average for the same period in 2015-2019. Data for Chile, Germany and Greece are compared against the average for 2016-2019. Those for Australia refer to doctor-certified deaths only. In all panels, the OECD average excludes Costa Rica, Ireland, Japan, Korea and Turkey.
Source: OECD calculations based on OECD (n.d.[13]) *COVID-19 Health Indicators* (database), https://stats.oecd.org/index.aspx?queryid=104676#.

StatLink https://stat.link/2kgqaj

Figure 3.4. In 2020, life expectancy in 29 OECD countries fell by 0.6 years on average

Life expectancy at birth, years, 2019 and 2020

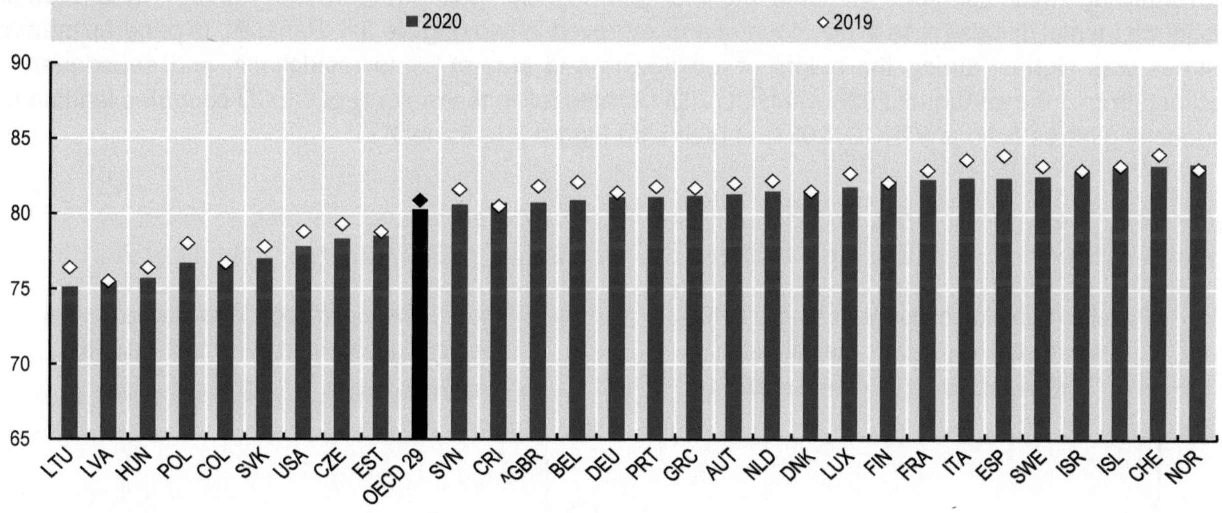

Note: ^GBR data refer to England, only. Data for Germany are provisional for 2020, and for Costa Rica in 2019 and 2020. 2020 data for the United States refer to January through June provisional estimates, only. The OECD average excludes Australia, Canada, Chile, Ireland, Japan, Korea, Mexico, New Zealand and Turkey.

Source: OECD (n.d.[14]), *Health Status* (database) https://stats.oecd.org/Index.aspx?DataSetCode=HEALTH_STAT; Arias, E., B. Tejada-Vera and F. Ahmad (2021[11]), "Provisional life expectancy estimates for January through June, 2020", *Vital Statistics Rapid Release*, Vol. 10, https://www.cdc.gov/nchs/data/vsrr/VSRR10-508.pdf; Public Health England (n.d.[15]), *Wider Impacts of COVID-19 on Health (WICH) Monitoring Tool* (database), https://analytics.phe.gov.uk/apps/covid-19-indirect-effects/; OECD (forthcoming[6]), *Health at a Glance 2021: OECD Indicators*, OECD Publishing, Paris; and the Israeli Central Bureau of Statistics (CBS), who provided data for Israel.

StatLink https://stat.link/dlc501

3.1.2. Depression, anxiety, eating disorders and deaths from suicide

Symptoms of anxiety and depression spiked across the OECD in 2020, and as of mid-2021, have not begun to recover on average, though recent evidence suggests a recovery in some countries

Over the course of 2020, mental health deteriorated across the OECD area, with rates of anxiety and depression doubling in a number of countries (OECD, 2021[16]). Experience from previous pandemics illustrates how these events often have significant impacts on population-level mental health, leading to an increase in feelings of depression, anxiety, insomnia, post-traumatic stress disorder and even suicide (Cénat et al., 2020[17]; Tzeng et al., 2020[18]; Yip et al., 2010[19]). Symptoms of psychological distress are not solely confined to the patients themselves, but also affect family members (Tsang, Scudds and Chan, 2004[20]). The COVID-19 virus combines a number of threats to mental health: of contracting the virus, spreading the virus to loved ones, death, disruptions to daily routines, school closures, and losing one's employment and livelihood, all while being forced to physically distance from friends and family (United Nations, 2020[21]).

Given that mental health conditions exist on a continuum, individuals who were previously able to cope may find that they are now struggling in the pandemic (Patel et al., 2018[22]). Prior to the pandemic, around 264 million people worldwide were affected by depression, and suicide was the second-largest cause of death for young people (United Nations, 2020[21]). The share of individuals feeling anxious, worried, depressed or taking little pleasure in everyday activities has been on the rise. From April through December 2020, 10.2% of respondents in 15 OECD countries had a Patient Health Questionnaire

(PHQ-4)[4] score indicating severe mental distress, and an additional 13.6% were at risk of moderate mental distress. From January to June 2021, those rates rose slightly, on average, to 10.6% and 13.8%, respectively (Figure 3.5). Rates of severe mental distress rose in six countries and declined only in two (in the remaining seven countries with data, the change was insignificant) (Figure 3.5, Panel A), and rates of moderate mental distress rose in one country and improved in two (Figure 3.5, Panel B). In general, mental distress was highest during the height of lockdowns and stay-at-home restrictions, and subsequently declined from June to August 2020 when COVID-19 rates fell in the majority of OECD countries leading to a loosening of restrictions (OECD, 2021[16]) (see also Figure 3.8, Panel A).

Figure 3.5. The share of those experiencing severe or moderate mental distress in 15 OECD countries rose slightly, on average, between the second half of 2020 and the first half of 2021

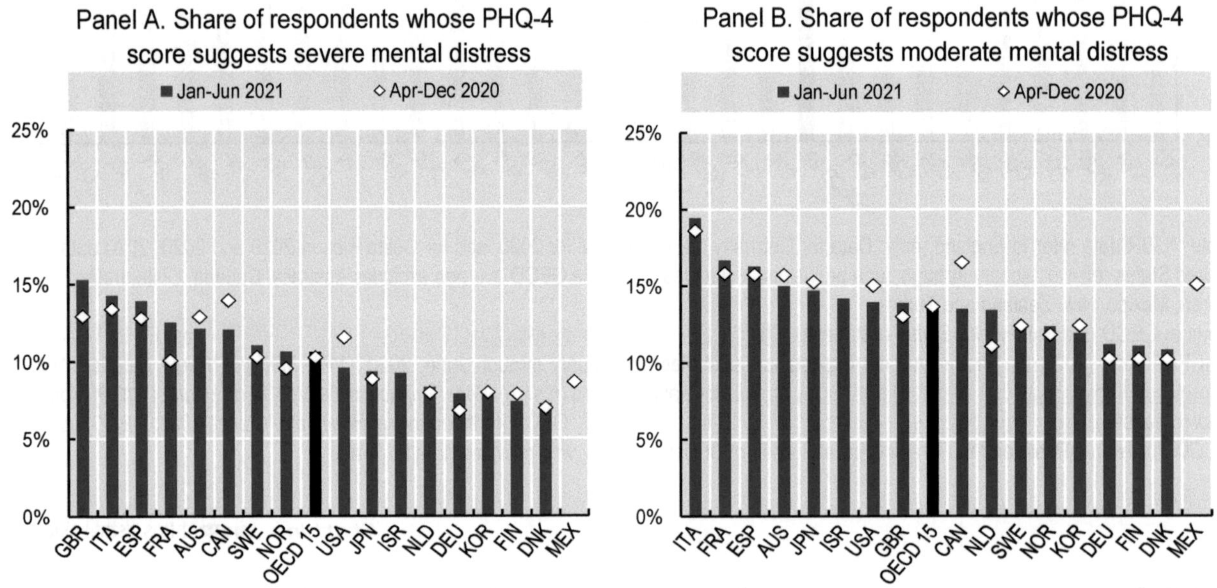

Note: Severity of mental distress is measured using the PHQ-4 survey. In both Panels A and B, 2020 pooled averages run from April through December, except for Mexico and the United States, which report pooled averages from April through September 2020. The 2021 data are pooled averages from January through June, aside from the United States (February through June), the Netherlands (January through February) and Finland (January only). The OECD average includes only those 15 countries with 2020-2021 data. In Panel A, changes in outcomes between 2020 and 2021 are significant at the 5% level for Canada, France, Germany, Italy, Norway, OECD 15, Spain, the United Kingdom and the United States. In Panel B, changes in outcomes between 2020 and 2021 are significant at the 5% level for Canada, Germany, the Netherlands, OECD 15 and the United Kingdom.

Source: OECD calculations based on Imperial College London YouGov (2020[1]), *Covid 19 Behaviour Tracker Data Hub* (database), https://github.com/YouGov-Data/covid-19-tracker.

StatLink https://stat.link/31klt6

Over one-quarter of respondents in 15 OECD countries were at risk of anxiety (25.0%) and depression (26.58%) in 2020; both rates increased slightly, but significantly, in the first half of 2021 (for anxiety to 26.6%, for depression to 26.64%, see Figure 3.6). For eight OECD countries with comparable baseline measures, the share of respondents at risk of depression by mid-2021 had risen significantly since 2014: by more than 20 percentage points in two European countries (Figure 3.7). While the source of the baseline data is different from the source of the pandemic-era data, implying that caution should be exercised in interpreting any individual country trajectory, both data sources use the same instrument (PHQ-2) to assess the risk of depression, therefore the overall trend of large deteriorations is likely to be true. See also OECD (2021[16]) for similar evidence of dramatic increases in the prevalence of mental health problems in 2020 compared to pre-pandemic baselines in OECD countries.

Data collected by national statistics offices across OECD countries corroborate these findings (see Box 3.1). The share of Canadians reporting fair or poor mental health during 24 April to 11 May 2020 was 24%, a significant increase from the 8% reported by the Canadian Community Health Survey (CCHS) for 2018 (Statistics Canada, 2020[23]). In Great Britain, data from the Opinions and Lifestyle Survey from June 2020 showed that 19% of Britons had some form of depression, as measured by the PHQ-8 questionnaire,[5] and that depression rates had almost doubled from the pre-pandemic baseline. Furthermore, the pandemic resulted in declining mental health among those who previously had no, or only mild, symptoms: 13% of adults in Great Britain developed moderate to severe symptoms over the course of 2020 (ONS, 2020[24]). In March 2020, 50% of Britons reported high levels of anxiety; however, unlike depression, there is evidence suggesting that anxiety levels have fallen since early lockdown (ONS, 2020[25]). Survey data collected by the Japanese Ministry of Health, Labour and Welfare in August showed that 6% of respondents reported feeling depressed all day every day over the past two weeks, while 9% reported having no interest in things or having lost interest in things that used to be enjoyable to them (LINE Research Official Blog, 2020[26]).[6]

Figure 3.6. More than a quarter of the population in 15 OECD countries are at risk of anxiety and depression, 2020-21

Share of respondents who are at risk for depression or anxiety disorders, Apr-Dec 2020 vs. Jan-Jun 2021

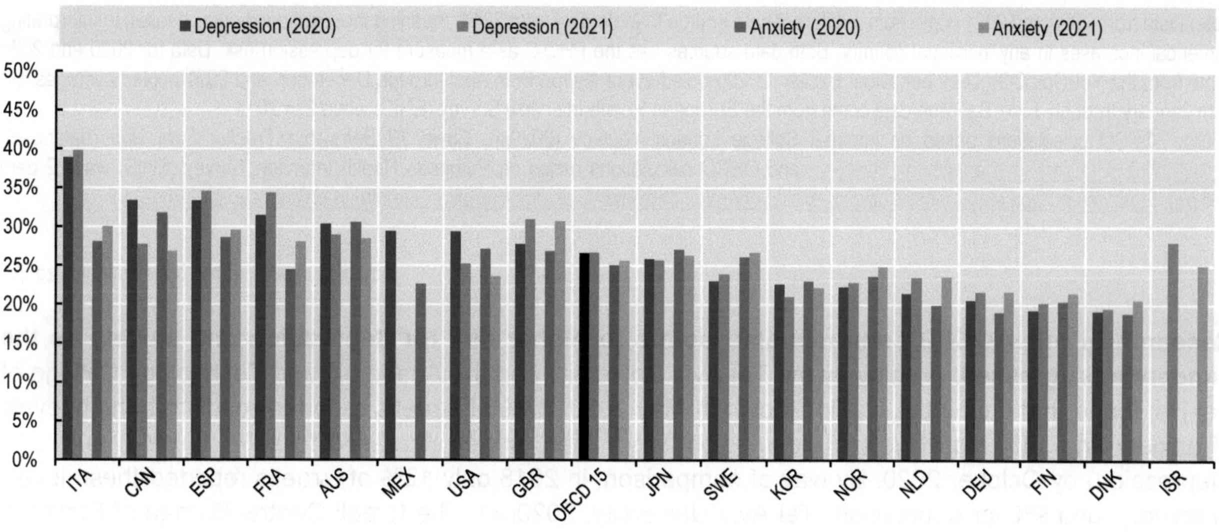

Note: Risk for depression and anxiety are measured using the PHQ-4 questionnaire. 2020 pooled averages run from April through December, except for Mexico and the United States, which report pooled averages from April through September 2020. The 2021 data are pooled averages from January through June, aside from the United States (February through June), the Netherlands (January through February) and Finland (January only). The OECD average includes only those 15 countries with 2020-2021 data. For all countries, as well as the OECD average, depression prevalence in 2020 and 2021 are the first two bars on the left, and anxiety prevalence in 2020 and 2021 are the right two bars. Changes in depression outcomes between 2020 and 2021 are significant at the 5% level for all countries, including OECD 15, aside from Denmark, Finland, Italy, Japan, the Netherlands, Norway and Sweden. Changes in anxiety outcomes between 2020 and 2021 are significant at the 5% level for all countries, including OECD 15, aside from Finland, Japan, Korea, Spain and Sweden.
Source: OECD calculations based on Imperial College London YouGov (2020[1]), *Covid 19 Behaviour Tracker Data Hub* (database), https://github.com/YouGov-Data/covid-19-tracker.

StatLink https://stat.link/1bej8g

Figure 3.7. The risk of depression has increased dramatically in eight European countries

Share of respondents at risk of depression, 2020 and 2021 vs. 2014

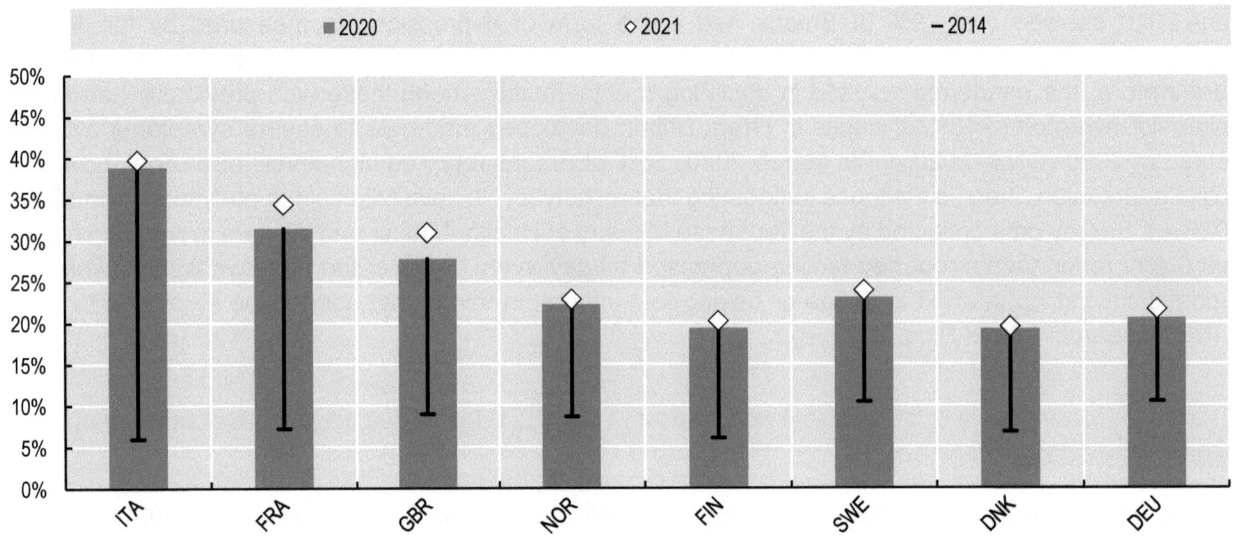

Note: Data from 2020 and 2021 come from a different data source than do data from 2014, meaning that caution should be taken in interpreting numerical increases in any individual country. Both data sources use the PHQ-2 as a measure for depression risk. Data for 2020 and 2021 come from the YouGov COVID-19 behaviour tracker: 2020 pooled averages run from April through December, and 2021 pooled averages run from January through June. Baseline data come from the European Health Interview Survey (EHIS) wave 2 in 2014.
Source: OECD calculations based on Imperial College London YouGov (2020[1]), *Covid 19 Behaviour Tracker Data Hub* (database), https://github.com/YouGov-Data/covid-19-tracker; and OECD calculations based on European Health Interview Survey (EHIS) wave 2 data (n.d.[27]), https://ec.europa.eu/eurostat/statistics-explained/index.php?title=Glossary:European_health_interview_survey_(EHIS).

StatLink https://stat.link/zd9jk1

Research in other OECD countries also points to higher risk for depression and anxiety as the pandemic progressed. A study by the Tel Aviv University and the Academic and Technology College of Tel-Hai found that during the first lockdown in May 2020, 23% of Israelis reported medium to high levels of anxiety and 14% high levels of depression, which had further increased to 29% (anxiety) and 20% (depression) by October 2020. By way of comparison, in 2018 only 12% of Israelis reported these levels of anxiety, and 9% for depression (Tel Aviv University, 2020[28]). The Israeli Central Bureau of Statistics (CBS) flash survey, the *Civilian Resilience during the Coronavirus Survey*, found similar results. The first round of data collection, from 26 April to 1 May 2020, showed that 16.2% of Israelis over the age of 21 felt depressed ("to a large extent"" or "to an extent") and 34.4% felt stress and anxiety (CBS, 2020[29]); these rates rose to 21% and 42%, respectively, during a follow-up survey conducted from 12 July to 16 July 2020 (CBS, 2020[30]). A Korean study published in May 2020 showed that 47% of respondents reported feelings of anxiety and/or depression because of the pandemic (Park and Yu, 2020[31]). The COVID-19 Social Survey in Chile (refer to Box 5.3 for survey details) found that 21.4% of adults reported moderate or severe symptoms of anxiety and/or depression based on the PHQ-4 scale from 24 June to 7 August 2020 (Ministerio Desarrollo Social y Familia, 2020[32]). An online survey[7] of mental health in Costa Rica found that risk for depression and anxiety (measured using the PHQ-4 scale) increased more than three-fold between March and October 2020 (UNED, 2021[33]).

Some country evidence suggests that although mental health declined precipitously in the early stages of the pandemic, it may have started to recover by mid-2021 in some instances. In Colombia, an online (non-representative) survey of more than 18 000 adults, running from 20 May to 20 June 2020 in the early days of the pandemic, found that 35% of respondents were at risk of depression (using PHQ-2) and 29% at risk of depression (using GAD-2);[8] the same survey also found that women and young adults were most at risk (Guzmán Mena and Tamayo, 2020[34]; Sanabria-Maxo et al., 2021[35]). Data collected by Colombia's statistical office (DANE) as a part of its Social Pulse survey (refer to Box 4.1 for methodological information) around the same time, July 2020, found that 22.5% of Colombians reported feeling sad over the past seven days, 40.4% preoccupied or nervous, and 4.9% that it was impossible to feel positive feelings. However one year later, in July 2021, these rates had improved to 14.8%, 38.1%, 0.9%, respectively (DANE, n.d.[36]). Similarly, data from the Australian Bureau of Statistics' Household Impacts of COVID-19 Survey collected in mid-April 2020 – when the country was experiencing peak levels of new COVID-19 cases – showed that 35.4% of respondents reported being nervous at least some of the time, up from 20.1% in 2017-18; and 41.8% felt restless or fidgety, compared to 23.7% pre-pandemic. Conversely, the rate of feeling "so depressed that nothing could cheer you up" remained more or less the same – 7.8% in 2017-18 vs. 7.5% in April 2020 (ABS, 2020[37]). However data from Australia National University's COVID-19 impact monitoring survey (ANUPoll) showed that by April 2021, levels of psychological distress had reverted to pre-pandemic levels, with the only exception of young people, whose rates of psychological distress remained significantly higher in April 2021 than they were before COVID-19 (AIHW, 2021[38]).

Box 3.1. Innovation: National Statistics Offices have launched COVID-19-specific surveys that capture changes in mental distress

United States: Household Pulse Survey and COVID Impact Survey

The US Census Bureau is leading a multi-agency push to collect experimental survey data on the socio-economic and health effects of COVID-19 on American households. Unlike other Census Bureau surveys, the Household Pulse Survey is designed to mobilise data quickly, with results released in a matter of weeks rather than months or years. The Household Pulse Survey began in April 2020 and encompasses three phases of data collection (US Census Bureau, n.d.[39]).[1] The first phase collected data on a weekly basis, however subsequent phases moved to a biweekly approach.

A total of 14 million Americans were contacted via email and text, inviting them to complete a 20-minute online questionnaire. The survey receives around 100 000 responses weekly. Data were initially published within eight days of collection (though in later phases this moved to once every 14 days), to provide a real-time snapshot of how COVID is affecting the lives of Americans. Data are weighted to be representative at the national and state levels; in addition, representative statistics are available for the fifteen largest Metropolitan Statistical Areas. The survey is not longitudinal, in that it does not track unique respondents over time, nor does it include pre-pandemic outcomes for individuals. However, many of the topics covered in the Pulse Survey are covered in the annual National Health Interview Survey (NHIS), which allows for baseline comparisons (CDC, 2020[40]).

The Data Foundation, a private non-profit organisation, introduced the COVID Impact Survey in April 2020, designed to be complementary to the Household Pulse Survey. The survey is conducted by the National Opinion Research Center (NORC) at the University of Chicago and uses an address-based random sampling design to be representative of the population aged 18 years and over at the national and regional (ten states and eight metropolitan areas) levels. Around 2 000 respondents are interviewed during each week of data collection: the first wave of data collection took place in April 2020, the second in May 2020 and the third in June 2020. Survey modules cover physical, social and mental health as well as financial and economic health (Wozniak et al., 2020[41]). Data from both the Pulse and Impact surveys are used in this publication.

Data collected in the first phase of the Household Pulse (from 23 April to 21 July) showed that rates of anxiety (measured using GAD-2) among Americans reached 36% in mid-July, and 37% in early November. Rates of depression peaked at 29.6% in mid-July and rose to 30.2% in December 2020 (Figure 3.8, Panel A). The weekly averages from April through December point to a large increase from baseline values. Comparable data from January-June 2019 showed only 8% of respondents with symptoms of an anxiety disorder, and 7% of respondents with symptoms of depression (National Center for Health Statistics, 2020[42]). A separate study using nationally representative survey data in the United States came to similar conclusions. By comparing data during the pandemic (from the COVID-19 and Life Stressors Impact on Mental Health and Well-being study, 31 March-13 April) with data from earlier periods (National Health and Nutrition Examination Survey, 2017-18), Ettman et al. (2020[43]) found that depressive symptoms (measured using the PHQ-9) increased more than threefold during the COVID crisis. Rates of depression increased for all levels of severity, with the greatest rises for the share of those with mild to moderate depression. However there is some suggestive evidence that rates of depression and anxiety may be dropping over the course of 2021: as can be seen in Figure 3.8 (Panel A), both measures have been steadily falling since the early months of 2021.

Germany: Socio-Economic Factors in and Consequences of the Spread of the Coronavirus in Germany (SOEP-CoV)

The German Socio-Economic Panel (SOEP) conducted by the German Institute for Economic Research (DIW Berlin) is a longitudinal survey of over 30 000 individuals in 20 000 households that has been running for more than three decades (Goebel et al., 2019[44]). Households remain in the study, which means their outcomes can be tracked over a lifetime. The questionnaire covers topics relating to household composition and demographics, employment and earnings, along with health and life satisfaction indicators. During the early stages of the pandemic in April 2020, SOEP collaborated with researchers from the Universität Bielefeld to initiate a new project entitled, "Socio-Economic Factors in and Consequences of the Spread of the Coronavirus in Germany (SOEP-CoV)" (SOEP-CoV, 2021[45]), which capitalises on the existing survey infrastructure to provide panel data on a representative sample of Germans during the pandemic. By integrating with the existing SOEP, the new SOEP-CoV has comparable baseline (i.e. pre-pandemic) measures for a wide range of well-being outcomes.[2]

Two rounds of telephone interviews ran from 1 April to 28 June 2020, and from January to February 2021. Participating households were selected from the overall SOEP sample and randomly divided into nine tranches, in such a way that the complex design information of the existing SOEP subsamples was preserved (Kühne et al., 2020[46]). Tranches 1-5 were surveyed with a time difference of two weeks between each tranche. This difference was shortened to one week after tranche 5. 12 000 households were invited to participate in telephone interviews, and 6 700 households completed surveys. Reported data are weighted to account for non-responses. All individuals interviewed in the first wave were re-interviewed in 2021. Because all selected households participate in the longitudinal study, it is possible to track their outcomes before, during and after the pandemic (Kühne et al., 2020[46]).

The survey captures mental health, including anxiety and depression, through the PHQ-4 questionnaire. According to this survey, rates of severe and moderate depression remained relatively stable in Germany from 2016 through 2019, 2020 and 2021, however the share of those with mild depression increased significantly from 2019 to 2020 (Figure 3.8, Panel B). Yet by the subsequent year, this increased prevalence appears to have dissipated; in 2021 the share of the population reporting symptoms of mild depression, along with overall prevalence of anxiety and depression, were not significantly different from any pre-pandemic year (Figure 3.8, Panel B) (Entringer and Kröger, 2021[47]).

Figure 3.8. Anxiety and depression rates spiked in the United States in July and again in December 2020, while in Germany declines in mental health have been less marked

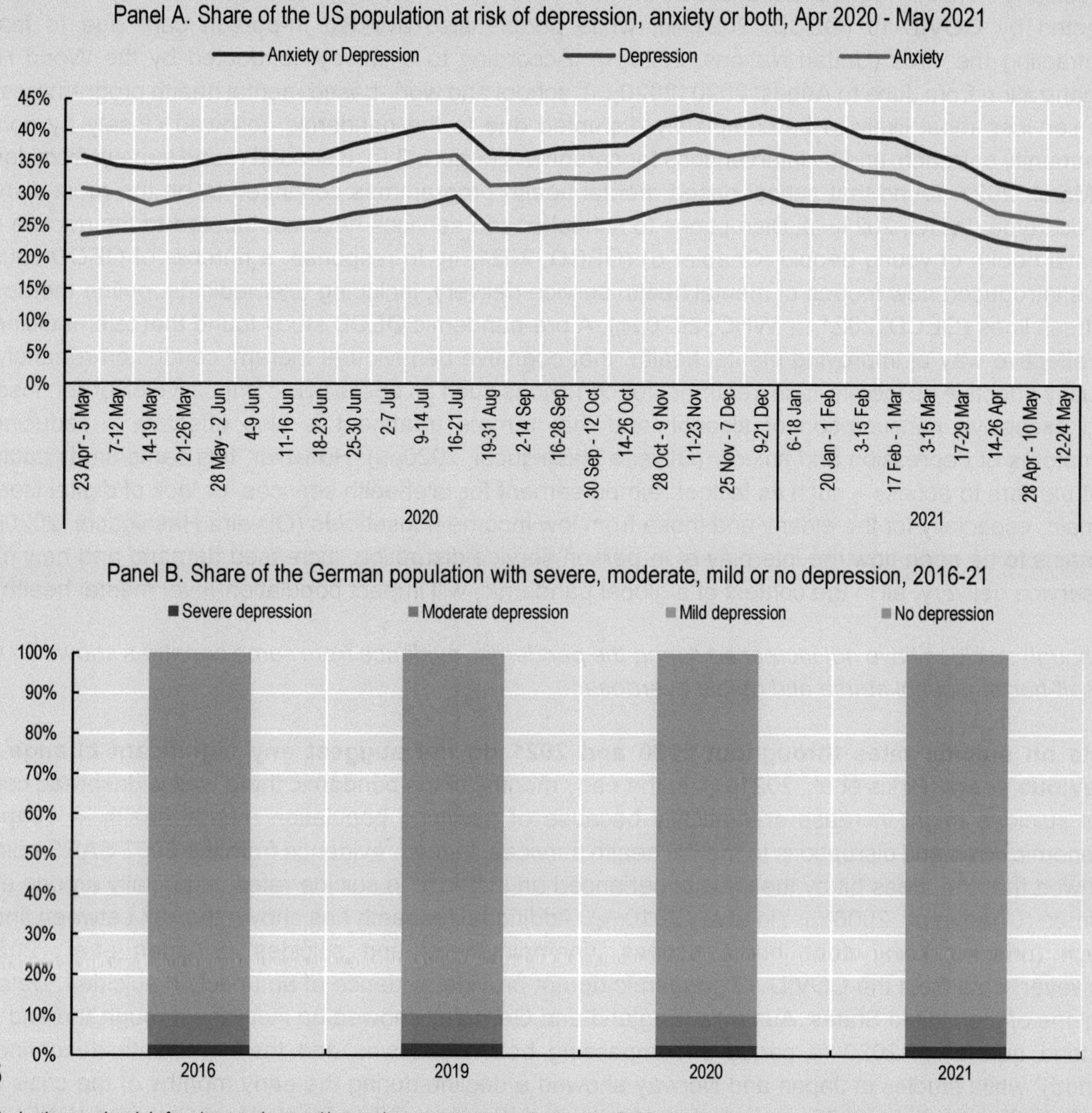

15

Note: In both panels, risk for depression and/or anxiety are measured with the PHQ-4 questionnaire. In Panel A, data were collected from April 2020 to May 2021. In Panel B, 2020 data were collected from April to June; 2021 data were collected in January and February.

Source: US Census Bureau (n.d.[39]), *Measuring Household Experiences during the Coronavirus Pandemic* (database), https://www.census.gov/householdpulsedata (Panel A); and Kühne et al. (2020[46]), "The need for household panel surveys in times of crisis: The case of SOEP-CoV", *Survey Research Methods*, Vol. 14/2, pp. 195-203, https://doi.org/10.18148/srm/2020.v14i2.7748 (Panel B).

StatLink https://stat.link/zqx70v

Notes:

1. Phase 1: 23 Apr - 21 Jul 2020; Phase 2: 19 Aug - 26 Oct 2020; Phase 3: 28 Oct 2020 - 1 Mar 2021 (with a break in data collection from 21 Dec 2020 - 6 Jan 2021); Phase 3.1: 14 Apr - 5 Jul 2021; Phase 3.2: 21 Jul - 11 Oct 2021.
2. The project is funded by the German Federal Ministry of Education and Research (BMBF).

The pandemic has disrupted access to mental health services (Figure 3.9)**.** Access to mental health services was already limited before the pandemic: 67% of working-age adults with mental distress who wanted mental health care reported having difficulties accessing it (OECD, 2021[48]). In 2020, hospitals in particularly hard-hit regions used beds normally reserved for mental health patients to care for those infected by COVID-19 (OECD, 2021[16]), while people also avoided in-person care due to fears of contracting the virus (United Nations, 2020[21]). According to a survey conducted by the World Health Organization from June to August 2020 (2020[49]), school and work-based mental health programmes were the services most likely to be completely disrupted due to the pandemic, followed closely by home or community outreach, and by interventions for caregivers (Figure 3.9); a second round survey, from January to March 2021, found that school-based mental health programmes continued to be the most disrupted service type (WHO, 2021[50]). Disruptions to school-based services have contributed to the decline in the mental health of young people (Chapter 6) (OECD, 2021[51]). In response, a number of OECD countries have introduced new modes of mental health service delivery, including telemedicine, online therapy and distress lines (OECD, 2021[16]; WHO, 2020[49]). A pre-pandemic OECD study found that telemedicine was an effective way of improving mental health; that cognitive behavioural therapy conducted remotely was equally effective as face-to-face treatment for conditions such as obsessive-compulsive disorder, insomnia and excessive consumption of alcohol; and that remote treatment is also effective in reducing the symptoms of depression and anxiety (Oliveira Hashiguchi, 2020[52]). However, this same study cautioned that barriers to access – such as lack of reimbursement for telehealth services, or lack of digital literacy – remain, especially for the elderly and those from low income households (Oliveira Hashiguchi, 2020[52]). It remains to be seen how the interplay of in-person service disruption, increased demand and new modes of service delivery, all in the context of a global pandemic, will impact population-level mental health.

Although suicides have not increased during the pandemic, evidence from some countries shows an uptick in self-harm, alcohol abuse and opioid overdoses

Data on suicide rates throughout 2020 and 2021 do not suggest any significant change from previous years (Pirkis et al., 2021[53]). In the early months of the pandemic there was widespread concern that suicides might increase dramatically because of declining population mental health, a deepening economic crisis and disruptions to mental health services. Indeed, evidence from the 2003 SARS epidemic showed that the areas hit by the virus experienced an increase in suicide rates, especially among elderly women (Chan et al., 2006[54]; Yip et al., 2010[19]). Additional research has shown the link between financial strain (encompassing debt, homelessness, unemployment) and suicides (Elbogen et al., 2020[55]). However, data from the COVID-19 pandemic do not provide evidence of an uptick in suicides. Data from regions of the United States, Australia, England and Germany showed no increase through the end of the second quarter of 2020 (a period encompassing both lockdowns and the immediate deconfinement period), while studies in Japan and Norway showed a decline during the early months of the crisis (John et al., 2020[56]; Knight, 2020[57]). Data from the United Kingdom Office for National Statistics (ONS) in fact found that suicides in England and Wales decreased during the first wave of the pandemic (Apr-Jul 2020), compared to previous years (ONS, 2021[58]). However, in the case of Japan, data from later in 2020 showed a subsequent increase (see Box 3.2). A study of 2 000 respondents in France in September 2020 showed that around 20% reported having suicidal thoughts. Although high, this was more or less the same level as 2016 (Gaubert, 2020[59]; Debout and Fourquet, 2016[60]). As the pandemic and its economic effects wear on, it will be important to monitor suicide risk (see Box 3.2): survey data from Belgium, France and the United Kingdom show that suicidal thoughts have increased among younger people, even if rates of actual suicides have not yet done so (OECD, 2021[51]). It is also important to measure suicide rates among sub-populations. In the United States, the overall number of suicides dropped by 5% between 2019 and 2020; however, suggestive evidence from some states, including Illinois, Maryland and Connecticut, suggests that suicides have risen for Black Americans (Rabin, 2021[61]).

Figure 3.9. School and work-related mental health programmes were the most likely to experience disruptions during the pandemic, across 21 OECD countries

Share of countries reporting disruptions to mental, neurological and substance abuse (MNS) services, Jun-Aug 2020

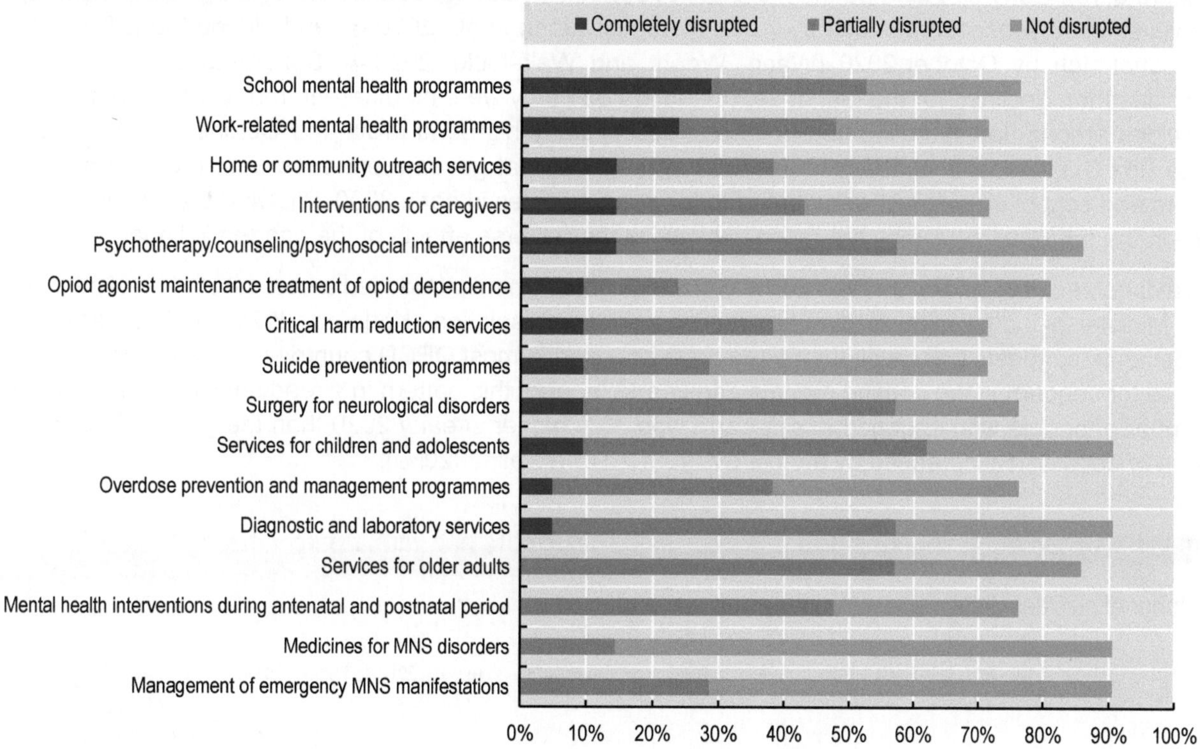

Note: Mental health focal points within the Ministry of Health in 130 countries were surveyed by the WHO; the above figure shows outcomes for the 21 OECD countries included in the report. The OECD average includes Australia, Austria, Belgium, Canada, Chile, Colombia, the Czech Republic, Denmark, Finland, Germany, Hungary, Ireland, Japan, Latvia, Lithuania, Mexico, the Netherlands, Norway, Poland, Slovenia and the United States. Totals may not sum to 100% due to missing values.
Source: WHO (2020[49]), *The Impact of COVID-19 on Mental, Neurological and Substance Use Services: Results of a Rapid Assessment*, World Health Organization, https://www.who.int/publications/i/item/978924012455.

StatLink https://stat.link/qsuxkw

In early April, the WHO issued a warning about the potential for excessive alcohol consumption during emergency situations such as the pandemic and ensuing lockdowns (WHO Regional Office for Europe, 2020[62]). Evidence from household surveys using online sampling suggests average measures of per capita alcohol consumption did not increase markedly, although more people reported drinking more since the start of the pandemic than those reporting drinking less (see Figures 9.3 and 9.4) (OECD, 2021[63]; OECD, 2021[64]). Increased alcohol consumption entails a number of health risks, including worse mental health outcomes, and it increases instances of domestic violence, along with a higher risk of disease or injury (OECD, 2021[63]).

Box 3.2. Spotlight: Suicides on the rise in Japan after falling in the first phase of the pandemic

Data from the Japanese National Police Agency show the dynamic nature of suicide rates in 2020 (Figure 3.10). Early on in the pandemic (April 2020) suicides in the country fell by 20% (Blair, 2020[65]); however, they subsequently rose by 7.7% in August (John et al., 2020[56]) and climbed to a five-year-seasonal-high by October 2020 (Wang, Wright and Wakatsuki, 2020[66]; Sakamoto et al., 2021[67]). Suicides then declined for the rest of 2020, and in 2021 they were no different from the five years prior. Suicides among Japanese women have been particularly high and drove the October 2020 increase (see Box 6.3). Tanaka and Okamoto (2021[68]) suggest that government subsidies, reduced working hours and school closures all contributed to lowering suicides in early 2020, implying that suicides may rise in the future as subsidies are rolled back while the adverse effects of the pandemic linger.

As a direct result of suicide increases, the Japanese government introduced a new cabinet-level position, the Minister of Loneliness, to diminish feelings of social isolation (Kodama, 2021[69]). The Japanese experience suggests that, even if suicides have not risen in most OECD countries to date, there may be cause for concern in the coming months and years. Indeed, this pattern in already evident in Korea: the number of people who engaged in self-harm was 36% higher in early 2020 than the year before, while rates of depression increased by almost 6% from 2019 (Ryall, 2020[70]).

Figure 3.10. Suicides in Japan fell in the early stages of the pandemic before rising in late 2020

Number of suicides, total

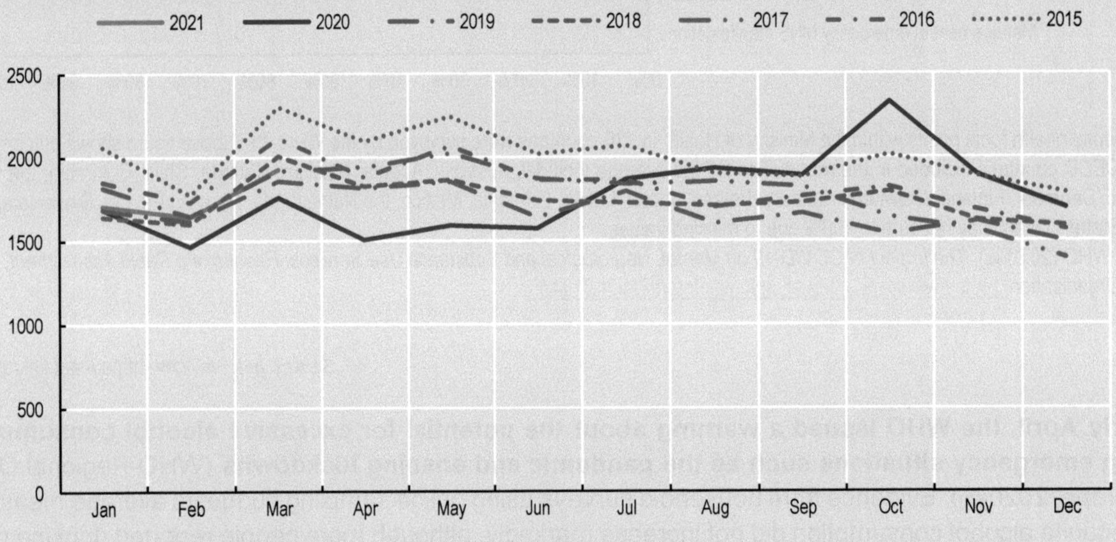

Source: Japanese National Police Agency (2021[71]), 令和２年中における自殺の状況, https://www.npa.go.jp/safetylife/seianki/jisatsu/R03/R02_jisatuno_joukyou.pdf.

StatLink https://stat.link/vr28xa

Evidence shows that opioid overdoses are on the rise in some countries. In the United States the Centers for Disease Control and Prevention (CDC) reported 93 331 opioid overdoses in 2020, a 30% increase from the year prior and the highest annual rate ever recorded (Ahmad and Rossen, 2021[72]; Katz and Sanger-Katz, 2021[73]): in addition, mental health and overdose calls to first responders (those first on the scene in case of emergency, such as EMTs (emergency medical technicians), firefighters, police officers, etc.) doubled in 2020, compared to the two years prior (Graham, 2021[74]). In Canada, 2020 also proved to be the deadliest year for opioid overdoses. In the province of Alberta, overdose deaths reached a peak of 142 in July, the highest rate since data collection began in 2016 (Government of Alberta Ministry of Health, n.d.[75]). The increase coincided with a decrease in treatment availability because of the pandemic: as a result of the decline in treatment adherence[9] in April (52.6%) and May (55.8%) 2020, the annual average treatment adherence decreased to 75.4% from 89.8% in 2019 (Government of Alberta Ministry of Health, 2020[76]).[10] Data from England and Wales show that the number of drug-related deaths in 2020 were the highest since record keeping began in 1993, and 3.8% higher than the year prior; however the ONS cautions that, due to delays in reporting, a large number of these deaths may have occurred in 2019, i.e. before the start of the pandemic (ONS, 2021[77]).

3.2. Subjective well-being

Life satisfaction remained fairly resilient on average, but outcomes are heavily dependent on the timing of data collection in relation to the progression of the pandemic

While material conditions and mental health deteriorated in the wake of the pandemic, trends in subjective well-being measures – such as life satisfaction and negative affect balance – are currently less clear-cut. Data from the Gallup World Poll show that life satisfaction deteriorated by a very small amount on average across OECD countries (from 6.71 in 2019 to 6.66 in 2020), but the pattern across countries is inconsistent (Figure 3.11, Panel A). Similarly, the share of people within a country reporting low levels of life satisfaction (defined as answering less than or equal to 4, on a scale from 0 "least satisfied" to 10 "most satisfied") has fallen in some countries but increased in others (Figure 3.12). Finally, the share of the population reporting a negative affect balance – the share of the population reporting more negative feelings (anger, sadness, worry) than positive feelings (enjoyment, laughing or smiling a lot, feeling well-rested) the day before being interviewed – has increased for OECD countries on average (from 12.9% in 2019 to 14% in 2020), although this increase has not been consistent across all OECD members (Figure 3.11, Panel B).

One factor explaining the lack of clear trends in life satisfaction is the sensitivity of the measure to the time when data are gathered. Context is always important for measurement, but when gauging the impacts of the pandemic on measures of subjective well-being, understanding the relationship between fieldwork timing and the progression of the pandemic in the national context is vital. Data from the Gallup World Poll were collected throughout 2020, with fieldwork taking place at different times in different countries (refer to Box 3.4 for full details). This, coupled with the fact that different countries experienced waves of the pandemic at different times, means that pooled national averages may mask substantial variations in life satisfaction over the course of 2020 (as shown in Box 3.3). For example, national data from France show that 2020 life satisfaction peaked in June/July as the country emerged from a strict lockdown, before falling dramatically as a second wave took hold in late 2020 (Figure 3.14, Panel C).

Figure 3.11. National averages show only small changes in life satisfaction and negative affect balance from 2019 to 2020

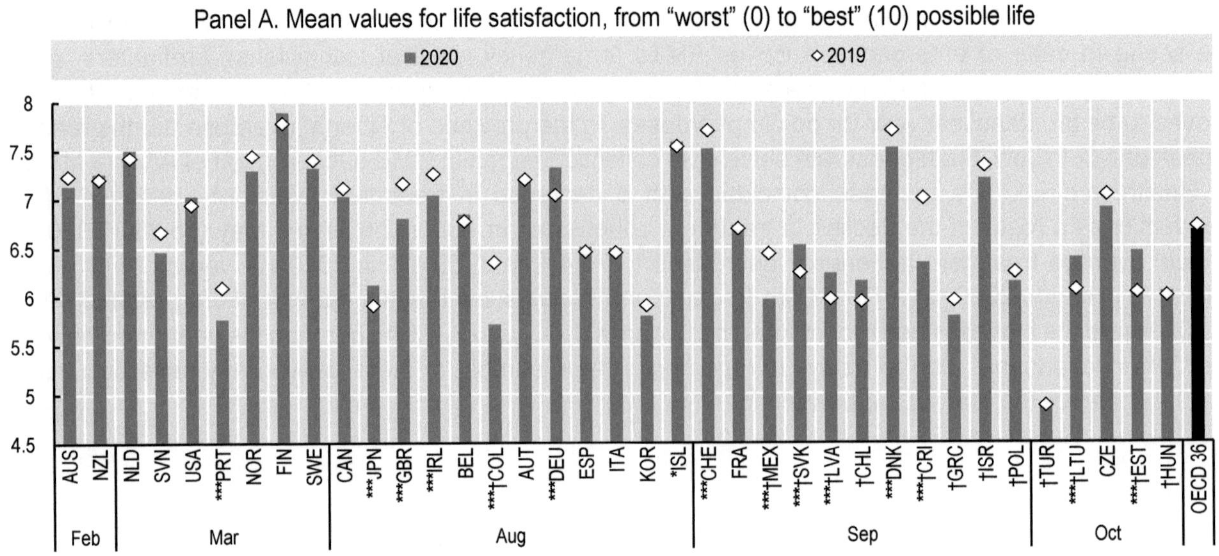

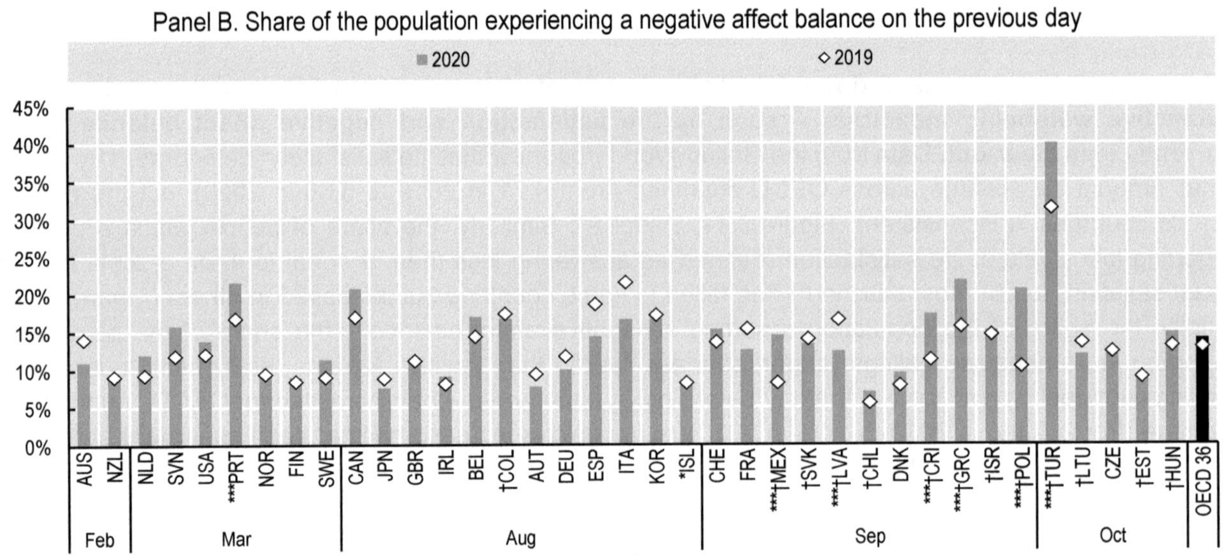

Note: In both panels, countries preceded by *** experienced statistically significant (at the 5% level) changes in outcomes from 2019 to 2020. † denotes countries in which the mode of data collection changed between 2019 and 2020 (generally, moving from face-to-face interviews to phone-based interviews). * denotes countries with between 301 and 500 observations. More than 500 observations are available for all other countries. The OECD average excludes Luxembourg (no data in 2020) and the Czech Republic (no data in 2019). The 2019 value for the Czech Republic refers to 2018. Countries are ranked by fieldwork start date (earliest to latest) in 2020. Refer to the Reader's Guide for a complete list of Gallup World Poll data collection dates in 2020, and to Box 3.4 for additional information about the data collection methodology.
Source: OECD calculations based on the *Gallup World Poll* (n.d.[78]) (database), https://www.gallup.com/178667/gallup-world-poll-work.aspx.

StatLink https://stat.link/816day

Figure 3.12. Deprivations in life satisfaction slightly increased on average in the OECD, with mixed patterns across countries

Share of the population rating their life satisfaction as 4 or lower (on a 0-10 scale), 2019-20

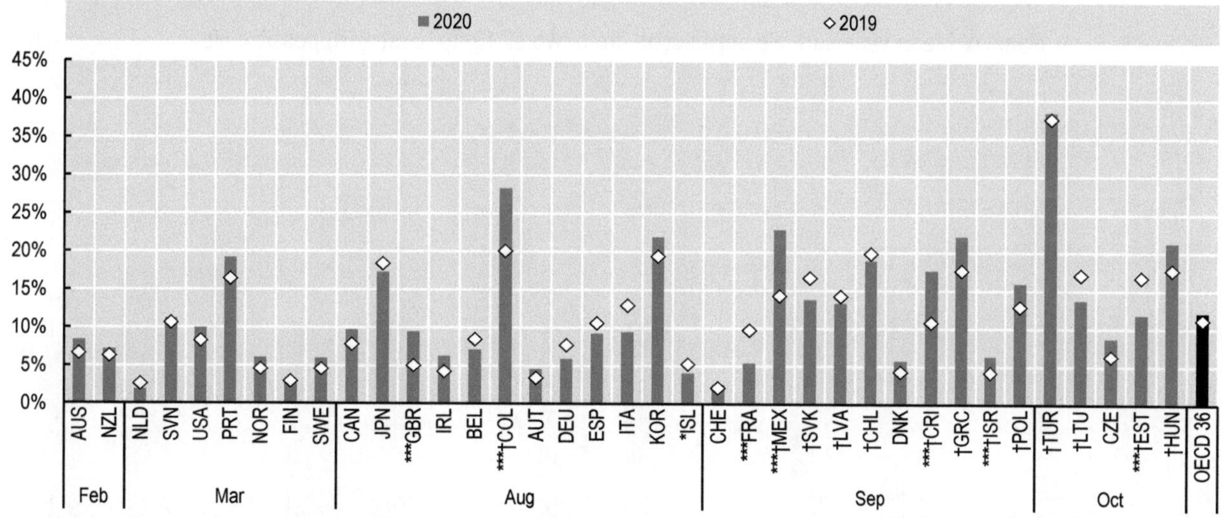

Note: Deprivation in life satisfaction is defined as answering 4 or less on the 0-10 Cantril ladder scale measuring life satisfaction. Countries preceded by *** experienced statistically significant (at the 5% level) changes in outcomes from 2019 to 2020. † denotes countries in which the mode of data collection changed between 2019 and 2020 (generally, moving from face-to-face interviews to phone-based interviews). * denotes countries with between 301 and 500 observations. More than 500 observations are available for all other countries. The OECD average excludes Luxembourg (no data in 2020) and the Czech Republic (no data in 2019). The 2019 value for the Czech Republic refers to 2018. Countries are ranked by fieldwork start date (earliest to latest) in 2020. Refer to the Reader's Guide for a complete list of Gallup World Poll data collection dates in 2020, and to Box 3.4 for additional information about the data collection methodology.

Source: OECD calculations based on the *Gallup World Poll* (n.d.[78]) (database), https://www.gallup.com/178667/gallup-world-poll-work.aspx.

StatLink https://stat.link/ivm67n

Countries that experienced worse than average pandemic outcomes, or severe COVID-19 situations that necessitated more stringent than average government responses, feature larger deteriorations in subjective well-being in 2020 than other countries (Figure 3.13). For example, countries that implemented more stringent than average lockdown policies had larger deteriorations in both life satisfaction and negative affect balance, than did countries with less stringent policies. Importantly, these measures are averages *during the period in which Gallup fieldwork was underway*, which differ across countries (refer to Box 3.4 for exact field dates). Similarly, countries with above-average excess death rates experienced a significant decline in life satisfaction, and countries with above-average stay-at-home measures experienced a significant deterioration in negative affect balance. The impact of economic support is somewhat more nuanced, with no significant differences in the subjective well-being outcomes for countries above the OECD average; however, negative affect balance significantly improved among countries with support below the OECD average. This is likely because the average outcomes for countries with low economic support includes both countries that were not, at the time, severely negatively impacted by the pandemic – thus not needing support – as well as countries that simply did not provide support. Similarly, respondents in countries that provided above-OECD average economic support likely experienced positive subjective well-being impacts from the support received, and negative subjective well-being impacts from necessitating the support in the first place (unemployment, job insecurity, etc.).

Figure 3.13. The pandemic context during fieldwork is key to understanding subjective well-being outcomes across OECD countries

Selected measures of subjective well-being by country groupings according to pandemic outcome and policy response, 2019-20

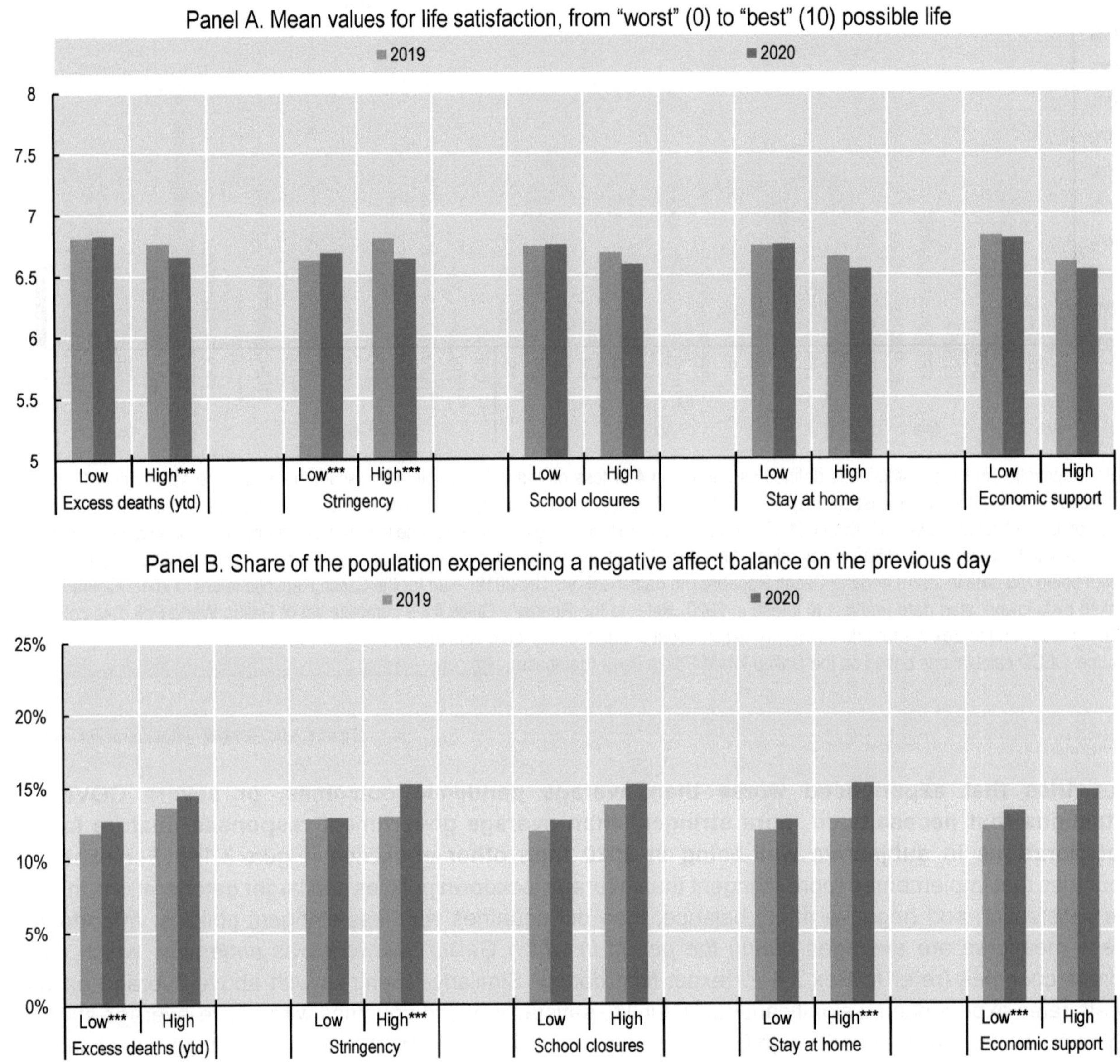

Note: Low and high groupings are made by grouping countries that have below (or above) the OECD average value during the duration of Gallup fieldwork. See the Reader's Guide for a complete list of Gallup World Poll data collection dates in 2020, and to Box 3.4 for additional information about the data collection methodology. Because the groups are relative, the countries included in low vs. high groupings vary by indicator.[11] The Czech Republic and Luxembourg are not included due to missing data in 2019 and 2020, respectively. Categories followed by *** experienced statistically significant (at the 5% level) changes in outcomes from 2019 to 2020.

Source: OECD calculations based on the *Gallup World Poll* (n.d.[78]) (database), https://www.gallup.com/178667/gallup-world-poll-work.aspx; OECD (n.d.[13]), *COVID-19 Health Indicators* (database), https://stats.oecd.org/index.aspx?queryid=104676#; and Hale et.al (2021[79]), "A global panel database of pandemic policies (Oxford COVID-19 Government Response Tracker)", *Nature Human Behaviour*, Vol. 5/4, pp. 529-538, http://dx.doi.org/10.1038/s41562-021-01079-8.

StatLink https://stat.link/9jyhbg

Another important explanation for lack of clear trends is that **averages in life satisfaction mask large inequalities within national populations:** while the pandemic has caused great suffering in some parts of the population, its effects have been far from uniform. Women (especially mothers), parents of school-age children, young people, those with financial and employment difficulties, and racial and ethnic minority groups reported greater drops in both life satisfaction and negative affect balance than their peers (refer to Chapter 6, as well as Chapters 5 and 7).

Box 3.3. Spotlight: Evidence from individual OECD countries shows both declines in life satisfaction as well as resilience in the face of the pandemic

Evidence from the Office for National Statistics (ONS) Annual Population Survey (APS) in Great Britain shows that life satisfaction dropped in the second quarter of 2020, erasing more than five years' worth of gains (Figure 3.14, Panel A) and ending a decade of small but steady improvements in subjective well-being (Hardoon, 2021[80]). As of September 2020, life satisfaction had not yet rebounded. Data from the German SOEP-CoV survey (see Box 3.1 for details) show a decline in life satisfaction in April-June 2020 relative to the previous year, but to levels not significantly different from recent years (i.e. 2017); however, a follow-up survey in 2021 showed that life satisfaction had fallen significantly, to the lowest levels since 2016 (Figure 3.14, Panel B).

Quarterly data from France show a different picture, at least in the early stages of the pandemic (Figure 3.14, Panel C). Subjective well-being data collected by the Observatoire du Bien-être of CEPREMAP beginning in 2016, based on a representative sample of 1 800 respondents, show that life satisfaction reached a four-year high in late May/early June 2020. This peak coincided with de-confinement measures introduced after several months of strict lockdown (CEPREMAP, n.d.[81]).This surprising result could reflect the mitigating effects of government policies to protect livelihoods during the lockdown, or to changing frames of reference: after months in confinement, the lifting of restrictions may have led to spikes in satisfaction. The relationship of the spike with lockdown measures seems likely, as data from March 2021 showed that life satisfaction had fallen to the lowest levels since data collection began: this coincided with the third national lockdown (Perona and Senik, 2021[82]).

Conversely, life satisfaction in New Zealand has remained more or less stable over the past few years (Figure 3.14, Panel D). Data indicate an average life satisfaction level of 7.9 in 2020, up from 7.7 in 2018. These increases were reasonably consistent across most population groups (gender, age, ethnicity, region) (New Zealand Government, 2021[83]). However, New Zealand was quick to react and contain the pandemic and as a result had fewer cases, fewer fatalities, and a shorter period of domestic restrictions overall in 2020, relative to many other OECD countries.

Life satisfaction trends in 2020 may also respond to non-pandemic events. Data from the ANU Poll found that life satisfaction in Australia fell from 6.9 in January 2020 to 6.5 in April 2020, but quickly rebounded to 6.8 by April and May; by November 2020, life satisfaction reached 7.1, which was not significantly different from levels in October 2019 (Biddle et al., 2020[84]; Biddle et al., 2020[85]). While ANU researchers suggested that increases in life satisfaction beginning in April and May could be the result of easing lockdown restrictions and declining COVID rates, they speculate that the low rates of life satisfaction in January 2020 (6.9, compared to 7.1 three months prior) are more likely to reflect the Black Summer Bushfire crisis than any pandemic-related event (Biddle et al., 2020[85]).

Figure 3.14. Changes to trends in life satisfaction in 2020 varied depending on OECD countries' experiences of the pandemic

Mean life satisfaction values, from "not at all" (0) to "completely satisfied" (10)

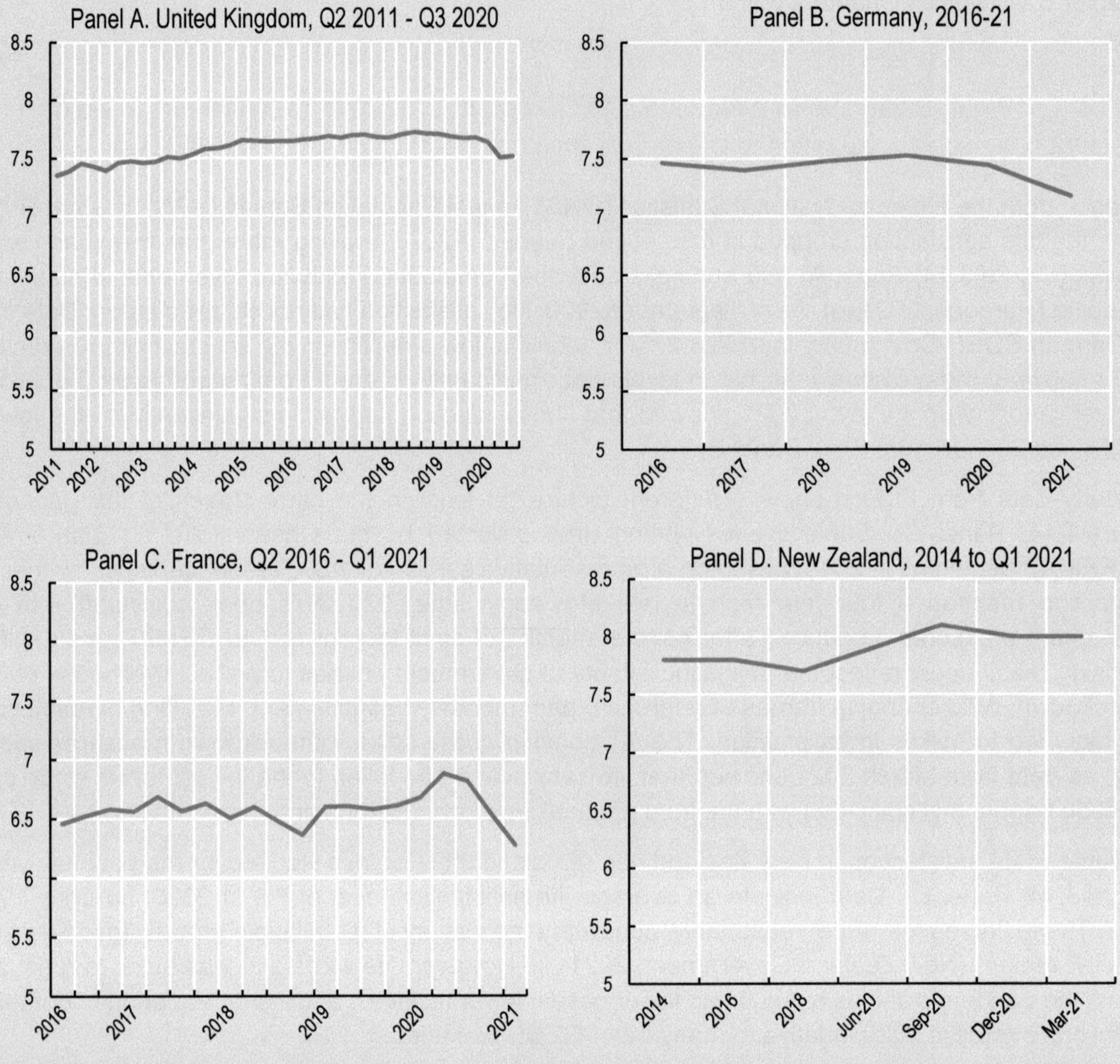

Note: In Panel A, data are seasonally adjusted quarterly estimates. The ONS changed data collection methods in March 2020 due to COVID-19, and data have been adjusted to make post-March 2020 data comparable. In Panel B, refer to Box 3.1 for more information on the SOEP-CoV survey. In Panel C, quarterly data are provided for a representative sample of 1 800 people. In Panel D, from June 2020 to March 2021, a selection of well-being questions were added to the regular household labour force survey (HLFS): one person aged 18+ was randomly selected from households to complete the questionnaire, and data were then weighted to be representative of the June 2020 population. Given methodological differences between the 2020-2021 data collection and the data collected from the General Social Survey (GSS) in preceding years, Stats NZ cautions against drawing strong conclusions comparing 2020-2021 outcomes with preceding years.

Source: ONS (n.d.[86]), *Quarterly Personal Well-being Estimates – Seasonally Adjusted* (database), Office of National Statistics, https://www.ons.gov.uk/peoplepopulationandcommunity/wellbeing/datasets/quarterlypersonalwellbeingestimatesseasonallyadjusted (Panel A); Kühne et al. (2020[46]), "The need for household panel surveys in times of crisis: The case of SOEP-CoV", *Survey Research Methods*, Vol. 14/2, pp. 195-203, https://doi.org/10.18148/srm/2020.v14i2.7748 (Panel B); CEPREMAP/INSEE (n.d.[81]), *Le Bien-être en France* (database), http://www.cepremap.fr/Duree.html (Panel C); and Stats NZ (n.d.[87]), *Wellbeing Statistics: March 2021 Quarter* (database), https://www.stats.govt.nz/information-releases/wellbeing-statistics-march-2021-quarter (Panel D).

StatLink https://stat.link/g2o5m6

Box 3.4. Methods: Gallup World Poll Data in 2020

The Gallup World Poll has been collecting nationally representative data in over 150 countries, including all 38 OECD countries, since 2007. The questionnaire includes a variety of topics, including business and economics, government and politics, and health (including mental health). Four of the headline indicators in the OECD's *How's Life?* report are measured using Gallup World Poll data, due to the absence of official data harmonised across member countries.[1] In general, Gallup World Poll data focus on people's opinions and perceptions. The survey is a repeated cross-section, meaning that respondents are sampled during each survey wave and are not tracked over time. Sample sizes vary by country, year and indicator type (from as small as 400 to as large as 13 000 and more), but average around 1 000 respondents. Gallup World Poll data in 2020 provide an opportunity to study the impacts of COVID-19 as they unfolded, in that fieldwork took place at different times in different countries, each of which experienced peaks and troughs of the virus at different times (Figure 3.15). Because of varying on-the-ground circumstances, each figure in this publication that presents Gallup data includes the timing of field work and ranks countries in chronological order of data collection.

Figure 3.15. Fieldwork timelines for the Gallup World Poll, 2020

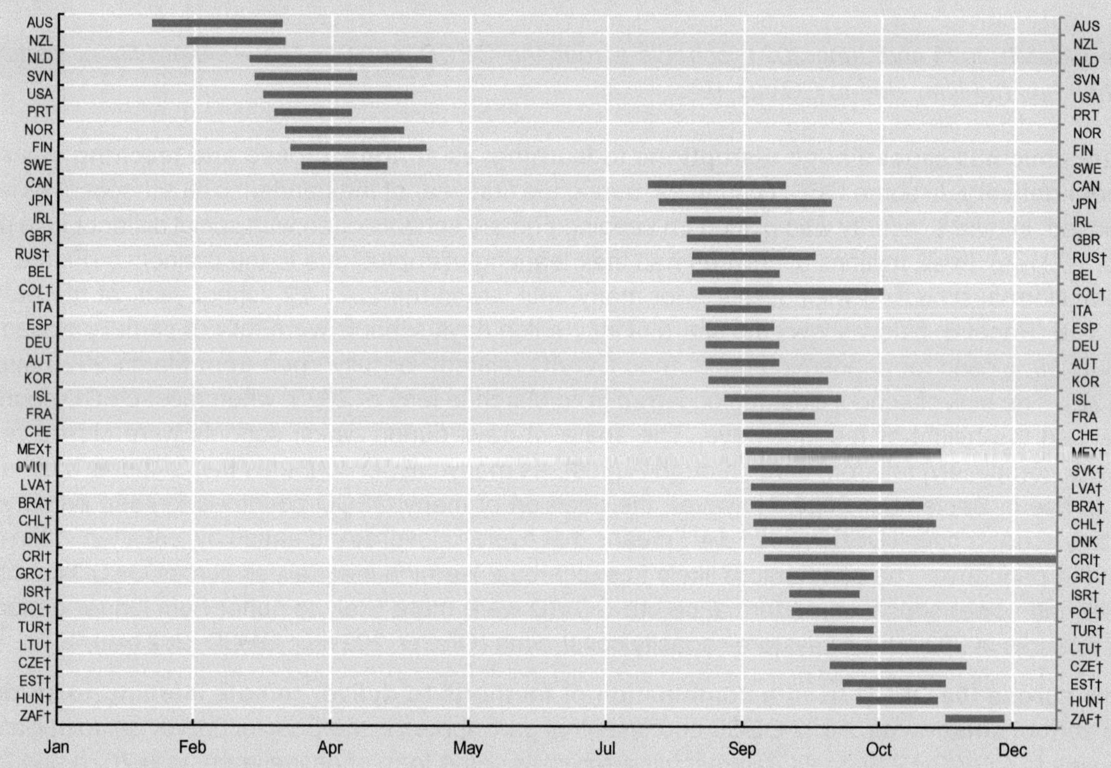

Note: † denotes countries in which the mode of data collection changed between 2019 and 2020 (generally, moving from face-to-face interviews to phone-based interviews).

Source: *Gallup World Poll* (n.d.[78]) (database), https://www.gallup.com/178667/gallup-world-poll-work.aspx.

StatLink https://stat.link/gkfnme

Gallup survey data are collected through a combination of face-to-face and telephone (mobile and/or landline) interviews, depending on the country. From around March 2020 onwards, all data collection transitioned to telephone interviewing. Prior to 2020, data in the majority of OECD countries were already collected entirely over the phone. However, in 14 OECD countries (Chile, Colombia, Costa Rica, the Czech Republic, Estonia, Greece, Hungary, Israel, Lithuania, Latvia, Mexico, Poland, the Slovak Republic and Turkey) and three partner countries (Brazil, the Russian Federation and South Africa), interviews previously conducted face-to-face were switched in 2020 to telephone-based, which may result in some mode effects. In this publication, all countries with data collection method switches are marked with † in figures.

Notes:

1. These comprise negative affect balance, gender gap in feeling safe at night, perceived lack of social support, and trust in national government. In general, three-year pooled averages are used when reporting Gallup Data in official OECD publications. This increases the number of observations within each country to allow for sufficiently large samples to estimate inequalities in gender, age and educational attainment outcomes. Not all countries are surveyed annually, therefore pooled averages also reduce the gaps in country coverage. This procedure is relaxed in the current publication, since the main aim is to detect 2019 to 2020 changes in outcomes.

3.3. Knowledge and skills

Between March 2020 and June 2021, schools across the OECD were closed – either fully or partially – more than half the time, due to COVID-19

The pandemic has caused huge disruptions to learning, as schools closed and teaching switched to remote delivery. In some OECD countries, during the first year of the pandemic all schools of all levels were closed; in others, priority was placed on keeping primary schools open with social distancing in place (OECD, 2021[88]). In all, millions of children had their learning disrupted due to the pandemic (Figure 3.16, Panel A). Normal schooling will not return for many until late in the 2021-22 school year, at the earliest. Figure 3.16 (Panel B) below shows the share of instruction days schools were fully or partially closed due to COVID-19, closed for academic breaks (non-COVID related), or fully open from March 2020 through June 2021. The bulk of school closures occurred from March to May of 2020, when most OECD countries experienced the height of the first wave. The share of days during which schools were closed (either partially or completely) fell from June through August, as many OECD countries had summer breaks, but began to rise in September 2020. However, the decision of many OECD countries to keep primary and secondary schools open (OECD, 2021[89])[12] means that overall closures increased by less than in the early days of the pandemic. The pandemic is likely to exacerbate learning inequalities across OECD countries: countries with lower education performance pre-COVID were more likely to suffer from longer periods of school closures in 2020 due to system capacity constraints (OECD, 2021[89]; OECD, 2021[88]).

Schools across the OECD used a combination of methods to deliver remote learning to students during school shutdowns. All 32 OECD countries that participated in the *Special Survey on Joint National Responses to COVID-19 School Closures*[13] implemented some form of online learning in 2020 and 2021. Online platforms were used for primary and secondary institutions in all countries aside from Sweden and the Russian Federation, where online solutions were not used in primary schools (OECD, 2021[90]). Take-home packages and television were the second-most common form of instructional delivery, with the first method more commonly used (by 84% of countries surveyed) in primary and lower-secondary schools (OECD, 2021[90]). Given the focus on online instruction, most OECD countries reported introducing measures to ensure inclusion in distance learning, including the introduction of self-paced coursework, partnering with mobile networks to increase access to the Internet, distributing or subsidising digital infrastructure, and providing economic support to low-income households (OECD, 2021[90]).

Figure 3.16. Millions of children across OECD countries had their schooling interrupted

Panel A. Share of instruction days when schools were closed (fully or partially) due to the pandemic, Mar 2020 – Jun 2021

Panel B. Share of instruction days when schools were closed (fully or partially) due to the pandemic, on academic break, or fully open, OECD, Mar 2020 – Jun 2021

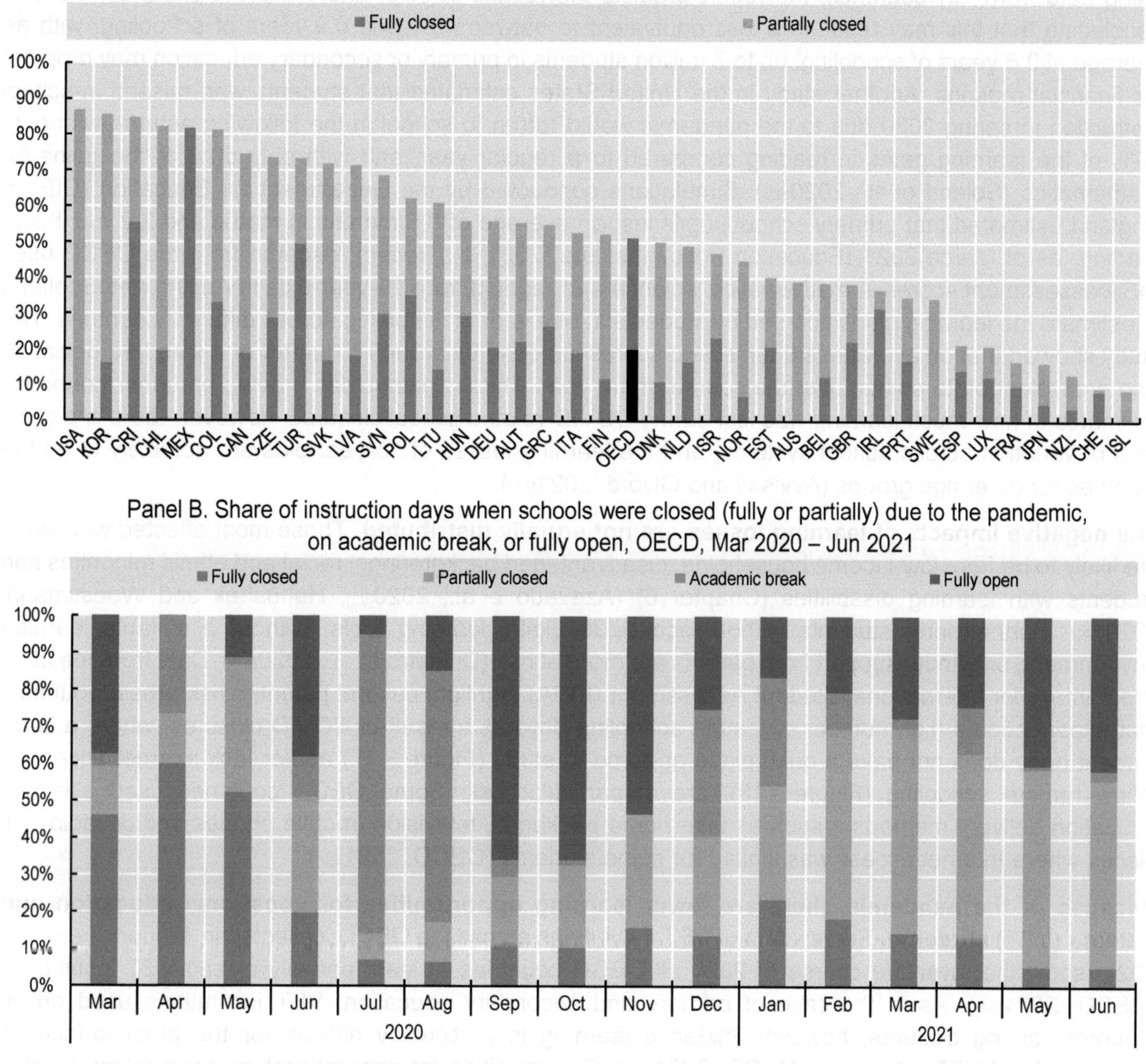

Note: "Fully closed" is defined as government-mandated closures of schools (pre-primary through upper secondary, ISCED levels 0 through 3) because of the COVID-19 pandemic. "Partially closed" refers to instances in which schools are closed in certain regions only, and/or are closed for some grade levels/age groups but not others, and/or are employing a hybrid (in-person combined with distance learning) approach. Panel A shows the share of days during which schools fully or partially closed due to COVID-19, as a share of the total number of all instruction days (i.e., excluding school holidays, public holidays and weekends), as a pooled average from March 2020 to June 2021. Panel B shows the OECD average of the share of days during which school was closed either fully or partially due to COVID-19, or was fully open, or was on academic break, during the same time period.

Source: UNESCO (n.d.[91]), *Global Monitoring of School Closures, COVID-19* (database), United Nations Educational, Scientific and Cultural Organization, https://en.unesco.org/covid19/educationresponse.

StatLink https://stat.link/txz1f5

Even temporary school closures are likely to lead to significant learning losses. The World Bank estimates that learning disruptions caused by the pandemic could lead to a 25% increase in the share of secondary students performing below PISA level 2 (Azevedo et al., 2020[92]). Through a series of models using data from 157 countries, the report predicts the results of 3, 5, and 7 months of school closure, concluding that this may result in a loss equivalent to between 0.3 and 0.9 years of schooling, with an average of 0.6 years of schooling; up to 7 million students in primary or secondary education may drop out for financial reasons. Another study in the United States estimated that students who missed in-school instruction in spring 2020 due to the pandemic would return to school in the following autumn with only 70% of the learning gains in reading compared to a regular year, and with only 50% of the gains for mathematics (Soland et al., 2020[93]). Simulations conducted by the Department for Education (DfE) in England estimated that primary school pupils lost an average of 3.5 months in maths and 2.2 months in reading, as of March 2021 (Education Policy Institute, 2021[94]). Recent research from the OECD uses PISA assessment scores in mathematics, science and reading from 15-year-olds in Austria and Scotland to estimate the learning gains accrued by students in one year of schooling across different countries. The study showed that on average, students' test scores increase by around a quarter of a standard deviation (the equivalent of 25 points) over the course of the year. These findings can provide an upper bound for estimates of how much learning was lost during COVID-related school closures; however, there is a great deal of variation across school systems, and the learning losses of 15-year-olds are not likely to be the same as for other age groups (Avvisati and Givord, 2021[95]).

The negative impacts of learning losses are not equally distributed. Those most affected worldwide are likely to be from low-income households, disadvantaged backgrounds, racial and ethnic minorities and students with learning disabilities (Chapter 6) (Azevedo et al., 2020[92]; Hanushek and Woessmann, 2020[96]). Furthermore, students without access to digital learning tools, without a suitable learning environment, or without support from parents are more at risk (Di Pietro et al., 2020[97]). Data from the 2018 Programme for International Student Assessment (PISA) highlight several potential risk areas: countries that experienced a high number of remote schooling days as a result of COVID closures, where a large student body does not have a quiet place at home to study (Figure 3.17) and/or lack Internet access to follow remote schooling (Figure 3.18), are at particular risk. Some OECD countries used alternate education delivery methods – such as take-home packages, television, mobile phones and/or radio – in places where Internet access was limited for some students (OECD, 2021[90]).

Because of the pandemic, there are fewer learning opportunities for vocational education and training (VET) students. Survey data of VET institutions across the OECD, collected in January-February 2021, show that over the course of 2020 all OECD countries at least partially closed VET institutions (OECD, 2021[98]). As in the case of primary and secondary education, VET institutions used online platforms during closures, however, distance learning is particularly difficult for the practice-focused components of VET education (OECD, 2021[98]). Opportunities for apprenticeships have fallen, limiting opportunities for VET students entering the workforce. Indeed, a survey of enterprises in 114 countries conducted by the International Labour Organization (ILO) from April to June 2020 found that 55% of firms reported that the training of apprentices had been completely disrupted by the pandemic, and another 31% indicated that this had been partially disrupted (ILO, 2021[99]). Shortages of work-based learning opportunities could mean fewer students able to graduate in the short term, but in the long term it may lead to fewer students choosing to enter VET programmes in the first place (OECD, 2021[98]). Given the difficulties in completing the work-based training components of VET, a number of programmes made adjustments to graduation requirements in 2020. Perhaps because of the relaxation of certain restrictions, in 8 of the 14 countries for which data are available, VET graduation rates increased in 2019-20 compared to the previous academic year (OECD, 2021[98]). However, given the changes to the programmes, there are some concerns as to how prepared these students will be in the long term. In general, these disruptions to VET training have a number of consequences, including potential long-term shortages of important skills in the labour market, along with an increase the share of youth not in education, employment or training (NEET) (OECD, 2021[100]).

Figure 3.17. OECD countries with high rates of school closures and large numbers of students without a suitable place to study at home are particularly at risk of falling behind in educational achievement

Share of instruction days when schools were fully or partially closed due to the pandemic, Mar 2020 – Jun 2021, and share of students with a desk and quiet place to study at home, 2018

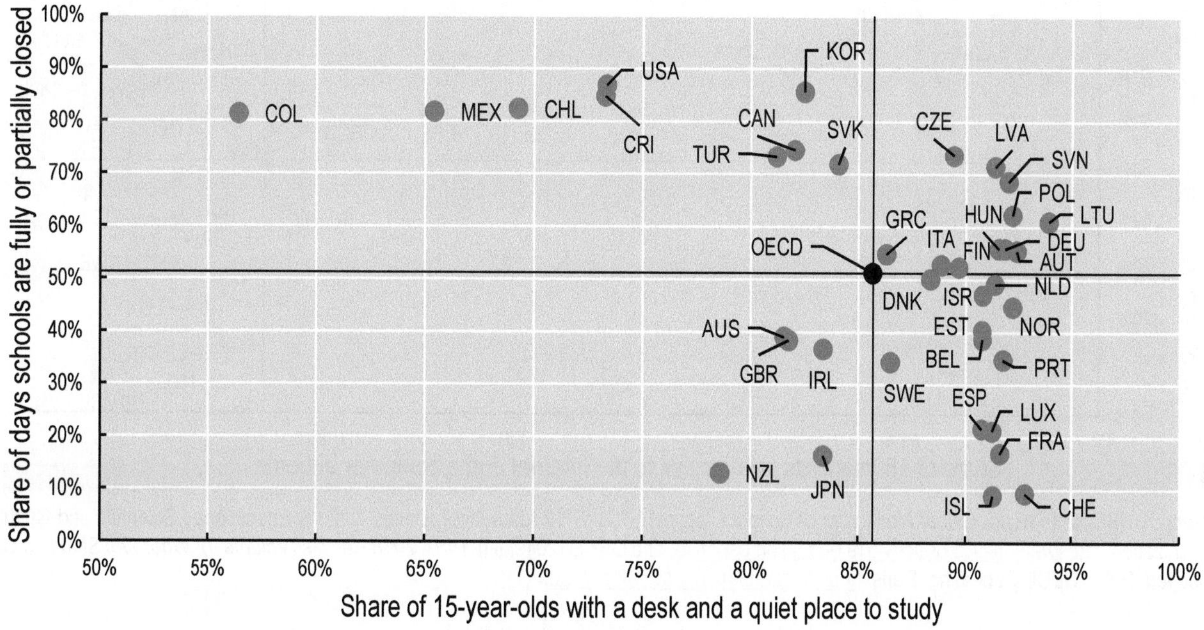

Source: UNESCO (n.d.[91]), *Global Monitoring of School Closures, COVID-19* (database), United Nations Educational, Scientific and Cultural Organization, https://en.unesco.org/covid19/educationresponse; and OECD (2019[101]), *PISA 2018 Results (Volume II): Where All Students Can Succeed*, PISA, OECD Publishing, Paris, https://doi.org/10.1787/b5fd1b8f-en.

StatLink https://stat.link/cljzf8

On-the-job training has also fallen during the pandemic. OECD data show that prior to COVID-19, workers across the OECD spent 4.9 hours per week, on average, in informal learning and 0.7 hours in non-formal learning.[14] Simulations show that, during the pandemic, these rates would have dropped to 3.7 hours and 0.6 hours, respectively, i.e. a notable learning loss (OECD, 2021[102]). It is also estimated that low-skilled adults would have been disproportionately affected, as their jobs could not be conducted remotely, and on-the-job learning (non-formal and informal) would have been interrupted entirely. Disruptions to work-based training may not dissipate in the near term. Survey data from the ILO show that 52% of enterprises agreed with the statement that they envisaged a reduction in investment in training and development due to financial constraints "following the pandemic": these rates were highest for micro, small and medium enterprises (61%) and for governmental and public organisations (52%) (ILO, 2021[99]).

Figure 3.18. Remote learning can be difficult if students lack access to digital tools

Share of instruction days when schools were fully or partially closed due to the pandemic, Mar 2020 – Jun 2021, and share of students with access to the Internet and a computer at home, 2018

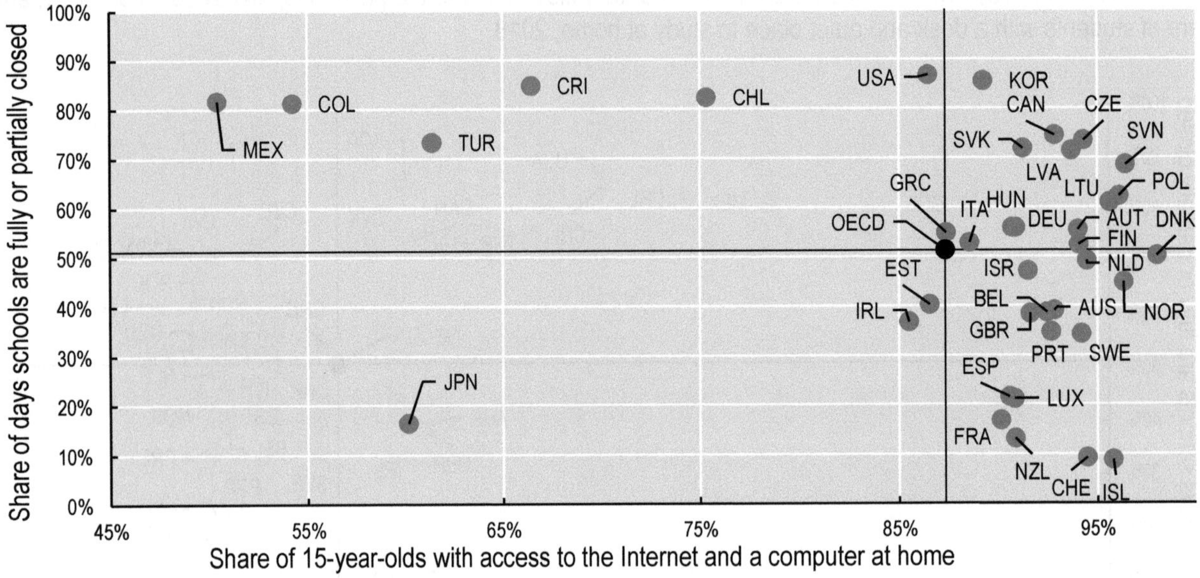

Source: UNESCO (n.d.[91]), *Global Monitoring of School Closures, COVID-19* (database), United Nations Educational, Scientific and Cultural Organization, https://en.unesco.org/covid19/educationresponse; and OECD (2019[101]), *PISA 2018 Results (Volume II): Where All Students Can Succeed*, PISA, OECD Publishing, Paris, https://doi.org/10.1787/b5fd1b8f-en.

StatLink https://stat.link/pnzm9d

3.4. Environmental quality

3.4.1. Air pollution and access to green space

Lockdowns did not bring hoped-for reductions in air pollution, and evidence shows no significant improvements in air quality over the course of 2020

The pandemic has had profound impacts for population groups impacted by climate change and natural disasters as well as on long-term natural capital (Chapter 11); but it has also affected the day-to-day environmental conditions of OECD residents. **Air pollution is a risk factor for COVID-19 infection and outcomes**. Recent research conducted in the first half of 2020 estimated that long-term exposure to air pollution contributed to around 15% of global COVID-19 deaths (Pozzer et al., 2020[103]). A study in the United States showed that individuals with long-term exposure to high levels of fine particulate matter ($PM_{2.5}$) in the air had more severe COVID-19 symptoms, including increased mortality rates (Wu et al., 2020[104]). A study in Canada corroborates this finding, showing a positive association between the incidence of COVID-19 and long-term $PM_{2.5}$ exposure (Stieb et al., 2020[105]). Conversely, a study by the Office for National Statistics in the United Kingdom found that once ethnicity was controlled for, long-term exposure to air pollution did not have a significant impact on COVID-19 deaths between 27 March and 12 June 2020 in England (ONS, 2020[106]). Even prior to the pandemic, research had demonstrated that exposure to elevated levels of $PM_{2.5}$ increased the risk of heart disease, stroke, respiratory diseases and respiratory infections (OECD, 2020[107]). Nearly two-thirds of people in OECD countries were exposed to dangerous levels of $PM_{2.5}$ in 2017 (OECD, 2020[108]).

The first lockdowns to curb the COVID-19 pandemic led to a temporary decrease in some forms of pollution and greenhouse gas emissions – primarily through lowered activity in the transport and industrial sectors (OECD, 2020[109]) (Chapter 11). While CO_2 and NO_2 emissions fell temporarily in most countries with strict business lockdown and confinement measures (Le Quéré et al., 2020[110]; Narain, 2020[111]; Berman and Ebisu, 2020[112]),[15] the impacts of confinement on $PM_{2.5}$ levels are ambiguous. Studies in the United States, China, India and Australia reported a modest decline in $PM_{2.5}$, especially in areas that are more urban, colder and more industrialised (Berman and Ebisu, 2020[112]; He, Pan and Tanaka, 2020[113]; Wang et al., 2020[114]; Kumari and Toshniwal, 2020[115]; Duc et al., 2021[116]). However, other cross-country studies found no impact on $PM_{2.5}$ levels (Narain, 2020[111]; Air Quality Expert Group, 2020[117]). The sources of $PM_{2.5}$ are multifaceted and include both human-induced factors, such as industrial activity, as well as climate-induced factors.[16]

The ambiguous relationship between $PM_{2.5}$ levels and confinement measures is shown in Figure 3.19 **below,** which shows $PM_{2.5}$ levels from January 2020 to August of 2021 for the capital cities of France, Germany, Italy and the United Kingdom. As can be seen, there is little noticeable trend in the data; rates in 2020 and 2021 all fall within the range of previous values observed on that day from 2017-19.

With people confined to their homes, concerns about the negative health impacts of indoor air pollution increased (Brunekreef, 2021[118]). According to the World Health Organization, around 4 million people die prematurely from illnesses stemming from household air pollution, including strokes, ischaemic heart disease and chronic obstructive pulmonary disease (COPD) (WHO, 2018[119]). Traditionally, indoor air pollution is associated with the use of cooking and heating fuels: those who have open flames in the home, or stoves fuelled by kerosene, biomass and/or coal, are most at risk. However, recent research suggests that the causes of indoor air pollution go well beyond the fuels themselves. Cooking large meals using modern stoves can cause spikes of indoor $PM_{2.5}$ concentrations as high as 250ugm-3 – a level comparable to the world's most polluted cities (Patel et al., 2020[120]). Living near heavily polluted roadways (EPA, n.d.[121]), as well as the use of household cleaning supplies, tobacco and the presence of mould, can also contribute to indoor pollution, with household ventilation playing an important moderating role (Twilley, 2019[122]). Preliminary research from King's College London suggests that levels of $PM_{2.5}$ exposure in the United Kingdom might have increased during lockdown periods, with the potential decline in outdoor $PM_{2.5}$ air pollution more than offset by an increase in exposure to indoor air pollution (Air Quality Expert Group, 2020[117]).

The mental health and well-being benefits of time spent in nature were all the more important when people were confined to their homes

Access to green space improves mental health and overall well-being. Research across a number of OECD countries has shown that those who spend more time in nature, and who have access to green spaces, are more likely to have higher levels of health (both self-reported and objective measures) (de Bell et al., 2020[123]; WHO Regional Office for Europe, 2016[124]), better psychological and emotional well-being (Mayer et al., 2008[125]; Engemann et al., 2019[126]; Crouse et al., 2021[127]; Astell-Burt and Feng, 2019[128]), and are more likely to live longer (Rojas-Rueda et al., 2019[129]). It is not just green space that provides well-being benefits: living and spending time near natural water features ("blue space") is also associated with reduced risks of mortality, especially for women and older adults (Crouse et al., 2018[130]).

Evidence from COVID-19 corroborates the relationship between time spent in nature and general well-being. Data collected in the People and Nature Survey for England in April through June 2020 found that 85% of adult respondents reported that being in nature made them happy, and that those who spent time in a natural place within the past week had higher levels of reported happiness than those who did not (Natural England, 2020[131]). Data from the first week of April in France showed that those with access to green space (either public or private) reported significantly higher levels of subjective well-being (Recchi et al., 2020[132]).[17] An online questionnaire of 3 000 Japanese respondents in June 2020 found that the frequency of greenspace use, and the existence of windows within the home overlooking greenspaces, was associated with higher levels of self-esteem, life satisfaction and happiness, and decreased levels of depression, anxiety and loneliness – even after controlling for socio-demographic characteristics and lifestyle variables (Soga et al., 2021[133]).

Figure 3.19. No clear link between pandemic lockdowns and PM2.5 levels in European cities throughout 2020 and 2021

PM2.5 daily levels from 3 Jan 2020 - 8 Aug 2021, compared to 2017-19 baseline averages

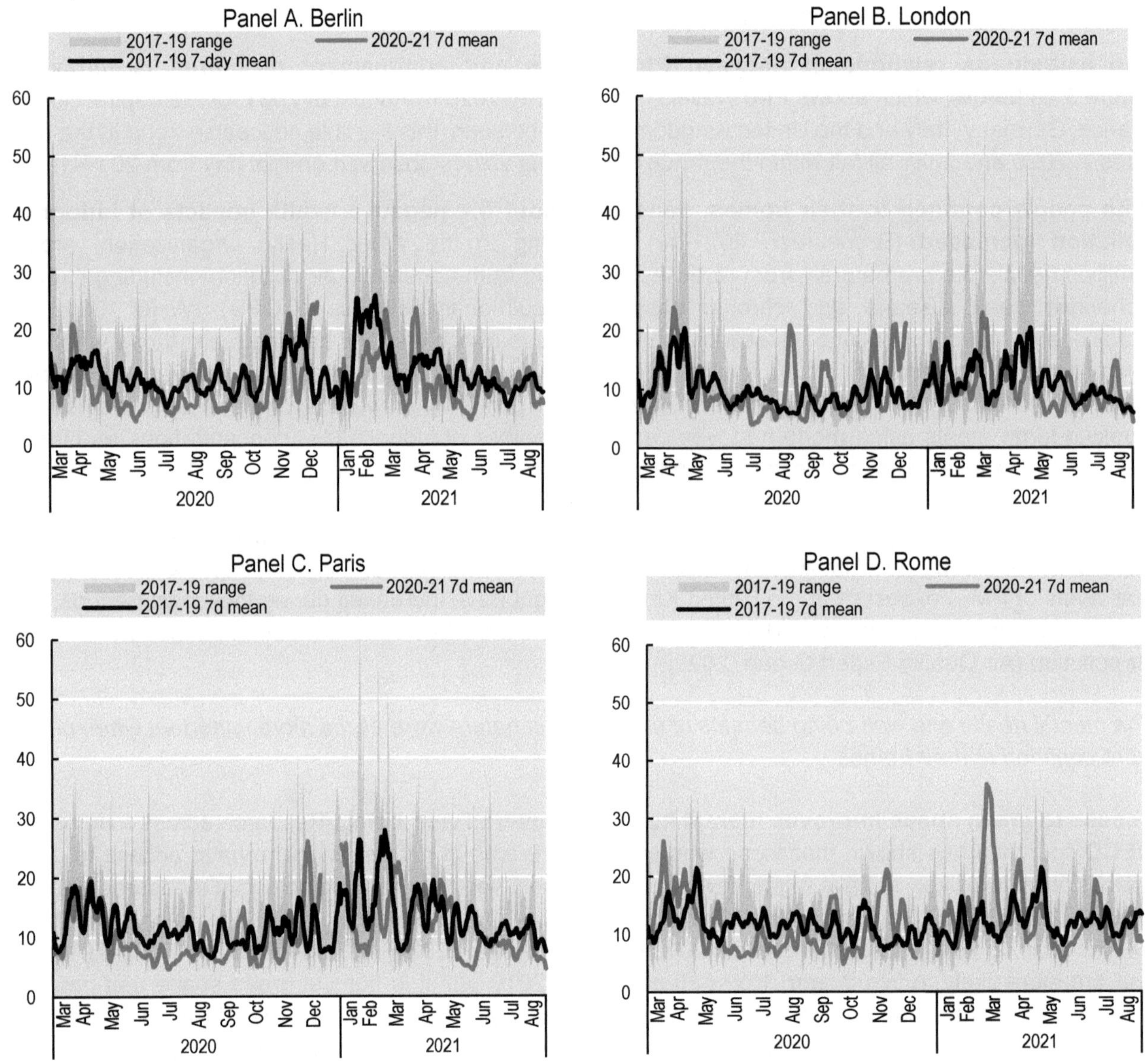

Note: All panels show the seven-day moving average of PM2.5 from March 2020 to August 2021 – shown in green – compared to the seven-day moving average during the baseline period (2017 to 2019), shown in black. The full range of PM2.5 values from the period 2017-2019 is shown in grey shading.

Source: CAMS (n.d.[134]), *European Air Quality Information in Support of the COVID-19 Crisis* (database), Copernicus Atmosphere Monitoring Service, https://atmosphere.copernicus.eu/european-air-quality-information-support-covid-19-crisis.

StatLink https://stat.link/5h8k1o

Box 3.5. Further reading

- OECD (forthcoming), *Health at a Glance 2021: OECD Indicators*, OECD Publishing, Paris
- Morgan et al. (2020), "Excess mortality: Measuring the direct and indirect impact of COVID-19", *OECD Health Working Papers*, No. 122, OECD Publishing, Paris, https://dx.doi.org/10.1787/c5dc0c50-en
- OECD (2021), "Tackling the mental health impact of the COVID-19 crisis: An integrated, whole-of-society response," *OECD Policy Responses to Coronavirus (COVID-19)*, OECD Publishing, Paris, https://doi.org/10.1787/0ccafa0b-en
- OECD (2021), *The State of Global Education: 18 Months into the COVID Pandemic*, OECD Publishing, Paris, https://doi.org/10.1787/1a23bb23-en
- OECD (2021), *Data Insights: Green Recovery*, OECD, Paris, http://www.oecd.org/coronavirus/en/data-insights

References

ABS (2020), *Household Impacts of COVID-19 Survey, 24-29 June 2020*, Australian Bureau of Statistics, https://www.abs.gov.au/statistics/people/people-and-communities/household-impacts-covid-19-survey/24-29-june-2020#emotional-and-mental-wellbeing. [37]

Ahmad, F. and L. Rossen (2021), *Provisional drug overdose death counts*, National Center for Health Statistics, https://www.cdc.gov/nchs/nvss/vsrr/drug-overdose-data.htm (accessed on 21 July 2021). [72]

AIHW (2021), *The first year of COVID-19 in Australia: Direct and indirect health effects, Summary*, Australian Institute of Health and Welfare, https://www.aihw.gov.au/reports/burden-of-disease/the-first-year-of-covid-19-in-australia/summary. [38]

Air Quality Expert Group (2020), *Estimation of changes in air pollution emissions, concentrations and exposure during the COVID-19 outbreak in the UK*, Department for Environment Food & Rural Affairs, https://uk-air.defra.gov.uk/library/reports.php?report_id=1005. [117]

Arias, E., B. Tejada-Vera and F. Ahmad (2021), "Provisional life expectancy estimates for January through June, 2020", *Vital Statistics Rapid Release*, Vol. 10, https://www.cdc.gov/nchs/data/vsrr/VSRR10-508.pdf (accessed on 3 March 2021). [11]

Astell-Burt, T. and X. Feng (2019), "Association of urban green space with mental health and general health among adults in Australia", *JAMA Network Open*, Vol. 2/7, pp. e198209-e198209, http://dx.doi.org/10.1001/jamanetworkopen.2019.8209. [128]

Avvisati, F. and P. Givord (2021), "The learning gain over one school year among 15-year-olds: An analysis of PISA data for Austria and Scotland (United Kingdom)", *OECD Education Working Papers*, No. 249, OECD Publishing, Paris, https://doi.org/10.1787/d99e8c0a-en. [95]

Azevedo, J. et al. (2020), *Simulating the potential impacts of the COVID-19 school closures on schooling and learning outcomes: A set of global estimates*, The World Bank, https://www.worldbank.org/en/topic/education/publication/simulating-potential-impacts-of-covid-19-school-closures-learning-outcomes-a-set-of-global-estimates. [92]

Berman, J. and K. Ebisu (2020), "Changes in U.S. air pollution during the COVID-19 pandemic", *Science of the Total Environment*, Vol. 739, p. 139864, http://dx.doi.org/10.1016/J.SCITOTENV.2020.139864. [112]

Biddle, N. et al. (2020), "Tracking outcomes during the COVID-19 pandemic (August 2020) – Divergence within Australia", *COVID-19 Briefing Paper*, ANU Centre for Social Research and Methods, Australian National University, https://csrm.cass.anu.edu.au/research/publications/tracking-outcomes-during-covid-19-pandemic-august-2020-divergence-within. [84]

Biddle, N. et al. (2020), "Tracking outcomes during the COVID-19 pandemic (November 2020) – Counting the costs of the COVID-recession", *COVID-19 Briefing Paper*, ANU Centre for Social Research and Methods, Australian National University, https://csrm.cass.anu.edu.au/research/publications/tracking-outcomes-during-covid-19-pandemic-november-2020-counting-costs-covid. [85]

Blair, G. (2020), "Japan suicides decline as COVID-19 lockdown causes shift in stress factors", *The Guardian*, https://www.theguardian.com/world/2020/may/14/japan-suicides-fall-sharply-as-covid-19-lockdown-causes-shift-in-stress-factors. [65]

Brunekreef, B. (2021), *Air pollution and COVID-19*, Policy Department for Economic, Scientific and Quality of Life Policies, https://www.europarl.europa.eu/RegData/etudes/STUD/2021/658216/IPOL_STU(2021)658216_EN.pdf. [118]

CAMS (n.d.), *European Air Quality Information in Support of the COVID-19 Crisis (database)*, Copernicus Atmosphere Monitoring Service, https://atmosphere.copernicus.eu/european-air-quality-information-support-covid-19-crisis (accessed on 18 August 2021). [134]

CBS (2020), *Civil resilience during the Coronavirus crisis among persons aged 21 and over*, Central Bureau of Statistics, https://www.cbs.gov.il/en/mediarelease/Pages/2020/Situation-Report-of-Civil-Resilience-during-the-Coronavirus-Crisis.aspx. [29]

CBS (2020), *Civil resilience during the Coronavirus crisis, findings from a follow-up survey*, Central Bureau of Statistics, https://www.cbs.gov.il/en/mediarelease/Pages/2020/Civil-Resilience-During-the-Coronavirus-Crisis-Findings-from-a-Follow-Up-Survey.aspx. [30]

CDC (2020), *Pulse Survey | COVID-19*, Centers for Disease Control and Prevention, https://www.cdc.gov/coronavirus/2019-ncov/communication/accomplishments/pulse-survey.html. [40]

Cénat, J. et al. (2020), "Prevalence of mental health problems in populations affected by the Ebola virus disease: A systematic review and meta-analysis", *Psychiatry Research*, Vol. 289, p. 113033, http://dx.doi.org/10.1016/J.PSYCHRES.2020.113033. [17]

CEPREMAP (n.d.), *Le Bien-être en France (database)*, http://www.cepremap.fr/Duree.html (accessed on 15 June 2021). [81]

Chan, S. et al. (2006), "Elderly suicide and the 2003 SARS epidemic in Hong Kong", *International Journal of Geriatric Psychiatry*, Vol. 21/2, pp. 113-118, http://dx.doi.org/10.1002/GPS.1432. [54]

Crouse, D. et al. (2018), "Associations between living near water and risk of mortality among urban Canadians", *Environmental Health Perspectives*, Vol. 126/7, http://dx.doi.org/10.1289/EHP3397. [130]

Crouse, D. et al. (2021), "Residential greenness and indicators of stress and mental well-being in a Canadian national-level survey", *Environmental Research*, Vol. 192, http://dx.doi.org/10.1016/j.envres.2020.110267. [127]

DANE (n.d.), *Encuesta Pulso Social (database)*, Departamento Administrativo Nacional de Estadística, https://www.dane.gov.co/index.php/estadisticas-por-tema/encuesta-pulso-social (accessed on 21 September 2021). [36]

de Bell, S. et al. (2020), "Spending time in the garden is positively associated with health and wellbeing: Results from a national survey in England", *Landscape and Urban Planning*, Vol. 200, p. 103836, http://dx.doi.org/10.1016/J.LANDURBPLAN.2020.103836. [123]

Debout, M. and J. Fourquet (2016), *Les Français et le suicide*, La Fondation Jean Jaurès, https://www.jean-jaures.org/publication/les-francais-et-le-suicide/. [60]

Di Pietro, G. et al. (2020), *The likely impact of COVID-19 on education: Reflections based on the existing literature and recent international datasets*, Publications Office of the European Union, https://op.europa.eu/en/publication-detail/-/publication/b48d50f6-b753-11ea-bb7a-01aa75ed71a1/language-en. [97]

Diaz Ramirez, M., P. Veneri and A. Lembcke (2021), "Where did it hit harder?: The geography of excess mortality during the COVID-19 pandemic", *OECD Regional Development Papers*, No. 21, OECD Publishing, Paris, https://doi.org/10.1787/ab4848a4-en. [9]

Duc, H. et al. (2021), "The effect of lockdown period during the COVID-19 pandemic on air quality in Sydney region, Australia", *International Journal of Environmental Research and Public Health 2021, Vol. 18, Page 3528*, Vol. 18/7, p. 3528, http://dx.doi.org/10.3390/IJERPH18073528. [116]

Education Policy Institute (2021), *EPI research for the Department for Education on pupil learning loss*, Education Policy Institute, https://epi.org.uk/publications-and-research/department-for-education-publishes-new-epi-research-on-pupil-learning-loss/. [94]

Elbogen, E. et al. (2020), "Financial strain and suicide attempts in a nationally representative sample of US adults", *American Journal of Epidemiology*, Vol. 189/11, pp. 1266-1274, http://dx.doi.org/10.1093/AJE/KWAA146. [55]

Engemann, K. et al. (2019), "Residential green space in childhood is associated with lower risk of psychiatric disorders from adolescence into adulthood", *Proceedings of the National Academy of Sciences of the United States of America*, Vol. 116/11, pp. 5188-5193, http://dx.doi.org/10.1073/pnas.1807504116. [126]

Entringer, T. and H. Kröger (2021), "Psychische Gesundheit im zweiten Covid-19 Lockdown in Deutschland", *SOEP Papers on Multidisciplinary Panel Research*, No. 1136, DIW SOEP, https://www.diw.de/documents/publikationen/73/diw_01.c.819601.de/diw_sp1136.pdf. [47]

EPA (n.d.), *Research on near roadway and other near source air pollution*, United States Environmental Protection Agency, https://www.epa.gov/air-research/research-near-roadway-and-other-near-source-air-pollution (accessed on 13 September 2021). [121]

Ettman, C. et al. (2020), "Prevalence of depression symptoms in US adults before and during the COVID-19 pandemic", *JAMA Network Open*, Vol. 3/9, p. e2019686, http://dx.doi.org/10.1001/JAMANETWORKOPEN.2020.19686. [43]

European Observatory on Health Systems and Policies & WHO (2020), "Managing health services on a seesaw: Balancing the delivery of essential health services whilst responding to COVID-19", *Eurohealth*, Vol. 26/2, https://apps.who.int/iris/handle/10665/336299. [3]

Eurostat (2021), *Excess mortality starting to fall back in 2021, after a large death toll*, Products Eurostat News, https://ec.europa.eu/eurostat/web/products-eurostat-news/-/ddn-20210416-2. [7]

Eurostat (n.d.), *European Health Interview Survey (EHIS) (database)*, https://ec.europa.eu/eurostat/statistics-explained/index.php?title=Glossary:European_health_interview_survey_(EHIS) (accessed on 16 June 2021). [27]

Gallup (n.d.), *Gallup World Poll (database)*, https://www.gallup.com/178667/gallup-world-poll-work.aspx (accessed on 18 June 2021). [78]

Gaubert, C. (2020), *Covid-19 : les suicides, la dernière vague que la crise pourrait déclencher*, https://www.sciencesetavenir.fr/sante/cerveau-et-psy/covid-19-une-crise-qui-menace-d-augmenter-le-risque-de-suicides_149069. [59]

Goebel, J. et al. (2019), "The German socio-economic panel (SOEP)", *Jahrbücher für Nationalökonomie und Statistik*, Vol. 239/2, pp. 345-360, http://dx.doi.org/10.1515/JBNST-2018-0022. [44]

Government of Alberta Ministry of Health (2020), *Alberta COVID-19 opioid response surveillance report Q2 2020*, http://open.alberta.ca/licence. [76]

Government of Alberta Ministry of Health (n.d.), *Substance Use Surveillance Data*, https://www.alberta.ca/substance-use-surveillance-data.aspx#jumplinks-0 (accessed on 17 June 2021). [75]

Graham, C. (2021), *America's crisis of despair: A federal task force for economic recovery and societal well-being*, The Brookings Institution, https://www.brookings.edu/research/americas-crisis-of-despair-a-federal-task-force-for-economic-recovery-and-societal-well-being/?utm_campaign=Brookings%20Brief&utm_medium=email&utm_content=111998200&utm_source=hs_email. [74]

Guzmán Mena, J. and A. Tamayo (2020), *Ansiedad y depresión, 'verdugos' de los jóvenes durante la pandemia*, Pontificia Universidad Javeriana Colombia, https://www.javeriana.edu.co/pesquisa/ansiedad-y-depresion-verdugos-de-los-jovenes-durante-la-pandemia/. [34]

Hale, T. et al. (2021), "A global panel database of pandemic policies (Oxford COVID-19 Government Response Tracker)", *Nature Human Behaviour*, Vol. 5/4, pp. 529-538, http://dx.doi.org/10.1038/s41562-021-01079-8 (accessed on 11 June 2021). [79]

Hanushek, E. and L. Woessmann (2020), "The economic impacts of learning losses", *OECD Education Working Papers*, No. 225, OECD Publishing, Paris, https://doi.org/10.1787/21908d74-en. [96]

Hardoon, D. (2021), *A decade of subjective wellbeing data*, What Works Wellbeing, https://whatworkswellbeing.org/blog/a-decade-of-subjective-wellbeing-data/?mc_cid=ca8e7d2523&mc_eid=19c16de127. [80]

He, G., Y. Pan and T. Tanaka (2020), "The short-term impacts of COVID-19 lockdown on urban air pollution in China", *Nature Sustainability 2020 3:12*, Vol. 3/12, pp. 1005-1011, http://dx.doi.org/10.1038/s41893-020-0581-y. [113]

ILO (2021), *Skilling, upskilling and reskilling of employees, apprentices & interns during the COVID-19 pandemic: Findings from a global survey of enterprises*, International Labour Organization, http://www.ilo.org/skills/areas/work-based-learning/WCMS_794569/lang--en/index.htm. [99]

Imperial College London YouGov (2020), *Covid 19 Behaviour Tracker Data Hub (database)*, https://github.com/YouGov-Data/covid-19-tracker (accessed on 13 July 2021). [1]

Japanese National Police Agency (2021), *令和２年中における自殺の状況*, https://www.npa.go.jp/safetylife/seianki/jisatsu/R03/R02_jisatuno_joukyou.pdf (accessed on 12 May 2021). [71]

John, A. et al. (2020), "Trends in suicide during the COVID-19 pandemic: Prevention must be prioritised while we wait for a clearer picture", *BMJ*, Vol. 371, p. m4352, http://dx.doi.org/10.1136/bmj.m4352. [56]

Jones, N. (2020), "How Coronavirus lockdowns stopped flu in its tracks", *Nature*, http://dx.doi.org/10.1038/D41586-020-01538-8. [4]

Katz, J. and M. Sanger-Katz (2021), "'It's Huge, It's Historic, It's Unheard-of': Drug Overdose Deaths Spike", *The New York Times*, https://www.nytimes.com/interactive/2021/07/14/upshot/drug-overdose-deaths.html. [73]

Knight, B. (2020), *Weniger Selbstmorde in Corona-Zeiten*, DW, https://www.dw.com/de/weniger-selbstmorde-in-corona-zeiten/a-53620594. [57]

Kodama, S. (2021), "Japan appoints 'minister of loneliness' to help people home alone", *Nikkei Asia*, https://asia.nikkei.com/Spotlight/Coronavirus/Japan-appoints-minister-of-loneliness-to-help-people-home-alone. [69]

Kroenke, K., R. Spitzer and J. Williams (2001), "The PHQ-9: Validity of a brief depression severity measure", *Journal of General Internal Medicine*, Vol. 16/9, pp. 606-613, http://dx.doi.org/10.1046/J.1525-1497.2001.016009606.X. [136]

Kroenke, K. et al. (2009), "An ultra-brief screening scale for anxiety and depression: The PHQ-4", *Psychosomatics*, Vol. 50/6, pp. 613-621, http://dx.doi.org/10.1176/APPI.PSY.50.6.613. [137]

Kühne, S. et al. (2020), "The need for household panel surveys in times of crisis: The case of SOEP-CoV", *Survey Research Methods*, Vol. 14/2, pp. 195-203, https://doi.org/10.18148/srm/2020.v14i2.7748 (accessed on 19 May 2021). [46]

Kumari, P. and D. Toshniwal (2020), "Impact of lockdown measures during COVID-19 on air quality– A case study of India", *International Journal of Environmental Health Research*, http://dx.doi.org/10.1080/09603123.2020.1778646. [115]

Le Quéré, C. et al. (2020), "Temporary reduction in daily global CO2 emissions during the COVID-19 forced confinement", *Nature Climate Change 2020 10:7*, Vol. 10/7, pp. 647-653, http://dx.doi.org/10.1038/s41558-020-0797-x. [110]

LINE Research Official Blog (2020), *第5回 新型コロナ対策のための全国調査*, LINE Research Official Blog, https://research-platform.line.me/archives/35785304.html?utm_source=lg&utm_medium=link&utm_campaign=covid19_survey#3. [26]

Mayer, F. et al. (2008), "Why is nature beneficial?: The role of connectedness to nature", *Environment and Behavior*, Vol. 41/5, pp. 607-643, http://dx.doi.org/10.1177/0013916508319745. [125]

Ministerio Desarrollo Social y Familia (2020), *Encuesta social COVID-19 (COVID-19 social survey)*, http://observatorio.ministeriodesarrollosocial.gob.cl/encuesta-social-covid19 (accessed on 20 May 2021). [32]

Morgan, D. et al. (2020), "Excess mortality: Measuring the direct and indirect impact of COVID-19", *OECD Health Working Papers*, No. 122, OECD Publishing, Paris, https://dx.doi.org/10.1787/c5dc0c50-en. [5]

Narain, U. (2020), *Air pollution: Locked down by COVID-19 but not arrested*, The World Bank, https://www.worldbank.org/en/news/immersive-story/2020/07/01/air-pollution-locked-down-by-covid-19-but-not-arrested. [111]

National Center for Health Statistics (2020), *Anxiety and depression: Household Pulse Survey - COVID-19*, https://www.cdc.gov/nchs/covid19/pulse/mental-health.htm. [42]

Natural England (2020), *The people and nature survey for England: Adult data Y1Q1 (April - June 2020) (experimental statistics)*, Natural England, https://www.gov.uk/government/statistics/the-people-and-nature-survey-for-england-adult-data-y1q1-april-june-2020-experimental-statistics/the-people-and-nature-survey-for-england-adult-data-y1q1-april-june-2020-experimental-statistics (accessed on 24 February 2021). [131]

New Zealand Government (2021), *Budget Policy Statement 2021*, New Zealand Treasury, https://www.treasury.govt.nz/sites/default/files/2021-02/bps21.pdf. [83]

OECD (2021), *A New Benchmark for Mental Health Systems: Tackling the Social and Economic Costs of Mental Ill-Health*, OECD Health Policy Studies, OECD Publishing, Paris, https://dx.doi.org/10.1787/4ed890f6-en. [48]

OECD (2021), "Adult Learning and COVID-19: How much informal and non-formal learning are workers missing?", *OECD Policy Responses to Coronavirus (COVID-19)*, OECD Publishing, Paris, https://doi.org/10.1787/56a96569-en. [135]

OECD (2021), *Education at a Glance 2021: OECD Indicators*, OECD Publishing, Paris, https://dx.doi.org/10.1787/b35a14e5-en. [89]

OECD (2021), *Implications of the COVID-19 Pandemic for Vocational Education and Training*, OECD Publishing, Paris, https://dx.doi.org/10.1787/55afea00-en. [98]

OECD (2021), *OECD Skills Outlook 2021: Learning for Life*, OECD Publishing, Paris, https://doi.org/10.1787/0ae365b4-en. [102]

OECD (2021), *Preventing Harmful Alcohol Use*, OECD Health Policy Studies, OECD Publishing, Paris, https://dx.doi.org/10.1787/6e4b4ffb-en. [63]

OECD (2021), "Supporting young people's mental health through the COVID-19 crisis", *OECD Policy Responses to Coronavirus (COVID-19)*, OECD Publishing, Paris, https://doi.org/10.1787/84e143e5-en. [51]

OECD (2021), "Tackling the mental health impact of the COVID-19 crisis: An integrated, whole-of-society response", *OECD Policy Responses to Coronavirus (COVID-19)*, OECD Publishing, Paris, https://doi.org/10.1787/0ccafa0b-en. [16]

OECD (2021), "Teaching and learning in VET: Providing effective practical training in school-based settings", *OECD Policy Responses to Coronavirus (COVID-19)*, OECD Publishing, Paris, https://doi.org/10.1787/64f5f843-en. [100]

OECD (2021), "The effect of COVID-19 on alcohol consumption, and policy responses to prevent harmful alcohol consumption", *OECD Policy Responses to Coronavirus (COVID-19)*, OECD Publishing, Paris, https://doi.org/10.1787/53890024-en. [64]

OECD (2021), *The race to vaccinate: Understanding the policy challenges around COVID-19 vaccines*, OECD, Paris, https://www.oecd.org/coronavirus/en/vaccines. [8]

OECD (2021), *The State of Global Education: 18 Months into the Pandemic*, OECD Publishing, Paris, https://doi.org/10.1787/1a23bb23-en. [88]

OECD (2021), *The State of School Education: One Year into the COVID Pandemic*, OECD Publishing, Paris, https://doi.org/10.1787/201dde84-en. [90]

OECD (2020), "COVID-19 and the low-carbon transition Impacts and possible policy responses", *OECD Policy Responses to the Coronavirus (COVID-19)*, OECD Publishing, Paris, https://doi.org/10.1787/749738fc-en. [109]

OECD (2020), *Data Insights: Despite temporary drop, global CO_2 emissions continue to grow*, OECD, Paris, http://www.oecd.org/coronavirus/en/data-insights/despite-temporary-drop-global-co2-emissions-continue-to-grow. [140]

OECD (2020), *Data Insights: Progress in reducing GHG emissions is insufficient to achieve the 2015 Paris Agreement*, OECD, Paris, http://www.oecd.org/coronavirus/en/data-insights/progress-in-reducing-ghg-emissions-is-insufficient-to-achieve-the-2015-paris-agreement. [139]

OECD (2020), *Environment at a Glance Indicators*, OECD Publishing, Paris, https://dx.doi.org/10.1787/ac4b8b89-en. [107]

OECD (2020), *How's Life? 2020: Measuring Well-being*, OECD Publishing, Paris, https://dx.doi.org/10.1787/9870c393-en. [108]

OECD (2020), *OECD Regions and Cities at a Glance 2020*, OECD Publishing, Paris, https://dx.doi.org/10.1787/959d5ba0-en. [10]

OECD (2019), *PISA 2018 Results (Volume II): Where All Students Can Succeed*, PISA, OECD Publishing, Paris, https://dx.doi.org/10.1787/b5fd1b8f-en. [101]

OECD (2017), *Health at a Glance 2017: OECD Indicators*, OECD Publishing, Paris, https://dx.doi.org/10.1787/health_glance-2017-en. [12]

OECD (n.d.), *COVID-19 Health Indicators (database)*, https://stats.oecd.org/index.aspx?queryid=104676# (accessed on 19 September 2021). [13]

OECD (forthcoming), *Health at a Glance 2021: OECD Indicators*, OECD Publishing, Paris. [6]

OECD (n.d.), *Health Status (database)*, https://stats.oecd.org/Index.aspx?DataSetCode=HEALTH_STAT (accessed on 28 September 2021). [14]

OECD/European Union (2020), *Health at a Glance: Europe 2020: State of Health in the EU Cycle*, OECD Publishing, Paris, https://dx.doi.org/10.1787/82129230-en. [2]

Oliveira Hashiguchi, T. (2020), "Bringing health care to the patient: An overview of the use of telemedicine in OECD countries", *OECD Health Working Papers, No. 116*, OECD Publishing, Paris, https://doi.org/10.1787/8e56ede7-en. [52]

ONS (2021), *Deaths from suicide that occurred in England and Wales*, Office for National Statistics, https://www.ons.gov.uk/peoplepopulationandcommunity/birthsdeathsandmarriages/deaths/articles/deathsfromsuicidethatoccurredinenglandandwales/aprilandjuly2020. [58]

ONS (2021), *Deaths related to drug poisoning in England and Wales*, Office for National Statistics, https://www.ons.gov.uk/peoplepopulationandcommunity/birthsdeathsandmarriages/deaths/bulletins/deathsrelatedtodrugpoisoninginenglandandwales/2020#measuring-the-data. [77]

ONS (2020), *Coronavirus and anxiety, Great Britain*, Office for National Statistics, https://www.ons.gov.uk/peoplepopulationandcommunity/wellbeing/articles/coronavirusandanxietygreatbritain/3april2020to10may2020. [25]

ONS (2020), *Coronavirus and depression in adults, Great Britain: June 2020*, Office for National Statistics, https://www.ons.gov.uk/peoplepopulationandcommunity/wellbeing/articles/coronavirusanddepressioninadultsgreatbritain/june2020. [24]

ONS (2020), *Does exposure to air pollution increase the risk of dying from the coronavirus (COVID-19)?*, Office for National Statistics, https://www.ons.gov.uk/economy/environmentalaccounts/articles/doesexposuretoairpollutionincreasetheriskofdyingfromthecoronaviruscovid19/2020-08-13. [106]

ONS (n.d.), *Quarterly Personal Well-being Estimates – Seasonally Adjusted (database)*, https://www.ons.gov.uk/peoplepopulationandcommunity/wellbeing/datasets/quarterlypersonalwellbeingestimatesseasonallyadjusted (accessed on 26 February 2021). [86]

Park, H. and S. Yu (2020), "Mental healthcare policies in South Korea during the COVID-19 epidemic", *Health Policy and Technology*, Vol. 9/3, pp. 279-280, http://dx.doi.org/10.1016/J.HLPT.2020.06.006. [31]

Patel, S. et al. (2020), "Indoor particulate matter during HOMEChem: Concentrations, size distributions, and exposures", *Environmental Science & Technology*, Vol. 54/12, pp. 7107-7116, http://dx.doi.org/10.1021/ACS.EST.0C00740. [120]

Patel, V. et al. (2018), "The Lancet Commission on global mental health and sustainable development"", *The Lancet Commissions*, Vol. 392/10157, pp. 1553-1598, https://www.thelancet.com/journals/lancet/article/PIIS0140-6736(18)31612-X/fulltext. [22]

Perona, M. and C. Senik (2021), *Note de l'Observatoire du Bien-être n°2021-04 : Le Bien-être des Français – Mars 2021*, CEPREMAP, http://www.cepremap.fr/en/2021/04/note-de-lobservatoire-du-bien-etre-n2021-04-le-bien-etre-des-francais-mars-2021/. [82]

Pirkis, J. et al. (2021), "Suicide trends in the early months of the COVID-19 pandemic: An interrupted time-series analysis of preliminary data from 21 countries", *The Lancet Psychiatry*, Vol. 8/7, pp. 579-588, http://dx.doi.org/10.1016/S2215-0366(21)00091-2. [53]

Pozzer, A. et al. (2020), "Regional and global contributions of air pollution to risk of death from COVID-19", *Cardiovascular Research*, Vol. 116/14, pp. 2247-2253, http://dx.doi.org/10.1093/CVR/CVAA288. [103]

Public Health England (n.d.), *Wider Impacts of COVID-19 on Health (WICH) Monitoring Tool (database)*, https://analytics.phe.gov.uk/apps/covid-19-indirect-effects/ (accessed on 4 June 2021). [15]

Rabin, R. (2021), "U.S. suicides declined over all in 2020 but may have risen among people of color", *The New York Times*, https://www.nytimes.com/2021/04/15/health/coronavirus-suicide-cdc.html. [61]

Recchi, E. et al. (2020), “Lockdown for all, hardship for some: Insights from the first wave of the CoCo project”, *HAL*, https://halshs.archives-ouvertes.fr/halshs-03070206/document. [132]

Rojas-Rueda, D. et al. (2019), “Green spaces and mortality: A systematic review and meta-analysis of cohort studies”, *The Lancet Planetary Health*, Vol. 3/11, pp. e469-e477, http://dx.doi.org/10.1016/S2542-5196(19)30215-3. [129]

Ryall, J. (2020), “South Korea's soaring suicide, self-harm rates pinned on pandemic”, *DW*, https://www.dw.com/en/south-koreas-soaring-suicide-self-harm-rates-pinned-on-pandemic/a-54931167. [70]

Sakamoto, H. et al. (2021), “Assessment of suicide in Japan during the COVID-19 pandemic vs previous years”, *JAMA Network Open*, Vol. 4/2, p. e2037378, http://dx.doi.org/10.1001/JAMANETWORKOPEN.2020.37378. [67]

Sanabria-Maxo, J. et al. (2021), *Psychometric properties of the online version of the Patient Health Questionnaire-4 in a large Colombian sample: Results from the PSY-COVID study*, PSY-COVID, https://www.researchgate.net/publication/354610035_Psychometric_properties_of_the_online_version_of_the_Patient_Health_Questionnaire-4_in_a_large_Colombian_sample_Results_from_the_PSY-COVID_study. [35]

SOEP-CoV (2021), *SOEP-CoV The spread of the coronavirus in Germany: Socio-economic factors and consequences*, Funded by the German Federal Ministry of Education and Research (BMBF); the data can be accessed via the research data center of the SOEP, https://www.soep-cov.de/Startseite/. [45]

Soga, M. et al. (2021), “A room with a green view: The importance of nearby nature for mental health during the COVID-19 pandemic”, *Ecological Applications*, Vol. 31/2, p. e2248, http://dx.doi.org/10.1002/eap.2248. [133]

Soland, J. et al. (2020), *The impact of COVID-19 on student achievement and what it may mean for educators*, The Brookings Institution, https://www.brookings.edu/blog/brown-center-chalkboard/2020/05/27/the-impact-of-covid-19-on-student-achievement-and-what-it-may-mean-for-educators/. [93]

Spitzer, R. et al. (2006), “A brief measure for assessing generalized anxiety disorder: The GAD-7”, *Archives of Internal Medicine*, Vol. 166/10, pp. 1092-1097, http://dx.doi.org/10.1001/ARCHINTE.166.10.1092. [138]

Statistics Canada (2020), *Canadians' mental health during the COVID-19 pandemic*, The Daily, https://www150.statcan.gc.ca/n1/daily-quotidien/200527/dq200527b-eng.htm. [23]

Stats NZ (n.d.), *Wellbeing Statistics: March 2021 Quarter (database)*, https://www.stats.govt.nz/information-releases/wellbeing-statistics-march-2021-quarter (accessed on 15 June 2021). [87]

Stieb, D. et al. (2020), “An ecological analysis of long-term exposure to PM2.5 and incidence of COVID-19 in Canadian health regions”, *Environmental Research*, Vol. 191, p. 110052, http://dx.doi.org/10.1016/j.envres.2020.110052. [105]

Tanaka, T. and S. Okamoto (2021), “Increase in suicide following an initial decline during the COVID-19 pandemic in Japan”, *Nature Human Behaviour 2021 5:2*, Vol. 5/2, pp. 229-238, http://dx.doi.org/10.1038/s41562-020-01042-z. [68]

Tel Aviv University (2020), *Israelis suffering from anxiety and depression at "disturbing" rates*, Tel Aviv University, https://english.tau.ac.il/news/depression-covid19. [28]

Tsang, H., R. Scudds and E. Chan (2004), "Psychosocial impact of SARS", *Emerging infectious diseases*, Vol. 10/7, pp. 1326-1327, http://dx.doi.org/10.3201/EID1007.040090. [20]

Twilley, N. (2019), "The hidden air pollution in our homes", *The New Yorker*, https://www.newyorker.com/magazine/2019/04/08/the-hidden-air-pollution-in-our-homes. [122]

Tzeng, N. et al. (2020), "What could we learn from SARS when facing the mental health issues related to the COVID-19 outbreak? A nationwide cohort study in Taiwan", *Translational Psychiatry 2020 10:1*, Vol. 10/1, pp. 1-9, http://dx.doi.org/10.1038/s41398-020-01021-y. [18]

UNED (2021), *Salud mental y COVID-19 Costa Rica 2020*, https://investiga.uned.ac.cr/2021/01/29/salud-mental-y-covid-19-costa-rica-2020/. [33]

UNESCO (n.d.), *Global Monitoring of School Closures, COVID-19 (database)*, United Nations Educational, Scientific and Cultural Organization, https://en.unesco.org/covid19/educationresponse (accessed on 5 October 2021). [91]

United Nations (2020), *COVID-19 and the Need for Action on Mental Health*, https://unsdg.un.org/sites/default/files/2020-05/UN-Policy-Brief-COVID-19-and-mental-health.pdf. [21]

US Census Bureau (n.d.), *Measuring Household Experiences during the Coronavirus Pandemic (database)*, https://www.census.gov/data/experimental-data-products/household-pulse-survey.html (accessed on 13 September 2021). [39]

Wang, S., R. Wright and Y. Wakatsuki (2020), "In Japan, more people died from suicide last month than from Covid in all of 2020", *CNN*, https://edition.cnn.com/2020/11/28/asia/japan-suicide-women-covid-dst-intl-hnk/index.html. [66]

Wang, Y. et al. (2020), "Four-month changes in air quality during and after the COVID-19 lockdown in six megacities in China", *Environmental Science & Technology Letters*, Vol. 7/11, pp. 802-808, http://dx.doi.org/10.1021/ACS.ESTLETT.0C00605. [114]

WHO (2021), *Second round of the national pulse survey on continuity of essential health services during the COVID-19 pandemic*, World Health Organization, https://www.who.int/publications/i/item/WHO-2019-nCoV-EHS-continuity-survey-2021.1. [50]

WHO (2020), *The Impact of COVID-19 on Mental, Neurological and Substance Use Services: Results of a Rapid Assessment*, World Health Organization, https://www.who.int/publications/i/item/978924012455 (accessed on 16 December 2020). [49]

WHO (2018), *Household Air Pollution and Health*, World Health Organization, https://www.who.int/news-room/fact-sheets/detail/household-air-pollution-and-health. [119]

WHO Regional Office for Europe (2020), *Alcohol does not protect against COVID-19; Access should be restricted during lockdown*, World Health Organization, https://www.euro.who.int/en/health-topics/disease-prevention/alcohol-use/news/news/2020/04/alcohol-does-not-protect-against-covid-19-access-should-be-restricted-during-lockdown. [62]

WHO Regional Office for Europe (2016), *Urban green spaces and health - A review of evidence*, World Health Organization, Copenhagen, https://www.euro.who.int/en/health-topics/environment-and-health/urban-health/publications/2016/urban-green-spaces-and-health-a-review-of-evidence-2016. [124]

Wozniak, A. et al. (2020), *COVID Impact Survey*, National Opinion Research Center, https://www.covid-impact.org/. [41]

Wu, X. et al. (2020), "Exposure to air pollution and COVID-19 mortality in the United States: A nationwide cross-sectional study", *Science Advances*, Vol. 6/45, http://dx.doi.org/10.1101/2020.04.05.20054502. [104]

Yip, P. et al. (2010), "The impact of epidemic outbreak: The case of severe acute respiratory syndrome (SARS) and suicide among older adults in Hong Kong", *Crisis*, Vol. 31/2, pp. 86-92, http://dx.doi.org/10.1027/0227-5910/A000015. [19]

Notes

[1] The first quarter of 2020 was mostly unaffected by COVID-19. Due to a mild 2019-20 influenza season, excess mortality in most European countries was below the 2015-19 average for the period January to early March 2020 (Morgan et al., 2020[5]).

[2] Data for some countries refer to the date a death is registered, rather then the date the death actually occurred. There may be variation across countries in delays in registration over holidays and weekends. In the longer term, data referring to date of registration can be retroactively amended to date of occurrence, however in the short-run weekly statistics may be influenced (Morgan et al., 2020[5]). Because all-cause mortality data are dynamic, changes (usually marginal) may be observed depending on when data were extracted, as data may be retroactively updated. All data for excess mortality figures in this report were extracted from the *COVID-19 Health Indicators* database (OECD, n.d.[13]) on 19 September 2021.

[3] The drops in life expectancy reported in 2020 for many countries are calculated based on the age-specific mortality rates in 2020, which were highly affected by COVID-19. Therefore it is unclear whether the 2020 drops in life expectancy will last in the long term, or quickly return to 2019 levels.

[4] The full Patient Health Questionnaire (PHQ) contains 59 questions, with modules focusing on mood, anxiety, alcohol, eating and somatoform disorders. The PHQ-4 screening tool is a short, four-question survey administered to respondents to gauge their mental condition, and to identify the presence and severity of depression and anxiety. PHQ-4 pulls two depression-related questions from the PHQ-9/8 (itself called the PHQ-2), and two anxiety-related questions from the Generalised Anxiety Disorder (GAD-7) questionnaire (itself called the GAD-2). Thus, the PHQ-4 is a combination of PHQ-2 and GAD-2. All question items are added together to provide a total score of mental distress: 0-2 normal, 3-5 moderate, 9-12 severe. A total score greater than or equal to 2 for the first two questions, pulled from the GAD-7, indicates that the respondent is at risk for anxiety. A total score greater than or equal to 2 for the final two questions, pulled from the PHQ-8, indicates that the respondent is at risk for depression (Kroenke et al., 2009[137]). The self-reported values from the PHQ surveys have been validated in separate studies comparing survey outcomes with actual diagnostic interviews with mental health professionals.

[5] The PHQ-8 and PHQ-9 questionnaires are a common shortened version of the full PHQ survey (see the above endnote for more information). PHQ-9 is a nine-question survey designed to detect the presence and severity of depression disorders. The PHQ-8 questionnaire is the same but removes the final question regarding suicidal ideation. In the PHQ-8 survey, all items are added together to provide a total score of depression severity: 0-4 none, 5-9 mild depression, 10-14 moderate depression, 15-19 moderately severe depression, 20-24 severe depression (Kroenke, Spitzer and Williams, 2001[136]).

[6] These rates are lower than those found in the YouGov Covid Data Hub survey; however, respondents were asked different questions. It is worth noting that the LINE data are preliminary and unweighted.

[7] Data were weighted post-hoc to be nationally representative by sex, age, education, labour market status, labour sector and province of residence.

[8] The Generalised Anxiety Disorder Questionnaire (GAD) identifies the risk of anxiety. Similar to the PHQ, data are self-reported. The validity of the tool has been backed by studies matching rates of clinical diagnoses of anxiety in respondents (Spitzer et al., 2006[138]).

[9] Treatment adherence refers to the extent to which an individual's behaviours are in compliance with the recommendations of their healthcare provider: taking medication, participating in counselling, instating lifestyle changes, etc.

[10] 2020 data refer to Q1 and Q2 only.

[11] Excess deaths are measured as the increase in the number of reported deaths from all causes in 2020 compared to the average from 2015-19 for the same period and are sourced from (OECD, n.d.[13]). Average values for "low excess deaths" refer to Australia, Austria, Denmark, Estonia, Finland, France, Germany, Greece, Hungary, Iceland, Latvia, Lithuania, Norway, New Zealand, Poland, Portugal, the Slovak Republic, Slovenia, Sweden and Switzerland; those for "high excess deaths" include Belgium, Canada, Chile, Colombia, Italy, Israel, Mexico, the Netherlands, Spain, the United Kingdom and the United States. The remaining indicators are all sourced from the COVID-19 Government Response Tracker (Hale et al., 2021[79]). The stringency index runs from 0 "least stringent" to 100 "most stringent", and combines data on school closures, workplace closures, cancellation of public events, restrictions on gatherings, closing of public transport, stay-at-home requirements, restrictions on internal movement and international travel controls. "Low stringency" includes Australia, Austria, Belgium, Denmark, Estonia, France, Germany, Greece, Hungary, Iceland, Italy, Japan, Korea, Latvia, Lithuania, New Zealand, Poland, the Slovak Republic and Switzerland; "high stringency" includes Canada, Chile, Colombia, Costa Rica, Finland, Ireland, Israel, Mexico, the Netherlands, Norway, Portugal, Slovenia, Spain, Sweden, Turkey, the United Kingdom, and the United States. "Low school closures" include Australia, Austria, Belgium, Denmark, Estonia, France, Germany, Greece, Hungary, Iceland, Japan, Korea, New Zealand, Poland, the Slovak Republic, Switzerland and the United Kingdom; "high school closures" include Canada, Chile, Colombia, Costa Rica, Latvia, Finland, Ireland, Israel, Italy, Lithuania, Mexico, Netherlands, Norway, Portugal, Slovenia, Spain, Sweden, Turkey and the United States. Stay at home policies refer to government policies on a scale from 0 (no restrictions) to 3 (most restrictions) that (1) recommend not leaving the house, (2) require not leaving the house aside from a range of exceptions, (3) or require not leaving the house aside for very minimal exceptions. "Low stay at home" includes Australia, Austria, Belgium, Estonia, France, Germany, Greece, Iceland, Ireland, Italy, Korea, Latvia, New Zealand, Norway, Poland, the Slovak Republic, Spain, Switzerland the United Kingdom; "high stay at home" includes Canada, Chile, Colombia, Costa Rica, Denmark, Finland, Hungary, Israel, Japan, Lithuania, Mexico, the Netherlands, Portugal, Slovenia, Sweden, Turkey and the United States. The economic support index also runs from 0 (least amount of support) to 100 (most amount of support) and encompasses financial support and debt relief to households. "Low economic support" includes Australia, Belgium, Canada, Costa Rica, Estonia, Finland, Germany, Hungary, Korea, Latvia, Lithuania, Mexico, New Zealand, Norway, Slovenia, Sweden, Switzerland and the United States; "high economic support" includes Austria, Chile, Colombia, Denmark, France, Greece, Iceland, Ireland, Israel, Italy, Japan, the Netherlands, Poland, Portugal, the Slovak Republic, Spain, Turkey and the United Kingdom.

[12] Many countries that placed a priority on keeping primary and secondary schools open did so while maintaining strict measures to limit or prevent social mixing in other contexts, such as in hospitality, retail and cultural sectors.

[13] The Survey on Joint National Responses to COVID-19 School Closures is a collaborative effort between the United Nations Educational, Scientific and Cultural Organization (UNESCO), the UNESCO Institute for Statistics (UIS), the United Nations Children's Fund (UNICEF), the World Bank (WB) and the OECD. The most recent round of data collection took place from January to February 2021.

[14] The OECD defines "non-formal" learning as participating in activities such as workshops and employer-provided trainings, and "informal learning" as learning from others, learning by doing and learning new things at work (OECD, 2021[135]).

[15] Although CO_2 emissions fell during lockdowns, the drop was only temporary, and global emissions are continuing to grow (OECD, 2020[140]). Similarly, lowered greenhouse gas emissions due to the pandemic will not be sufficient to reach the rates agreed in the 2015 Paris Agreement (OECD, 2020[139]).

[16] In the United Kingdom, $PM_{2.5}$ levels during the spring 2020 were higher than in the same period in 2019, primarily due to meteorological conditions (Air Quality Expert Group, 2020[117]).

[17] These findings come from the CoCo survey, a component of the "Coping with Covid-19: Social Distancing, Cohesion and Inequality in 2020 France" project. The CoCo survey is a part of the French Longitudinal Internet Studies for Social Sciences panel (ELIPSS), a panel survey maintained by the Centre de données socio-politiques (CDSP) at SciencesPo. ELIPSS is a panel of 1 400 French residents from 2012 through today. The sample is selected from census data. Responses are weighted to account for design effects, differential response refusal weights, and post-stratification weights for sex, age, education and region.

4 Community relations in the first year of COVID-19

COVID-19 has profoundly affected how people spend their time, how they relate to one another and their institutions, and how safe they are and feel. Social distancing multiplied and compounded feelings of loneliness and lack of connectedness during the first year of the pandemic. Working conditions in 2020 (including telework and contact restrictions in work locations outside the home) have worn people out. In addition, household and care tasks have multiplied. While overall crime levels (bar domestic violence) and road deaths have declined up to now amidst lockdowns, new types of cybercrime have emerged, and homicide rates are up in a few countries. Voter turnout in the first year of the pandemic was, for the most part, not held back as governments adapted special voting arrangements but a large share of the population feels increasingly left out of society.

4.1. Social connections

Limited social contact during the pandemic has left many feeling lonely…

Feelings of loneliness have been compounded over the first year of the pandemic. Between April and the beginning of June 2020, 1 in 7 respondents in European OECD countries, the majority of which implemented the first wave of lockdowns in that period, stated they felt lonely most or all of the time in the past two weeks – this share rose to almost 1 in 5 people by early 2021 (Figure 4.1, Panel A). When asked the same question in 2016, only 5.5% of respondents – less than one-third of the 2021 level –felt lonely (Eurofound, 2018[1]).[1] Countries with official data confirm this pattern: In Germany, different measures of social isolation between April-June 2020 at least doubled compared to 2017, and further intensified by January-February 2021 (Figure 4.2). And while there is no comparable pre-COVID data available in Great Britain, feelings of loneliness increased there too over the course of the first year of the pandemic: in the period October 2020-February 2021, 7.2% of the adult population said they often or always felt lonely, compared to 5% in April-May 2020 (ONS, 2021[2]) (Box 4.1).

Figure 4.1. Despite a temporary decline over the summer, loneliness increased during the multiple lockdowns

Loneliness and lockdown stringency in European OECD countries, 2016, Apr-Jun 2020 - Feb-March 2021

Panel A. Share of people feeling lonely most or all of the time in the past two weeks

Panel B. Share of people feeling lonely most or all of the time in the past two weeks (left axis) and lockdown stringency (right axis), OECD 22

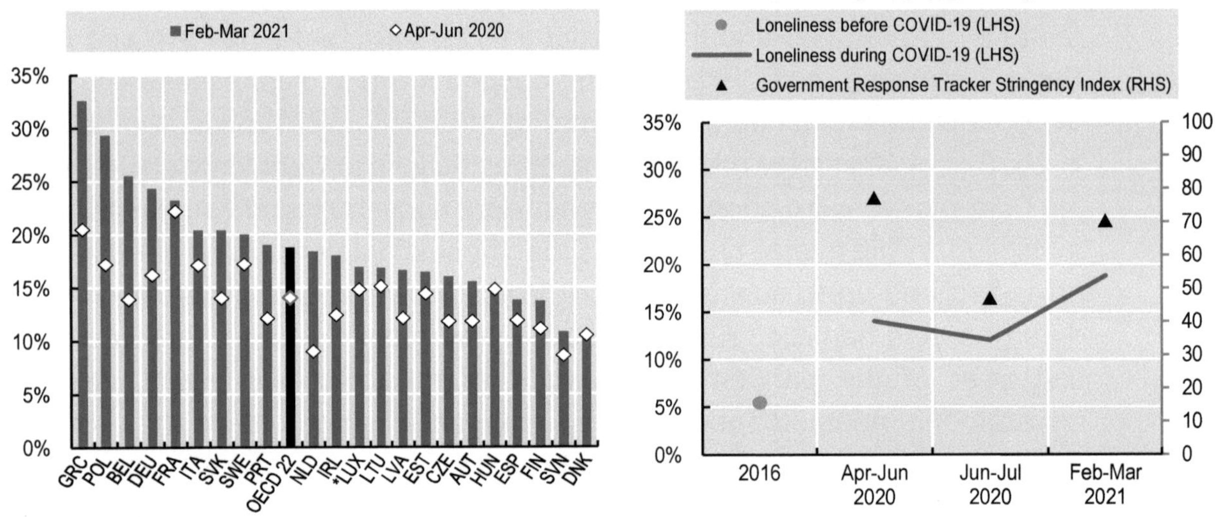

Note: In both panels, the OECD average includes only those 22 countries shown in Panel A. Changes in outcomes between April-June 2020 and February-March 2021 are significant at the 5% level for Belgium, the Czech Republic, Germany, Greece, Ireland, the Netherlands, OECD 22, Poland, Portugal and the Slovak Republic. Refer to Box 2.1 for methodological details on the Living, working and COVID-19 survey. In Panel A, * denotes countries with between 301 and 500 observations for at least one time period. More than 500 observations are available for all other countries. In Panel B, the stringency index by the University of Oxford Coronavirus Government Response Tracker considers containment and closure policies (closing of schools, universities, workplaces, cancellation of public events, limits on private gatherings, stay-at-home orders, restrictions on internal movement and international travel). A higher score (0-100) indicates higher strictness and more universal policy targeting.
Source: Eurofound (2018[1]), *European Quality of Life Survey 2016*, https://www.eurofound.europa.eu/publications/report/2017/fourth-european-quality-of-life-survey-overview-report; Eurofound (n.d.[3]), *Living, working and COVID-19 e-survey* (database), http://eurofound.link/covid19data; and University of Oxford (n.d.[4]), *Coronavirus Government Response Tracker* (database), https://www.bsg.ox.ac.uk/research/research-projects/coronavirus-government-response-tracker.

StatLink https://stat.link/pv45f8

Official regulations limiting social contact are directly linked to loneliness, but feelings of loneliness have remained elevated even when restrictions were eased for a time. In European OECD countries, loneliness temporarily declined in June-July 2020, alongside the strictness of government containment measures as governments moved out of lockdown over the summer (Figure 4.1, Panel B). Loneliness levels nevertheless remained more than double compared to double compared to 2016. In New Zealand, 3.8% of the population said they felt lonely most or all of the time after the first lockdown in June 2020, a similar level as in 2018 (StatsNZ, 2020[5]) (Box 4.1). However, 1 in 5 people continued to feel lonely at least some of the time in the past month (in 2018, 1 in 6 felt this way), and this remained stable through to the March 2021 quarter (StatsNZ, n.d.[6]; StatsNZ, 2020[5]; Stats NZ, 2021[7]) (Box 4.1).[2] Indeed, although official restrictions on contact were lifted, people continued to limit their interactions with others, teleworked, and were prevented from seeing family members living abroad due to travel restrictions. For instance, 45.7% of employed people in European OECD countries were working from home in June-July 2020, and between April and September more than half of respondents from 16 OECD countries said they were always or frequently avoiding small social gatherings (Eurofound, 2020[8]; Imperial College London YouGov, 2020[9]) (Box 4.2).[3]

Figure 4.2. Feelings of social isolation have markedly increased in Germany

Share of people in Germany reporting that they very often or often ..., 2017, Apr-Jun 2020, Jan-Feb 2021

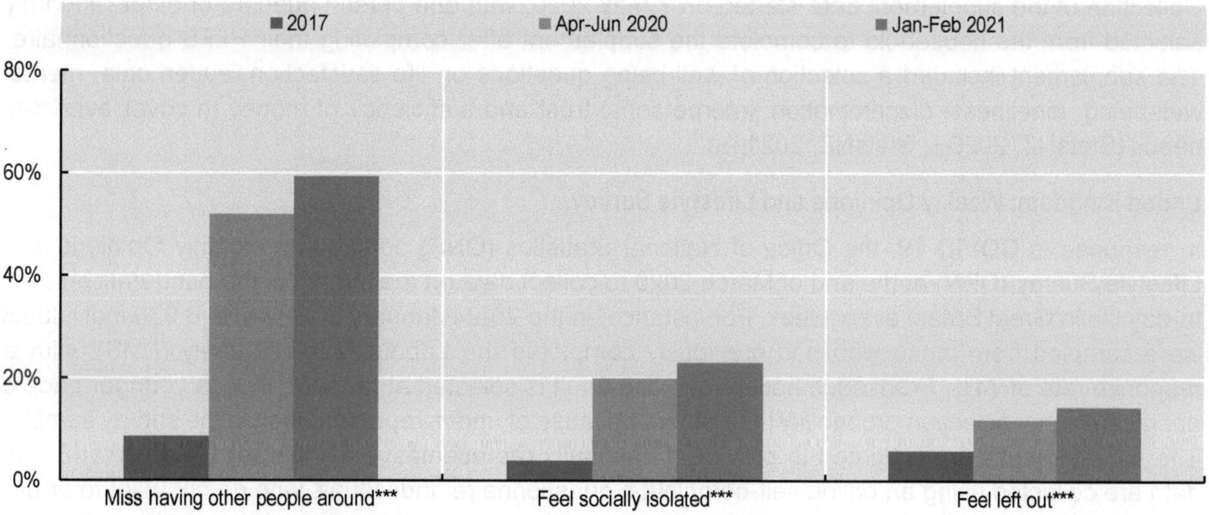

Note: Socially isolated is defined as the share of respondents who say they feel socially isolated very often or often. Categories followed by *** saw statistically significant (at the 5% level) changes from 2017-2021. Funded by the German Federal Ministry of Education and Research (BMBF). The data can be accessed via the research data centre of the SOEP. Refer to Box 3.1 for methodological details.
Source: Kühne et al. (2020[10]), "The need for household panel surveys in times of crisis: The case of SOEP-CoV", *Survey Research Methods*, Vol. 14/2, pp. 195-203, https://doi.org/10.18148/srm/2020.v14i2.7748.

StatLink https://stat.link/jsay8m

Box 4.1. Innovation: National Statistics Offices are increasing the frequency of well-being data collections through weekly and quarterly surveys

Colombia: Social Pulse Survey

In order to capture statistical information during the pandemic, the National Statistical Office of Colombia (DANE) began conducting a monthly Social Pulse Survey (SPS) in July 2020. The SPS relies on CATI (Computer Assisted Telephone Interview) to collect data, capturing around 10 000 respondents each month. The survey is representative of 23 regional capitals and their metropolitan areas. By using a subsample of the existing Great Integrated Household Survey, responses to SPS can be linked to existing information on income and labour market outcomes. Topics covered include multiple well-being dimensions such as household consumption, subjective well-being, trust, child and adolescent well-being, care networks, access to social protection, as well as women's experiences during menstruation (DANE, n.d.[11]).

New Zealand: Household Labour Force Survey

StatsNZ's General Social Survey (GSS) is the official source of well-being data in New Zealand and was last collected over April 2018 - March 2019. Since the GSS has been delayed until April 2021 due to the pandemic, a selection of well-being questions from GSS was included as part of a supplement to the household labour force survey (HLFS) from June 2020 until at least the March 2021 quarter. Collection of the supplement data started on 7 May 2020, with one person aged 18 or older randomly selected from the household to complete the supplement after completing their HLFS questionnaire. The supplement included a selection of well-being questions on life satisfaction, eudemonia, mental well-being, loneliness, discrimination, interpersonal trust and sufficiency of money to cover everyday needs (StatsNZ, 2020[5]; StatsNZ, 2021[12]).

United Kingdom: Weekly Opinions and Lifestyle Survey

In response to COVID-19, the Office of National Statistics (ONS) adapted its monthly Opinions and Lifestyle Survey (OPN) at the end of March 2020 to collect data on the impact of the pandemic on day-to-day life in Great Britain every week. For instance, in the 20-24 January 2021 wave, 6 030 individuals were sampled from those who had previously completed the Labour Market Survey (LMS), with a response rate of 74%. From each household, one adult is selected at random, though younger people are given higher selection probability than others because of under-representation in the survey sample. The survey results are weighted to provide a nationally representative sample for Great Britain, with data are collected using an online self-completion questionnaire. Individuals who do not want to or are unable to complete the survey online have the possibility to take part over the phone (ONS, 2021[13]).

...but COVID-19 might have also led to a re-evaluation of existing support networks

Despite the rise in loneliness, a large majority of people in 2020 said they have someone they can count on in an emergency. Across OECD countries, the share of respondents stating that they have no friends and family to count on in times of need in 2020 remained stable at 8.5% compared to the previous year (Figure 4.3). Only a handful of countries have experienced changes in perceived social support in 2020 compared to 2019 that would be considered meaningful (i.e.at least 3 percentage points), with more people feeling a lack of social support during COVID-19 in Austria, Colombia, Costa Rica, Greece and Mexico, and with social support improving in Italy, Korea, Poland and Turkey.[4] Additional evidence suggests that, during the pandemic, people reached out more to their existing friends and family, and that vulnerable people may have received more support during lockdowns than they would have otherwise: a quarter of people across the OECD stated in September 2020 that they had provided assistance, such as running an errand or providing childcare for friends, neighbours or co-workers without expecting anything in return (Imperial College London YouGov, 2020[9]) (Box 4.2).

Figure 4.3. Feelings of social support have changed little in most OECD countries

Share of people stating they have no friend or family to count on in times of need, 2019-20

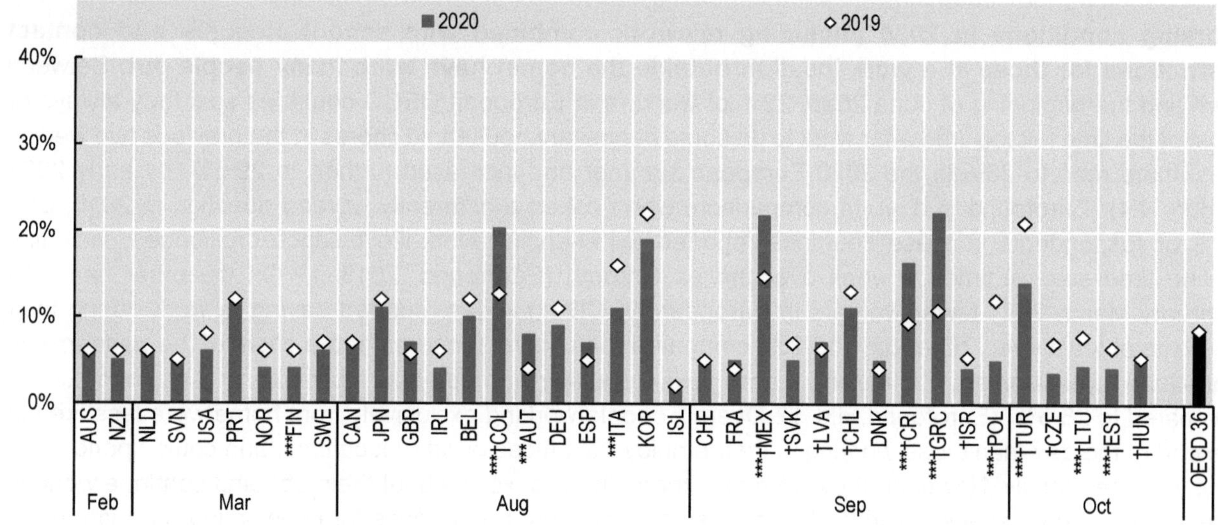

Note:. † denotes countries in which the mode of data collection changed between 2019 and 2020 (generally, moving from face-to-face interviews to phone-based interviews). Countries preceded by *** saw statistically significant (at the 5% level) changes from 2019-2020. The OECD average excludes Luxembourg (no data in 2020) and the Czech Republic (no data in 2019). The 2019 value for the Czech Republic refers to 2018. Countries are ranked by fieldwork start date (earliest to latest) in 2020. Refer to the Reader's Guide for a complete list of Gallup World Poll data collection dates in 2020, and to Box 3.4 for additional information about the data collection methodology.

Source: OECD calculations based on the *Gallup World Poll* (n.d.[14]) (database), https://www.gallup.com/178667/gallup-world-poll-work.aspx.

StatLink https://stat.link/vgof4a

Box 4.2. Methods: Imperial College London and YouGov COVID-19 behaviour tracker

YouGov, a global public opinion company, partnered with the Institute of Global Health Innovation at Imperial College London to gather global insights into people's behaviours, experiences and feelings in response to COVID-19. Starting on 31 March 2020, around 21 000 people complete online surveys or are interviewed via the phone each week across 29 countries, including 16 OECD members (Australia, Canada, Denmark, Finland, France, Germany, Italy, Japan, Mexico, the Netherlands, Norway, Korea, Spain, Sweden, the United Kingdom and the United States). The sample frame of the survey is drawn from YouGov's existing online research panel of over six million panellists worldwide and is designed to be nationally representative. Data collection is currently expected to continue at least until the middle of October 2021. Anonymised respondent level data are publicly available (Imperial College London YouGov, 2020[9]).

4.2. Work-life Balance

Many workers have felt progressively more exhausted

Working conditions in 2020 (including telework combined with school closures and contact restrictions for those at a work location outside the home) have worn many people out. Between April and the beginning of June 2020, 22% of workers in European OECD countries said they always or most of the time felt too tired after work to do some necessary household chores in the previous two weeks. This share rose to 28% in the 2020 European summer and increased further, to 29.5%, by early 2021 (Figure 4.4) (Eurofound, n.d.[3]). In comparison, when asked a differently worded question in 2016, only 20% of respondents in these countries reported experiencing work-life balance challenges, including feeling tired several times a week over the past month (Eurofound, 2018[1]).[5] On the other hand, by February-March 2021 fewer workers in European OECD countries reported having to work during their free time at least every other day (15.2%) compared to the level recorded at the onset of the pandemic in April-June a year earlier (17.8%), and slightly fewer regularly worried about work when not working (23.8% compared to 26.5%) (Eurofound, n.d.[3]). Overall, people working exclusively from home were less tired at the end of the day than those working at their employers' offices or other locations, and could spend more time with their family. However, they were also more likely to worry about their jobs and continue working after hours (see Chapters 5 and 7). Regardless experiences, preferences for teleworking are high: more than 1 in 3 employed people in European countries (44%) interviewed between June 2020 and March 2021 would like to work from home at least several times a week after COVID-19 subsides (Eurofound, n.d.[3]) (see Chapter 2 and 7).

Figure 4.4. A year into the pandemic, more workers feel tired

Share of people stating they always or most of the time felt too tired after work to do some of the necessary household chores in the past two weeks, Apr-Jun 2020 - Feb-Mar 2021

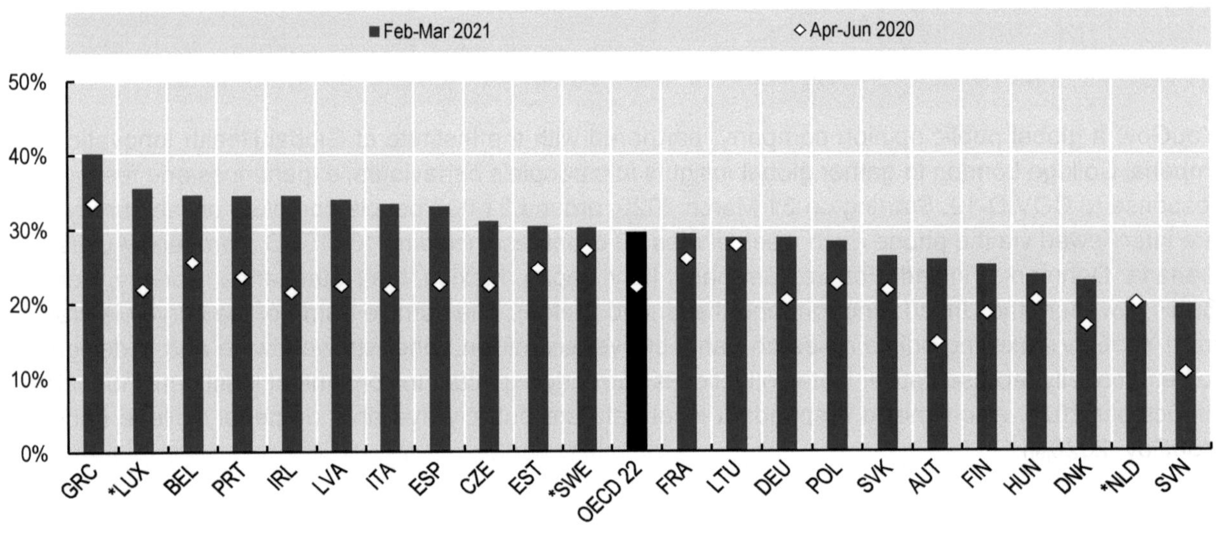

Note: The OECD average includes only those 22 countries shown. * denotes countries with between 300 and 500 observations for at least one time period. More than 500 observations per time period are available for all other countries. Refer to Box 2.1 for methodological details on the Living, working and COVID-19 survey.

Source: Eurofound (n.d.[3]), Living, working and COVID-19 e-survey (database), http://eurofound.link/covid19data.

StatLink https://stat.link/p4hjw3

Household and care tasks have multiplied during lockdowns

Whenever more people were at home due to pandemic-related measures including school and day-care closures, as well as interruptions in domestic help services, household and care tasks increased. For instance, between mid-June and early July 2020, one in six Australians (16%) spent more time on unpaid domestic activities compared to before COVID-19 restrictions, and one in three (36%) of those with unpaid caring responsibilities increased their time spent caring for others (ABS, 2020[15]). Similarly, evidence from UN Women Rapid Gender Assessment Surveys conducted in April 2020 in Chile, Mexico and Turkey suggests that both women and men reported an increase in time spent on both unpaid domestic work and care work since COVID-19 began (with stronger rises for women, who have continued to bear the main burden of such work during the pandemic) (see Chapter 7). Evidence from Germany shows that, a year into the pandemic, people were satisfied with how they spent their time in some ways but not in others. While fewer people reported being dissatisfied with the time they spent sleeping in early 2021 (compared to 2019), the share of those dissatisfied with family time nearly doubled, and it more than doubled regarding leisure time (Figure 4.5).

Figure 4.5. Compared to 2019, Germans were less satisfied with their leisure and family time in the first year of the pandemic, but felt better about their time spent sleeping

Share of people in Germany dissatisfied with the time spent in selected areas, 2019, Apr-Jun 2020, Jan-Feb 2021

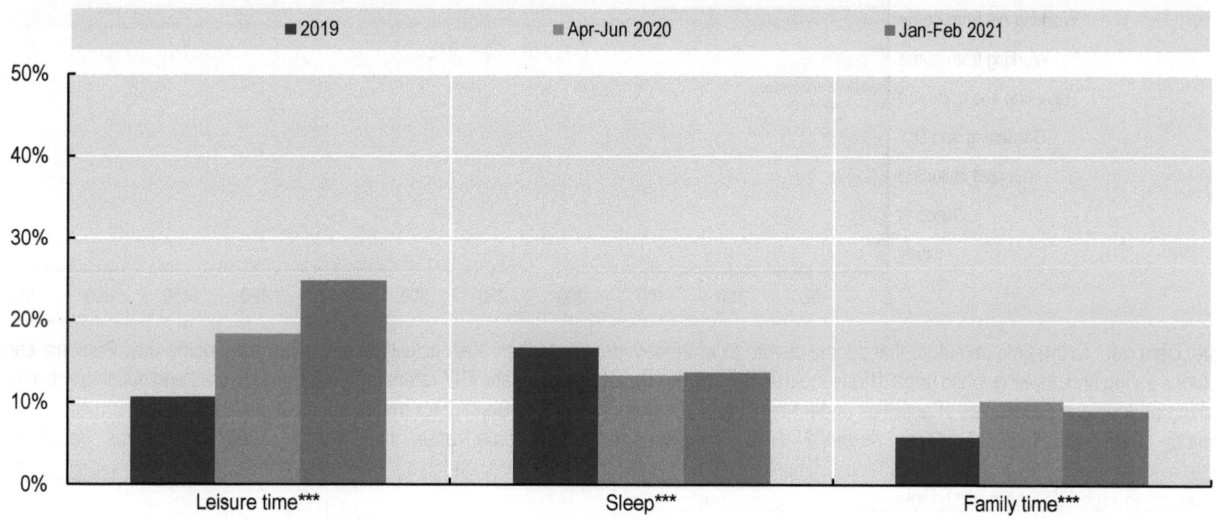

Note: Data refer to those who answered 4 or less on a scale of 0 (not at all satisfied) to 10 (completely satisfied) for each area of time use. Categories followed by *** saw statistically significant (at the 5% level) changes from 2019 to 2021. Funded by the German Federal Ministry of Education and Research (BMBF). The data can be accessed via the research data centre of the SOEP. Refer to Box 3.1 for methodological details.

Source: Kühne et al. (2020[10]), "The need for household panel surveys in times of crisis: The case of SOEP-CoV", *Survey Research Methods*, Vol. 14/2, pp. 195-203, https://doi.org/10.18148/srm/2020.v14i2.7748.

StatLink https://stat.link/jkiwuq

Not all lifestyle changes are likely to be permanent

Evidence from the United Kingdom also suggests that, apart from working from home, many behaviours have returned to pre-pandemic levels by the third quarter of 2020. Time-use data from Great Britain capture the first national lockdown in March-April 2020 as well as further (comparatively less strict) restrictions six months later. They highlight substantial lifestyle changes during the first lockdown:

compared to 2014-15, people spent less time on travel, work outside the home and personal care, and more time on unpaid childcare, gardening and "do it yourself" (DIY) activities, working from home, entertainment and sleep. However, most habits returned to pre-pandemic levels by September-October 2020, as people resumed spending more time with family and friends, increased their overall working time and most likely had finished the longstanding gardening and DIY chores performed in early 2020 (ONS, 2021[16])(Figure 4.6).[6] Indeed, working from home is the only activity category that had not moved back to pre-pandemic levels by September 2020.

Figure 4.6. In Great Britain, except for working from home, people returned to pre-lockdown habits by September 2020

Minutes spent on an average day per activity for adults aged 18 or over, 2014-15 for the United Kingdom, Mar-Apr 2020 and Sep-Oct 2020 for Great Britain

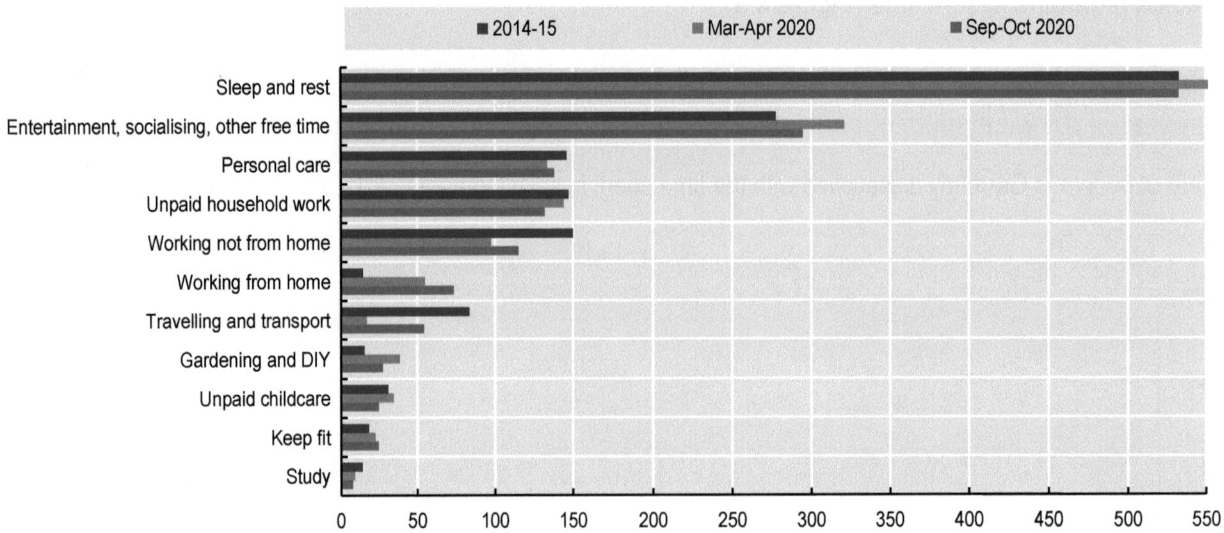

Note: Data refer to the time (minutes) that people devote to what they identify as their main activity at any given point of the day. Personal care includes eating and drinking, while unpaid household work excludes travel and childcare. DIY refers to ""do it yourself" craft and building activities; walking or driving are examples of activities under travelling and transport. Refer to Box 7.2 for methodological details.

Source: ONS (2021[16]), *A "new normal"? How people spent their time after the March 2020 coronavirus lockdown*, https://www.ons.gov.uk/peoplepopulationandcommunity/healthandsocialcare/conditionsanddiseases/articles/anewnormalhowpeoplespenttheirtimeafterthemarch2020coronaviruslockdown/2020-12-09.

StatLink https://stat.link/4arfql

4.3. Safety

Road fatalities as well as burglaries, pickpocketing and theft dropped in 2020…

With lower mobility, the number of road fatalities fell during the first months of 2020. Preliminary data show that road deaths in April 2020 decreased by almost 30% year-on-year, while traffic contracted by almost 50% in OECD countries with available data (Figure 4.7, Panel A). Only two countries – the Netherlands and Sweden – did not have severe mobility restrictions in place during the first lockdown. However, some countries, among them Chile, the Czech Republic, Denmark, France, Greece, Spain and Poland, registered increases in average speed and in the severity of road crashes, possibly due to less traffic intensity during usual rush hours (International Transport Forum, 2020[17]). There is evidence, however, that road fatalities, while below their 2019 levels, started to rise again from the second quarter of 2020 onward (Figure 4.7, Panel B).

Figure 4.7. In 2020, road deaths declined when mobility restrictions were in place

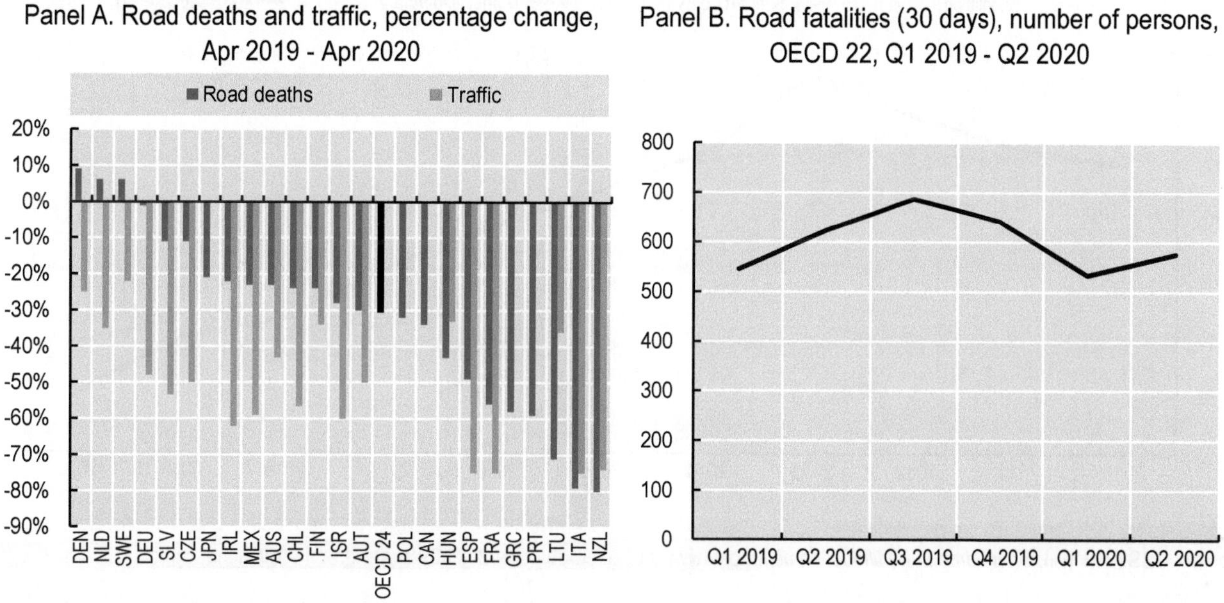

Note: In Panel A, the OECD average includes only those 24 countries shown. Traffic figures for Chile refer to Santiago only. In Panel B, the OECD average includes the Czech Republic, Estonia, Finland, France, Germany, Greece, Hungary, Iceland, Ireland, Israel, Japan, Latvia, Lithuania, Luxembourg, New Zealand, Norway, Poland, Slovenia, Sweden, Switzerland, the United Kingdom and the United States.
Source: International Transport Forum (2020[17]), *Road Safety Annual Report*, https://www.itf-oecd.org/road-safety-annual-report-2020 (Panel A); and International Transport Forum (n.d.[18]), *Short Term Indicators* (database), https://stats.oecd.org/index.aspx?queryid=73641 (Panel B).

StatLink https://stat.link/fu4l0w

Data from a limited number of OECD countries suggest that domestic burglaries, pickpocketing and thefts in 2020 have fallen overall. Most countries will not publish comparable crime statistics until after the publication of this report, making it difficult to get an overall picture of the impact of the pandemic on various crimes. However, evidence suggests that, with fewer people on the streets, criminal activities typically carried out in groups, outdoor crowds as well as in otherwise empty homes have declined. In the Netherlands, the total number of crimes registered by police in 2020 was down by 2% on the previous year, with pickpocketing (-47%), domestic burglary (-23%), shoplifting (-13%) and street robbery (-7.6%) dropping sharply (Figure 4.8) (CBS, 2021[19]). Similarly, New Zealand police recorded 14.6% fewer burglaries and 10.1% fewer theft victimisations in 2020 compared to 2019 (New Zealand Police, 2021[20]). In Germany, domestic burglaries in 2020 declined 13.9% year-on-year (BKA, 2021[21]). In the United States, the FBI's 2020 annual report *Crime in the United States* shows a 7.8% decline in property crimes and a 9.3% decline in robbery offenses compared to 2019 (FBI, 2021[22]). In Israel, 2.7% of adults declared being a victim of theft from a building in 2020, down from 3.5% in 2019 (CBS, 2021[23]).

These types of crime have been especially low during lockdown periods. In 17 OECD countries, the number of theft offenses fell significantly in March and April 2020, but rose again in June and July (Figure 4.9). In England and Wales, where total police-recorded crimes for the 12-month period ending December 2020 decreased by 8%, this was mostly driven by falls during the periods of national lockdown and mainly concerned theft offences (ONS, 2021[24]). Overall, property and contact crime rates are predicted to return to pre-pandemic levels in the medium term, and could increase further in case of economic downturn, replicating a trend observed during other major economic crises (UNODC, 2020[25]).

Figure 4.8. In the Netherlands, shoplifting, street robbery, burglary and pickpocketing were already on a long-term downward trend and dropped further in 2020

Registered crimes in the Netherlands, 2010=100

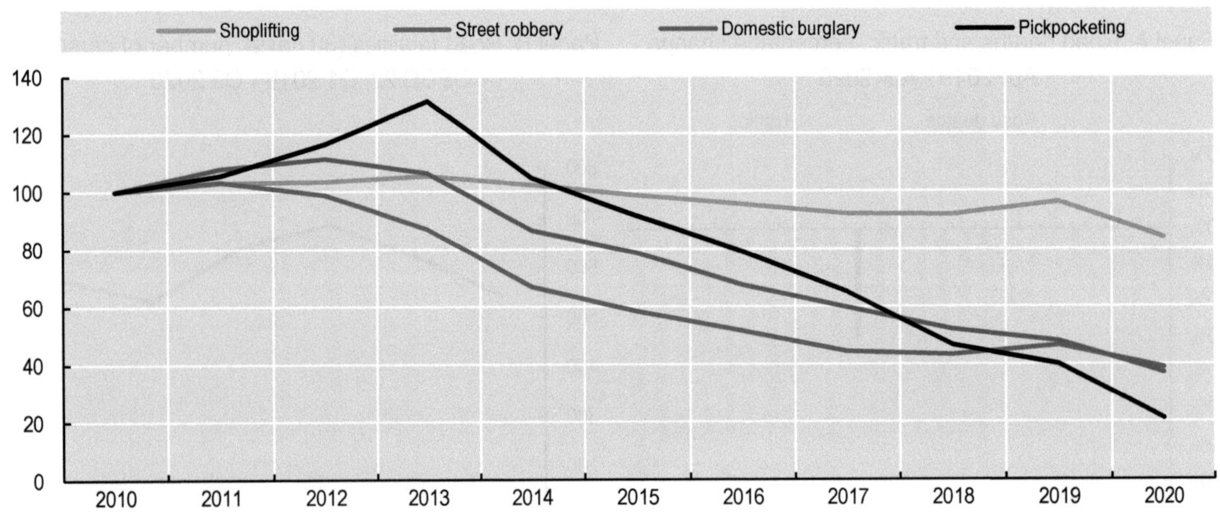

Note: Data for 2019 and 2020 are provisional.
Source: CBS (2021[19]), *Sharp drop in traditional crime*, https://www.cbs.nl/en-gb/news/2021/09/sharp-drop-in-traditional-crime.

StatLink https://stat.link/2fznbv

Figure 4.9. In the first half of 2020, theft in 17 OECD countries declined during lockdown periods

Theft, number of recorded offences, OECD 17, Oct 2019 – Aug 2020

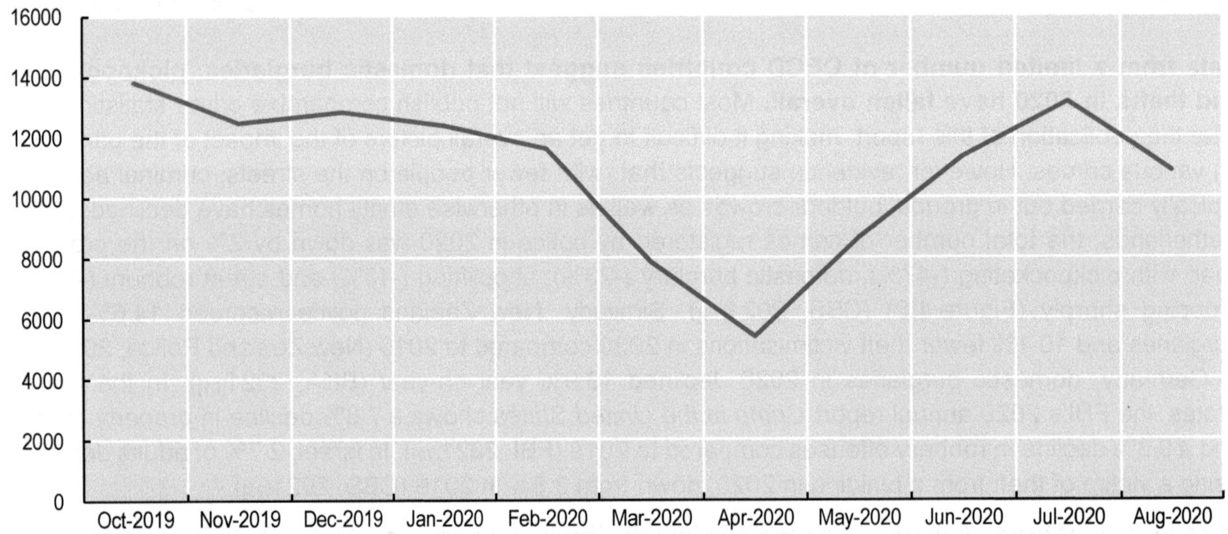

Note: The OECD average includes Colombia, Chile, the Czech Republic, Denmark, Finland, Greece, Hungary, Iceland, Italy, Latvia, Lithuania, Mexico, New Zealand, Poland, Portugal, the Slovak Republic and Sweden.
Source: UNODC (n.d.[26]), *Crime during COVID-19 pandemic* (database), https://dataunodc.un.org/content/covid-19.

StatLink https://stat.link/41c2mv

... but the downfall in criminal activity does not apply to domestic violence and homicide, and the pandemic provided new opportunities for cybercrime

In 2020, reports of domestic violence have risen in most countries, and shootings and homicide have increased in some. Lockdowns, isolation, school closures and job losses during COVID-19 have created fertile conditions for domestic abuse, and intimate partner violence against women and girls worldwide has intensified since the pandemic outbreak (see Chapter 7) (OECD, 2020[27]). Other data show that in some countries, certain types of violent crime increased in 2020: although rape offenses in the United States were down 12% in 2020 compared to 2019, the FBI also recorded a 12.1% increase in the number of aggravated assault offences and a record 29.4% rise for murder and non-negligent manslaughter (the largest yearly increase since records began in the 1960s) (FBI, 2021[22]). Assault victimisations in New Zealand in 2020 also increased by 12.4% relative to the previous 12 months (New Zealand Police, 2021[20]). Mexico meanwhile recorded 3 000 homicides in March 2020, one of the highest monthly totals on record (UNODC, 2020[25]). On the other hand, homicide rates in European countries did not change much in early 2020 compared to pre-pandemic levels (or even decreased in the short term), while in Colombia there were 32% fewer homicide victims in April 2020 compared with the average level recorded for that month over the period 2015–19 (though the number of victims returned to the pre-COVID-19 baseline by June 2020) (UNODC, 2020[25]).

Like many statistics coming out of the pandemic, crime data must be interpreted with some caution. First, they refer to reported crimes, and the pandemic might have changed people's willingness to come forward in person – although some evidence suggests that the (property) crime trends described in this chapter largely reflect decreases in the number of crimes committed rather than changes in reporting (UNODC, 2020[25]). Second, legal changes occurred in 2020, e.g. more lenient drug laws were introduced in some United States jurisdictions and new family violence offences were added in New Zealand, which influenced what is recognised and recorded as crime. Relatedly, the focus of police work can change recorded crimes: in the United Kingdom, a 15% increase in drug offences in 2020 compared to 2019 is partly explained by proactive police activity in crime hotspots (ONS, 2021[24]). Lastly, homicides remain rare events and rates can easily be inflated by single incidents.[7] Overall, people's perceptions of safety in 2020 remained stable compared to 2019 in most OECD countries (Figure 4.10).

COVID-19 has also led to new opportunities for organised crime in the cyberspace and medical products market. The threat posed by counterfeit medicines increased dramatically between 2019 - 20, and is continuing in 2021, with organized crime groups taking advantage of high demand for medicines, personal protection and hygiene items (including fake negative COVID-19 test certificates). This led to a record number of fake online pharmacies being shut down by authorities (Interpol, 2020[28]; Europol, 2021[29]; Interpol, 2021[30]). Due to increases in working from home and remote access to business resources, many individuals and businesses who may have been less active online before the crisis have become a lucrative target for cybercriminals employing phishing, online scams and fake news more generally (Europol, 2020[31])). The detection of online child sexual abuse material has also spiked at a time when restrictions prevented offenders from travelling (Interpol, 2020[32]).

Figure 4.10. Feelings of safety have remained stable

Share of people feeling safe walking alone at night in the neighbourhood where they live, 2019-20

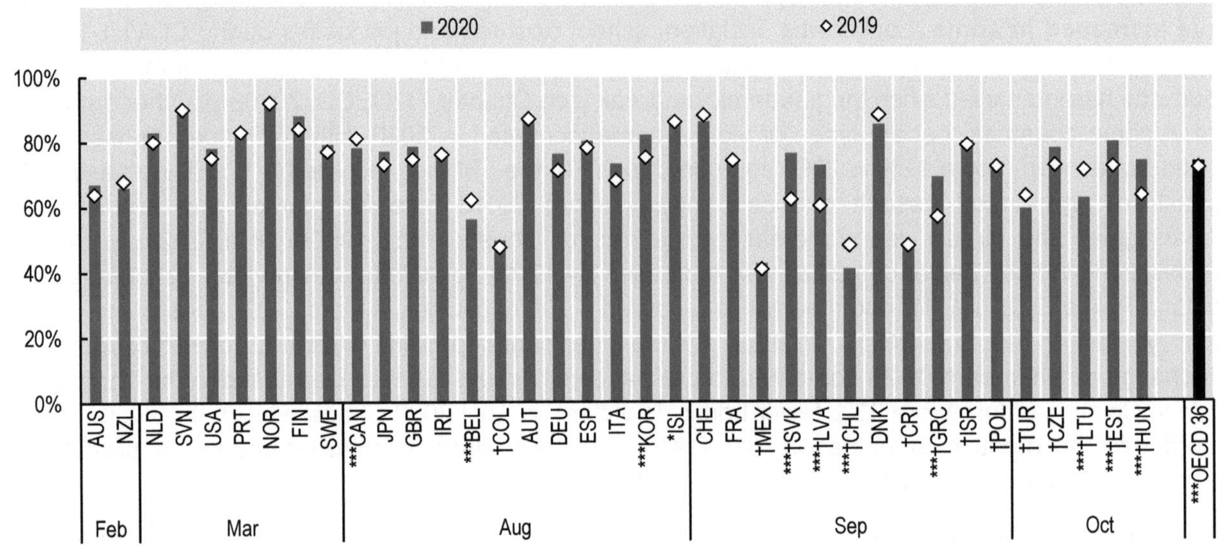

Note: † denotes countries in which the mode of data collection changed between 2019 and 2020 (generally, moving from face-to-face interviews to phone-based interviews). * denotes countries with between 301 and 500 observations. More than 500 observations are available for all other countries. Countries preceded by *** saw statistically significant (at the 5% level) changes from 2019-2020. The OECD average excludes Luxembourg (no data in 2020) and the Czech Republic (no data in 2019). The 2019 value for the Czech Republic refers to 2018. Countries are ranked by fieldwork start date (earliest to latest) in 2020. Refer to the Reader's Guide for a complete list of Gallup World Poll data collection dates in 2020, and to Box 3.4 for additional information about the data collection methodology.
Source: OECD calculations based on the *Gallup World Poll* (n.d.[14]) (database), https://www.gallup.com/178667/gallup-world-poll-work.aspx.

StatLink https://stat.link/ih7tby

4.4. Civic Engagement

Voter turnout in the first year of the pandemic was mostly not held back as many governments introduced special voting arrangements, but participation was lower in locations hit hardest by COVID-19

Despite the pandemic, people exercised their right to vote in 2020 and early 2021. With some exceptions, voter turnout in most OECD countries with national elections in 2020 and 2021 was not hindered by COVID-19. While voter turnout in Iceland and Portugal decreased by almost 10 percentage points compared to the previous election, the share of people casting a ballot increased by more than 5 percentage points in Poland, Korea and the Slovak Republic (Figure 4.11). Timing and political context partly explain this pattern: the Slovak Republic, Ireland and Israel (for the March 2020 vote) held their elections at the beginning of 2020, at a time when no COVID-19 cases had been reported in their territories, while voters in Poland and the United States were motivated to cast their ballot by closely contested and highly polarised electoral races.[8]

Figure 4.11. COVID-19 has not prevented people from expressing their political voice

Share of votes cast among the population registered to vote in national elections, 2020-21 and year of previous election

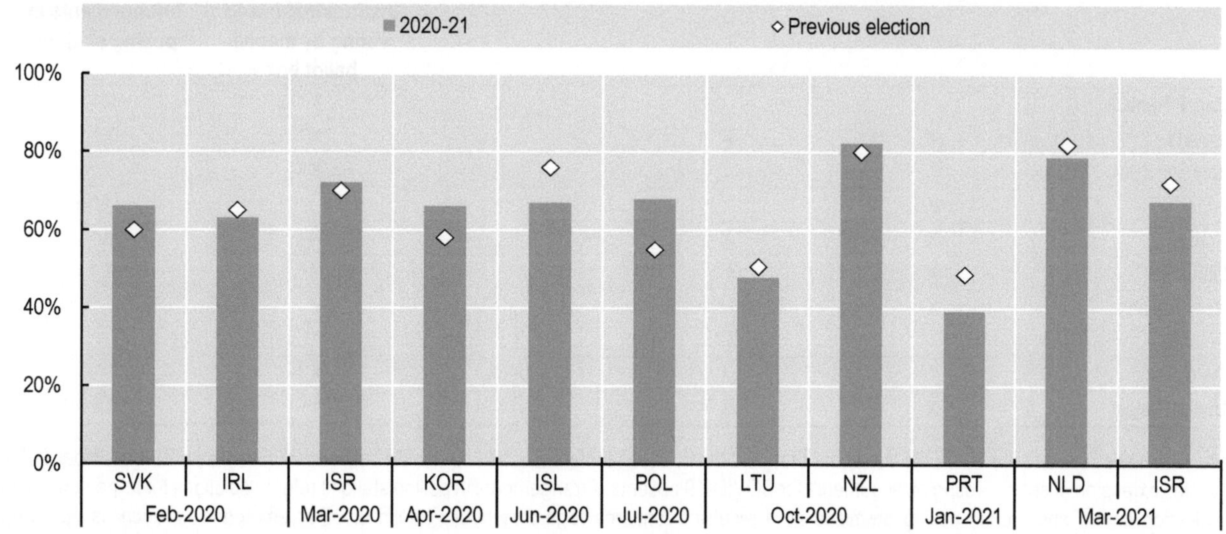

Note: National elections refer to presidential elections in Iceland, Poland and Portugal, and to parliamentary elections for the rest of countries shown. Previous elections were held in 2019-2020 in Israel, 2017 in the Netherlands and New Zealand, 2015 in Poland, and 2016 in all other countries.
Source: IDEA (n.d.[33]), *Voter turnout* (database), https://www.idea.int/data-tools/data/voter-turnout.

StatLink https://stat.link/xd73ck

In several contexts, processes for both national elections and referenda were adapted in 2020 to cope with health restrictions imposed by the pandemic. These included new special voting arrangements and changes in existing practices to reduce crowds and implement social distancing on election day, as well ensuring access for vulnerable groups and allowing people with COVID-19 or in quarantine to vote (Table 4.1). The lessons of these arrangements during 2020 will be significant both during the pandemic and beyond.[9] The only special voting arrangement that was reduced rather than expanded in 2020 and early 2021 was out-of-country voting (OCV) or voting from abroad. For instance, Korea's Electoral Commission cancelled the planned OCV arrangements, disenfranchising about 87 000 potential voters living abroad who could no longer vote by mail, while in Portugal the lower voter turnout in January 2021 can be partly attributed to changes in how to account for voters abroad (Gomes, 2021[34]; IDEA, 2021[35]) (Figure 4.11).

While voter turnout in national elections has not generally declined, there is evidence of differential impacts of the pandemic by the location and age of voters (Santana, Rama and Bertoa, 2020[36]). Most of the available data so far stems from municipal elections: for instance, during the March 2020 French municipal elections, the participation rate decreased with the city's proximity to COVID-19 clusters and with its proportion of elderly (Noury et al., 2021[37]). In Italy, a 1 percentage point increase in the elderly mortality rate decreased the voter turnout in the September-October 2020 municipal elections by 0.5 percentage points, with stronger effects in densely populated municipalities (Santolini and Picchio, 2021[38]).

Table 4.1. Many OECD countries expanded voting arrangements in 2020

Special voting arrangements used in 2020 national elections and referenda by country

	Early voting	Postal voting	Proxy voting	Home and institutional-based voting by mobile ballot box	COVID-19 related arrangements in polling stations
Czech Republic				X*	X*
Iceland	X	X		X*	X*
Italy				X*	
Israel	X				X*
Korea	X	X		X*	X*
Lithuania	X	X*		X*	X*
New Zealand	X	X (from abroad)			
Poland		X*	X		
Switzerland		X	X	X*	
United States	X	X			X (Idaho)*

Note: This table refers to the 10 OECD members that held direct national elections and referenda between 21 February - 31 December 2020. *denotes extension of special voting arrangements for COVID-19 patients. Arrangements in polling stations refer to solutions for in-person voting on election day in and around polling premises as a result of concerns regarding public health or other emergencies, such as reserving designated times or creating special polling stations for voters infected with COVID-19 or in quarantine, as well as drive-through/curb-site voting.
Source: IDEA (2021[35]) , *Elections and Covid-19: How special voting arrangements were expanded in 2020*, https://www.idea.int/news-media/news/elections-and-covid-19-how-special-voting-arrangements-were-expanded-2020.

A large share of people increasingly feel disconnected from society

Throughout the first year of the pandemic, many people have been feeling increasingly disconnected from communal life. Civic engagement is also about feeling able to shape the society one lives in and about having influence on politics. Yet, in June-July 2020, when economies were slowly reopening, almost 1 in 5 of respondents in European OECD countries agreed with the statement that they felt left out of their societies, while a year later nearly 1 in 3 people felt this way (Figure 4.12, Panel A). When asked the same question in the 2016 wave of the European Quality of Life Survey, only 7.8% of respondents in European OECD countries voiced this sentiment (Figure 4.12, Panel B).[10] Already pre-COVID 19, in 2018, on average only 35% of people in European OECD countries reported feeling confident participating in politics, and only 40% believed the political system in their countries allowed people like them to have a say in what the government does (OECD, 2021[39]).

Figure 4.12. Societal alienation increased between mid-2020 and early 2021

Share of people in European OECD countries agreeing or strongly agreeing with the statement "I feel left out of society", 2016, Jun-Jul 2020, Feb-Mar 2021

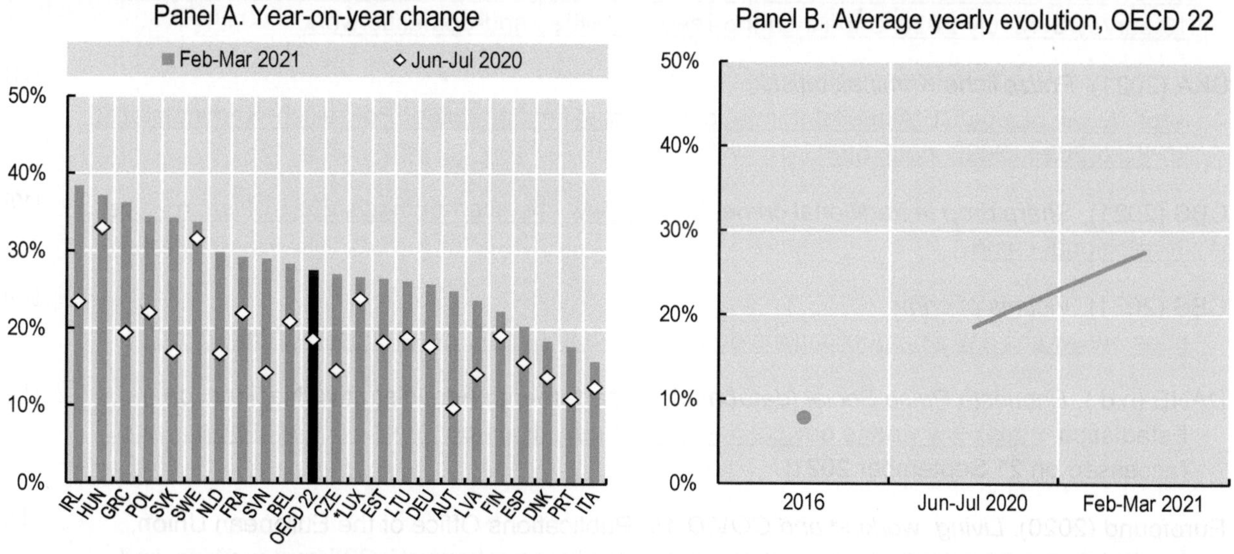

Note: In both panels, the OECD average includes only those 22 countries shown in Panel A. Changes in outcomes between June-July 2020 and February-March 2021 are significant at the 5% level for all countries, including OECD 22, except for Denmark, Finland, Hungary, Italy, Luxembourg, Spain and Sweden. * denotes countries with between 300 and 500 observations for at least one of the time periods. More than 500 observations are available for all other countries. Refer to Box 2.1 for methodological details on the Living, working and COVID-19 e-survey.
Source: Eurofound (2018[1]), *European Quality of Life Survey 2016*, https://www.eurofound.europa.eu/publications/report/2017/fourth-european-quality-of-life-survey-overview-report; and Eurofound (n.d.[3]), *Living, working and COVID-19 e-survey* (database), http://eurofound.link/covid19data.

StatLink https://stat.link/5kjlgf

Box 4.3. Further reading

- OECD (2021), "All the lonely people: Education and loneliness", *Trends Shaping Education Spotlights*, No. 23, OECD Publishing, Paris, https://doi.org/10.1787/23ac0e25-en
- OECD (2020), *Taking Public Action to End Violence at Home: Summary of Conference Proceedings*, OECD Publishing, Paris, https://doi.org/10.1787/cbff411b-en
- OECD (2020), "COVID-19: Protecting people and societies", *OECD Policy Responses to Coronavirus (COVID-19)*, OECD Publishing, Paris, https://doi.org/10.1787/e5c9de1a-en
- Eurofound (2021), Living, working and COVID-19, *COVID-19 series*, Publications Office of the European Union, Luxembourg, https://www.eurofound.europa.eu/publications/report/2021/living-working-and-covid-19-update-april-2021-mental-health-and-trust-decline-across-eu-as-pandemic
- IDEA (2021), *Global overview of COVID-19: Impact on elections*, https://www.idea.int/news-media/multimedia-reports/global-overview-covid-19-impact-elections

References

ABS (2020), *Household Impacts of COVID-19 Survey*, https://www.abs.gov.au/statistics/people/people-and-communities/household-impacts-covid-19-survey/6-10-july-2020#unpaid-caring-responsibilities-and-domestic-work. [15]

BKA (2021), *Polizeiliche Kriminalstatistik*, https://www.bka.de/DE/AktuelleInformationen/StatistikenLagebilder/PolizeilicheKriminalstatistik/PKS2020/pks2020_node.html. [21]

CBS (2021), *Sharp drop in traditional crime*, https://www.cbs.nl/en-gb/news/2021/09/sharp-drop-in-traditional-crime. [19]

CBS (2021), *Victims of crime*, https://www.cbs.gov.il/he/publications/doclib/2021/8.shnatoncrimeandjustice/st08_03.pdf. [23]

DANE (n.d.), *Encuesta Pulso Social (database)*, Departamento Administrativo Nacional de Estadística, https://www.dane.gov.co/index.php/estadisticas-por-tema/encuesta-pulso-social (accessed on 21 September 2021). [11]

Eurofound (2020), *Living, working and COVID-19*, Publications Office of the European Union, Luxembourg, https://www.eurofound.europa.eu/publications/report/2020/living-working-and-covid-19. [8]

Eurofound (2018), *European Quality of Life Survey 2016*, Publications Office of the European Union, Luxembourg, https://www.eurofound.europa.eu/publications/report/2017/fourth-european-quality-of-life-survey-overview-report. [1]

Eurofound (n.d.), *Living, working and COVID-19 dataset*, https://www.eurofound.europa.eu/data/covid-19 (accessed on 21 August 2021). [3]

Europol (2021), *The illicit sales of false negative COVID-19 test certificates*, https://www.europol.europa.eu/sites/default/files/documents/ewn_-_illicit_sales_of_false_negative_covid-19_test_certificates.pdf. [29]

Europol (2020), *Internet Organised Crime Threat Assessment*, https://www.europol.europa.eu/newsroom/news/covid-19-sparks-upward-trend-in-cybercrime. [31]

FBI (2021), *FBI Releases 2020 Crime Statistics*, https://www.fbi.gov/news/pressrel/press-releases/fbi-releases-2020-crime-statistics. [22]

Gallup (n.d.), *Gallup World Poll (database)*, https://www.gallup.com/178667/gallup-world-poll-work.aspx (accessed on 18 June 2021). [14]

Gomes, C. (2021), *Portuguese Presidential Elections In-Depth: Strange Bedfellows, a Landslide Victory and Signs of Political Realignment*, https://europeelects.eu/2021/02/04/portugal-presidential-election-result-and-signs-of-change/. [34]

IDEA (2021), *Elections and Covid-19: How special voting arrangements were expanded in 2020*, https://www.idea.int/news-media/news/elections-and-covid-19-how-special-voting-arrangements-were-expanded-2020. [35]

Imperial College London YouGov (2020), *Covid 19 Behaviour Tracker Data Hub*, https://github.com/YouGov-Data/covid-19-tracker. [9]

International Institute for Democracy and Electoral Assistance (n.d.), *Voter turnout database*, https://www.idea.int/data-tools/data/voter-turnout (accessed on 26 September 2021). [33]

International Transport Forum (2020), *Road Safety Annual Report 2020*, https://www.itf-oecd.org/road-safety-annual-report-2020. [17]

International Transport Forum (n.d.), *Short term indicators - Road*, https://stats.oecd.org/index.aspx?queryid=73641 (accessed on 1 July 2021). [18]

Interpol (2021), *Thousands of fake online pharmacies shut down in INTERPOL operation*, https://www.interpol.int/en/News-and-Events/News/2021/Thousands-of-fake-online-pharmacies-shut-down-in-INTERPOL-operation. [30]

Interpol (2020), *Covid-19: child sexual exploitation and abuse threats and trends*, https://www.interpol.int/en/News-and-Events/News/2020/INTERPOL-report-highlights-impact-of-COVID-19-on-child-sexual-abuse. [32]

Interpol (2020), *COVID-19: the global thread of fake medicines*, https://www.interpol.int/content/download/15305/file/20COM0356%20-%20IGGH_COVID-19%20threats%20to%20medicines_2020-05_EN.pdf?inLanguage=eng-GB. [28]

Kühne, S. et al. (2020), "The need for household panel surveys in times of crisis: The case of SOEP-CoV", *Survey Research Methods*, Vol. 14/2, pp. 195-203, https://doi.org/10.18148/srm/2020.v14i2.7748. [10]

Morris, K. and P. Miller (2021), "Voting in a Pandemic: COVID-19 and Primary Turnout in Milwaukee, Wisconsin", *Urban Affairs Review*, http://dx.doi.org/10.1177/10780874211005016. [40]

New Zealand Police (2021), *Crime at a glance*, https://www.police.govt.nz/sites/default/files/publications/crime-at-a-glance-dec2020.pdf. [20]

Noury, A. et al. (2021), "How does COVID-19 affect electoral participation? evidence from the French municipal elections", *PLOS ONE*, Vol. 16/2, http://dx.doi.org/10.1371/journal.pone.0247026. [37]

OECD (2021), *Government at a Glance 2021*, OECD Publishing, Paris, https://dx.doi.org/10.1787/1c258f55-en. [39]

OECD (2020), *Taking Public Action to End Violence at Home: Summary of Conference Proceedings*, OECD Publishing, Paris, https://dx.doi.org/10.1787/cbff411b-en. [27]

OECD (2017), *How's Life? 2017: Measuring Well-being*, OECD Publishing, Paris, https://dx.doi.org/10.1787/how_life-2017-en. [41]

ONS (2021), *A "new normal"? How people spent their time after the March 2020 coronavirus lockdown*, https://www.ons.gov.uk/peoplepopulationandcommunity/healthandsocialcare/conditionsanddiseases/articles/anewnormalhowpeoplespenttheirtimeafterthemarch2020coronaviruslockdown/2020-12-09. [16]

ONS (2021), *Coronavirus and the social impacts on Great Britain: 29 January 2021*, https://www.ons.gov.uk/peoplepopulationandcommunity/healthandsocialcare/healthandwellbeing/bulletins/coronavirusandthesocialimpactsongreatbritain/29january2021#measuring-the-data. [13]

ONS (2021), *Crime in England and Wales: year ending December 2020*, https://www.ons.gov.uk/peoplepopulationandcommunity/crimeandjustice/bulletins/crimeinenglandandwales/yearendingdecember2020#perception-and-nature-of-crime-during-the-coronavirus-pandemic. [24]

ONS (2021), *Mapping loneliness during the coronavirus pandemic*, https://www.ons.gov.uk/peoplepopulationandcommunity/wellbeing/articles/mappinglonelinessduringthecoronaviruspandemic/2021-04-07. [2]

Santana, A., J. Rama and F. Bertoa (2020), "The Coronavirus Pandemic and Voter Turnout: Addressing the Impact of Covid-19 on Electoral Participation", https://osf.io/preprints/socarxiv/3d4ny/. [36]

Santolini, R. and M. Picchio (2021), "The COVID-19 Pandemic's Effects on Voter Turnout", No. 14241, IZA Discussion Papers, https://www.iza.org/publications/dp/14241/the-covid-19-pandemics-effects-on-voter-turnout. [38]

Stats NZ (2021), *Wellbeing statistics: March 2021 quarter*, https://www.stats.govt.nz/information-releases/wellbeing-statistics-march-2021-quarter. [7]

StatsNZ (2021), *Wellbeing statistics: A year in review (June 2020 to March 2021 quarter)*, https://www.stats.govt.nz/reports/wellbeing-statistics-a-year-in-review-june-2020-to-march-2021-quarter#worse. [12]

StatsNZ (2020), *Wellbeing statistics: June 2020 quarter*, https://www.stats.govt.nz/information-releases/wellbeing-statistics-june-2020-quarter#most. [5]

StatsNZ (n.d.), *Wellbeing data for New Zealanders - Loneliness*, https://wellbeingindicators.stats.govt.nz/en/loneliness/ (accessed on 26 March 2021). [6]

University of Oxford (n.d.), *Coronavirus Government Response Tracker*, University of Oxford, https://www.bsg.ox.ac.uk/research/research-projects/coronavirus-government-response-tracker (accessed on 20 May 2021). [4]

UNODC (2020), *UNODC Research Reveals Drop in Reported Property Crime and Homicide During COVID-19 Lockdown Is Only Short-Lived*, https://www.unodc.org/unodc/en/frontpage/2020/December/unodc-research-reveals-drop-in-reported-property-crime-and-homicide-during-covid-19-lockdown-is-only-short-lived.html. [25]

UNODC (n.d.), *Crime during COVID-19 pandemic*, https://dataunodc.un.org/content/covid-19 (accessed on 26 July 2021). [26]

Notes

[1] The 2020-21 and 2016 data, from the Eurofound Living, working and Covid-19 e-survey and the European Quality of Life Survey respectively, are not directly comparable due to different sampling designs, but similar county rankings lend face validity to the results.

[2] Some caution needs to be exercised when comparing 2020 data from the HLFS supplement (Box 4.1) with estimates produced from the General Social Survey, as differences in collection method, sampled population, reporting periods, and restrictions on face-to-face interviewing, among other things, may all impact on comparability.

[3] These answers about behaviour have to be interpreted in light of potential social desirability bias (i.e. the perceived socially accepted response to questions about social isolation). This implies that rates of actual avoidance of contact might be slightly lower in reality.

[4] Three percentage points are typically considered to be the minimum threshold to denote meaningful change for this indicator between two points in time, as outlined in *How's Life? 2017* (OECD, 2017[41]).

[5] The 2018 European Quality of Life Survey question asked in a single question about being too tired after work to do household chores, difficulty fulfilling family responsibilities because of time spent at work, and difficulty concentrating at work because of family responsibilities.

[6] People with a paid job reported a 20% increase in time worked on an average day in September-October 2020 since the April 2020 lockdown. And, as schools re-opened by September-October 2020, parents were doing more paid work on average (up by 54 minutes), while at the same time spending less time on childcare and unpaid housework (down by 51 minutes on average) (ONS, 2021[16]).

[7] For example, the police recorded a 12% decrease in homicides in England and Wales (excluding Greater Manchester) in the year ending December 2020 compared with the previous year. These latest homicide figures include 39 people whose bodies were found in a lorry in Essex in October 2019 – without this single incident, the number of victims would have decreased by only 6%.

[8] Official data on voter turnout for the United States 2020 elections had not been published as of 26 September 2021.

[9] These also include potential negative effects: for instance, polling place consolidation in Milwaukee during the presidential primary election in April 2020 disproportionally reduced voter turnout of Black people in the city, even when accompanied by widespread absentee voting (Morris and Miller, 2021[40]).

[10] The 2020-21 and 2016 data, from the Eurofound Living, working and Covid-19 e-survey and the European Quality of Life Survey respectively, are not directly comparable due to different sampling designs.

5 Inclusion, material conditions and COVID-19

The pandemic's consequences for jobs and incomes are weighing heavily on already vulnerable population groups. Industries that were most affected by lockdowns typically include higher shares of younger, lower-educated and lower-paid workers. Across the OECD, the employment gap between young people and other working-age adults widened, and the youth unemployment rate reached twice that of other working-age adults in Q2 2020. On average across EU countries, the labour income loss between 2019 and 2020 was four times higher for workers in the bottom income quintile, relative to workers in the top quintile. Women, mothers, immigrants and those belonging to racial/ethnic minorities and LGBTQ+ communities were more likely to lose their jobs and are now facing particular financial strain. Housing challenges were also exacerbated, with vulnerable groups struggling to access affordable and quality housing.

5.1. Work and Job Quality

Lower-paid and less-educated workers were more likely to stop working during the pandemic, and those who remained in employment were less able to telework

Lower-paid and less-educated workers were most exposed to the pandemic's immediate impacts on the labour market. These workers are less likely to be in roles that are amenable to teleworking (Box 5.1), making them both more adversely impacted by pandemic-related business closures and more likely to be in roles involving higher social contact and infection risk (OECD, 2020[1]). In 22 European OECD countries, low-wage earners make up a much higher share of those who lost their jobs in 2020 (Figure 5.1). It is therefore not surprising that, across the EU 27, it is estimated that the average loss of employment income between 2019 and 2020 was four times higher for workers in the bottom income quintile compared to those in the top income quintile (-10.2% vs. -2.5%) (Eurostat, 2021[2]).[1] Evidence from a separate survey conducted in 25 OECD countries in September-October 2020 also shows that people from low-income households were more likely than those in medium- or high-income households to report a job loss or a job-related disruption (OECD, n.d.[3]).[2]

Figure 5.1. In 22 European OECD countries, low-wage earners accounted for at least 40% of job losses in 2020

Share of people who lost their job by income group, 2020

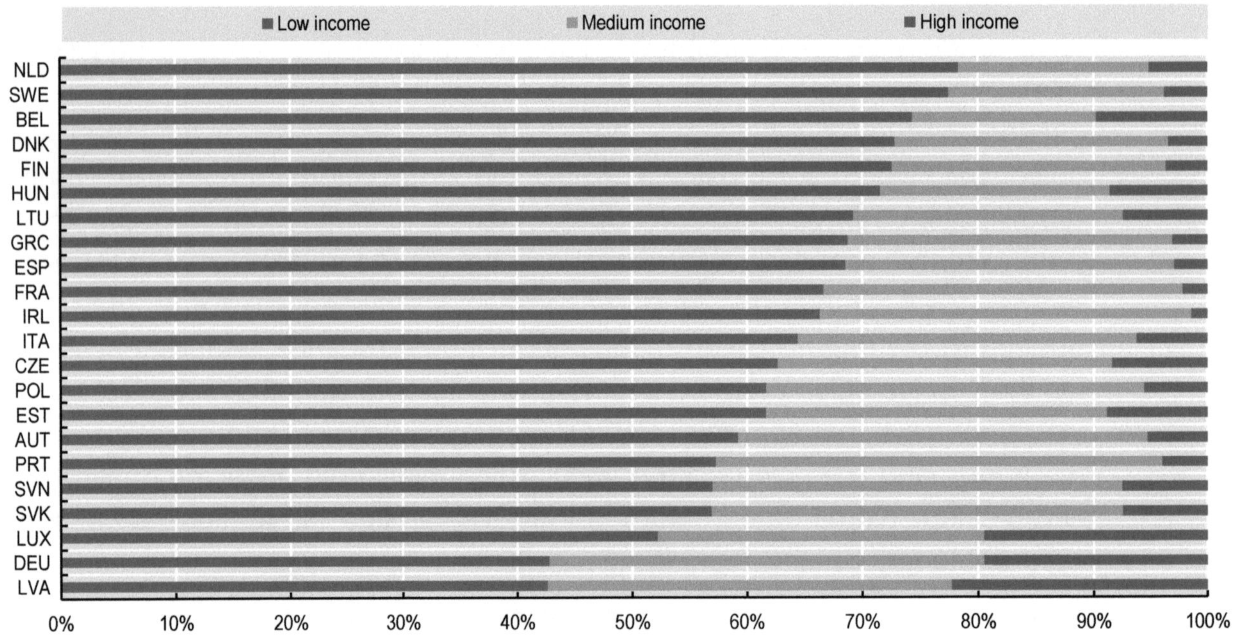

Note: All figures are part of the experimental statistics produced by Eurostat in the frame of advanced estimates on income inequality and poverty indicators. Low-income earners comprise individuals in deciles 1, 2 and 3; middle-income earners comprise individuals in deciles 4, 5, 6 and 7; and high-income earners comprise individuals in deciles 8, 9 and 10.

Source: Eurostat (2020[4]), *Impact of COVID-19 on employment income - advanced estimates*, https://ec.europa.eu/eurostat/statistics-explained/index.php?title=Impact_of_COVID-19_on_employment_income_-_advanced_estimates#A_sharp_decrease_in_the_median_employment_income.

StatLink https://stat.link/ldvywf

On average in 34 OECD countries, workers with tertiary education experienced a smaller rise in unemployment in 2020 relative to their less-educated peers. Nevertheless, education gaps related to the change in unemployment between 2019 and 2020 did vary across OECD countries, with some experiencing a greater widening of the education gap than others (Figure 5.2). Evidence from the United States indicates that the magnitude of this education gap also varies by sector (Box 5.2).

Figure 5.2. People with less than a tertiary education experienced larger increases in unemployment in 34 OECD countries

Share of the total labour force aged 25-64 who are unemployed, by education level, year-on-year percentage point change, 2019-20

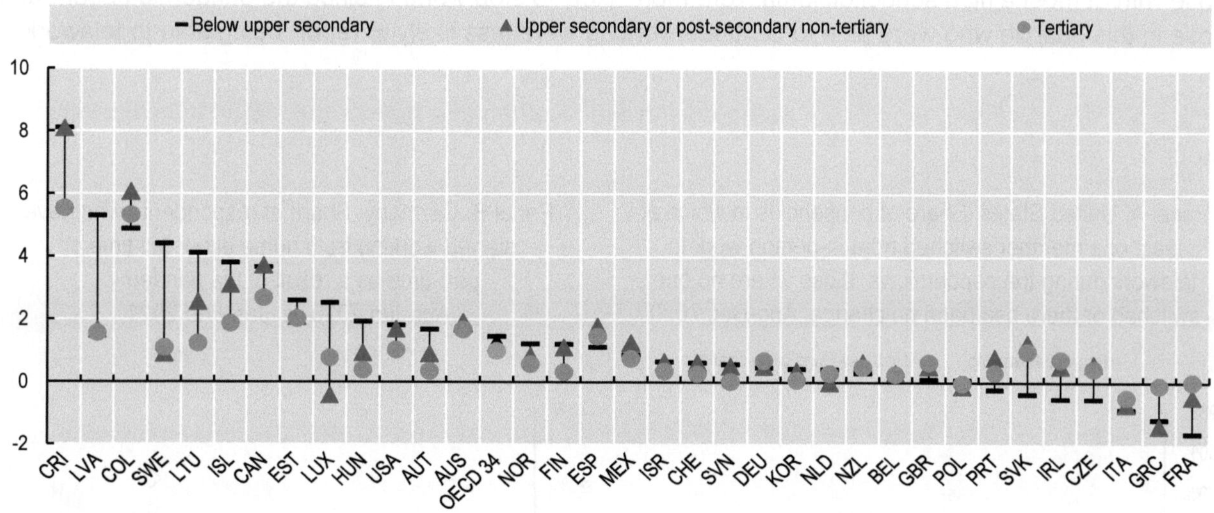

Note: The OECD average excludes Chile, Denmark, Japan and Turkey. Data for Germany in 2020 are provisional and might be subject to low reliability due to technical issues with the introduction of the new German system of integrated household surveys.
Source: OECD (n.d.[5]), *OECD Education statistics* (database), https://doi.org/10.1787/889e8641-en.

StatLink https://stat.link/u9sixo

Box 5.1. Methods: Teleworking by income and education – evidence from the United States Census Bureau Household Pulse, the German Socio-Economic Panel, and the REPEAT survey

Data from the US Census Bureau Household Pulse survey (see Box 3.1 for methods) collected between 19 August and 21 December 2020 show that the propensity to switch from in-person work to telework increased with education level: those with a university degree are more than three times as likely to have started working from home during the pandemic, compared to those with only a high school degree (Figure 5.3, Panel A). Data collected as part of Germany's Socio-Economic Panel (see Box 3.1 for methods) in April-June 2020 meanwhile found that those with higher levels of education are more than four times as likely to report working from home (Figure 5.3, Panel B). This is true both for employees who are able to work from home full-time (18% for high education, 4% for low), as well as for those who work from home only part-time (16% vs. 3%). A subsequent round of data collection in January-February 2021 suggests even greater disparities: 19% of those with higher levels of education were able to work from home full-time, compared to only 2% of those with lower levels of education.

The REpresentations, PErceptions and ATtitudes on COVID-19 (REPEAT) survey collects data on attitudes and behavioural responses to COVID-19, as well as labour market outcomes, in eighteen countries. The survey is a part of a larger project, "Citizens' Attitudes towards COVID-19", housed at Sciences Po Paris. Data are collected at four different points in time in each country, so that outcomes can be tracked over the course of the pandemic. Each survey wave samples around 1 000 respondents. Surveys are conducted online; data are then weighted to account for gender, age, occupation, geographic location and political orientation.

The data used in Figure 5.4 were gathered during the second wave of data collection, in mid-April 2020 (see figure note for exact dates per country). In total, surveys were administered to 15 045 respondents in twelve countries: Australia, Austria, Brazil, Canada, France, Germany, Italy, New Zealand, Poland, Sweden, the United Kingdom and the United States. Employees from the bottom earnings quartile and those with at most a high school diploma were more likely to stop working since the pandemic began; and those in this quartile who were able to continue working were less likely to report being able to telework.

Figure 5.3. The ability to work from home during the pandemic is highly correlated with workers' education level

Panel A. United States: Share of households in which at least one member switched from in-person work to telework during the pandemic vs. those where no one switched or there had been no change, Aug-Dec 2020

Panel B. Germany: Share of respondents who have started working from home either full-time or part-time as a result of the pandemic, Apr-Jun 2020 vs. Jan-Feb 2021

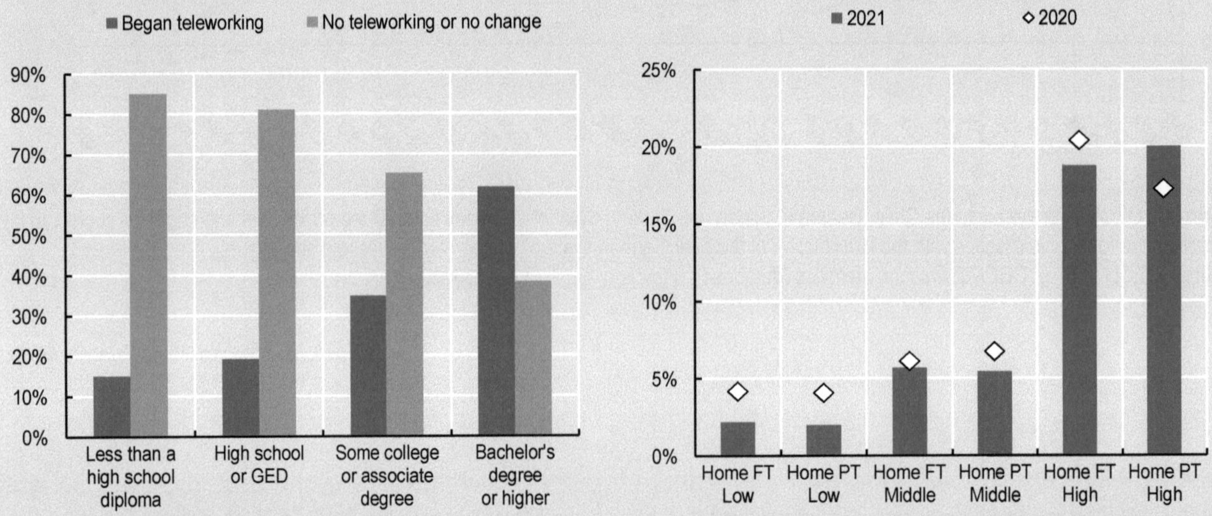

Note: Panel B shows the share of respondents who report working from home either full-time (FT) or part-time (PT), by education level (low, middle, high), in 2020 vs. 2021. The educational categories are defined as follows: "Low" refers to below upper-secondary education (i.e. less than primary, primary and lower secondary education), "Middle" refers to upper secondary education (i.e. secondary and post-secondary non-tertiary education), and "High" refers to tertiary education. Funded by the German Federal Ministry of Education and Research (BMBF). The data can be accessed via the research data centre of the SOEP.

Source: Marshall, J., C. Burd and M. Burrows (2021[6]), *Working From Home During the Pandemic*, US Census Bureau, https://www.census.gov/library/stories/2021/03/working-from-home-during-the-pandemic.html (Panel A); and Kühne et al. (2020[7]), "The need for household panel surveys in times of crisis: The case of SOEP-CoV", *Survey Research Methods*, Vol. 14/2, pp. 195-203, https://doi.org/10.18148/srm/2020.v14i2.7748 (Panel B).

StatLink https://stat.link/ijtehp

Figure 5.4. While higher-earning and higher-educated employees often worked from home, lower-earning and lower-educated employees had to stop working

Share of employees working from home, working in the workplace, or who stopped working, Apr-May 2020

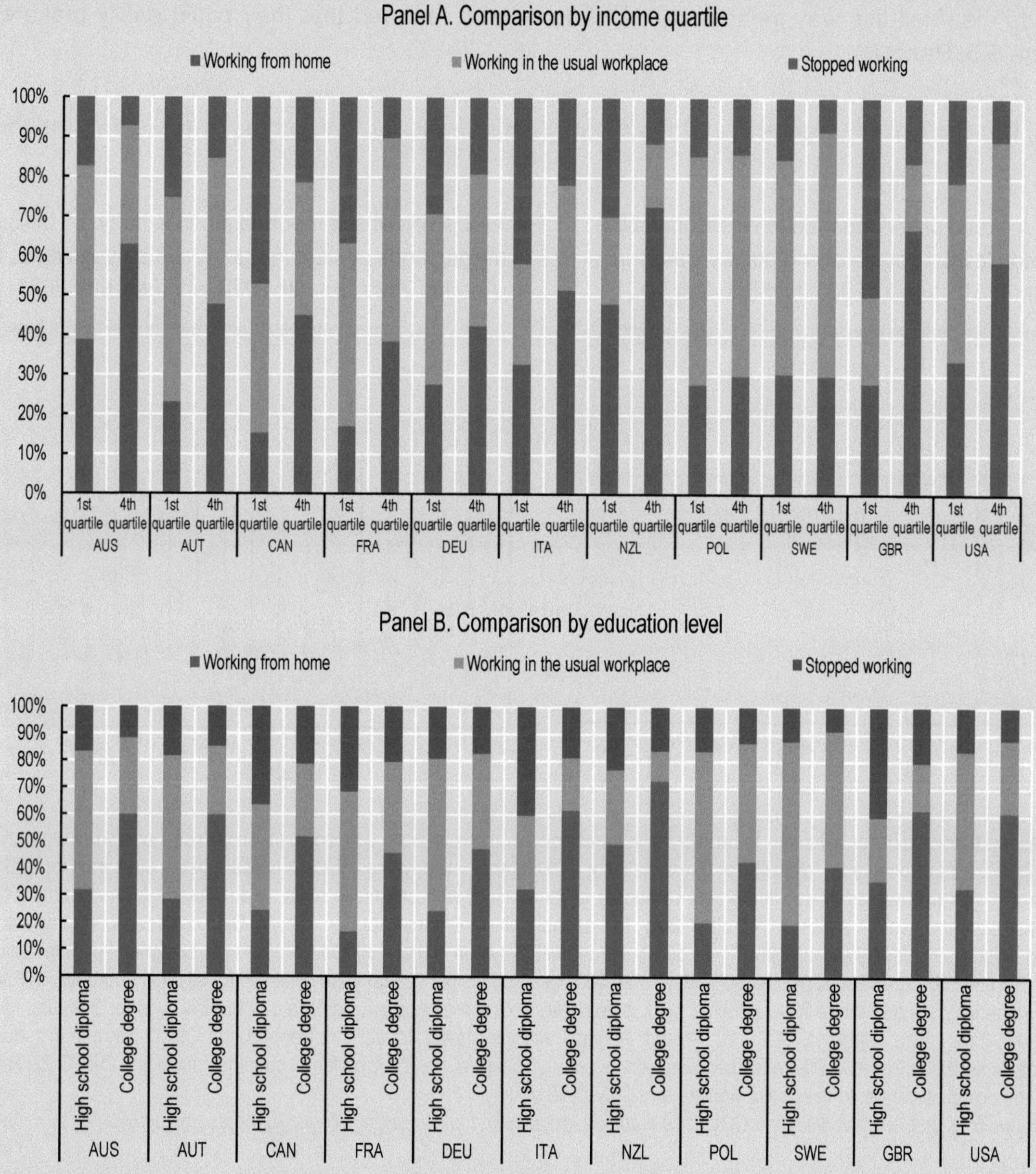

Note: Data are from the REPEAT (REpresentations, PErceptions and ATtitudes on the COVID-19) survey. Data were collected: 15-20 April (Australia); 15-18 April (Austria and New Zealand); 30 April-2 May (Poland); 14-17 April (Canada); 15-16 April (France); 16-18 April (Germany and the United States); 15-17 April (Italy and the United Kingdom); and 16-17 April (Sweden). No data are available on service workers in Australia, New Zealand or the United States, on self-employed in Australia, and on the type of occupation in Canada.

Source: Galasso, V. and M. Foucault (2020[8]), *Working during COVID-19: Cross-country evidence from real-time survey data*, OECD Social, Employment and Migration Working Papers, No. 246, OECD Publishing, Paris, https://doi.org/10.1787/34a2c306-en.

StatLink https://stat.link/latm70

Workers with lower levels of education and people facing financial difficulties were most worried about losing their jobs between April-June 2020 and February-March 2021. Data for 22 European OECD countries indicate that 13% of those with a secondary education or less reported that it was "very likely" or "likely" that they would lose their jobs within the next three months, compared to 9% of those with a tertiary or above education level (Figure 5.5, Panel A). Similarly, 29% of people who are having difficulty making ends meet felt this way, relative to 7% of those who reported that they could easily make ends meet (Figure 5.5, Panel B).

Figure 5.5. Less-educated workers and people facing financial difficulties feel more insecure about their jobs, selected European countries

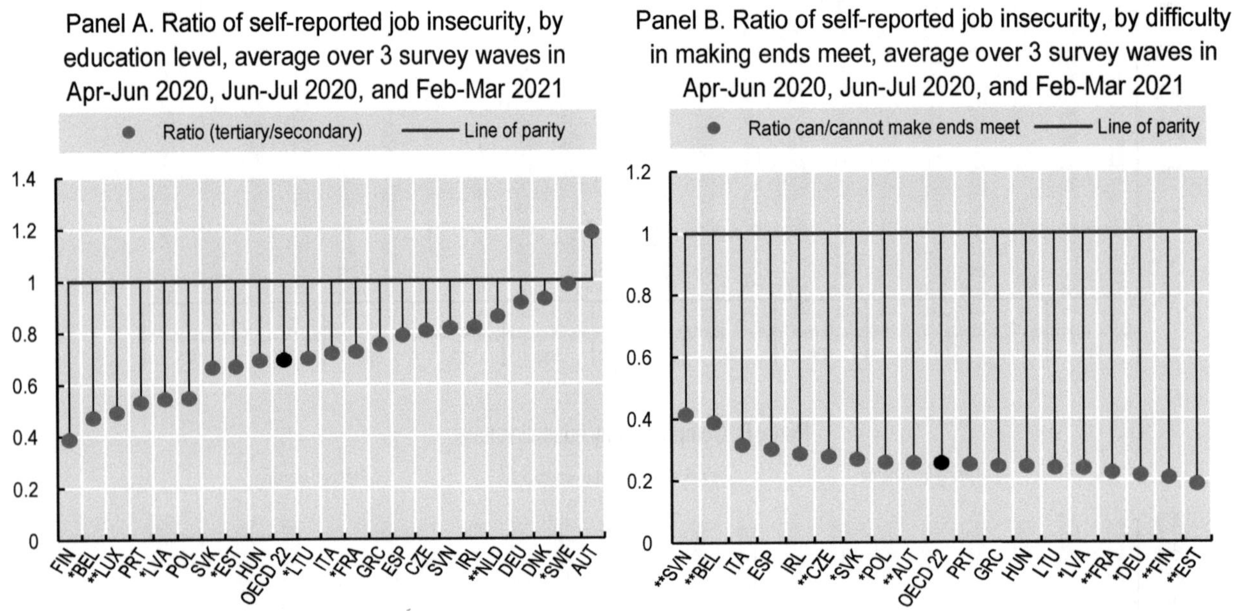

Note: Ratios above 1 indicate better outcomes for workers with lower education levels (here, defined as those with secondary or below levels of education) or for workers who reported "difficulty" or "great difficulty" making ends meet; values below 1 indicate better outcomes for those with higher education levels (defined as those with tertiary or above) or for workers who can make ends meet "easily". Job insecurity refers to respondents indicating they were "very likely" or "rather likely" to lose their job within the next three months. Data are not reported where fewer than 100 observations per category are available. ** denotes countries with between 100 and 300 observations per category; * denotes countries with between 301 and 500 observations per category. More than 500 observations per category are available for all other countries. In Panel A, the OECD average includes only those 22 countries shown. Differences between groups are significant at the 5% level for Belgium, Finland, Greece, Hungary, Italy, Latvia, Lithuania, OECD 22, Poland, Portugal and the Slovak Republic. In Panel B, the OECD average includes only those 22 countries shown in Panel A. Difference between groups are significant at the 5% level for all countries, including OECD 22. Refer to Box 2.1 for methodological details on the Living, working and COVID-19 survey.
Source: Eurofound (n.d.[9]), *Living, working and COVID-19 e-survey* (database), https://www.eurofound.europa.eu/data/covid-19.

StatLink https://stat.link/g0fepk

Box 5.2. The relationship between unemployment, education and industry during the pandemic

In the United States, across all selected industries, workers with lower levels of education had higher unemployment rates than those with a university degree between January 2020 and February 2021. However, in the hardest hit sector of leisure and hospitality, the difference in unemployment rates between the two groups was considerably smaller than (for example) in manufacturing (Figure 5.6).

Figure 5.6. The leisure and hospitality sector was particularly hard-hit, with high unemployment rates for those with both secondary and tertiary degrees in the United States

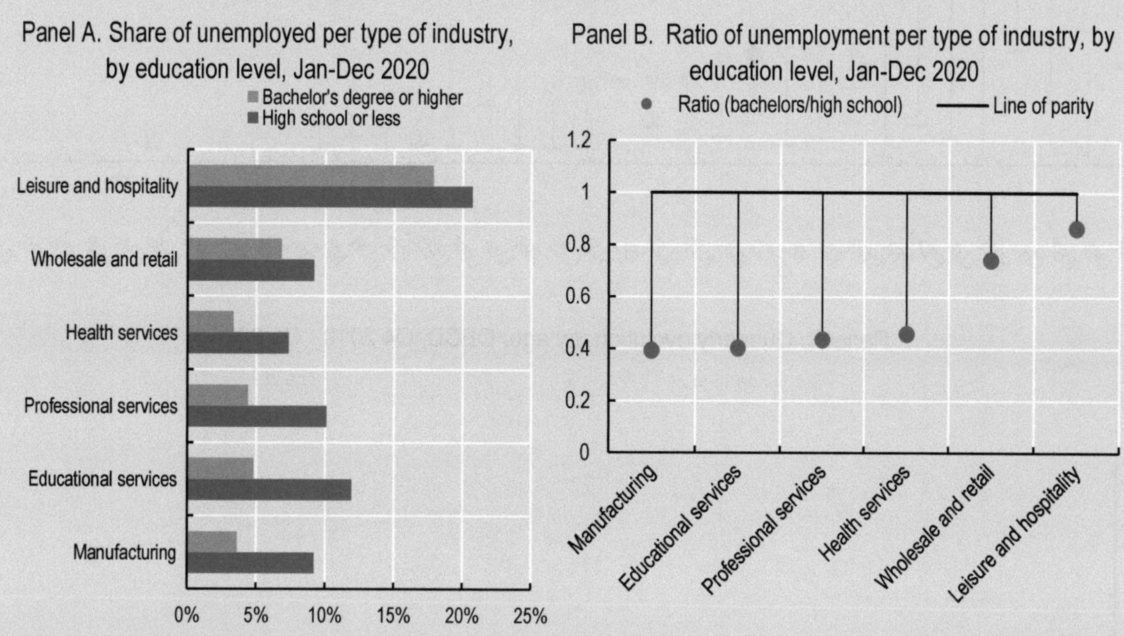

Note: Unemployment rates are expressed as a cumulative average of January-December 2020. In Panel B, ratios above 1 indicate better outcomes for those with lower education levels (high school or less); values below 1 indicate better outcomes for those with higher education levels (bachelor's degree or higher).

Source: Georgetown University (n.d.[10]), Tracking COVID-19 Unemployment and Job Losses, https://cew.georgetown.edu/cew-reports/jobtracker/#unemployment-tracking.

StatLink https://stat.link/jbwoys

Younger workers have been further disadvantaged by the pandemic, experiencing higher job and earnings losses than older workers

Young people aged 15 to 24 experienced a higher risk of job loss than workers aged 25 or over during the pandemic. Indeed, young people are more likely to hold less secure and lower skill jobs and are highly represented in sectors more severely exposed to government lockdowns (OECD, 2021[11]). In nearly all OECD countries, young workers experienced higher rises in unemployment compared to older workers between 2019 and 2020 (Figure 5.7, Panel A). In Q2 2020, the OECD average unemployment rate for workers aged 15-24 was 18.5%, more than twice as high as that of workers aged 25 or over (7.4%) (Figure 5.7, Panel B).

Figure 5.7. Young workers experienced higher rises in unemployment in 2020, peaking in Q2

Share of the labour force who are unemployed

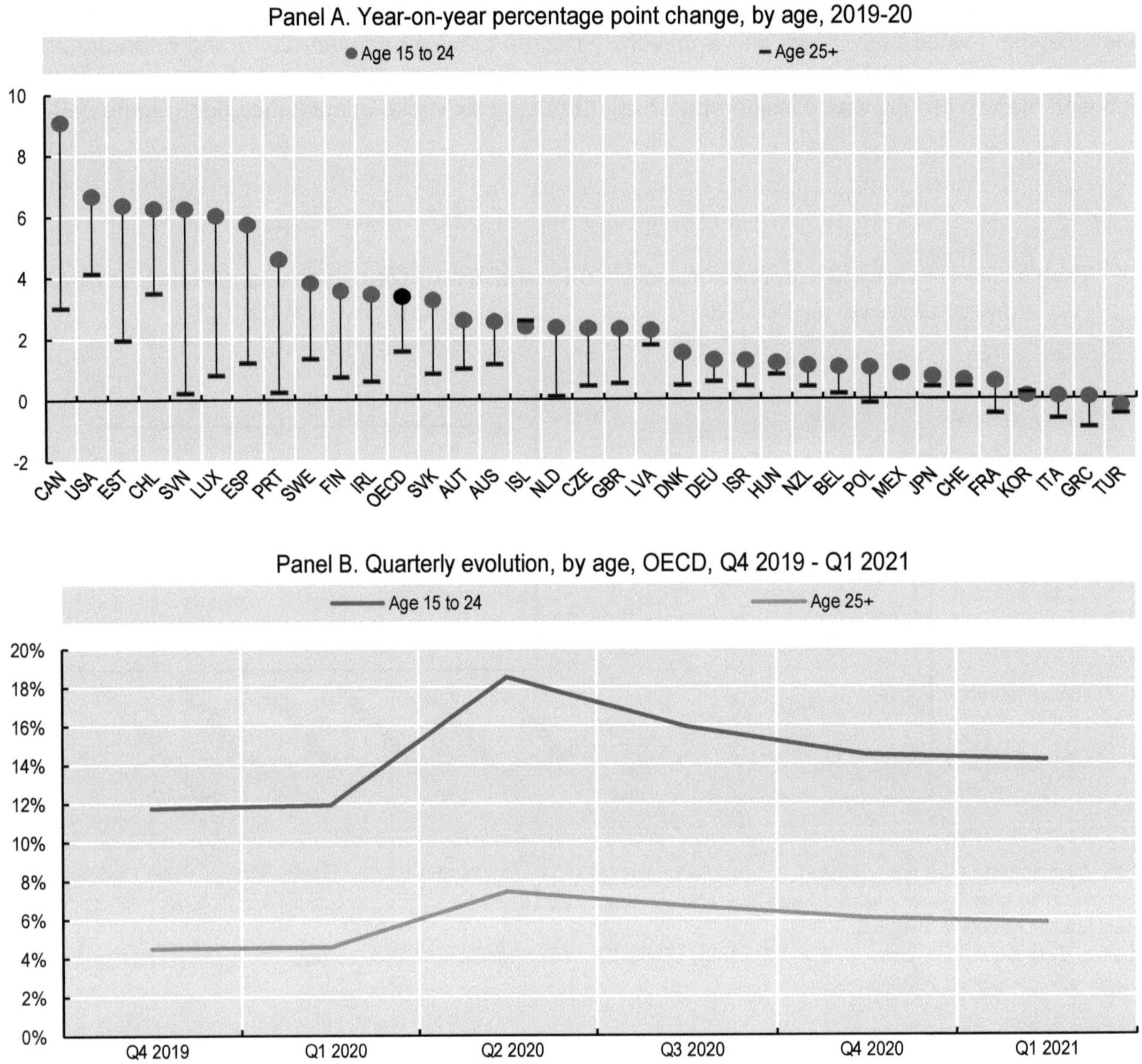

Note: The OECD unemployment rate is calculated as the total number of unemployed people in all OECD countries, as a percentage of the total labour force (i.e. the unemployed plus those in employment). Data for Germany in 2020 are provisional and might be subject to low reliability due to technical issues with the introduction of the new German system of integrated household surveys.
Source: OECD (n.d.[12]), *Main Economic Indicators* (database), https://doi.org/10.1787/data-00046-en.

StatLink https://stat.link/rhlg5y

The COVID-19 crisis has reversed the decade-long improvement in the number of young people not in education, employment or training (NEET). At the end of 2019, prior to the COVID-19 outbreak, just over 1 in every 10 young people aged 15 to 29 were NEET (OECD, 2021[11]). By the second quarter of 2020, however, the NEET rate increased by 2.9 percentage points year-on-year across the OECD, with a high share of the increase concentrated in inactivity (Figure 5.8). Despite having decreased in the third quarter of 2020, the share of inactive NEET youth remained elevated in the majority of countries in Q4 2020 (OECD, 2021[11]). Periods of inactivity have proved to be very damaging for young people's career prospects, and the high levels of NEET present during the pandemic are likely to result in longer-term scarring effects (see (OECD, 2021[11]) and Chapter 9 for more information on youth NEET during the pandemic).

Figure 5.8. The pandemic reversed the decade-long decrease in the number of youth NEET

Share of the youth aged 15 to 29 not in employment, education or training (NEET), year-on-year percentage point change, Q2 2019 - Q2 2020

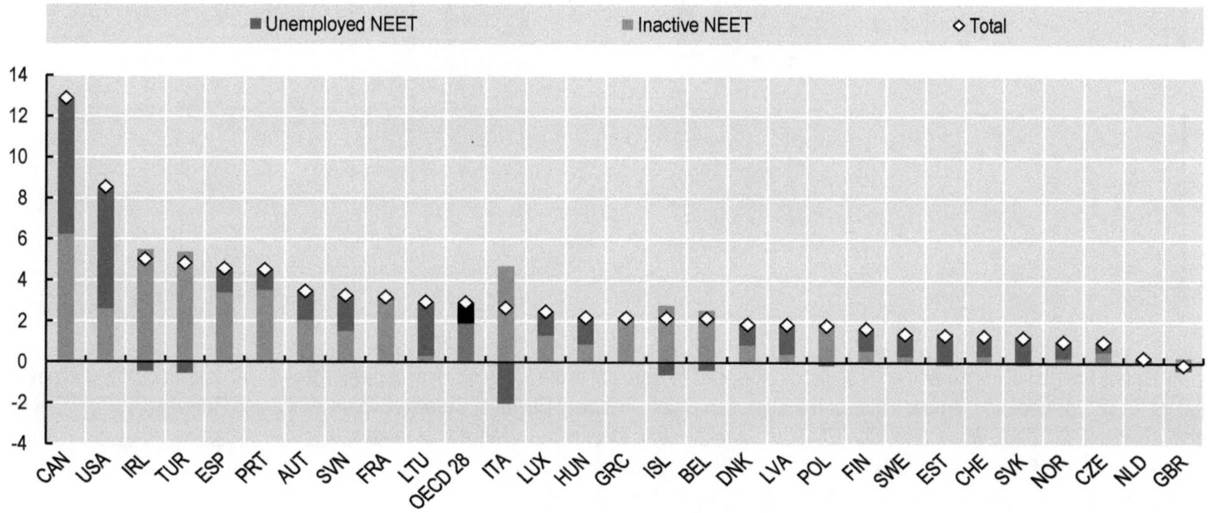

Note: The OECD average excludes Australia, Chile, Colombia, Costa Rica, Germany, Israel, Japan, Korea, Mexico and New Zealand. In Canada, the large increase in NEET rates in Q2 2020 was driven, in large part, by school closures and the large numbers of youth who, as a result, reported that they were not attending school. See https://www150.statcan.gc.ca/n1/pub/81-599-x/81-599-x2020001-eng.htm for more details. Elsewhere, data refer to enrolment rather than attendance and are, as a result, unaffected by school closures. See OECD (2021[11]) for more information on NEET during the pandemic.

Source: OECD (2021[11]), *OECD Employment Outlook 2021: Navigating the COVID-19 Crisis and Recovery* OECD Publishing, Paris, https://doi.org/10.1787/5a700c4b-en.

StatLink https://stat.link/glp4wn

Young people were also more exposed to greater falls in earnings and higher rates of job insecurity during 2020. It is estimated that, in the EU 27, younger workers aged 16-34 suffered higher losses in earnings compared to workers aged 35-65 between 2019 and 2020 – respectively 5.8% and 4.5% (Figure 5.9). The younger age group experienced higher losses in employment income in 20 EU Member States, with declines ranging from 15% to 2% compared with 2019. Nevertheless, income support by governments is estimated to have reduced the losses for both age groups (Eurostat, 2021[2]). In addition, data from 22 European OECD countries collected between April-June 2020 and February-March 2021 suggest that job insecurity was also higher among younger workers on average. Specifically, 19% of young people (aged 18 to 24) felt they were likely to lose their job in the following three months, compared to 11% of people aged 25 or over (Figure 5.10).

Figure 5.9. Young workers are estimated to have experienced higher earnings losses than their older peers

Employment income (before compensation schemes), by age, year-on-year percentage change, EU 27, 2019-20

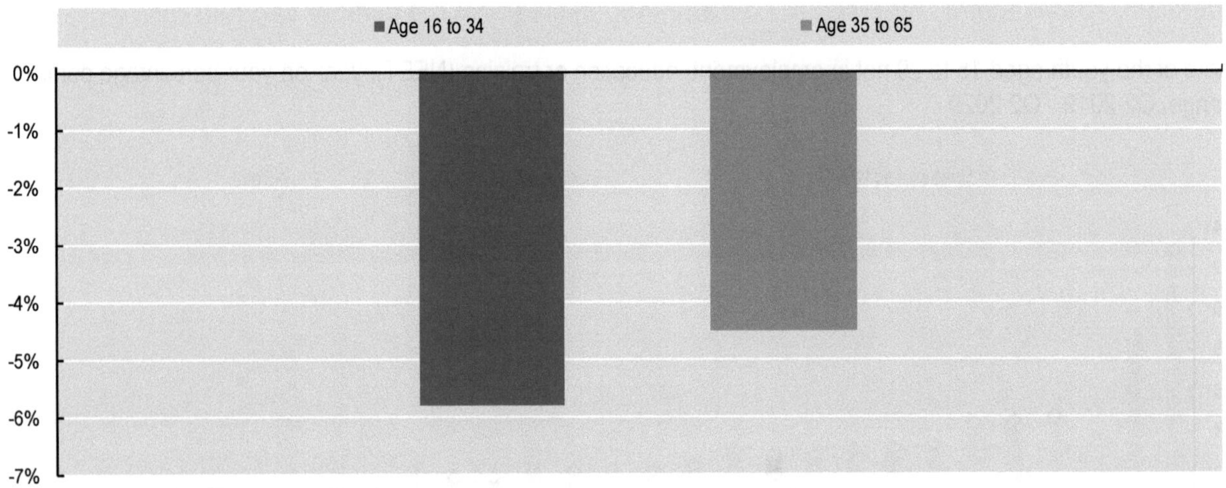

Note: All figures are part of the experimental statistics produced by Eurostat in the frame of advanced estimates on income inequality and poverty indicators. EU 27 includes all member states of the European Union, including Bulgaria, Croatia, Cyprus, Malta and Romania.
Source: Eurostat (2020[4]), *Impact of COVID-19 on employment income - advanced estimates*, https://ec.europa.eu/eurostat/statistics-explained/index.php?title=Impact_of_COVID-19_on_employment_income_-_advanced_estimates#A_sharp_decrease_in_the_median_employment_income.

StatLink https://stat.link/bojk2l

Figure 5.10. On average across 22 OECD countries, more young workers felt they were likely to lose their jobs within the next 3 months

Ratio of self-reported job insecurity, by age, average over 3 survey waves in Apr-Jun 2020, Jun-Jul 2020 and Feb-Mar 2021

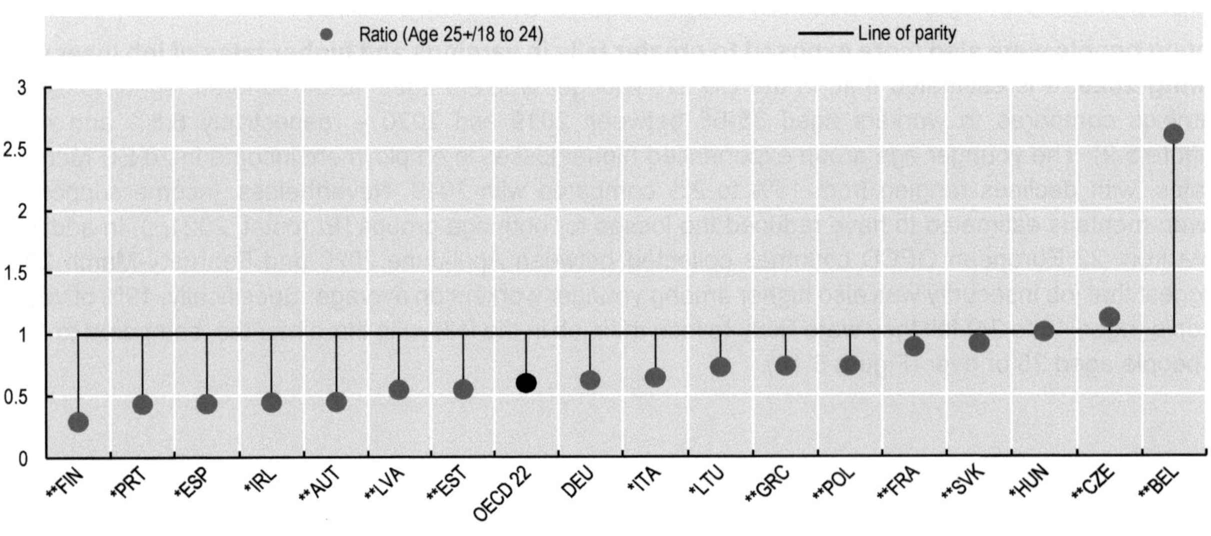

Note: Ratios above 1 indicate better outcomes for workers aged between 18 and 24; values below 1 indicate better outcomes for those aged 25 or over. Job insecurity refers to respondents indicating they were "very likely" or "rather likely" to lose their job within the next three months. Data are not reported where fewer than 100 observations per age category are available. ** denotes countries with between 100 and 300 observations per category; * denotes countries with between 301 and 500 observations per category. More than 500 observations per category are available for all other countries. The OECD average includes Austria, Belgium, the Czech Republic, Denmark, Estonia, Finland, France, Germany, Greece, Hungary, Ireland, Italy, Latvia, Lithuania, Luxembourg, the Netherlands, Poland, Portugal, the Slovak Republic, Slovenia, Spain and Sweden. Differences between groups are significant at the 5% level for Belgium, Finland, Ireland, OECD 22, Portugal and Spain. Refer to Box 2.1 for methodological details on the Living, working and COVID-19 survey.
Source: Eurofound (n.d.[9]), *Living, working and COVID-19 e-survey* (database), https://www.eurofound.europa.eu/data/covid-19.

StatLink https://stat.link/q6dwhe

COVID-19 also risks compounding existing labour market inequalities between young people. In the 2007-2008 financial crisis, young people with educational attainment below upper secondary level suffered the most from unemployment and inactivity, which persisted during the recovery. Indeed, in 2017, young people with no more than lower-secondary education were three times more likely to be not in employment, education or training (NEET) compared to those with a university degree (OECD, 2020[13]).

Young women were particularly affected by job and income losses during COVID-19. On average across the OECD, the youth unemployment rate for women aged 15 to 24 increased by 3.9 percentage points between 2019 and 2020, while the unemployment rate for young men grew by 2.9 percentage points (Figure 5.11). In addition, among EU 27 countries, young women (aged 16 to 24) are estimated to have experienced higher labour income losses between 2019 and 2020 compared to young men (12.7% versus 11.3%) (Eurostat, 2021[2]).

Figure 5.11. Young women experienced a greater increase in unemployment than young men

Share of the youth labour force aged 15 to 24 who are unemployed, year-on-year percentage point change, 2019-20

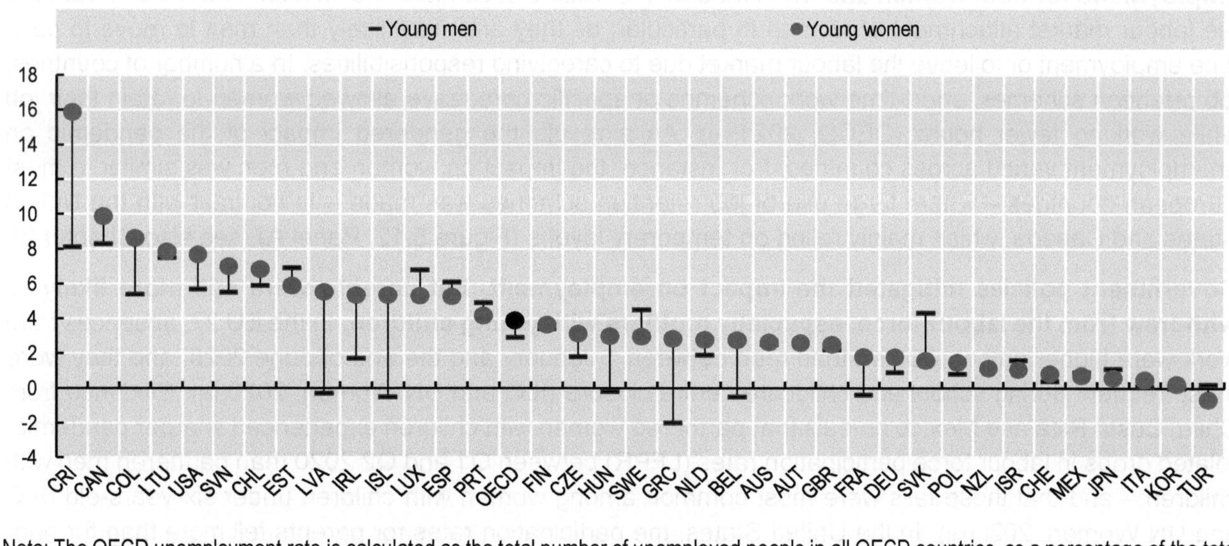

Note: The OECD unemployment rate is calculated as the total number of unemployed people in all OECD countries, as a percentage of the total labour force (i.e. the unemployed plus those in employment). Data for Germany in 2020 are provisional and might be subject to low reliability due to technical issues with the introduction of the new German system of integrated household surveys.
Source: OECD (n.d.[12]), *Main Economic Indicators* (database), https://doi.org/10.1787/data-00046-en.

StatLink https://stat.link/gjr5vn

The pandemic has affected both men and women negatively in terms of employment, but women, especially mothers, face a number of additional vulnerabilities and challenges

A number of factors have made women more vulnerable to job and income loss during the COVID-19 crisis. First, women tend to be less firmly attached to the labour force than men; they also tend to work fewer hours and to have lower wages (OECD, 2021[11]). Second, women are over-represented in the services sector, including retail, catering and hospitality, which were hit the hardest by government lockdown measures. In 2019, the share of employed women in the services sector across 26 OECD countries was 84.1% on average, 22.8 percentage points higher than that of men (61.3%).

Nevertheless, women make up a large share of workers in the sectors defined as essential, including health care and education. As such, women have been facing exceptional work demands and are more likely to be exposed to COVID-19 while working (OECD, 2021[11]). In addition, the pandemic's impact on employment has been partly shaped by whether people's jobs enable them to telework, which tends to be possible in both male and female-dominated sectors (e.g. education) (see Box 5.5 for information on teleworking experiences for different population groups) (OECD, 2021[11]).

Therefore, on average across the OECD, women and men experienced similar rises in unemployment in 2020 (respectively by 1.8 and 1.6 percentage points) (Figure 5.12, Panel A). Indeed, while in Q2 2020, right after the onset of the crisis, average unemployment rose slightly more for women than for men, the average gender unemployment gap went back to pre-pandemic levels by Q4 2020 and Q1 2021 (Figure 5.12, Panel B). Patterns vary across countries, however (see Box 5.3 for evidence from Chile and (OECD, 2021[11]) for more information) (Refer to Chapter 7 for information on how the pandemic impacted unpaid work for women and men). Eurostat estimates meanwhile indicate that, at the EU 27 level, there were no substantial differences in labour income losses between women and men (Eurostat, 2021[2]).

In many OECD countries, reduced work hours cushioned the impact of school closures on employment, for both women and men. Indeed, the closure of schools and childcare facilities threatened the labour market attachment of women in particular, as they are more likely than men to move to part-time employment or to leave the labour market due to caregiving responsibilities. In a number of countries, job retention schemes, short-time work schemes or specific care leave allowed women to retain their job while working fewer hours (OECD, 2021[11]). As a result, the gendered impact of the pandemic on unemployment varied across countries. For instance, the impact on women and men was similar in most European countries – where large use of job retention schemes was made – in contrast with the United States and Canada, which mainly relied on temporary layoffs (Figure 5.12, Panel A) (see also Chapter 2).

Government policies mitigated the impact on employment, but parents were still more likely to withdraw from the labour force, especially mothers with young children. In the EU 27, absences from work were higher among women than men between 1 January and the end of June 2020, and they were most frequent during school and childcare centre closure (ILO and UN Women, 2020[14]). Evidence from Chile, Costa Rica and Mexico reveals that partnered women with children experienced sharper pandemic-related drops in labour force participation rates (LFPR) between Q1 and Q2 2020 than partnered men with children – and that these falls were most common among women with children under six-years-old (ILO and UN Women, 2020[14]). In the United States, the participation rates for parents fell more than for non-parents during the first year of the pandemic, and mothers' participation rates fell more than for fathers. The LFPR of mothers overall was about 3.5 percentage points lower in March 2021 than in January 2020. By contrast, fathers' LFPR was down only by 1 percentage point. In particular, in March 2021, the LFPR of single mothers and mothers with children under 12 was lower than that for mothers with teenage children (Figure 5.13). Moreover, in the United States in October-November 2020, about 14% of unmarried mothers and mothers whose youngest child was under age 6 reported that they left their job due to child-care responsibilities in 2020, compared with 8% of mothers with children aged 6 to 12 (Bauer, 2021[15]).

On average in 14 OECD countries, the gender wage gap narrowed from 13.7% to 10.4% in 2020 (Figure 5.14). One possible explanation for this is compositional: women are over-represented in low-paid occupations in the sectors hardest hit by the pandemic, and therefore were more exposed to job loss in 2020. As a result of the missing lowest-paid women, the gender wage gap narrowed (Institute for Women's Policy Research, 2021[16]).

Figure 5.12. In 2020, women and men experienced similar rises in unemployment

Share of the labour force who are unemployed

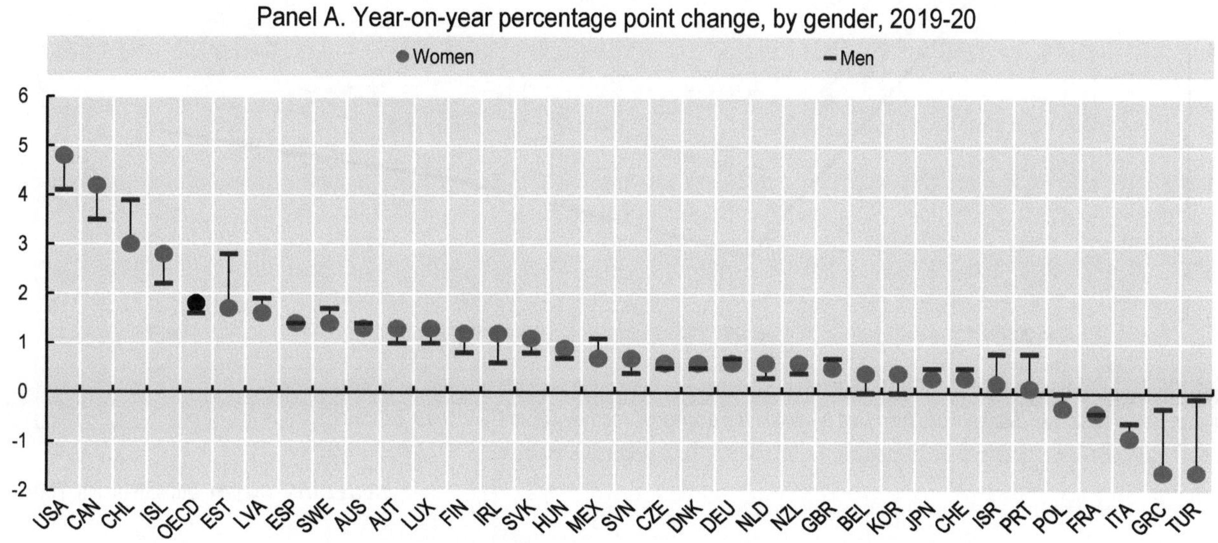

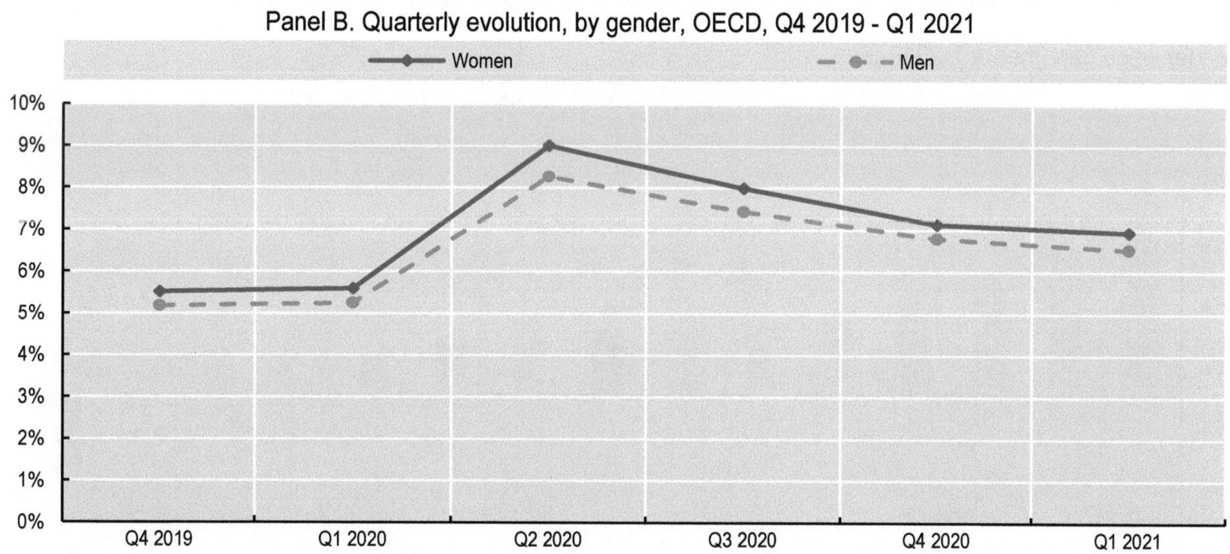

Note: The OECD unemployment rate is calculated as the total number of unemployed people in all OECD countries, as a percentage of the total labour force (i.e. the unemployed plus those in employment). Data for Germany in 2020 are provisional and might be subject to low reliability due to technical issues with the introduction of the new German system of integrated household surveys.
Source: OECD (n.d.[12]), *Main Economic Indicators* (database), https://doi.org/10.1787/data-00046-en.

StatLink https://stat.link/ilet1x

Figure 5.13. In the US, mothers showed lower labour force participation rates in March 2021

Share of the working age population aged 25 to 54 reporting to be working or actively seeking employment, by living situation, percentage point change, Jan 2020 - Mar 2021

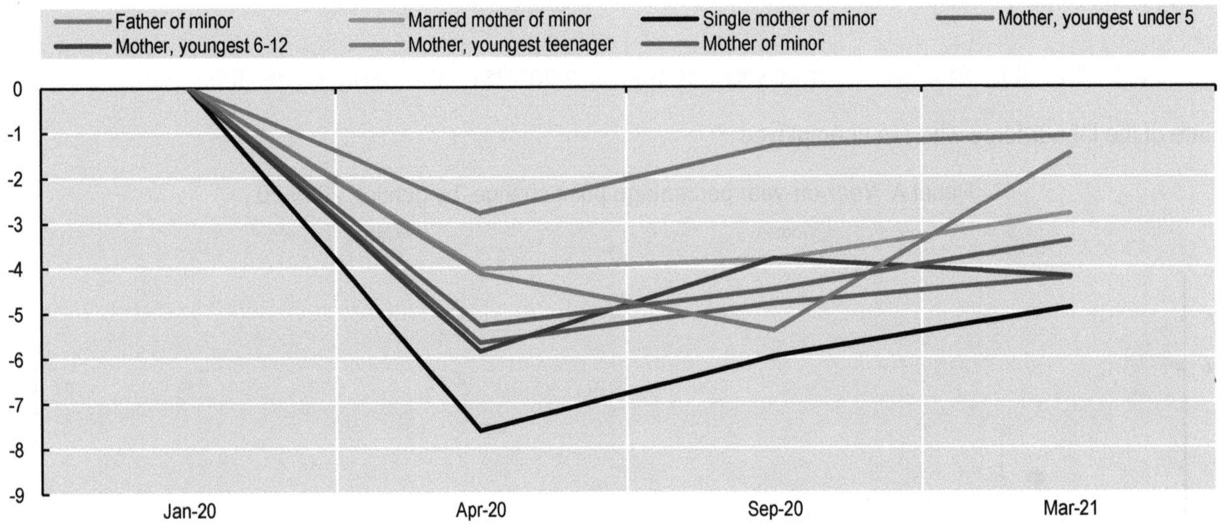

Note: The figure shows outcomes for mothers/fathers according to their marital status and age of their children.
Source: Bauer (2021[15]), *Mothers are being left behind in the economic recovery from COVID-19*, Brookings, https://www.brookings.edu/blog/up-front/2021/05/06/mothers-are-being-left-behind-in-the-economic-recovery-from-covid-19/.

StatLink https://stat.link/709khw

Figure 5.14. On average in 14 OECD countries, the gender wage gap decreased in 2020

Gender wage gap (median), 2019-20

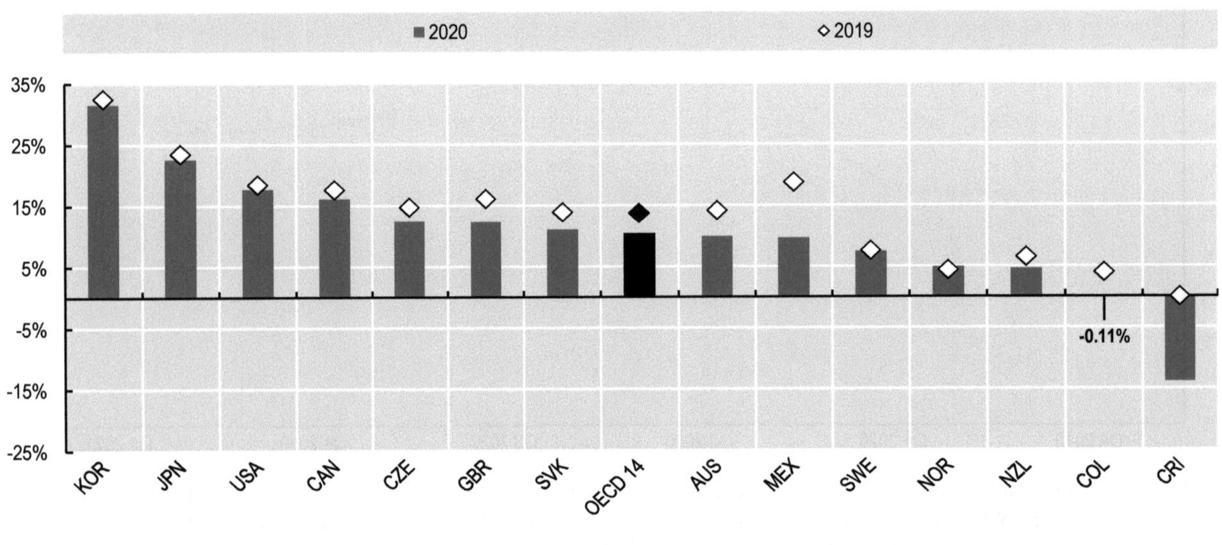

Note: The gender wage gap is calculated as the difference between the median earnings of men and women relative to the median earnings of men. The OECD average includes only those 14 countries shown.
Source: OECD (n.d.[17]), *Employment and Labour Market Statistics* (database), https://doi.org/10.1787/data-00302-en.

StatLink https://stat.link/xcdtbi

Box 5.3. Innovation: Instituto Nacional de Estadísticas (INE) and the COVID-19 Social Survey – in Chile, COVID-19 widened inequalities in material well-being between genders and income groups

The Chilean COVID-19 Social Survey (Encuesta Social COVID-19) is an initiative of the United Nations Development Program (UNDP), in conjunction with the National Institute of Statistics (INE) and in partnership with the Ministry of Social Development and Family (MDSF). Currently, two rounds of the survey have been conducted: the first in July 2020 and the second in November 2020. 13 648 people were surveyed in the first round, and 10 344 in the second round. For both rounds, the survey took place through a phone interview conducted with a web questionnaire. The survey is made up of the following modules: characterisation of the household economic impact, access to help from third parties, care, income, mental health and availability of information. The second round also included information about the presence of children and adolescents in the households.

According to the COVID-19 Social Survey, women and low-income households fared worse on a number of material well-being indicators. For instance, both the share of households with no employed members and the share of households who felt their income was insufficient were higher among women-led households and for those in the bottom income quintile in November 2020 (Figure 5.15).

Figure 5.15. In November 2020, 26% of women-led households and 33% of households in the bottom income quintile in Chile had no employed members

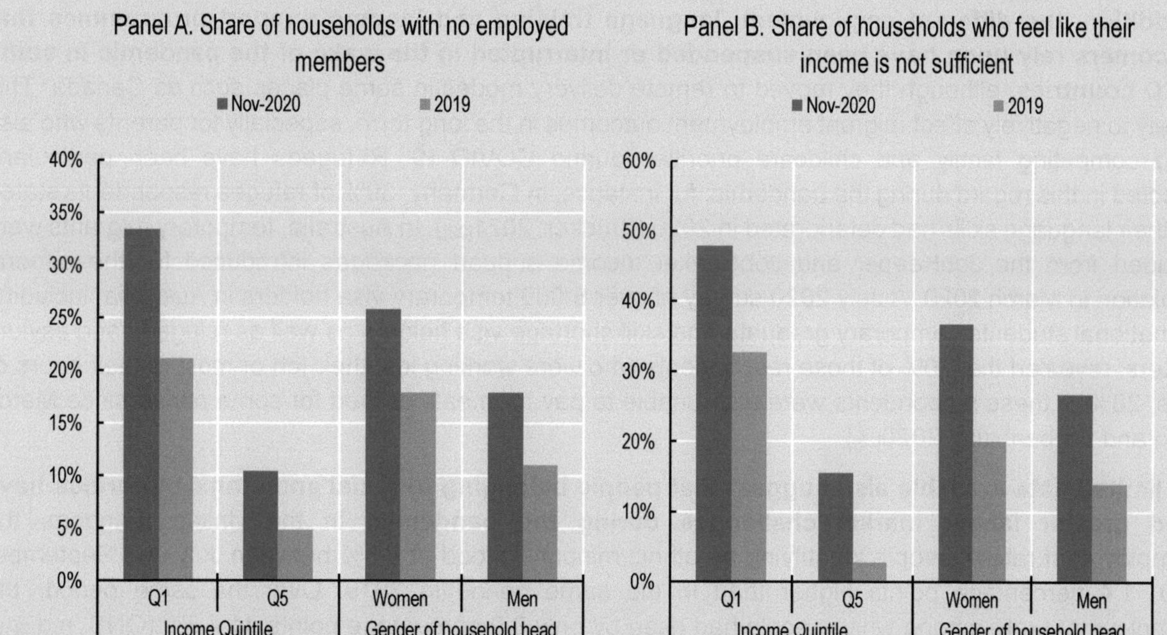

Source: Ministerio Desarrollo Social y Familia (n.d.[18]), *Encuesta Social COVID-19 (COVID-19 Social Survey)*, http://observatorio.ministeriodesarrollosocial.gob.cl/encuesta-social-covid19.

StatLink https://stat.link/ecudak

Immigrants and people belonging to racial/ethnic minorities were often the first to lose their jobs at the beginning of the pandemic

Although it is still too early to gauge the full labour market effects of the pandemic – especially in European OECD countries, where job retention schemes have cushioned the immediate impact of the lockdowns – initial evidence shows a disproportionate toll throughout 2020 on migrants in all countries where data are currently available (OECD, 2020[19]).[3] Overall, employment trajectories for native- and foreign-born individuals followed similar trends for 23 OECD countries – they dropped sharply in the second quarter of 2020 and slightly recovered in the third. Unlike that of native-borns, however, employment among migrant workers declined again in the last quarter of 2020 (Figure 5.16, Panel A and B). In the first quarter of 2021, the employment rate decreased more for foreign-born than for native-born individuals (Figure 5.16, Panel A). Some care is needed in interpreting the latest developments in the OECD employment rate, as methodological changes to the EU Labour Force Survey blur the comparison between the fourth quarter of 2020 and the first quarter of 2021 for EU countries.[4] Migrants were also more affected by unemployment, particularly in the first half of 2020 (OECD, 2020[19]).

Migrants face a number of vulnerabilities in the labour market. They are over-represented among employees with temporary contracts and low wages, in cyclical sectors and in service sectors (such as hospitality, security and cleaning) which were particularly affected by the pandemic (Statistics Canada, 2020[20]; OECD, 2020[19]). In the EU, migrants account for about 12% of the population, but for more than a quarter of employment in the hospitality industry (OECD, 2020[21]). Migrants have fewer networks to rely upon in times of economic downturn, and there is some evidence that discrimination is more pronounced in times of slack labour markets (OECD, 2020[19]).

In addition, the different employment, language training and income support programmes that newcomers rely upon have been suspended or interrupted in the wake of the pandemic in some OECD countries, although they moved to remote delivery modes in some places such as Canada. This is likely to negatively affect migrant employment outcomes in the long term, especially for parents who also faced competing family and childcare priorities during COVID-19. Refugees have been particularly impacted in this regard during the pandemic: for instance, in Germany, 39% of refugee respondents stated that their language skills had deteriorated in 2020 (Brücker, 2021[22]). In Australia, temporary migrants were excluded from the JobKeeper and JobSeeker income support packages introduced for the general population in March 2020. A July 2020 survey of over 6 000 temporary visa holders in Australia, including international students, temporary graduate and skill shortage visa holders as well as refugees and asylum seekers, revealed that 70% of those respondents who were working lost their job or most of their hours or shifts; 28% of these respondents were also unable to pay for meals or food for some period since March (Berg and Farbenblum, 2020[23]).

The limited data available also suggest that people belonging to racial and ethnic minorities have faced greater labour market challenges during the pandemic. In the United Kingdom, the unemployment rate of people identifying as ethnic minority[5] stood at 8.5% between July and September 2020, 1.4 percentage points higher than in the same period in 2019. Over the same period, the unemployment rate among white people had risen by only 0.9 percentage points, to 4.5% (ONS, n.d.[24]). Indeed, industries such as transport and storage as well as accommodation and food sectors in which ethnic minority workers are over-represented announced the most redundancies over the summer (ONS, 2020[25]; Powell, Francis-Devine and Foley, 2020[26]). Ethnic minority workers were also less likely to have been placed on job retention schemes, and more likely to have permanently lost their jobs, relative to white British people in April, while their average household earnings fell by slightly more than for white workers between February and April (8.4% compared to 8%) (Benzeval et al., 2020[27]; Hu, 2020[28]). In the United States, while by April 2021 unemployment rates had fallen from their April 2020 heights for all racial/ethnic groups, gaps between white and Black as well as Hispanic/Latino communities markedly widened compared to end 2019 (doubling for the former and tripling for the latter group) (Figure 5.17) (see Box 5.4

for information on the pandemic's impact on racial/ethnic minority-owned SMEs). In Canada, experimental estimates from the Labour Force Survey suggest that from January 2020 to January 2021, the unemployment rate increased by 5.3 percentage points among Black Canadians, compared to 3.7 percentage points among non-visible minority[6] Canadians (excluding Indigenous people). In the three months ending in January 2021, the unemployment rate among Black Canadians (13.1%) was about 70% higher than that among non-visible minority Canadians (7.7%) (Statistics Canada, 2021[29]).

Figure 5.16. Migrants' employment has declined by more than that of native-borns in almost one-third of OECD countries

Share of the total population who are employed, by place of birth

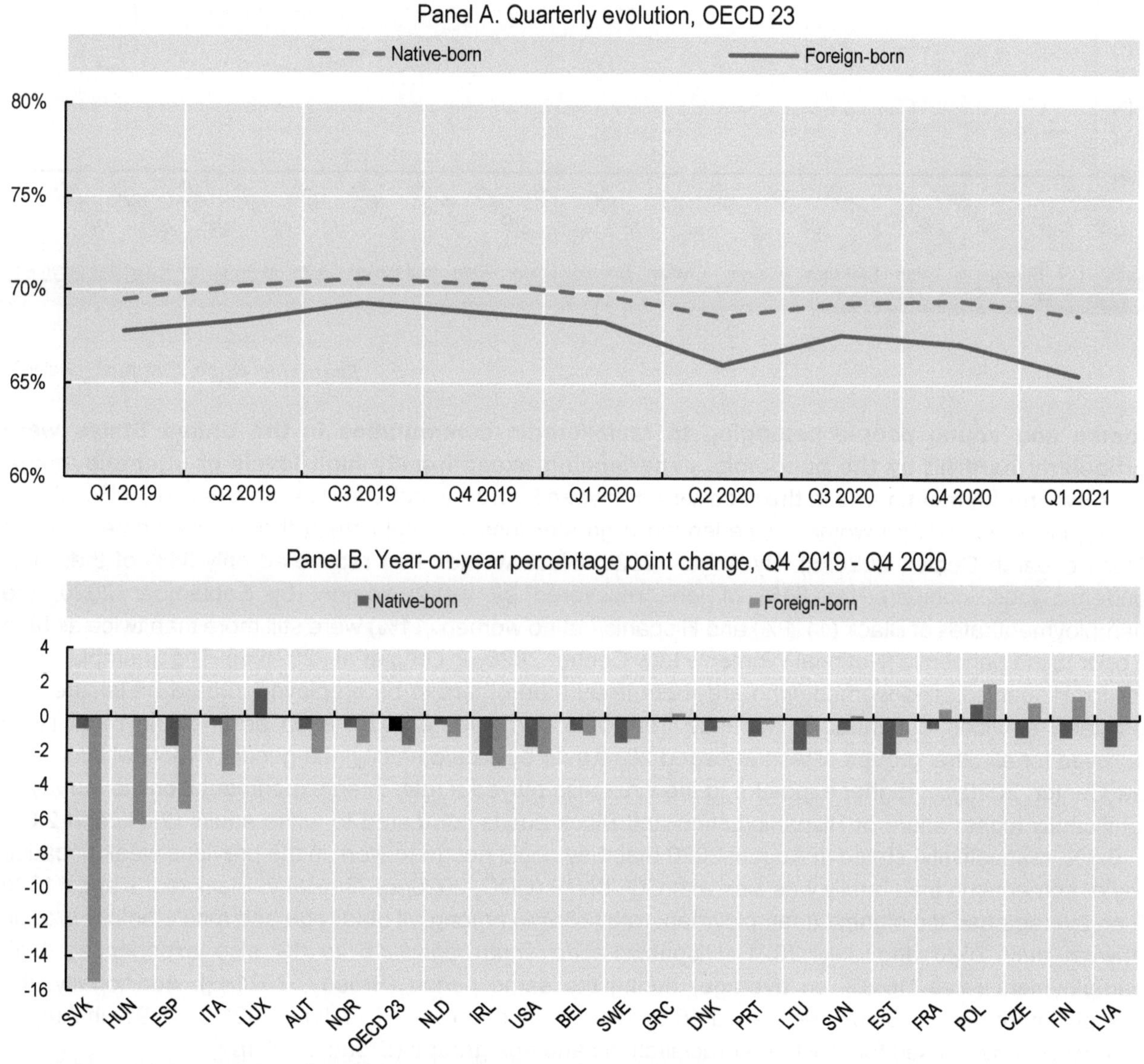

Note: In both panels, the OECD average includes only those 23 countries shown in Panel B.

Source: Eurostat (n.d.[30]), *Employment rates by sex, age and country of birth (%)* (database), https://ec.europa.eu/eurostat/web/lfs/data/database; and US Bureau of Labor Statistics (n.d.[31]), *Employment status of the civilian population by nativity and sex, not seasonally adjusted* (database), https://www.bls.gov/webapps/legacy/cpsatab7.htm.

StatLink https://stat.link/i65nh1

Figure 5.17. Unemployment in the United States has fallen from the 2020 peak, but gaps between racial/ethnic groups have widened

Share of the total population who are unemployed, by race/ethnicity, Nov 2019 - Apr 2021

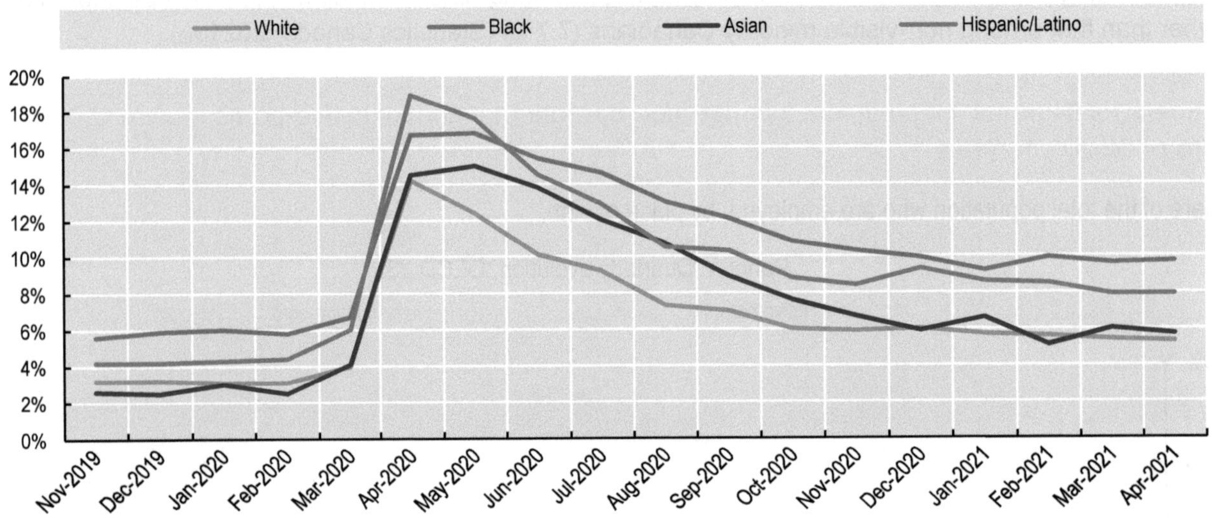

Source: US Bureau of Labor Statistics (n.d.[32]), *Civilian Unemployment Rate* (database), https://www.bls.gov/charts/employment-situation/civilian-unemployment-rate.htm.

StatLink https://stat.link/gjap07

Women and young people belonging to racial/ethnic communities in the United States were particularly hard hit by the pandemic, experiencing exceptionally high levels of unemployment, and slow employment gains in the recovery. Between February and May, Hispanic/Latino (-21%), Asian (-19%) and Black (-17%) women experienced a greater loss in employment than white women (-13%) (Pew Research Center, 2020[33]). By August 2020, Black women had recovered only 34% of their pre-pandemic jobs, compared to 61% of jobs recovered by white women; by September 2020, the unemployment rates of Black (11.1%) and Hispanic/Latino women (11%) were still more than twice as high as prior to the pandemic (National Women's Law Center, 2020[34]; Long et al., 2020[35]). The unemployment rate for Hispanic/Latino women, who are more likely than others to be employed in hard-hit leisure and hospitality services, continued to increase from 10.5% in August 2020, even as unemployment rates improved for all other groups of workers aged 20 or over by race/ethnicity and gender (National Women's Law Center, 2020[34]). Higher exposure to the virus also played a role: in an experimental online survey, a significantly higher share of Hispanic/Latino and Black adults compared to white adults (2.8% and 2.6% vs. 0.3%, respectively) stated in August 2020 that they could not go to work in the previous week because they or someone in their family was sick with COVID-19 (CDC, 2020[36]). Similarly, Black teens aged 16 to 19 on average had the highest unemployment rate (18.9%) among all other age and race/ethnicity groups between July 2020 and July 2021. Hispanic/Latino youth aged 16 to 19 also experienced high unemployment rates (16.8% on average) during the same period (Broady, 2021[37]). Additionally, the unemployment rate for Black teens aged 16 to 19 increased from 9.3% in June 2021 to 17.9% in August 2021, while it decreased for most other racial/ethnic and age groups (Broady, 2021[37]).

Emerging evidence also suggests that the crisis may have longer-lasting consequences among some more disadvantaged groups. In Canada, Indigenous and non-Indigenous people were similarly impacted in terms of unemployment initially, but greater disparities appeared as the pandemic progressed. From the three months ending in February to the three months ending in May 2020, the unemployment rate of Indigenous people living off reserve and non-Indigenous people both increased by a similar amount and stood at 16.6% and 11.7%, respectively. However, employment among Indigenous people has been slower to recover. Year-on-year, the employment rate in June-August 2020 was down 6.9 points among Indigenous people living off reserve and down 5.0 points among non-Indigenous people (Statistics Canada, 2020[38]). During the same months, Indigenous women's employment rate (for those living off reserve) was further away from pre-pandemic levels than the one for Indigenous men (Statistics Canada, 2020[38]).

Box 5.4. The pandemic has disproportionately hit women and racial/ethnic minority entrepreneurs

The COVID-19 crisis hit businesses owned by women, racial/ethnic minority and younger entrepreneurs disproportionately. Their businesses tend to be concentrated in the most affected sectors and are on average smaller and younger. Being typically self-funded or funded by friends and family, these businesses have fewer financial assets and more limited access to diversified sources of finance. Women and racial/ethnic minority entrepreneurs have faced higher risks of unemployment and income loss than other categories, and government support has been less effective at reaching their businesses. As far as women entrepreneurs are concerned, increasing household and care responsibilities also played a role in shaping these developments (OECD, 2021[39]).

Women-led SMEs were seven percentage points more likely to close compared to men-led SMEs, according to data collected in May 2020 by Facebook, the OECD and the World Bank. This pattern varies across regions, with the largest gender disparity in business closures to be found in North and Latin America (14 and 11 percentage points respectively). All regions in the world have at least a 6 percentage point gender disparity in business closure rates (OECD, 2021[40]). Other studies confirm the higher impact of the crisis on women entrepreneurs. In the United States, the number of women business owners declined by 10%, compared to 7% of men business owners (Fairlie, 2020[41]). In Germany, self-employed women were 35% more likely to experience revenue loss than men (Graeber, Kritikos and Seebauer, 2021[42]). Lastly, in Canada, 62% of women-owned businesses laid off more than 80% of their workers, against 45% on average for the small business population at large (OECD, 2021[40]).

Racial/ethnic minority entrepreneurs were significantly affected as well, according to evidence from the United States. Between February and April 2020, the number of Black and Hispanic/Latino businesses dropped by 41% and 32% respectively, compared to the general 22% decrease in active business owners (Fairlie, 2020[41]). In addition, a survey among small businesses conducted by the US Chamber of Commerce in the first half of November 2020 revealed that 74% of owners needed further government assistance to navigate the crisis. This share rises to 81% for racial/ethnic minority-owned businesses. Evidence from a US Federal Reserve Survey indicates that racial/ethnic minority-owned businesses are experiencing a slower recovery. In early 2021, 79% of Asian-owned, 77% of Black-owned and 66% of Hispanic/Latino-owned businesses described their financial situation as "fair" or "poor", compared to 54% of white-owned firms (OECD, 2021[40]).

Members of LGBTQ+ communities have experienced very large job and income losses since the pandemic began

The demographic composition of LGBTQ+ communities and their prevalence in the sectors most affected by government containment measures – such as hospitality, arts and entertainment – makes them more vulnerable to job and income loss (Wenham, 2020[43]). In Canada, in 2018, LGBTQ2+[7] Canadians were generally younger than non-LGBTQ2+ Canadians and were significantly less likely to identify as male (Prokopenko and Kevins, 2020[44]). A majority (53%) of LGBTQI2S[8] households in Canada have been affected by lay-offs and reduced hours as a result of the pandemic, compared to 39% of overall Canadian households (Innovative Research Group, 2020[45]).[9] In the United States, according to a survey conducted in July-August 2020, 64% of LGBTQ households experienced employment loss compared to 45% of non-LGBTQ households (this included losing their jobs, having their hours or wages reduced, having been furloughed, or taking a mandatory unpaid leave) (Movement Advancement Project, 2020[46]). This share rises to 71% of Hispanic/Latino LGBTQ households and 68% of lower-income LGBTQ households (< USD 30 000 per year) (Movement Advancement Project, 2020[46]). Compounding these difficulties, LGBTQ people report higher rates of employment discrimination generally and may struggle to find new jobs.[10]

Box 5.5. COVID-19 and teleworking

Even for those who can telework, the pandemic has brought disruptions to their working lives. Parents working from home faced challenges juggling work and childcare responsibilities, particularly in the face of school and nursery closures. In the United States in October 2020, parents were more likely than non-parents to report not being able to meet deadlines and not having the right space and equipment to work from home. In addition, half of teleworking parents with children younger than 18 said it's been difficult for them to be able to get their work done without interruptions, while only 20% of parents who do not have minor children reported the same (Parker, Menasce Horowitz and Minkin, 2020[47]).[1] In the United States, teleworkers younger than 50 have been significantly more likely than older workers to say it's been difficult for them to be able to get their work done without interruptions (38% versus 18%) (Parker, Menasce Horowitz and Minkin, 2020[47]).

Teleworking is having mixed impacts on work-life balance, enabling more flexibility and family time, but bringing more worry and workaholism. In 22 European OECD countries, in July 2020, respondents who worked exclusively from home were slightly more likely to worry about work when not working (24%) compared to those who worked at their employer's premises or other locations (20%). At that same time in the EU 27, 22% of parents working exclusively from home reported finding it hard to focus on work due to family, compared to only 8% of parents working at other locations and 5% of teleworkers with no children (Eurofound, 2020[48]). Younger workers struggled too: according to the qualitative study run by the European Commission Joint Research Centre in Italy, France and Spain in April-May 2020, "workaholism" was more common among younger workers living alone (Fana et al., 2020[49]). However, many appreciate the flexibility and additional family time that come with teleworking. In the EU 27, teleworkers with children under 12 were less likely to report that their job prevents them from spending time with family (32%) than those working at other locations (38%) in July 2020 (refer to Chapter 4 for more information on work-life balance) (Eurofound, 2020[48]). In the United States, in October 2020, 29% of teleworkers said they now have more flexibility to choose when to put in their work hours, and 38% of them said it is now easier for them to balance work with family responsibilities (Parker, Menasce Horowitz and Minkin, 2020[47]). Indeed, additional evidence from the United States suggests that workers with children under 18 have the strongest preferences to continue working from home, at least two or three times a week (64% compared to 49% of workers with no children). This preference is also more common among women than men (57.8% versus 54.1%) and among workers with a four-year college degree (58% versus 53% of employees without a four-year college degree) (Barrero, Bloom and Davis, 2021[50]).[2]

Work generally has been more stressful and draining since the beginning of the pandemic, including for teleworkers. COVID-19 has put additional pressure on workers, as anxiety or job insecurity affect many of them (refer to Chapter 2), and those working from home have not been spared this experience. According to a survey conducted in nine countries worldwide by the Capgemini

Research Institute, in September-October 2020, over half of the surveyed employees felt burnt out as a result of working remotely, and the figure rises to 61% for younger employees aged 31-40.[3] Moreover, 56% of surveyed employees feared the stresses and demands of being "always on" (Capgemini Research Institute, 2020[51]).

There is a significant age gap in the extent to which workers are facing motivational challenges in their virtual work lives. In October 2020 in the United States, while the majority of teleworkers (six-in-ten) said it has been "very or somewhat easy" to feel motivated to do their work since the pandemic started, 53% of those between aged 18-29 compared to 20% of those over 50 found it "difficult" (Parker, Menasce Horowitz and Minkin, 2020[47]). In 22 European OECD countries, in July 2020, it was less likely for teleworkers to feel like they are doing a useful job "always" or "most of the time" (71%) compared to those who work at other locations (76%) (Eurofound, 2020[48]).

In addition, some workers miss in-person contact and have been feeling isolated while teleworking. According to an Ipsos study conducted in 28 countries in November-December 2020, nearly half of those who worked from home said they have felt lonely or isolated when they did (Ipsos, 2020[52]).[4] In the EU 27, 12% of all employees felt isolated at work "always" or "most of the time" in July 2020. This affected a larger share of younger respondents (15% of those aged 18-34), but only 12% of those aged 35-49, and just 9% of 50+ year-olds. Isolation is also reported by a larger share of those exclusively working from home (15%) compared to those working from other locations (10%) (Eurofound, 2020[48]).

Young workers and newcomers feel disconnected from their teams. 56% of the employees surveyed by the Capgemini Research Institute felt disconnected from their organisation due to remote working in September-October 2020. Of the employees who feel disconnected, 41% fall in the 31-40 age bracket, but in the over-50s, this drops to 8% (Capgemini Research Institute, 2020[51]). The experience of teleworking has been particularly difficult for newcomers in this respect. In fact, 50% of these new joiners say that they would not continue with the organisation if they had to work only from a remote location, and 55% of them do not feel integrated into the organisation due to the impersonal nature of interactions (Capgemini Research Institute, 2020[51]).

Notes:

1. Data collected between 13 and 19 October 2020. Sample size: 5 858, national, random sampling of residential addresses. The survey is weighted to be representative of the United States adult population by gender, race, ethnicity, partisan affiliation, education and other categories.
2. Data are from the June 2021 Survey of Working Arrangements and Attitudes. Sample size: 2 232. Raw responses were re-weighted to match population shares in the 2010 to 2019 CPS.
3. The Remote Workforce Survey was conducted in France, India, Italy, Germany, the Netherlands, Spain, Sweden, the United Kingdom and the United States. The survey included 500 organisations, 5 016 employees and 500 executives.
4. Study conducted in Argentina, Australia, Belgium, Brazil, Canada, Chile, China (mainland), Colombia, France, Germany, Hungary, India, Italy, Japan, Malaysia, Mexico, the Netherlands, Peru, Poland, Russia, Saudi Arabia, South Africa, South Korea, Spain, Sweden, Turkey, the United Kingdom and the United States. Average sample size per country: 458.

Younger, lower-paid and less-educated employees have lost the highest number of hours worked, mostly due to joblessness rather than reduced working time

Working hours fell for different reasons among people of different ages, incomes and education levels: while some lost their jobs, others remained in employment but worked fewer or zero hours (OECD, 2021[11]). Despite the widespread use of job retention schemes in many OECD countries, joblessness accounted for the majority of the hours lost among less-educated, lower-paid and younger workers (OECD, 2021[11]). For example, in Q2 2020 compared to Q2 2019, average hours worked fell by 8.5% among those with a tertiary education, compared to 24.3% among those holding a lower-secondary diploma or less. In addition to having experienced a higher reduction in hours worked, in Q2 2020, half of the total hours lost among less-educated employees was due to joblessness (Figure 5.18, Panel A). By contrast, for people with a tertiary education, net losses in total hours worked are all attributable to reduced working time, while remaining in employment (Figure 5.18, Panel B). Educational disparities were reinforced across the third and the fourth quarters of 2020, when many high-educated employees returned to work, while joblessness persisted among the low-educated (Figure 5.18).

Figure 5.18. Joblessness largely drove the reduction in hours worked among less-educated employees

Total hours worked, by education level, year-on-year percentage change, OECD 29, 2019-20

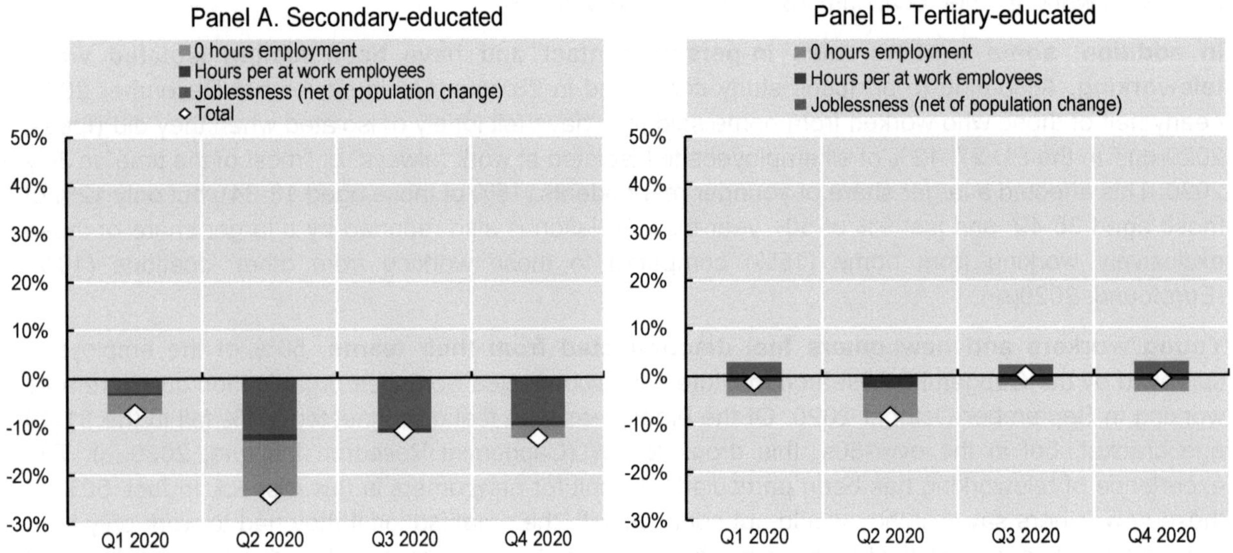

Note: The figure reports the contribution of each category to the change in total hours. The change in hours is decomposed in (1) the change in the average hours worked for at-work employees, (2) the net change in the level of 0-hour employees and (3) the net change in the level of jobless individuals (inactive and unemployed). Positive values for "joblessness" indicate net job creation. See Annex 1.A in OECD (2021[11]) for further details on the decomposition. The OECD average excludes Australia, Colombia, Costa Rica, Iceland, Germany, Israel, Japan, Korea and New Zealand.

Source: OECD (2021[11]), *OECD Employment Outlook 2021: Navigating the COVID-19 Crisis and Recovery* OECD Publishing, Paris, https://doi.org/10.1787/5a700c4b-en.

StatLink https://stat.link/ho8wvf

Similarly, younger employees lost a higher number of working hours compared to their older peers. In Q2 2020, across the OECD, young people aged 15-24 saw their working hours reduced by 26.3%, while the working hours of those aged 25 and over decreased by 15% compared to Q2 2019. The reduction in working hours of employees over 25 was largely driven by reduced working time in employment, while for younger workers, joblessness was the primary cause (Figure 5.19). Even when young workers lost their hours due to reduced working time, this largely consisted of zero-hours employment (Figure 5.19) (OECD, 2021[11]).

Figure 5.19. Younger workers mainly lost working hours due to joblessness or zero-hours employment

Total hours worked, by age, year-on-year percentage change, OECD 32, Q2 2019 - Q2 2020

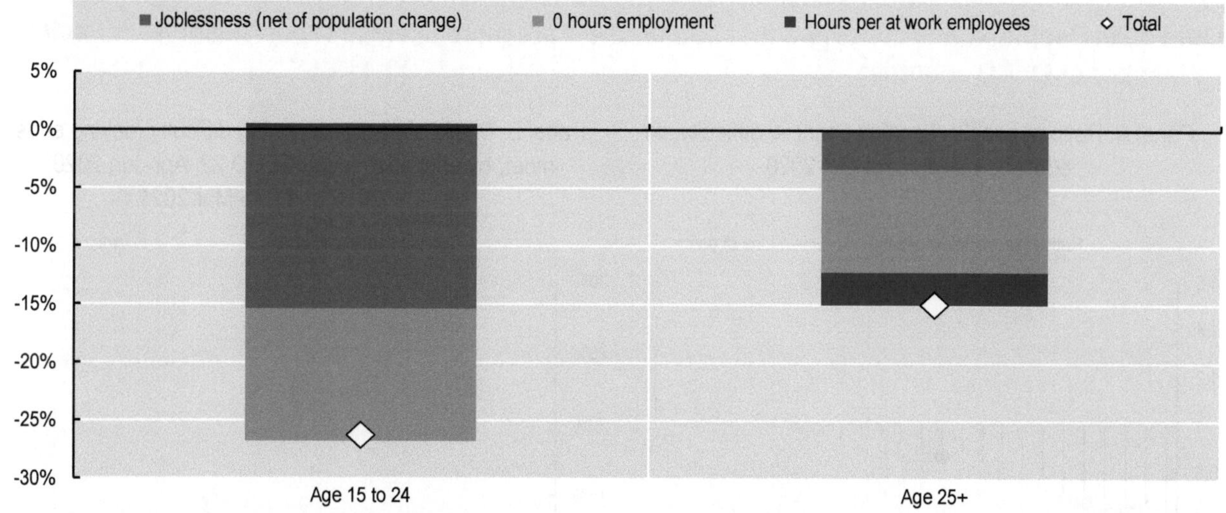

Note: The figure reports the contribution of each category to the change in total hours. The change in hours is decomposed in (1) the change in the average hours worked for at-work employees, (2) the net change in the level of zero-hour employees and (3) the net change in the level of jobless individuals (inactive and unemployed). Positive values for "joblessness" indicate net job creation. See Annex 1.A in OECD (2021[11]) for further details on the decomposition. The OECD average excludes Australia, Colombia, Costa Rica, Israel, Korea and New Zealand.

Source: OECD (2021[11]), *OECD Employment Outlook 2021: Navigating the COVID-19 Crisis and Recovery* OECD Publishing, Paris, https://doi.org/10.1787/5a700c4b-en.

StatLink https://stat.link/gkiprz

5.2. Income and Wealth

People who lost their jobs and those with lower levels of educational attainment have been facing particular financial strain

The year 2020 has been characterised by widespread financial difficulty, especially for the less educated and the unemployed, who tend to have less of a financial safety net. Indeed, those who lost their jobs as a result of the COVID-19 crisis tend to belong to more financially vulnerable groups (e.g. young, low-income, racial/ethnic minorities). Similarly, people with higher levels of education typically have greater household wealth to rely upon in times of need and more financial security. Around 2016, data from 28 OECD countries showed that, on average, median wealth among households headed by someone with a tertiary education was around double that of households headed by someone with a below upper secondary education (OECD, 2020[53]). At the same time, 26% of tertiary-headed households on average were financially insecure (measured as having liquid financial wealth to support their household above the poverty threshold for more than three months), while over 35% of households headed by a person lacking tertiary education faced this risk (OECD, 2020[53]).

Given the lower wealth of the less educated before the COVID-19 crisis, it is not surprising that they report greater financial difficulties. Across 25 OECD countries, 33% of respondents with less than a tertiary education reported that they or someone in their household had experienced some form of financial difficulty, compared to 28% of those with at least a tertiary education in September-October 2020 (see note to Figure 5.20 for the full list of financial difficulties) (Figure 5.20, Panel A). Separate evidence collected in 22 European OECD countries reveals that between April-June 2020 and February-March 2021 the share of people with a secondary or lower education facing difficulty in making ends meet increased at a higher rate compared to that of people with a tertiary education (by 1.6 and 0.7 percentage points respectively) (Figure 5.20, Panel B).

Figure 5.20. People with secondary education or lower are more likely to report financial difficulty in a number of OECD countries

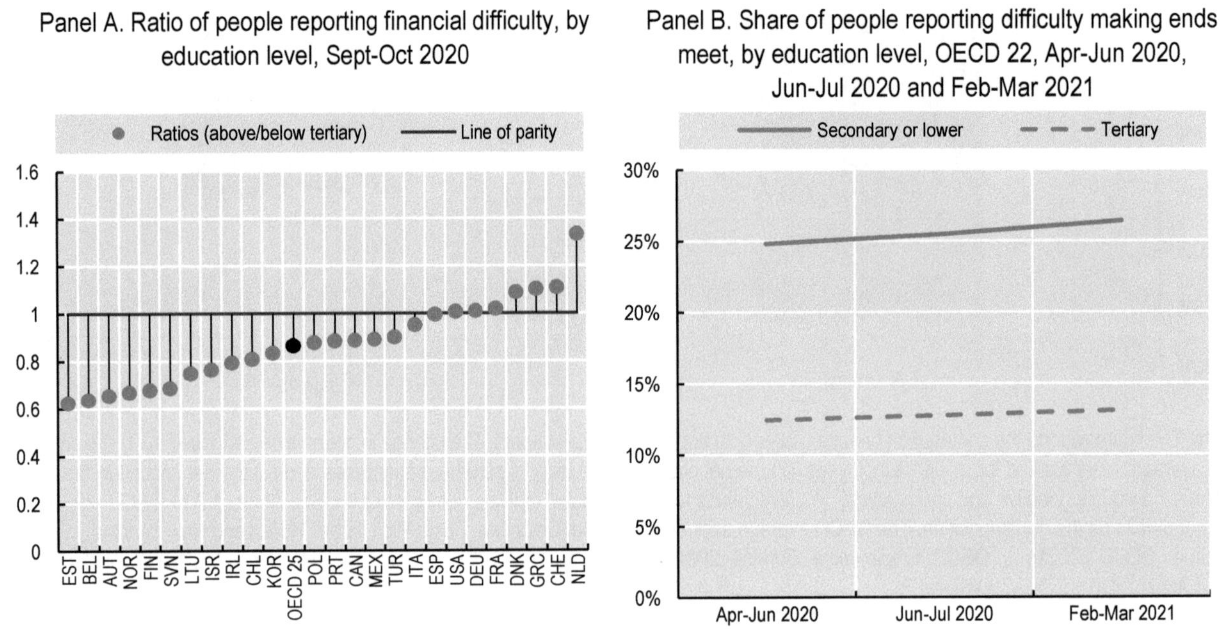

Note: In Panel A, ratios with values above 1 indicate better outcomes for those with less than a tertiary education; values below 1 indicate better outcomes for those with at least a tertiary education. Respondents were asked whether, at any time since the start of the COVID-19 pandemic, they (or their household) had experienced one or more of a range of specific finance-related events. Options included: failed to pay a usual expense; took money out of savings or sold assets to pay for a usual expense; took money from family or friends to pay for a usual expense; took on additional debt or used credit to pay for a usual expense; asked a charity or non-profit organisation for assistance because they could not afford to pay; went hungry because they could not afford to pay for food; lost their home because they could not afford the mortgage or rent; or declared bankruptcy or asked a credit provider for help. Respondents could select all the options that applied. The OECD average includes only those 25 countries shown. In Panel B, the OECD average includes Austria, Belgium, the Czech Republic, Denmark, Estonia, Finland, France, Germany, Greece, Hungary, Ireland, Italy, Latvia, Lithuania, Luxembourg, the Netherlands, Poland, Portugal, the Slovak Republic, Slovenia, Spain and Sweden. Differences between groups are significant at the 5% level in April-June 2020, June-July 2020 and February-March 2021. Refer to Box 2.1 for methodological details on the Living, working and COVID-19 survey.

Source: OECD (n.d.[3]), *Risks That Matter Survey*, http://oe.cd/RTM (Panel A); and Eurofound (n.d.[9]), *Living, working and COVID-19 e-survey* (database), https://www.eurofound.europa.eu/data/covid-19 (Panel B).

StatLink https://stat.link/ln01sm

In 25 OECD countries in September-October 2020, those who experienced job loss during the pandemic were more than twice as likely to report financial difficulties. Of people reporting that they or someone else in their household had lost their job, 68% had at least one form of financial difficulty during the pandemic (Figure 5.21, Panel A, see the figure note for the full list of financial difficulties). This compares to an average of 26.3% of people who did not experience job loss. Moreover, almost three-quarters (74%) of those who lost their job during COVID-19 were somewhat or very concerned about their household not being able to pay all expenses and make ends meet in the next year or two, compared to 60% of those who did not report job loss (OECD, 2021[54]).

In 22 European OECD countries, the crisis has widened inequalities in financial difficulties between employment groups. In April-June 2020, on average, 51% of unemployed respondents in 22 European OECD countries reported difficulties in making ends meet, compared to only 17% of the employed. Data from 2018 imply that the percentage of unemployed people who could not make ends meet in the same countries increased by 3.9 percentage points between 2018 and April-June 2020, while the share of employed people in the same condition increased by only 2.2 percentage points. What is more, while the share of employed respondents reporting difficulties to make ends meet decreased to 16% by February-March 2021, that of unemployed respondents in the same condition increased to 57% (Figure 5.21, Panel B).

Figure 5.21. People who lost their jobs have been experiencing particular financial struggles

Panel A. Share of respondents reporting at least one financial difficulty since the start of the COVID-19 pandemic, by reported experience of job loss in the household, 2020

Panel B. Share of respondents with difficulties in making ends meet, European Statistics on Income and Living Conditions (2018), and Living, Working, and COVID-19 e-survey (Apr-Jun 2020, Jun-Jul 2020 and Feb-Mar 2021), OECD 22

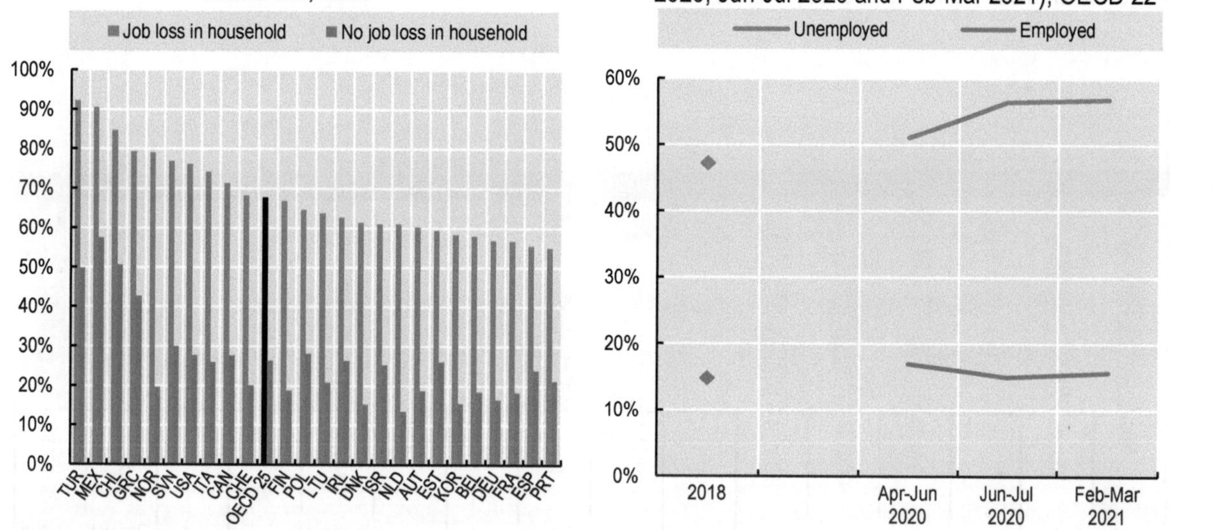

Note: In Panel A, respondents were asked whether, at any time since the start of the COVID-19 pandemic, they (or their household) had experienced one or more of a range of specific finance-related events. Options included: failed to pay a usual expense; took money out of savings or sold assets to pay for a usual expense; took money from family or friends to pay for a usual expense; took on additional debt or used credit to pay for a usual expense; asked a charity or non-profit organisation for assistance because they could not afford to pay; went hungry because they could not afford to pay for food; lost their home because they could not afford the mortgage or rent; or declared bankruptcy or asked a credit provider for help. Respondents could select all the options that applied. "Job loss in household" refers to respondents reporting that either they or any member of their household have/has either "Lost their job or been laid off permanently by their employer" and/or "Lost their self-employed job or their own business", since the start of the COVID-19 pandemic. The OECD average includes only those 25 countries shown. In Panel B, the OECD average includes Austria, Belgium, the Czech Republic, Denmark, Estonia, Finland, France, Germany, Greece, Hungary, Ireland, Italy, Latvia, Lithuania, Luxembourg, the Netherlands, Poland, Portugal, the Slovak Republic, Slovenia, Spain and Sweden. Differences between groups are significant at the 5% level in April-June 2020, June-July 2020 and February-March 2021. Refer to Box 2.1 for methodological details on the Living, working and COVID-19 survey.

Source: OECD (n.d.[3]), *Risks That Matter Survey*, http://oe.cd/RTM (Panel A); data from 2018 are from the Eurostat (n.d.[55]), *EU Survey on Income and Living Conditions* (database), https://ec.europa.eu/eurostat/web/income-and-living-conditions/data/database; and data from 2020-2021 are from Eurofound (n.d.[9]), *Living, working and COVID-19 e-survey* (database), https://www.eurofound.europa.eu/data/covid-19 (Panel B).

StatLink https://stat.link/416tw2

Young people, parents and those from low-income households have been most likely to run into financial difficulties…

In 25 OECD countries, young people, people with children under 18 and those from low-income households have been more likely to be experiencing some kind of financial difficulty in September-October 2020 (Figure 5.22). This reflects the disproportionate job and income losses experienced by these groups since the beginning of the crisis. In particular, as expected, respondents in low-income households – regardless of employment status – were on average the most likely to report having financial trouble (39%), while high-income households were least likely (25%) (Figure 5.22) (see Box 5.6 for evidence from France).

Figure 5.22. In 25 OECD countries, over 30% of parents, young adults and those from low-income households have been suffering financially since the start of the pandemic

Share of respondents reporting at least one financial difficulty since the start of the COVID-19 pandemic, by selected socioeconomic characteristics, OECD 25, Sep-Oct 2020

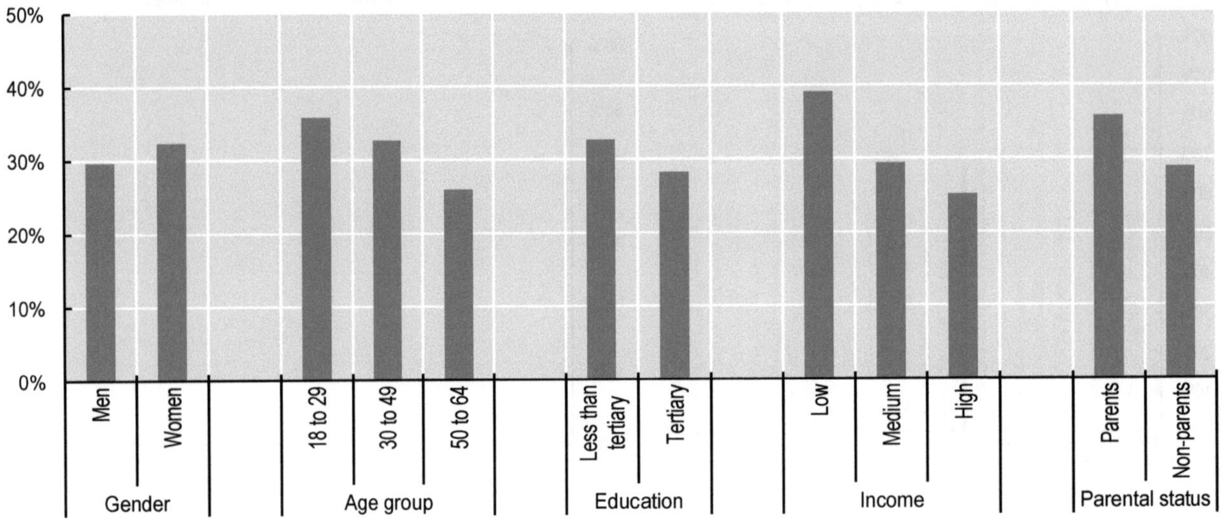

Note: Respondents were asked whether, at any time since the start of the COVID-19 pandemic, they (or their household) had experienced one or more of a range of specific finance-related events. "Less than tertiary" indicates respondents with less than a tertiary education, "tertiary" indicates respondents with a tertiary education. "Low income" households are those with an equivalised disposable income (for 2019) in the bottom three deciles of the national disposable income distribution, "medium income" households those in the middle four deciles, and "high income" households those in the top three deciles. Parents are defined as respondents with at least one own child under age 18 living in the same household. The OECD average includes Austria, Belgium, Canada, Chile, Denmark, Estonia, Finland, France, Germany, Greece, Ireland, Israel, Italy, Korea, Lithuania, Mexico, the Netherlands, Norway, Poland, Portugal, Slovenia, Spain, Switzerland, Turkey and the United States.
Source: OECD (n.d.[3]), *Risks That Matter Survey*, http://oe.cd/RTM.

StatLink https://stat.link/vnbuo4

Box 5.6. Innovation: INSEE and Inserm EpiCov survey – Consequences of lockdown measures on different socio-economic groups in France

The Epidemiology and Living Conditions (EpiCov) survey was set up by Drees, Inserm, Santé Publique France and INSEE (France's national statistics office) in order to study the impact of the pandemic and associated confinement measures on living conditions. The first wave of the survey took place between

2 May and 2 June 2020. 135 000 people aged 15 or over living in mainland France, Martinique, Guadeloupe and Reunion were selected in the Fidéli 2018 database of INSEE and interviewed online or by phone. The EpiCov survey includes questions on respondents' financial situation, employment situation, working conditions (especially teleworking) and working time. According to the EpiCov survey, in May 2020, 23% of households declared that their financial situation had deteriorated since the start of confinement. Conversely, only 2% say their financial situation has improved, while for two-thirds it remained stable. Among households within the lowest decile of a standard of living measure based on equivalised income, 35% declared that their financial situation had deteriorated since the start of confinement, compared to 16% of households in the top decile. In addition, people with children were more likely to say that the financial situation of their household has deteriorated (33%) since the confinement, than people without children (18%) (Figure 5.23).

Figure 5.23. In France, poorer households and parents were hit the hardest by the financial impact of the virus

Share of people who reported that their financial situation had deteriorated since the confinement, by socio-economic characteristics, May-2020

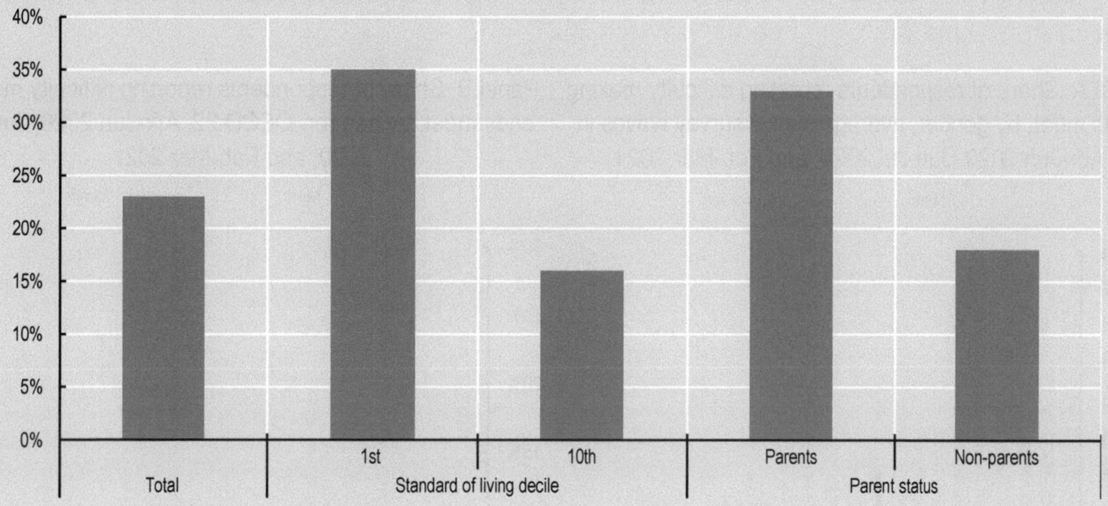

Note: The standard of living is equal to the disposable income of the household divided by the number of consumption units (CU). The standard of living is therefore the same for all individuals in the same household. Consumption units are generally calculated according to the OECD equivalence scale, which assigns 1 CU to the first adult in the household, 0.5 CU to other persons 14 years of age or over, and 0.3 CU to children under 14 years old.

Source: Givord and Silhol (2020[56]), *Containment: unequal economic consequences according to households*, Insee, https://www.insee.fr/fr/statistiques/4801313#consulter.

StatLink https://stat.link/b1ru3k

A survey conducted in the United States revealed that low-income households with children were facing high rates of financial difficulty in April 2020. 76% reported concerns about financial stability, 69% about food availability, 43% about employment and 31% about housing stability. What is more, 94% of the families reported being food insecure, with a 22-percentage point increase since the final months of 2019.[11] Food insecurity was higher among Hispanic/Latino respondents (95%), relative to other racial/ethnic groups (Sharma et al., 2020[57]) (see also Box 5.7).[12]

Findings from the United Kingdom and the United States indicate that people with lower personal incomes face greater difficulty in meeting both unexpected and routine household costs. In the

United Kingdom, between March and July 2020, 37.9% of people with total annual income below GBP 10 000 were unable to pay an unexpected expense of GBP 850 compared to 10.5% of people with an annual income of GBP 40 000 or over (ONS, 2020[58]). In the United States, among lower-income adults, 46% say they have had trouble paying their bills since the pandemic started, and 32% say they have been struggling to pay rent/mortgage. By contrast only 5% and 3% of people from the upper-income group have been struggling to pay bills and rent/mortgage respectively. In addition, 35% of lower-income adults say they have received food from a food bank/organisation, compared to only 12% of middle-income and 1% of upper-income adults (Parker, Minkin and Bennett, 2020[59]).[13]

... and women had more financial difficulties than men

Women were more likely than men to experience difficulties in making ends meet. Across 22 European countries, between April-June 2020 and February-March 2021, the share of women reporting difficulties in making ends meet was 23%, which was 3 percentage points higher than for men (Figure 5.24, Panel A). Between June-July 2020 and February-March 2021, the share of women reporting such difficulties increased by 2 percentage points, while that of men remained stable (Figure 5.24, Panel B).

Figure 5.24. Over a quarter of women in 22 European OECD countries could not make ends meet between April-June 2020 and February-March 2021

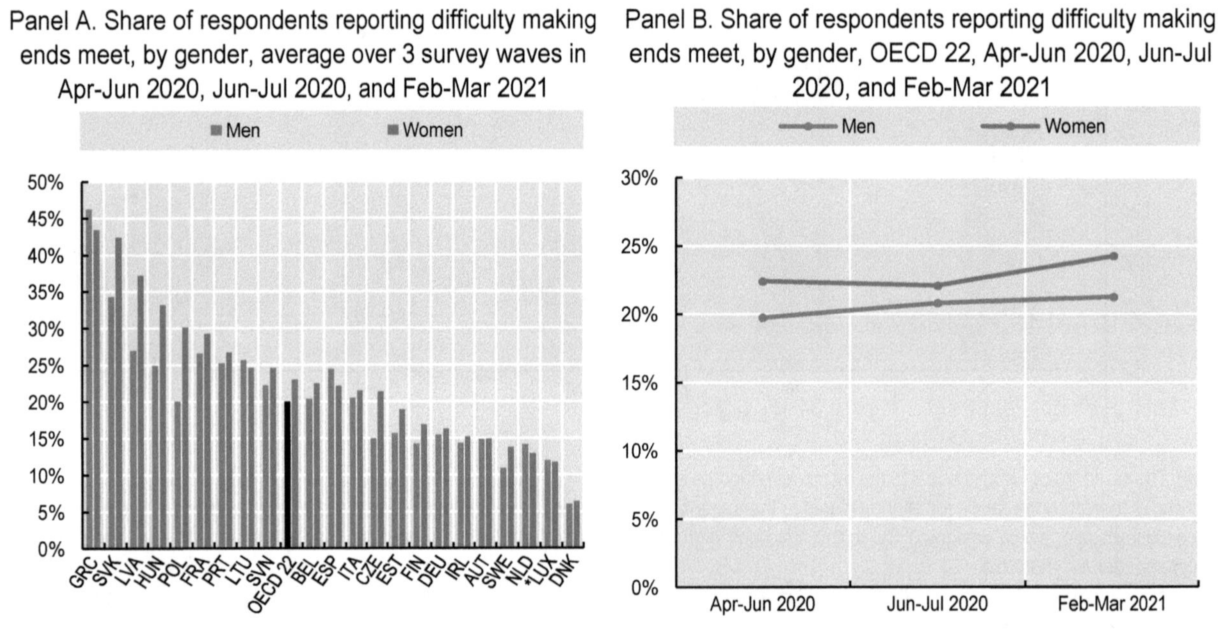

Note: In Panel A, data are not reported where fewer than 100 observations per gender category are available. * denotes countries with between 301 and 500 observations per category. More than 500 observations per category are available for all other countries. The OECD average includes only those 22 countries shown. Differences between groups are significant at the 5% level for the Czech Republic, Hungary, Latvia, OECD 22, Poland and the Slovak Republic. In Panel B, the OECD average includes only those 22 countries shown in Panel A. Refer to Box 2.1 for methodological details on the Living, working and COVID-19 survey.
Source: Eurofound (n.d.[9]), *Living, working and COVID-19 e-survey* (database), https://www.eurofound.europa.eu/data/covid-19.

StatLink https://stat.link/0n5f47

Box 5.7. In Chile and the United States, food insecurity hit vulnerable population groups the hardest, including mothers and racial/ethnic minorities

In Chile, moderate-severe food insecurity was most common among vulnerable households in November 2020. In particular, it was most prevalent in households which "felt like their income was not enough" and those with no employed members (Figure 5.25).

Figure 5.25. Vulnerable households in Chile have been facing higher rates of food insecurity

Share of respondents reporting moderate-severe food insecurity, Nov-2020

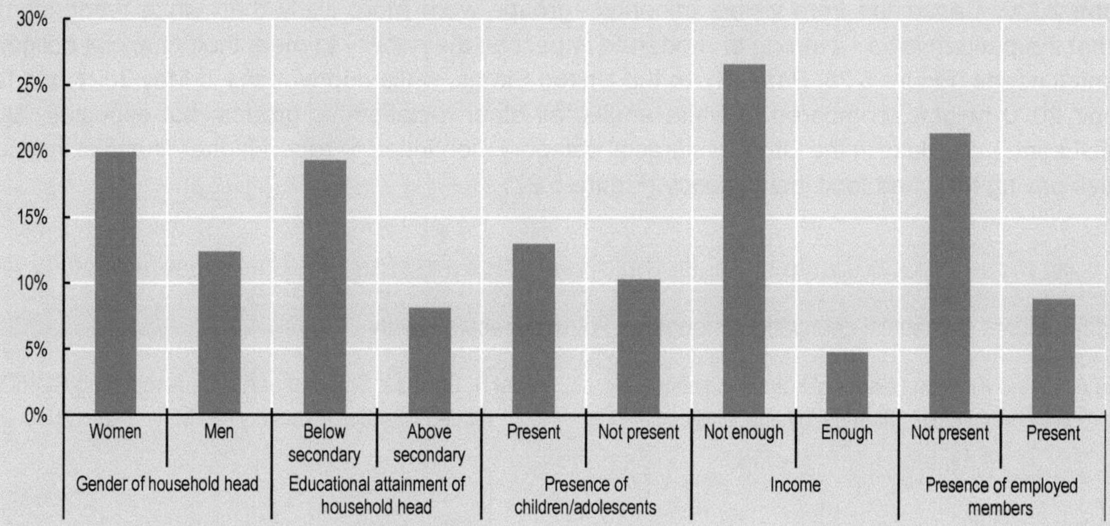

Note: People who face uncertainties in their abilities to acquire food or who are forced to buy less/lower-quality food than usual are said to face moderate food insecurity, and people who often run out of food or that go one or more days without eating are said to face severe food insecurity.

Source: Ministerio Desarrollo Social y Familia (n.d.[18]), *Encuesta Social COVID-19 (COVID-19 Social Survey)* (database), http://observatorio.ministeriodesarrollosocial.gob.cl/encuesta-social-covid19.

StatLink https://stat.link/qhfc0i

Evidence from the United States reveals similar trends. In June 2020, 20% of households indicated that they often or sometimes ran out of food before having enough money to buy more. Food insecurity was more widespread among individuals without a high school diploma (45%), households with less than USD 30 000 in annual income (40%), Hispanic/Latino households (33%) and households with children (27%) (Wozniak et al., 2020[60]) (refer to Box 3.1 for methods). Evidence from 12-24 May 2021 confirms that American adults in households with children were more likely to report that the household sometimes or often did not have enough to eat in the previous seven days (11%), compared to those in households without children (7%). In addition, 9% of all households living with children reported that the *children* sometimes or often in the previous seven days were "not eating enough because we just couldn't afford enough food" (US Census Bureau, n.d.[61]). Notably, the prevalence of food insecurity among households differed by race/ethnicity (Figure 5.27). As of late March 2021, single mothers experienced elevated levels of food insecurity (35%), higher than other respondents with children (23%), and higher than the pandemic peak for all respondents on average (24%) (Bauer, 2021[15]).

COVID-19 has also exacerbated the material hardship of racial/ethnic minorities

COVID-19 has exacerbated the material hardship of racial/ethnic minorities in the United Kingdom, Canada, and the United States. In the United Kingdom, prior to the pandemic, households headed by someone of Black African or Other Black ethnicity were significantly less likely to have enough financial assets to cover a drop in employment income than those from most other ethnic groups (ONS, 2020[62]). In April 2020, over a quarter of those from Black, African, Caribbean or Black British ethnic groups reported finding it very or quite difficult to get by financially; this level was significantly higher than those from other ethnic backgrounds, with a 5 percentage point increase compared to 2019 (Figure 5.26, Panel A). All other ethnic groups except for white Irish, also experienced increases in financial insecurity. In May, households that included at least one adult who identifies as ethnic minority also experienced levels of food insecurity at least 50% higher than their white peers (Equality and Human Rights Commission, 2020[63]). Similarly, in May-June 2020, Canadians from visible minority[14] groups were more likely than white respondents to report that the pandemic had a strong or moderate impact on their ability to meet their financial obligations or essential needs (Figure 5.26, Panel B). In the United States, while deprivations in May 2021 had fallen from their 2020 heights, compared to white adults, all other racial/ethnic groups, but especially Black, Hispanic/Latino and adults in the Other/Multiracial category, continued to report higher financial insecurity, difficulties paying rent, and food insufficiency (Figure 5.27).

Figure 5.26. In the UK and Canada, racial/ethnic minorities are struggling the most financially

Selected measures of financial deprivation throughout 2020, by race/ethnicity

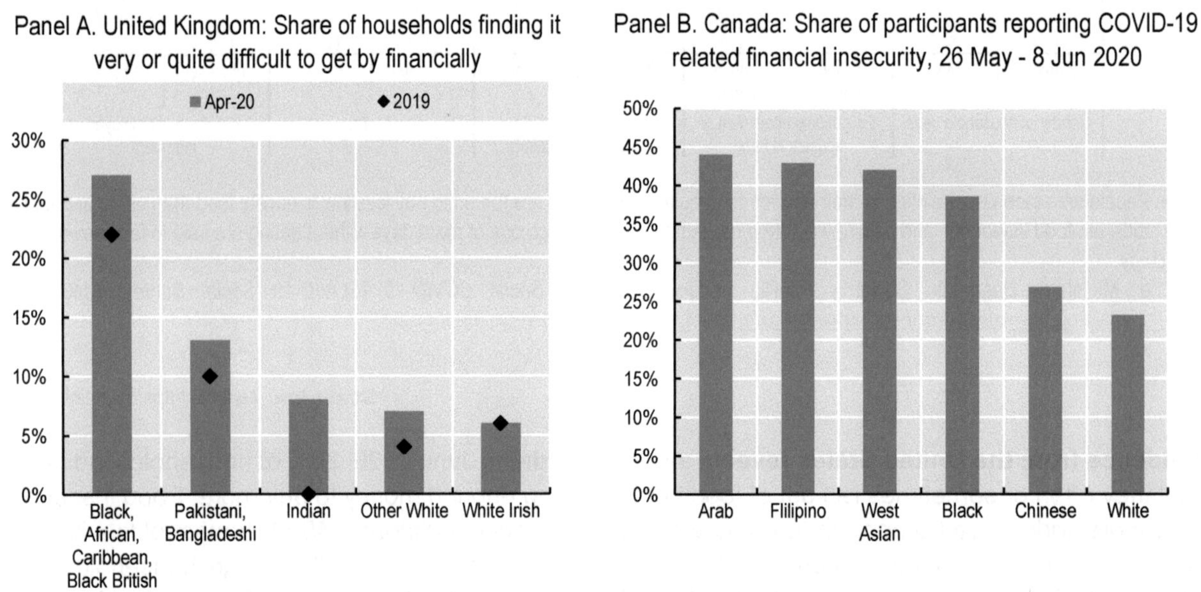

Note: In Panel A, no 2019 data are available for Indian households. Ethnicity is defined as the ethnicity reported by the head of the household. In Panel B, the question refers to participants who reported that COVID-19 has had a strong or moderate impact on their ability to meet their financial obligations or essential needs such as rent or mortgage payments, utilities, and groceries. Since this is sourced from an experimental crowd-sourced survey that does not apply a probabilistic sampling design, inferences about the overall Canadian population or its subgroups should not be made.

Source: ONS (2020[62]), *Coronavirus and the social impacts on different ethnic groups in the UK: 2020*, Office for National Statistics, https://www.ons.gov.uk/peoplepopulationandcommunity/culturalidentity/ethnicity/articles/coronavirusandthesocialimpactsondifferentethnicgroupsintheuk/2020 (Panel A); and Statistics Canada (2020[64]), *Economic impact of COVID-19 among visible minority groups*, https://www150.statcan.gc.ca/n1/pub/45-28-0001/2020001/article/00042-eng.htm (Panel B).

StatLink https://stat.link/h9aigd

Figure 5.27. Racial/ethnic minorities in the United States reported higher financial insecurity, difficulties paying rent, and food insufficiency

Selected measures of financial deprivation throughout 2020-21, by race/ethnicity

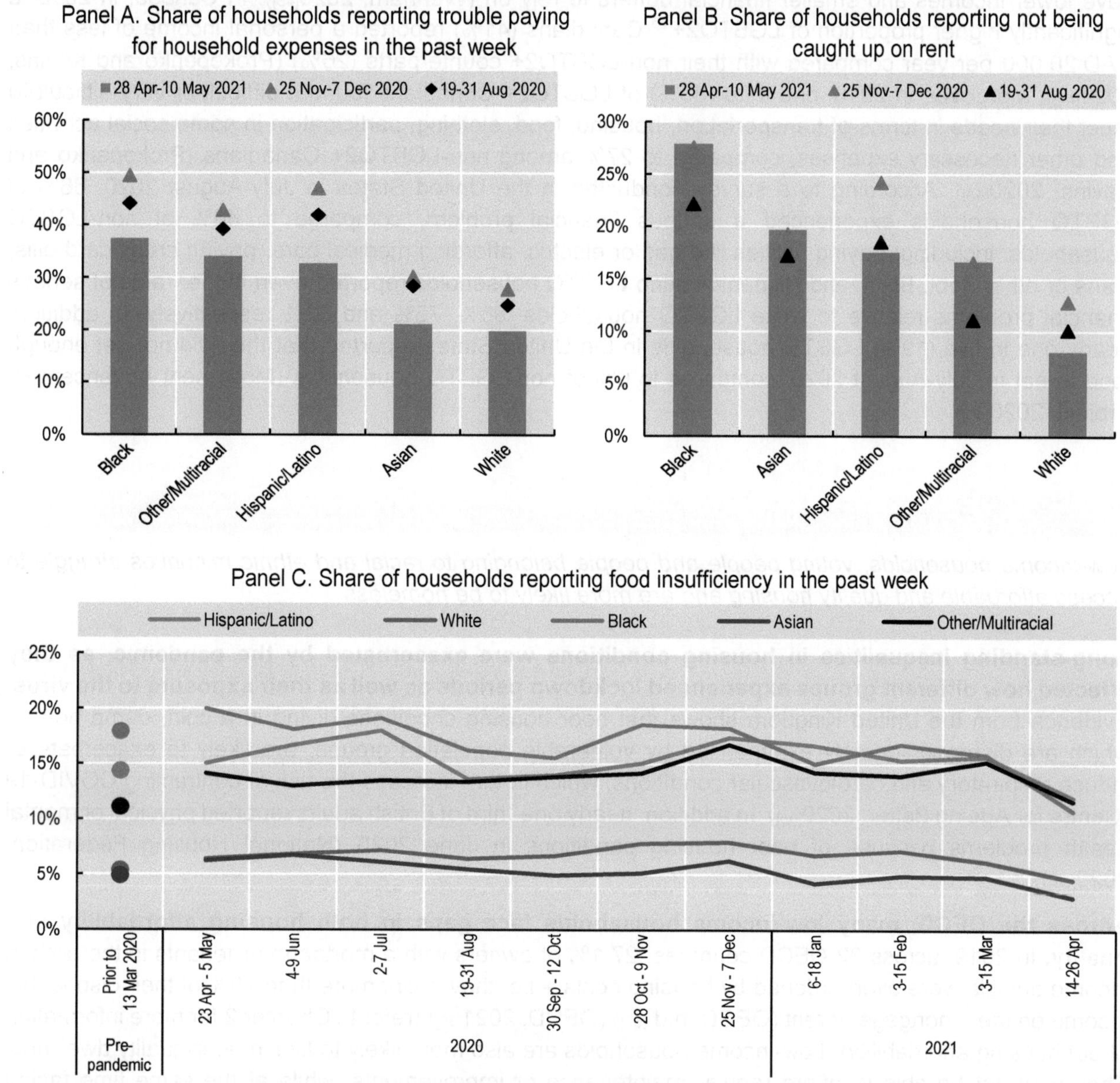

Note: In Panels A and B, "Other/Multiracial" refers to people identifying as American Indian, Alaska Native, Native Hawaiian or Pacific Islander, or more than one race. Percentages do not include non-responses. In Panel A, items refer to the share of adults in the United States reporting that it was somewhat or very difficult for their household to pay for usual expenses in the last seven days, in Panel B, that their household is not caught up on rent (share of adult renters only), and in Panel C, that their household sometimes or often did not have enough to eat in the last seven days. In Panel C, "Pre-pandemic" includes data from a self-reported recall question (asked between 23 April - 5 May 2020) about food insufficiency prior to 13 March 2020, in addition to the previous seven days. This limits direct comparability with subsequent data points.

Source: US Census Bureau (n.d.[61]), *Measuring household experiences during the coronavirus pandemic* (database), https://www.census.gov/householdpulsedata (refer to Box 3.1 for methodological details).

StatLink https://stat.link/ou3586

In countries with available data, the pandemic worsened the financial situation for LGBTQ+ communities

LGBTQ+ people are particularly vulnerable to financial difficulty in times of crisis. During the pandemic, LGBTQ+ people have been experiencing considerable employment losses. They also tend to have lower incomes and smaller financial buffers to rely on (Wenham, 2020[43]). In Canada, in 2018, a significantly higher proportion of LGBTQ2+[15] Canadians (41%) reported a personal income of less than CAD 20 000 per year compared with their non-LGBTQ2+ counterparts (26%) (Prokopenko and Kevins, 2020[44]). Moreover, in 2018, one-third (33%) of LGBTQ2+ Canadians found it difficult or very difficult to meet their needs in terms of transportation, housing, food, clothing, participation in some social activities and other necessary expenses, compared to 27% among non-LGBTQ2+ Canadians (Prokopenko and Kevins, 2020[44]). According to a survey conducted in the United States in July-August 2020, 66% of LGBTQ households experienced a serious financial problem, compared to 44% of non-LGBTQ households, including: paying utilities like gas or electric, affording medical care, paying credit card bills, loans or other debt. Black and Hispanic/Latino LGBTQ households reported even higher rates of serious financial problems relative to white LGBTQ households: 95%, 75% and 62% respectively. In addition, nearly one in five (19%) LGBTQ households in the United States reported that they did not get enough food to eat in July-August 2020, compared to 6% of non-LGBTQ households (Movement Advancement Project, 2020[46]).

5.3. Housing

Low-income households, young people and people belonging to racial and ethnic minorities struggle to access affordable and quality housing and are more likely to be homeless

Long-standing inequalities in housing conditions were exacerbated by the pandemic, as they affected how different groups experienced lockdown periods as well as their exposure to the virus. Evidence from the United Kingdom shows that poor housing conditions (living in a cold, damp home), which are disproportionately experienced by vulnerable population groups, are likely to exacerbate or induce respiratory and cardiovascular conditions, which in turn increase the risk of contracting COVID-19 (Centre for Ageing Better, 2020[65]). In addition, nearly one-third of British adults reported physical or mental health problems because of poor housing conditions in June 2020 (National Housing Federation, 2020[66]).[16]

Across the OECD, many low-income households face gaps in both housing affordability and quality. In 2019, across 32 OECD countries, 27.1% of owners with a mortgage or tenants in the bottom income quintile were overburdened by housing costs – i.e. they spent more than 40% of their disposable income on their mortgage or rent (OECD, n.d.[67]) (OECD, 2021[68]) (refer to Chapter 2 for more information about housing affordability). Low-income households are also more likely to live in poor-quality dwellings. They may not be able to afford regular maintenance or improvements, while at the same time facing barriers to move to better-quality housing. On average, households in the bottom income quintile show a higher share of overcrowding than those in the middle- or top-income quintiles (15.5%, 10.0% and 5.8% respectively) (Figure 5.28) (OECD, n.d.[67]) (OECD, 2021[68]). In addition, within the low-income population, children are more likely to live in overcrowded housing than other age groups (OECD, 2021[68]). In the United Kingdom, over 20% of children from households in the bottom income tertile live in overcrowded conditions, compared to less than 5% of children from households in the top income tertile (Judge and Rahman, 2020[69]).[17]

Young people have been facing significant difficulties in accessing affordable and quality housing in recent years. In particular, low-income youth face even bigger challenges than their higher-income peers in securing good-quality housing, often because they are not able to rely on their family resources for support (OECD, 2021[68]). For instance, in the United Kingdom, 6% of people aged 16-24 live in a damp home, compared to 2% of people aged 65 or over (Judge and Rahman, 2020[69]). The COVID-19 pandemic is likely to exacerbate these challenges, given the disproportionate impact of the crisis on young people's jobs and incomes. Indeed, in September-October 2020, in 25 OECD countries 53.4% of young people (aged 18 to 29) reported that they were concerned about not being able to find/maintain adequate housing in the next year or two, compared to 44.1% of the total population (Figure 5.29).

People belonging to ethnic minority groups in the United Kingdom are more likely to live in poor-quality housing. On average, households belonging to ethnic minority groups are larger than white British households, and therefore more likely to live in overcrowded conditions (12% of people from ethnic minority groups live in households of five people or more, compared to 5% of people from white groups) (Haque, Becares and Treloar, 2020[70]).[18] In particular, one-quarter of people under age 15 belonging to ethnic minority groups live in overcrowded housing, compared to fewer than 10% of white people (Judge and Rahman, 2020[69]). Furthermore, the proportion of households with no garden is a lot higher among ethnic minorities, as Black people in England are four times as likely as white British people to have no outdoor space at home (37% compared to 10%) (ONS, 2020[71]).[19]

Figure 5.28. Low-income households are more likely to live in overcrowded conditions

Share of overcrowded households, by income quintile, 2019 or latest year available

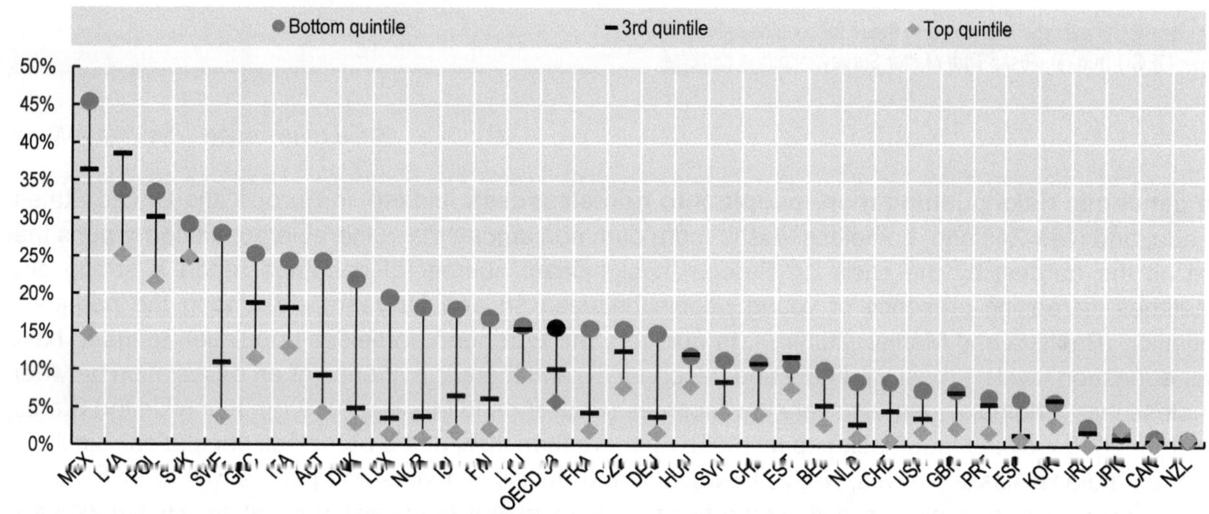

Note: Low-income households are households in the bottom quintile of the (net) income distribution. In Chile, Mexico, Korea and the United States gross income is used due to data limitations. For Chile, Mexico, Denmark, the Netherlands and the United States, no information on subsidised tenants is available due to data limitations. A household is considered overcrowded if it does not have at its disposal a minimum number of rooms equal to: one room for the household; one room per adult couple in the household; one room for each single person aged 18 or over; one room per pair of single persons of the same sex between 12 and 17 years of age; one room for each single person between 12 and 17 years of age and not included in the previous category; or one room per pair of children under 12 years of age. See section "Data and comparability issues" of Indicator HC2.1 in OECD (n.d.[67]) on limits to comparability across countries due to the definition of rooms. Data for Japan are available only on the respondent level due to data limitations. Results therefore refer to the population, rather than to households. Data for Canada are adjusted by Statistics Canada based on the assumption of the presence of a kitchen in dwellings where it is expected, while income quintiles are based on adjusted after-tax household income. The OECD average excludes Australia, Colombia, Costa Rica, Israel and Turkey.

Source: OECD (n.d.[67]), *Affordable Housing* (database), https://www.oecd.org/housing/data/affordable-housing-database/; and Statistics New Zealand, who provided data for New Zealand.

StatLink https://stat.link/ve1jdy

Figure 5.29. Young people are particularly worried about their housing conditions

Share of respondents reporting being either "somewhat concerned" or "very concerned" about not being able to find/maintain adequate housing, by age, Sept-Oct 2020

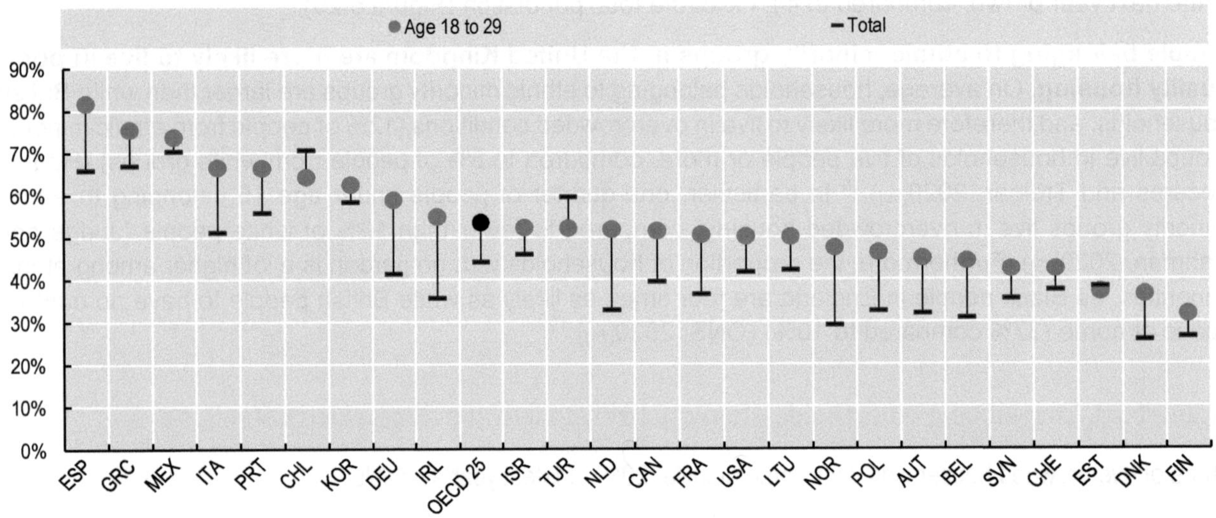

Note: The OECD average includes only those 25 countries shown.
Source: OECD (n.d.[3]), *Risks That Matter Survey*, http://oe.cd/RTM.

StatLink https://stat.link/0onit4

The pandemic risks pushing more people into homelessness. Indeed, in Europe, the United States, Canada, and New Zealand, homelessness is more common among the vulnerable population groups that were hit the hardest by the crisis. In Europe, a significant number of countries report a strong and sometimes increasing presence of young people between 15 and 29 years old among the homeless population (Baptista and Marlier, 2019[72]). In addition, the European homeless population tends to have lower education levels – mostly primary and secondary – and there is evidence of an association between homelessness, unemployment and very low incomes (Baptista and Marlier, 2019[72]). In the United States, data from 2019 indicate that Black people make up more than 40% of the homeless population. Similarly, American Indians/Alaska Natives, Native Hawaiians and Pacific Islanders and people who identify as two or more racial groups make up a disproportionate share of the homeless population. Hispanic/Latino people constitute a share of the homeless population approximately equal to the general population, while white and Asian people are significantly under-represented (National Alliance to End Homelessness, 2020[73]).[20] In Canada, young people aged 13-24 make up about 20% of those experiencing homelessness, and Indigenous people (including First Nations, Métis and Inuit peoples) are over-represented among those experiencing homelessness in urban centers (Gaetz et al., 2013[74]). People from LGBTQ+ communities are also more likely to be homeless or housing insecure. In Canada, 27% of people identifying as LGBTQ2+ reported experiencing some type of homelessness in their lifetime (Prokopenko and Kevins, 2020[44]). In the United States, 25% of LGBTQ people surveyed in July-August 2020 reported that their home has serious heating or cooling problems, mold problems, pest problems, problems with unsafe drinking water, or other serious environmental problems, compared to 10% of non-LGBTQ people (Movement Advancement Project, 2020[46]). Lastly, in New Zealand, data from 2018 indicate that severe housing deprivation particularly affects ethnic minorities and the youth: Māori and Pacific people are respectively four and six times more likely to be severely housing deprived than people of European descent, and people under 25 make up 48.3% of the total housing deprived population (Amore, 2021[75]).[21]

COVID-19 has also exacerbated the impact of the digital divide in housing, as households without Internet access have greater difficultly in teleworking or participating in distance learning. Across OECD regions, there is a clear urban-rural divide in access to high-speed broadband. On average in 26 OECD countries, 63.6% of households in rural areas have access to high-speed broadband, compared to 87% of all households. Digital divides also exist between income and racial/ethnic groups. In the United Kingdom, only 51% of households earning GBP 6 000-10 000 a year had Internet access at home in 2014, compared to 99% of households with an income of over GBP 40 000 (ONS, 2019[76]). In Canada, 97.9% of households in the top income quartile had Internet access at home in 2012, while 54.9% of households in the bottom quartile had such access (Statistics Canada, 2017[77]). In 2021, in the United States, roughly six-in-ten adults living in households earning USD 100 000 or more a year (63%) reported having home broadband services, a smartphone, a desktop or laptop computer and a tablet, compared to 23% of those living in lower-income households (earning less than USD 30 000 a year) (Figure 5.30, Panel A) (Vogels, 2021[78]). In addition, 80% of white adults reported having a broadband connection at home, while smaller shares of Black and Hispanic/Latino adults said the same – 71% and 65% respectively. White adults in the United States are also more likely to own a computer than Black or Hispanic/Latino adults (80%, 69% and 67% respectively) (Figure 5.30, Panel B) (Atske and Perrin, 2021[79]).[22] Access to the Internet and electronic devices can severely impact educational outcomes for vulnerable children. Across the OECD, children under the age of 15 from the bottom economic social and cultural status quartile were least likely to have a computer and access to the Internet at home in 2018 (76.9% versus 97.1% for children in the top quartile).[23] Similarly, 76.9% of children whose parents have less than a secondary education and 86.6% of immigrant students had access to a computer and to the Internet at home, compared to 91.6% of children whose parents have at least a tertiary degree and 90.2% of non-immigrant students (OECD, n.d.[80]).

Figure 5.30. In the United States, lower-income households, Black and Hispanic/Latino adults are less likely to have broadband access at home

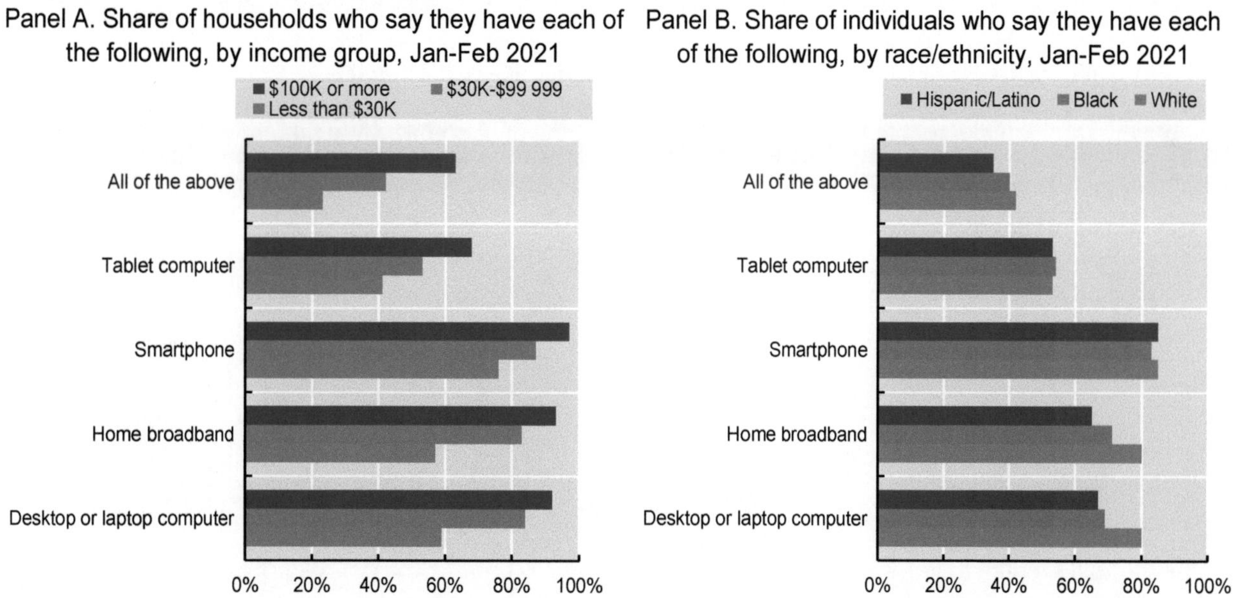

Source: Vogels (2021[78]), *Digital divide persists even as Americans with lower income make gains in tech adoption*, Pew Research Center, https://www.pewresearch.org/fact-tank/2021/06/22/digital-divide-persists-even-as-americans-with-lower-incomes-make-gains-in-tech-adoption/ (Panel A); and Atske and Perrin (2021[79]), *Home broadband adoption, computer ownership vary by race, ethnicity in the U.S.*, Pew Research Center, https://www.pewresearch.org/fact-tank/2021/07/16/home-broadband-adoption-computer-ownership-vary-by-race-ethnicity-in-the-u-s/ (Panel B).

StatLink https://stat.link/mad9c0

Box 5.8. Further reading

- OECD (2021), *Brick by Brick: Building Better Housing Policies*, OECD Publishing, Paris, https://dx.doi.org/10.1787/b453b043-en
- OECD (2021), *Building for a better tomorrow: Policies to make housing more affordable*. Employment, Labour and Social Affairs Policy Briefs, OECD Publishing, Paris, http://oe.cd/affordable-housing-2021
- OECD (2021), OECD *Employment Outlook 2021: Navigating the COVID-19 Crisis and Recovery*, OECD Publishing, Paris, https://dx.doi.org/10.1787/5a700c4b-en
- OECD (2021), *OECD SME and Entrepreneurship Outlook 2021*, OECD Publishing, Paris, https://dx.doi.org/10.1787/97a5bbfe-en
- OECD (2020), *International Migration Outlook 2020*, OECD Publishing, Paris, https://dx.doi.org/10.1787/ec98f531-en
- OECD (2020), *OECD Employment Outlook 2020: Worker Security and the COVID-19 Crisis*, OECD Publishing, Paris, https://dx.doi.org/10.1787/1686c758-en
- OECD (n.d.), *Affordable Housing database*, http://www.oecd.org/housing/data/affordable-housing-database/ (accessed 15 June 2021)

References

Amore, K. (2021), *Severe housing deprivation in Aotearoa New Zealand, 2018*, https://www.hud.govt.nz/assets/News-and-Resources/Statistics-and-Research/2018-Severe-housing-deprivation-estimate/Severe-Housing-Deprivation-2018-Estimate-Report.pdf. [75]

Atske, S. and A. Perrin (2021), *Home broadband adoption, computer ownership vary by race, ethnicity in the U.S.*, Pew Research Center, https://www.pewresearch.org/fact-tank/2021/07/16/home-broadband-adoption-computer-ownership-vary-by-race-ethnicity-in-the-u-s/. [79]

Baptista, I. and E. Marlier (2019), *Fighting homelessness and housing exclusion in Europe: A study of national policies*, European Commission, Directorate-general for Employment, Social Affairs, and Inclusion, https://op.europa.eu/en/publication-detail/-/publication/2dd1bd61-d834-11e9-9c4e-01aa75ed71a1/language-en. [72]

Barrero, J., N. Bloom and S. Davis (2021), *Let me work from home, or I will find another job*, VOX.org CEPR Policy Portal, https://voxeu.org/article/let-me-work-home-or-i-will-find-another-job. [50]

Bauer, L. (2021), *Mothers are being left behind in the economic recovery from COVID-19*, Brookings, https://www.brookings.edu/blog/up-front/2021/05/06/mothers-are-being-left-behind-in-the-economic-recovery-from-covid-19/?utm_campaign=brookings-comm&utm_medium=email&utm_content=125828433&utm_source=hs_email. [15]

Benzeval, M. et al. (2020), *The idiosyncratic impact of an aggregate shock: The distributional consequences of COVID-19*, Understanding Society Working Paper Series, No. 2020-09, https://www.understandingsociety.ac.uk/sites/default/files/downloads/working-papers/2020-09.pdf. [27]

Berg, L. and B. Farbenblum (2020), *As if we weren't humans - the abandonment of temporary migrants in Australia during COVID-19*, Migrant Worker Justice Initiative, https://apo.org.au/sites/default/files/resource-files/2020-09/apo-nid308305.pdf. [23]

Broady, K. (2021), *July's jobs report shows Black teens struggling with the highest unemployment rate*, Brookings, https://www.brookings.edu/blog/the-avenue/2021/08/09/julys-jobs-report-shows-black-teens-struggling-with-the-highest-unemployment-rate/. [37]

Brücker, H. (2021), *Special COVID-19 Survey of IAB-BAMF-SOEP Refugee Survey*, https://www.slideshare.net/StatsCommunications/impact-of-covid19-on-migrant-health-and-labour-market-outcomes-herbert-brcker. [22]

Capgemini Research Institute (2020), *The Future of Work: From remote to hybrid*, https://www.capgemini.com/it-it/research/the-future-of-work/. [51]

CDC (2020), *Loss of Work Due to Illness from COVID-19*, Centers for Disease Control and Prevention, https://data.cdc.gov/NCHS/Loss-of-Work-Due-to-Illness-from-COVID-19/qgkx-mswu (accessed on 10 February 2021). [36]

Centre for Ageing Better (2020), *Homes, health and COVID-19*, https://www.ageing-better.org.uk/sites/default/files/2020-09/Homes-health-and-COVID-19.pdf. [65]

Department of Finance Canada (2021), *Budget 2021: A Recovery Plan for Jobs, Growth, and Resilience, Annex 4: Gender, Diversity, and Quality of Life Statement*, https://www.budget.gc.ca/2021/report-rapport/anx4-en.html (accessed on 17 June 2021). [81]

Equality and Human Rights Commission (2020), *How coronavirus has affected equality and human rights*, https://www.equalityhumanrights.com/sites/default/files/equality_and_human_rights_commission_how_coronavirus_has_affected_equality_and_human_rights_2020.pdf. [63]

Eurofound (2020), *Living, working and COVID-19 series*, Publications Office of the European Union, Luxembourg, https://www.eurofound.europa.eu/sites/default/files/ef_publication/field_ef_document/ef20059en.pdf. [48]

Eurofound (n.d.), *Living, working and COVID-19 database*, https://www.eurofound.europa.eu/data/covid-19 (accessed on 13 August 2021). [9]

Eurostat (2021), *Early estimates of income inequalities during the 2020 pandemic*, https://ec.europa.eu/eurostat/statistics-explained/index.php?title=Early_estimates_of_income_inequalities_during_the_2020_pandemic (accessed on 13 August 2021). [2]

Eurostat (2020), *Impact of COVID-19 on employment income - advanced estimates*, https://ec.europa.eu/eurostat/statistics-explained/index.php?title=Impact_of_COVID-19_on_employment_income_-_advanced_estimates#A_sharp_decrease_in_the_median_employment_income. [4]

Eurostat (n.d.), *Employment rates by sex, age and country of birth (%) database*, https://ec.europa.eu/eurostat/web/lfs/data/database (accessed on 13 August 2021). [30]

Eurostat (n.d.), *EU Survey on Income and Living Conditions database*, https://ec.europa.eu/eurostat/web/income-and-living-conditions/data/database (accessed on 20 May 2021). [55]

Fairlie, R. (2020), *The impact of COVID-19 on small business owners: Evidence from the first three months after widespread social-distancing restrictions*, Journal of Economics & Management Strategy, http://dx.doi.org/10.1111/jems.12400. [41]

Fana, M. et al. (2020), *Telework, work organisation and job quality during the COVID-19 crisis: a qualitative study*, European Commission Joint Research Centre, http://dx.doi.org/JRC122591. [49]

Gaetz, S. et al. (2013), *The state of homelessness in Canada*, Canadian Homelessness Research Network Press, Toronto, https://www.homelesshub.ca/SOHC2016. [74]

Galasso, V. and M. Foucault (2020), *Working during COVID-19: Cross-country evidence from real-time survey data*, OECD Social, Employment and Migration Working Papers, OECD Publishing, Paris, https://dx.doi.org/10.1787/34a2c306-en. [8]

Georgetown University (n.d.), *Tracking COVID-19 Unemployment and Job Losses*, Georgetown University Center on Education and the Workforce, https://cew.georgetown.edu/cew-reports/jobtracker/#unemployment-tracking (accessed on 21 May 2021). [10]

Givord, P. and J. Silhol (2020), *Containment: unequal economic consequences depending on the household*, Insee, https://www.insee.fr/fr/statistiques/4801313#consulter. [56]

Graeber, D., A. Kritikos and J. Seebauer (2021), *COVID-19: A crisis of the female selfemployed*, Global Labor Organisation (GLO), https://www.econstor.eu/bitstream/10419/230677/1/GLO-DP-0788.pdf. [42]

Haque, Z., L. Becares and N. Treloar (2020), *Over-exposed and under-protected: The devastating impact of COVID-19 on Black and Minority Ethnic communities in Great Britain*, Runnymede Trust and ICM, http://www.runnymedetrust.org/uploads/Runnymede%20Covid19%20Survey%20report%20v3.pdf. [70]

Hu, Y. (2020), *Intersecting ethnic and native–migrant inequalities in the economic impact of the COVID-19 pandemic in the UK*, Research in Social Stratification and Mobility, http://dx.doi.org/10.1016/j.rssm.2020.100528. [28]

ILO and UN Women (2020), *Fallout of COVID-19: Working moms are being squeezed out of the labour force*, International Labour Organisation, https://ilostat.ilo.org/fallout-of-covid-19-working-moms-are-being-squeezed-out-of-the-labour-force/. [14]

Innovative Research Group (2020), *Impact of COVID-19: Canada's LGBTQI2S community in focus*, https://egale.ca/wp-content/uploads/2020/04/Impact-of-COVID-19-Canada%E2%80%99s-LGBTQI2S-Community-in-Focus-2020-04-06.pdf. [45]

Institute for Women's Policy Research (2021), *Equal Pay Day 2021: The Results of a COVID-Impacted Economy*, https://iwpr.org/media/in-the-lead/equal-pay-day-2021-the-results-of-a-covid-impacted-economy/#:~:text=Equal%20Pay%20Day%202021%3A%20The%20Results%20of%20a%20COVID%2DImpacted%20Economy,-For%20many%20women&text=Today%2C%20IWPR%20CEO%20and%20President%20C.&. [16]

Ipsos (2020), *The COVID-19 pandemic's impact on workers' lives*, https://www.ipsos.com/sites/default/files/ct/news/documents/2020-12/impact-of-the-covid-19-pandemic-on-workers-lives-report.pdf. [52]

Judge, L. and F. Rahman (2020), *Lockdown living: Housing quality across the generations*, Resolution Foundation, https://www.resolutionfoundation.org/app/uploads/2020/07/Lockdown-living.pdf. [69]

Kühne, S. et al. (2020), "The need for household panel surveys in times of crisis: The case of soep-cov", *Survey Research Methods*, Vol. 14/2, pp. 195-203. [7]

Long, H. et al. (2020), *The covid-19 recession is the most unequal in modern U.S. history*, The Washington Post, https://www.washingtonpost.com/graphics/2020/business/coronavirus-recession-equality/. [35]

Marshall, J., C. Burd and M. Burrows (2021), *Working From Home During the Pandemic*, US Census Bureau, https://www.census.gov/library/stories/2021/03/working-from-home-during-the-pandemic.html. [6]

Ministerio Desarrollo Social y Familia (n.d.), *Encuesta Social COVID-19 (COVID-19 Social Survey)*, http://observatorio.ministeriodesarrollosocial.gob.cl/encuesta-social-covid19 (accessed on 20 May 2021). [18]

Movement Advancement Project (2020), *The disproportionate impacts of COVID-19 on LGBTQ households in the U.S.*, http://www.lgbtmap.org/2020-covid-lgbtq-households. [46]

National Alliance to End Homelessness (2020), *Racial Inequalities in homelessness, by the numbers*, https://endhomelessness.org/resource/racial-inequalities-homelessness-numbers/. [73]

National Housing Federation (2020), *Poor housing causing health problems for nearly a third of brits during lockdown*, https://www.housing.org.uk/news-and-blogs/news/poor-housing-causing-health-problems-for-nearly-a-third-of-brits-during-lockdown/. [66]

National Women's Law Center (2020), *Four times more women than men dropped out of the labour force in September*, https://nwlc.org/resources/four-times-more-women-than-men-dropped-out-of-the-labor-force-in-september/. [34]

OECD (2021), "An in-depth analysis of one year of SME and entrepreneurship policy responses to COVID-19: Lessons learned for the path to recovery", *OECD SME and Entrepreneurship Papers*, No. 25, OECD Publishing, Paris, https://dx.doi.org/10.1787/6407deee-en. [40]

OECD (2021), *Building for a better tomorrow: Policies to make housing more affordable*, Employment, Labour and Social Affairs Policy Briefs, OECD Publising, Paris, http://oe.cd/affordable-housing-2021. [68]

OECD (2021), *OECD Employment Outlook 2021: Navigating the COVID-19 Crisis and Recovery*, OECD Publishing, Paris, https://dx.doi.org/10.1787/5a700c4b-en. [11]

OECD (2021), *OECD SME and Entrepreneurship Outlook 2021*, OECD Publishing, Paris, https://dx.doi.org/10.1787/97a5bbfe-en. [39]

OECD (2021), "Risks that matter 2020: The long reach of COVID-19", *OECD Policy Responses to Coronavirus (COVID-19)*, OECD Publishing, Paris, https://dx.doi.org/10.1787/44932654-en. [54]

OECD (2020), *How's Life? 2020: Measuring Well-being*, OECD Publishing, Paris, https://dx.doi.org/10.1787/9870c393-en. [53]

OECD (2020), *International Migration Outlook 2020*, OECD Publishing, Paris, https://dx.doi.org/10.1787/ec98f531-en. [21]

OECD (2020), *OECD Employment Outlook 2020: Worker Security and the COVID-19 Crisis*, OECD Publishing, Paris, https://doi.org/10.1787/1686c758-en. [1]

OECD (2020), "What is the impact of the COVID-19 pandemic on immigrants and their children?", *OECD Policy Responses to Coronavirus (COVID-19)*, OECD Publishing, Paris, https://dx.doi.org/10.1787/e7cbb7de-en. [19]

OECD (2020), "Youth and COVID-19: Response, recovery and resilience", *OECD Policy Responses to Coronavirus (COVID-19)*, OECD Publishing, Paris, https://dx.doi.org/10.1787/c40e61c6-en. [13]

OECD (n.d.), *Employment and Labour Market Statistics database*, https://doi.org/10.1787/data-00302-en (accessed on 13 August 2021). [17]

OECD (n.d.), *Main Economic Indicators database*, https://doi.org/10.1787/data-00046-en (accessed on 13 August 2021). [12]

OECD (n.d.), *OECD Affordable Housing database*, http://www.oecd.org/housing/data/affordable-housing-database/ (accessed on 15 June 2021). [67]

OECD (n.d.), *OECD Child Well-Being Data Portal*, https://www.oecd.org/social/family/child-well-being/data/education/ (accessed on 13 August 2021). [80]

OECD (n.d.), *OECD Education Statistics database*, https://doi.org/10.1787/889e8641-en (accessed on 24 September 2021). [5]

OECD (n.d.), *Risks That Matter Survey*, https://www.oecd.org/social/risks-that-matter.htm (accessed on 13 August 2021). [3]

ONS (2020), *Coronavirus and the social impacts on different ethnic groups in the UK: 2020*, Office for National Statistics, https://www.ons.gov.uk/peoplepopulationandcommunity/culturalidentity/ethnicity/articles/coronavirusandthesocialimpactsondifferentethnicgroupsintheuk/2020. [62]

ONS (2020), *One in eight British households has no garden*, Office for National Statistics, https://www.ons.gov.uk/economy/environmentalaccounts/articles/oneineightbritishhouseholdshasnogarden/2020-05-14. [71]

ONS (2020), *Personal and economic well-being in Great Britain: September 2020*, Office for National Statistics, https://www.ons.gov.uk/peoplepopulationandcommunity/wellbeing/bulletins/personalandeconomicwellbeingintheuk/june2020. [58]

ONS (2020), *Unemployment by ethnic background*, Office for National Statistics, https://commonslibrary.parliament.uk/research-briefings/sn06385/ (accessed on 9 February 2021). [25]

ONS (2019), *Exploring the UK's digital divide*, Office for National Statistics, https://www.ons.gov.uk/peoplepopulationandcommunity/householdcharacteristics/homeinternetandsocialmediausage/articles/exploringtheuksdigitaldivide/2019-03-04. [76]

ONS (n.d.), *A09: Labour market status by ethnic group*, Office for National Statistics, https://www.ons.gov.uk/employmentandlabourmarket/peopleinwork/employmentandemployeetypes/datasets/labourmarketstatusbyethnicgroupa09 (accessed on 9 February 2021). [24]

Parker, K., J. Menasce Horowitz and R. Minkin (2020), *How the Coronavirus outbreak has – and hasn't – changed the way americans work*, Pew Research Center, https://www.pewresearch.org/social-trends/2020/12/09/how-the-coronavirus-outbreak-has-and-hasnt-changed-the-way-americans-work/. [47]

Parker, K., R. Minkin and J. Bennett (2020), *Economic fallout from COVID-19 continues to hit lower-income Americans the hardest*, Pew Research Center, https://www.pewresearch.org/social-trends/2020/09/24/economic-fallout-from-covid-19-continues-to-hit-lower-income-americans-the-hardest/. [59]

Pew Research Center (2020), *Hispanic women, immigrants, young adults, those with less education hit hardest by COVID-19 job losses*, https://www.pewresearch.org/fact-tank/2020/06/09/hispanic-women-immigrants-young-adults-those-with-less-education-hit-hardest-by-covid-19-job-losses/. [33]

Powell, A., B. Francis-Devine and N. Foley (2020), *Unemployment by ethnic background*, House of Commons Library, https://commonslibrary.parliament.uk/research-briefings/sn06385/ (accessed on 10 February 2021). [26]

Prokopenko, E. and C. Kevins (2020), *Vulnerabilities related to COVID-19 among LGBTQ2+ Canadians*, Statistics Canada, https://www150.statcan.gc.ca/n1/pub/45-28-0001/2020001/article/00075-eng.htm. [44]

Sharma, S. et al. (2020), *Social determinants of health-related needs during COVID-19 among low-income households with children*, Centers for Disease Control and Prevention, https://www.cdc.gov/pcd/issues/2020/20_0322.htm. [57]

Statistics Canada (2021), *Study: A labour market snapshot of Black Canadians during the pandemic*, https://www150.statcan.gc.ca/n1/daily-quotidien/210224/dq210224b-eng.htm. [29]

Statistics Canada (2020), *Economic impact of COVID-19 among visible minority groups*, https://www150.statcan.gc.ca/n1/pub/45-28-0001/2020001/article/00042-eng.htm. [64]

Statistics Canada (2020), *Labour market impacts of COVID-19 on Indigenous people: March to August 2020*, https://www150.statcan.gc.ca/n1/daily-quotidien/201102/dq201102c-eng.htm (accessed on 3 March 2021). [38]

Statistics Canada (2020), *Transitions into and out of employment by immigrants during the COVID-19 lockdown and recovery*, https://www150.statcan.gc.ca/n1/pub/45-28-0001/2020001/article/00070-eng.htm. [20]

Statistics Canada (2017), *Household access to the Internet at home, by household income quartile and geography*, https://www150.statcan.gc.ca/t1/tbl1/en/tv.action?pid=2210000701 (accessed on 13 August 2021). [77]

US Bureau of Labor Statistics (n.d.), *Civilian unemployment rate*, https://www.bls.gov/charts/employment-situation/civilian-unemployment-rate.htm (accessed on 13 August 2021). [32]

US Bureau of Labor Statistics (n.d.), *Employment status of the civilian population by nativity and sex, not seasonally adjusted*, https://www.bls.gov/news.release/empsit.t07.htm (accessed on 13 August 2021). [31]

US Census Bureau (n.d.), *Measuring household experiences during the coronavirus pandemic*, https://www.census.gov/data/experimental-data-products/household-pulse-survey.html (accessed on 13 September 2021). [61]

Vogels, E. (2021), *Digital divide persists even as Americans with lower incomes make gains in tech adoption*, Pew Research Center, https://www.pewresearch.org/fact-tank/2021/06/22/digital-divide-persists-even-as-americans-with-lower-incomes-make-gains-in-tech-adoption/. [78]

Wenham, C. (2020), *The gendered impact of the COVID-19 crisis and post-crisis period*, European Parliament, Brussels, http://www.europarl.europa.eu/supporting-analyses. [43]

Wozniak, A. et al. (2020), *COVID Impact Survey*, National Opinion Research Center, https://www.covid-impact.org/ (accessed on 9 August 2021). [60]

Notes

[1] Employment income includes wages and self-employment income. Quintiles are based on people's ranking in terms of their equivalised disposable income.

[2] The OECD Risks that Matter (RTM) survey is a cross-national survey examining people's perceptions of the social and economic risks they face and how well they think their government addresses those risks. The survey was conducted for the first time in two waves in 2018. The 2020 survey, conducted in September-October 2020, draws on a representative sample of over 25 000 people aged 18 to 64 in the 25 OECD countries that agreed to participate: Austria, Belgium, Canada, Chile, Denmark, Estonia, Finland, France, Germany, Greece, Ireland, Israel, Italy, Korea, Lithuania, Mexico, the Netherlands, Norway, Poland, Portugal, Slovenia, Spain, Switzerland, Turkey and the United States.

[3] Consistent with OECD practice (e.g. in the Migration Outlook), this report uses the words "migrants", "immigrants" and "foreign-born" synonymously. Unless mentioned otherwise, these include all persons born abroad, regardless of their migration category, legal status or nationality. Likewise, unless mentioned otherwise, native-born includes all persons born in the country, regardless of the country of birth of their parents.

[4] The main changes involved by the new regulation are: persons on parental leave, and who are either receiving job-related income or benefits, or whose parental leave is expected to last three months or less, are counted as employed; persons raising agricultural products for own-consumption are excluded from employment; seasonal workers outside the season are classified as employed if they still regularly perform tasks and duties for the job or business during the off-season; and people with a job or business who were temporarily not at work during the reference week of the survey but with strong attachment to their job are still considered as employed. In the particular context of the COVID-19 crisis and of the measures applied to combat it, national specificities exist in the assessment of the job attachment; not employed people are considered to be searching for a job only if they use an active search method. The new regulation also achieved further harmonisation in the implementation of questions and modernisation of the nation surveys.

[5] For example, people stating their ethnicity as "Mixed", "Indian", "Pakistani", "Bangladeshi", "Chinese", "Black/African/Caribbean" or "Other".

[6] The term "visible minority" is used here because it is the official demographic category defined by the Canadian Employment Equity Act and is used by Statistics Canada in their surveys. The Employment Equity Act defines visible minorities as "persons, other than Aboriginal peoples, who are non-Caucasian in race or non-white in colour". The visible minority population consists mainly of the following groups: South Asian, Chinese, Black, Filipino, Latin American, Arab, Southeast Asian, West Asian, Korean and Japanese. The question of appropriate terminology is currently being reviewed in Canada, in the context of a task force on modernising the Employment Equity Act (Department of Finance Canada, 2021[81]).

[7] LGBTQ2+ is the official acronym used by the Government of Canada across its programmes and policies. At Statistics Canada, the LGBTQ2+ acronym is used in order to reflect the broad scope of gender and sexual identities that exist in society. Respondents were included in the LGBTQ2+ population on the basis of self-reported sexual orientation (lesbian, gay, bisexual or another minority sexual identity such as asexual, pansexual or queer) or gender identity (transgender, including respondents with non-binary identities like genderqueer, gender fluid or agender).

[8] The term LGBTQI2S indicates Lesbian, Gay, Bisexual, Transgender, Queer (or Questioning), Intersex, and Two-Spirit.

[9] Findings of an Innovative Research Group (INNOVATIVE) online poll conducted from 24 to 29 March, 2020. Each survey is administered to a series of randomly selected samples from the panel. Additional respondents were recruited from online advertisements on Facebook and Instagram. The sample has been weighted by age, gender, region and sexual orientation using Statistics Canada's 2016 Census data and the 2016 General Social Survey to reflect the actual demographic composition of the Canadian and LGBTQI2S populations, resulting in an overall representative national sample size of 2 000 Canadians and representative national LGBTQI2S sample size of 300.

[10] This report's findings are based on a polling series called The Impact of Coronavirus on Households, conducted by NPR, the Robert Wood Johnson Foundation and the Harvard T.H. Chan School of Public Health (NPR/RWJF/Harvard). As reported by Harvard, "Interviews were conducted online and via telephone (cellphone and landline), July 1-August 3, 2020, among a nationally representative, probability-based sample of 3 454 adults age 18 or older in the US". The poll included a question allowing respondents to identify as LGBTQ. The figures compare respondents who identified as LGBQ and/or transgender to those who identified as both heterosexual and cisgender (i.e., "non-LGBTQ"). Of the total sample, 353 identified as LGBTQ. Findings from the series, as well as additional methodological information, are available at www.hsph.harvard.edu/horp/npr-harvard.

[11] The parent or another adult in the family used the 2-item Hunger Vital Sign screening questionnaire to report household food security status during the COVID-19 pandemic. It is a 2-question screening tool, suitable for clinical or community outreach use, that identifies families with young children as being at risk for food insecurity if they answer that either or both of the following two statements is "often true" or "sometimes true" (vs. "never true"): "Within the past 12 months we worried whether our food would run out before we got money to buy more"; "Within the past 12 months the food we bought just didn't last and we didn't have money to get more."

[12] An electronic survey was distributed in April 2020 to 16 435 families in 4 geographic areas, and 1 048 responded. The survey asked families enrolled in a co-ordinated school-based nutrition programme about their social needs, COVID-19–related concerns, food insecurity, and diet-related behaviours during the pandemic. Three variables (food insecurity, frequency of eating out, and frequency of shopping for produce) in the responses were compared on similar items in data collected from 3 880 families in the same 4 locations in fall 2019. The Autumn 2019 survey and the April 2020 survey used similar questions for the 3 variables.

[13] Pew Research Center conducted this study to understand Americans' assessments of their personal financial situation during the coronavirus outbreak. For this analysis, Pew surveyed 13 200 US adults in August 2020. Everyone who took part in the survey is a member of Pew Research Center's American Trends Panel (ATP), an online survey panel that is recruited through national, random sampling of residential addresses. This way nearly all US adults have a chance of selection. The survey is weighted to be representative of the United States adult population by gender, race, ethnicity, partisan affiliation, education and other categories.

[14] See endnote 6 (above).

[15] See endnote 7 (above).

[16] The figure is from a YouGov survey of 4 116 adults. Fieldwork was undertaken between 11 and 15 June 2020. The survey was carried out online. The figures have been weighted and are representative

of all Great Britain adults (aged 18+). This percentage was applied to the latest ONS mid-year estimate for the total number of adults in Great Britain.

[17] These figures are based on author calculations from the English Housing Survey. This is a continuous national survey commissioned by the Ministry of Housing, Communities and Local Government (MHCLG). It collects information about people's housing circumstances and the condition and energy efficiency of housing in England. Each year a sample of addresses is drawn at random from a list of private addresses held by the Royal Mail.

[18] In the summer of 2020, the polling company ICM administered a survey on behalf of Runnymede Trust to 2 585 adults (aged 18+) in Great Britain. The survey covered people's experiences of the coronavirus pandemic and lockdown and explored the impact of COVID-19 on physical and mental health, work, finances, relationships, childcare and schooling, as well as the understanding of the government's COVID-19 social and economic measures. A total of 750 people in the sample belonged to an ethnic minority, including Chinese, Indian, Pakistani, Bangladeshi, Black Caribbean and Black African ethnic groups.

[19] ONS used a combination of data sources to look into how many people have access to a garden and how far they are from the nearest park. ONS used Natural England's Monitor for Engagement in the Natural Environment (MENE) survey to examine differences by personal characteristics (such as ethnicity, age and socio-economic group). The MENE survey covers England only. Fieldwork started in March 2009 with around 800 respondents interviewed every week across England using an in-home interview format. Every year at least 45 000 interviews are undertaken.

[20] Data are from the Annual Homeless Assessment Report to Congress, Part 1, 2020.

[21] Severe housing deprivation is synonymous with homelessness. It refers to people living in severely inadequate housing due to a lack of access to minimally adequate housing. This means not being able to access a private dwelling to rent or own that has all basic amenities. Housing that lacks at least two of the three core dimensions of housing adequacy – habitability, security of tenure, and privacy and control – is deemed severely inadequate.

[22] The Pew Research Centre surveyed 1 502 US adults from 25 January to 8 February 2021 by mobile phone and landline. The survey was conducted by interviewers under the direction of Abt Associates, and is weighted to be representative of the United States adult population by gender, race, ethnicity, education and other categories.

[23] The PISA index of economic, social and cultural status (ESCS) is a composite measure used to estimate a student's socio-economic background. The index is derived from several variables related to students' family background: parents' education, parents' occupations, a number of home possessions that can be taken as proxies for material wealth, and the number of books and other educational resources available in the home. The index itself is a composite score derived from these indicators via Principal Component Analysis (PCA). Here, however, students are divided into quartiles according to their position in the distribution of ESCS scores in their country or economy.

6 Inclusion, quality of life and COVID-19

The impacts of COVID-19 on quality of life have not been distributed evenly across the populations of OECD countries. While men and the elderly were more likely to die from the virus, women and young people have been more likely to suffer a deterioration in mental health and life satisfaction. People on lower incomes or without employment and/or members of racial and ethnic minority groups are more likely to experience worse physical and mental health outcomes. Children from disadvantaged households are at risk of being left behind as schools shift to remote learning, widening existing gaps in knowledge and skills. Inequalities in access to green space, which helps bolster mental well-being, further disadvantage low socio-economic and racial and ethnic minority groups during lockdowns.

6.1. Physical and mental health

6.1.1. Excess mortality

Men, the elderly, racial and ethnic minorities and those from lower socio-economic status had the highest rates of excess mortality over the first year of the pandemic

The risk of death from COVID-19 is slightly lower for women than for men. Statistics on the total number of deaths from 29 OECD countries show that deaths for men increased by 15% over the first year of the pandemic, compared to 2015-19 averages, compared to only 12% for women.[1] The same pattern of higher excess deaths for men holds in 26 of the 29 OECD countries for which data are available (Figure 6.1, Panel A). Across the OECD, excess deaths first peaked in April 2020, before subsiding from May to September, and then steadily rising again through the end of 2020; the overall pattern is similar across genders, though male rates are higher for all months (Figure 6.2). Even though women are at a lower risk of death, they are more likely to suffer long-term symptoms of COVID, including extreme tiredness, shortness of breath and chest pain (often termed "long COVID"). For example, two studies in the United Kingdom found that women aged 40-60 were more likely to have worse long-term health outcomes than men who had also contracted COVID, even if they did not have any pre-existing health problems (Kelland, 2021[1]). Similarly, a hospital in France reported that, among the 30 cases of long COVID treated from May to July 2020, female patients outnumbered males by 4 to 1 (Chinnappan, 2021[2]). Data from the United Kingdom Office for National Statistics show that long COVID is most common in women, those aged 35 to 69, those from low-income areas and those with pre-existing medical conditions (see Box 6.1).

Especially in the early stages of the pandemic, the elderly had much higher excess mortality rates than other age cohorts (Figure 6.2). The population aged 65 and over had the highest increase in total deaths over the first year of the pandemic in all but two OECD countries with data (Figure 6.1, Panel B).[2] The gaps in excess death rates between those aged 65 and over and those aged 45-64 peaked in April 2020 before dropping sharply from May through September 2020 – a period that coincided with an overall drop in COVID-19 cases in many OECD countries.[3] However, the gap increased again, surpassing the initial peak, from October to December 2020 (Figure 6.2). As of the beginning of 2021, the gaps in excess death rates between age cohorts have diminished, which may in part be a result of increasing vaccination rates in the older populations beginning early in 2021 (Lu, 2021[3]).

Already pre-COVID, there was ample evidence that those with lower levels of education and income had shorter lives (OECD, 2020[4]; Marmot et al., 2010[5]; Chetty et al., 2016[6]). People with lower levels of education and income are also more likely to suffer from medical conditions that put them at greater risk of COVID infections, such as diabetes (OECD, 2017[7]). Once the pandemic struck, these groups suffered mortality rates higher than the general population. A population-based cohort study in Sweden found that a low level of education also increases the risk of death from COVID-19, even when controlling for other risk factors (Drefahl et al., 2020[8]). According to this evidence, those with only a primary or secondary education may be twice as likely to die from the pandemic. In Germany, data from the second wave of the pandemic (Q4 2020 through Q1 2021) showed that mortality rates in socially disadvantaged regions were 50 to 70% higher than in regions with low levels of social disadvantage (Robert Koch Institut, 2021[9]). Studies in the United States and France, and cross-country studies in Europe, have also shown that poorer regions experienced higher COVID-19 mortality rates (Stantcheva, 2021[10]). A study in Ontario, Canada found that people with a recent experience of homelessness were more likely to contract COVID-19, and once positive, 20 times more likely to be admitted to a hospital, 10 times more likely to need intensive care and 5 times more likely to die of the virus (Richard et al., 2021[11]).

Figure 6.1. Excess deaths in the first year of the pandemic were highest for men and older-age cohorts in most OECD countries

Excess mortality, percentage change in total number of deaths from week 11 2020 to week 18 2021, compared with 2015-19 average

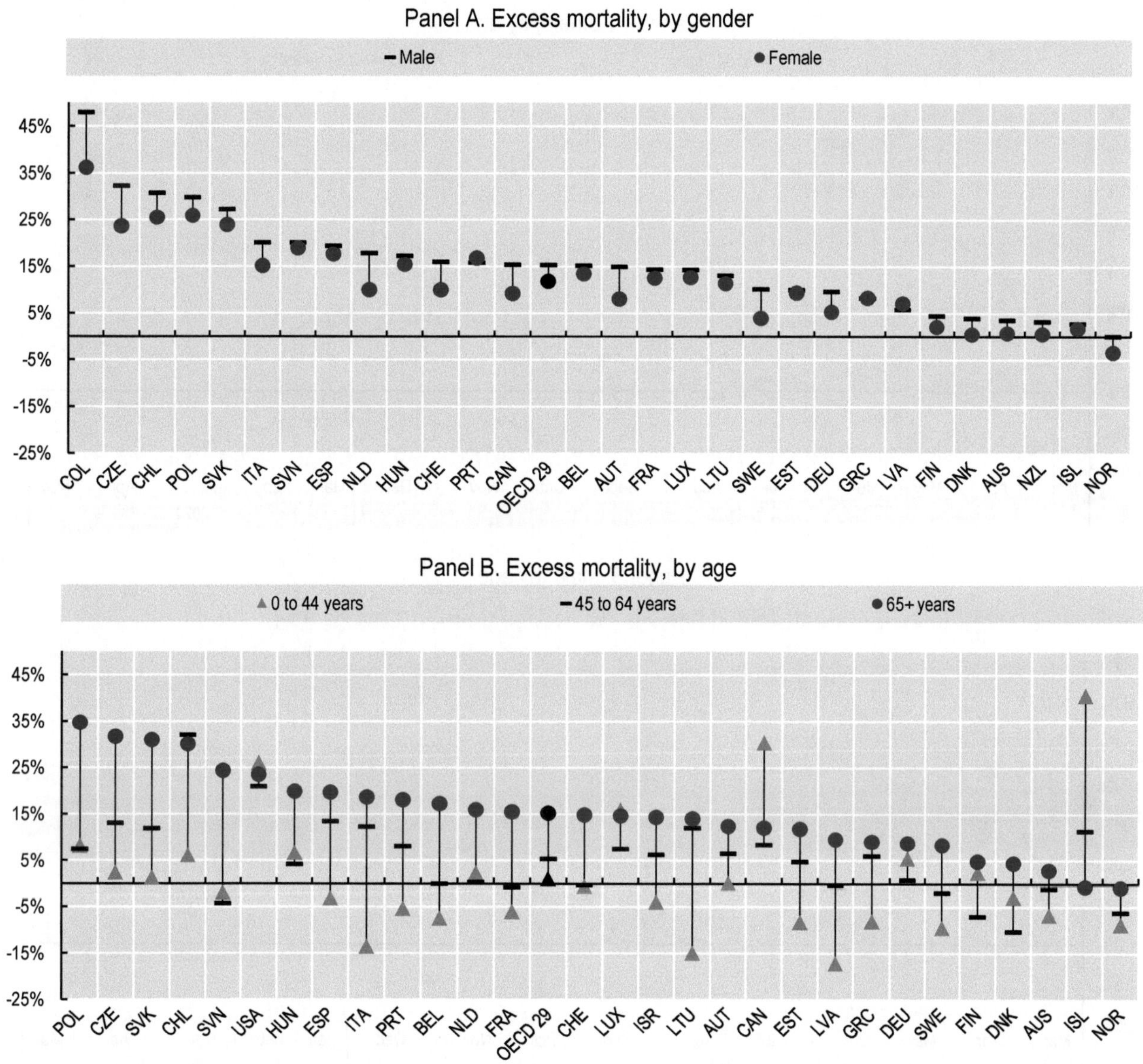

Note: The figure shows the increase in the number of reported deaths from all causes for the period March 2020 (week 11) to early May 2021 (week 18), compared to the average from 2015-2019 for the same period. In Panel A, the OECD average excludes Costa Rica, Ireland, Israel, Japan, Korea, Mexico, Turkey, the United Kingdom and the United States. In Panel B, the OECD average excludes Colombia, Costa Rica, Ireland, Japan, Korea, Mexico, New Zealand, Turkey and the United Kingdom. Data for Chile, Germany and Greece are compared against the average for 2016-2019. Those for Australia refer to doctor-certified deaths only. Deaths for the most recent weeks may be under-reported and subject to revision. Data from week 53 of 2020 are excluded from the overall average.

Source: OECD calculations based on OECD (n.d.[12]), *COVID-19 Health Indicators* (database), https://stats.oecd.org/index.aspx?queryid=104676#.

StatLink https://stat.link/e05a7v

Figure 6.2. Excess deaths first peaked in March and April 2020, and again from October to December 2020, for both men and women aged 65 and older

Excess mortality, OECD 26, percent change in total number of deaths from week 11 2020 to week 18 2021, compared with 2015-19 average

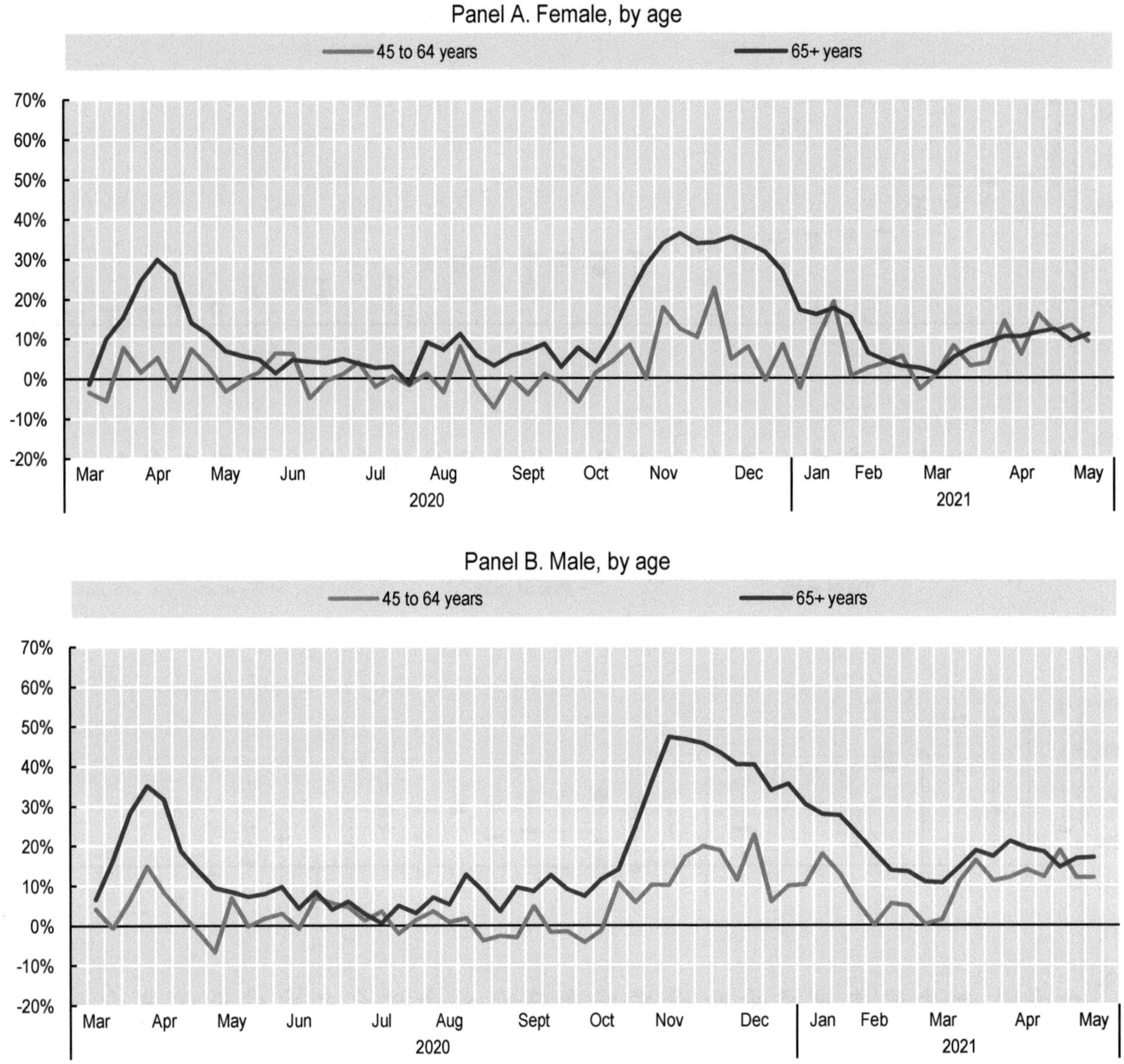

Note: Both panels show excess deaths from March (week 11) 2020 to early May (week 18) 2021. Data refer to outcomes for people aged 45-64, and those aged 65 and over. The OECD average includes Australia, Austria, Belgium, Canada, Chile, the Czech Republic, Denmark, Estonia, Finland, France, Germany, Greece, Hungary, Iceland, Italy, Latvia, Lithuania, Luxembourg, the Netherlands, Norway, Poland, the Slovak Republic, Slovenia, Spain, Switzerland and the United States.
Source: OECD calculations based on OECD (n.d.[12]), *COVID-19 Health Indicators* (database), https://stats.oecd.org/index.aspx?queryid=104676#.

StatLink https://stat.link/5m7vih

Box 6.1. Innovation: United Kingdom Coronavirus (COVID-19) Infection Survey

The United Kingdom's Office for National Statistics (ONS) administered the Coronavirus (COVID-19) Infection Survey in April-May 2021 to measure the prevalence of long COVID and identify its symptoms. 339 707 individuals over two-years-old living in private households were interviewed from 4 April to 2 May 2021. Parents and/or carers completed the survey for children under 12-years-old. Responses are weighted to be representative by age group, sex and region, and account for non-responses. Prevalence of long COVID was defined as having symptoms that persisted for more than four weeks after the initial onset of infection and that could not be otherwise explained. The data are self-reported, rather than clinical diagnoses, and thus may reflect differences in reporting between socio-demographic groups.

Data from the survey show that as of early May 2021, an estimated 1 million people (around 1.6% of the private household population) were experiencing self-reported symptoms of long COVID-19. The prevalence (and severity) of symptoms was greatest (and most severe) for women (Figure 6.3, Panel A), people aged 35 to 69 (Figure 6.3, Panel B), those living in deprived areas and those with pre-existing conditions. In September 2021, the ONS published updated information, taking into account data up to 1 August 2021, which found that the prevalence of long COVID may be lower than initially thought: 643 000 people in private households may have experienced symptoms of long COVID (rather than 1 million), with anywhere between 3-12% (depending on the measurement approach used) of those who had previously been infected with coronavirus still showing symptoms after 12 weeks. Women continue to have higher prevalence of self-reported long COVID-19, compared to men (ONS, 2021[13]).

Figure 6.3. Women and those aged 35-49 in the UK were most likely to report long COVID

Share of people living in private households in the United Kingdom with self-reported long COVID-19 symptoms by activity limitation, Apr-May 2021

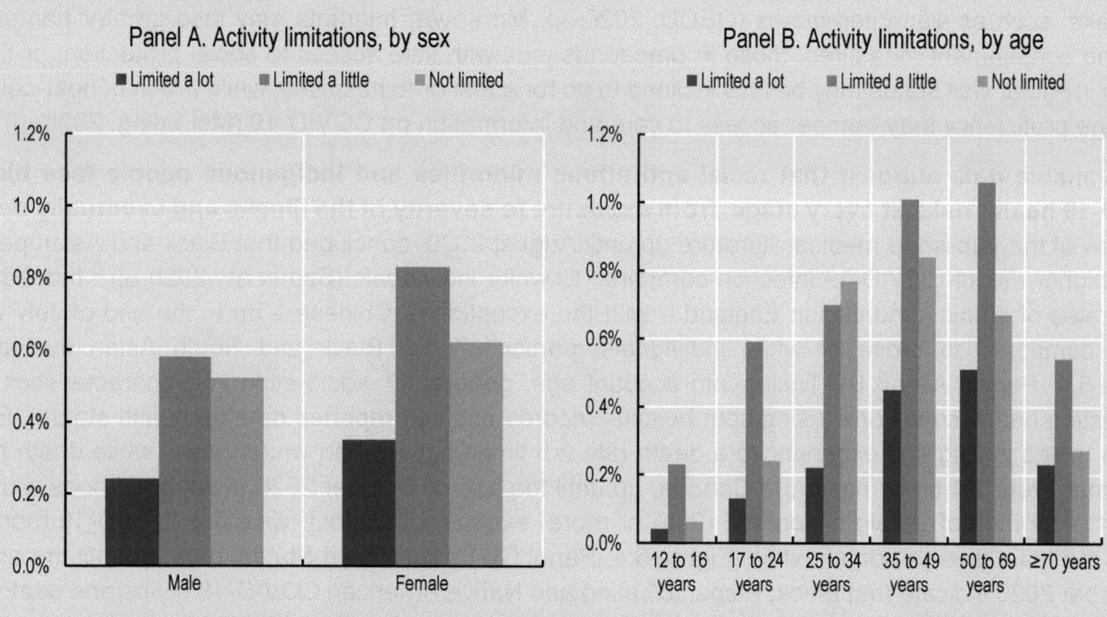

Source: ONS (2021[14]), *Prevalence of ongoing symptoms following coronavirus (COVID-19) in the UK* (database), Office for National Statistics, https://www.ons.gov.uk/peoplepopulationandcommunity/healthandsocialcare/condisionsanddiseases/bulletins/prevalenceofongoingsymptomsfollowingcoronaviruscovid19infectionintheuk/4june2021.

StatLink https://stat.link/vz6wir

The jobs held by low-income, low-education workers also put them at higher risk of infection. In addition to having more pre-existing risk factors, these workers are much less likely to be in roles that enable teleworking (Chapter 5) and much more likely to be working in fields (e.g. essential retail, transport, cleaning and other service jobs) that require them to commute and work in contact with others throughout the pandemic (Finch and Hernández Finch, 2020[15]; Eichenbaum, Rebelo and Trabandt, 2020[16]). A study in the United States found that frontline workers – who were required to continue working in person – have lower levels of education than the population at large: around 70% had less than a university degree (Rho, Brown and Fremstad, 2020[17]). A study on frontline workers in Toronto, Canada found that neighbourhoods with the highest concentration of frontline workers had cumulative per-capita rates of death from COVID-19 that were 2.5 times higher than neighbourhoods with the lowest concentration (Rao et al., 2021[18]).

The (sparse) available data[4] on COVID-19 mortality rates of migrants show that they are over-represented in terms of both incidence and severity, despite having a younger age on average. Migrants[5] made up a larger share of confirmed COVID-19 cases in Norway, Sweden, Denmark and Canada compared to their share of the population (OECD, 2020[19]). Mortality estimates in France and Sweden indicate that excess mortality among migrants between March and April 2020 was twice that of non-migrants and that the share of migrants among all deaths increased by between 2-4 percentage points compared to 2015-19 (OECD, 2020[19]). Data from Canada early in the pandemic (March to July 2020) show that COVID-19 mortality rates for migrants were much higher than migrant's share of the Canadian population, especially for men under the age of 65 (Statistics Canada, 2021[20]).

Migrants' working and living conditions make them more susceptible to COVID-19 exposure and infection, including: higher rates of relative poverty; a higher likelihood of using public transportation and living in sub-standard accommodation, in overcrowded dwellings and in higher density buildings (e.g. collective housing for asylum seekers, which complicates social distancing and increases the likelihood of infection) (OECD, 2020[19]). In three-quarters of OECD countries, migrants also have fewer options to telework (the share of those able to do so is at least 5 percentage points below that of their native counterparts), and they are over-represented in domestic services and workplaces linked to cluster outbreaks, such as slaughterhouses (OECD, 2020[19]). Moreover, migrants may face greater barriers to following containment measures: those in precarious jobs with little access to social protection, or those with an irregular visa status may be less inclined to go for a test or to hospitals, while a lack of host-country language proficiency may hamper access to care and information on COVID-19 (McFarling, 2020[21]).

The available data suggest that racial and ethnic minorities and Indigenous people face higher COVID-19 health risks at every stage, from exposure to severity of the illness and eventually death. A review of the published medical literature up until August 2020, concluded that Black and Asian people had a higher risk of COVID-19 infection compared to white individuals (Sze et al., 2020[22]).[6] Indeed, the death rates of ethnic minorities in England – with the exception of Chinese – up to the end of July were higher compared to those of white individuals, particularly for Black and South Asian individuals (Figure 6.4, Panels A and B). Taking into account age, geography, socio-economic characteristics and pre-existing health conditions (using both hospital records and self-reported data on health status), Black African males in England experienced a death rate 2.5 times higher than white males, while death rates for women were 2.1 times higher. In Canada, up until the end of October 2020, neighbourhoods with the highest proportion of visible minorities[7] (25% or more) experienced about twice the COVID-19 mortality rate of the least diverse communities (Figure 6.4, Panel C). In the United States, data up until the end of November 2020 indicate that Black, Hispanic/Latino and Native American COVID-19 cases and deaths by far exceeded their respective proportions of the population (Figure 6.4, Panel D). While life expectancy for the United States population as a whole dropped by a full year in the first half of 2020 (see Chapter 3), Black and Hispanic/Latino men suffered a 2.7 year and 2.4 year decline, respectively, over the same period (Arias, Tejada-Vera and Ahmad, 2021[23]). This large decline means that the gap in life expectancy between white and Black Americans – which had been narrowing in recent years – has now widened further (Tavernise and Goodnough, 2021[24]).

Figure 6.4. In England, the United States and Canada, racial and ethnic minorities and Indigenous people are bearing the heaviest health burden of COVID-19

Selected measures of COVID-19-related health outcomes throughout 2020, by population group

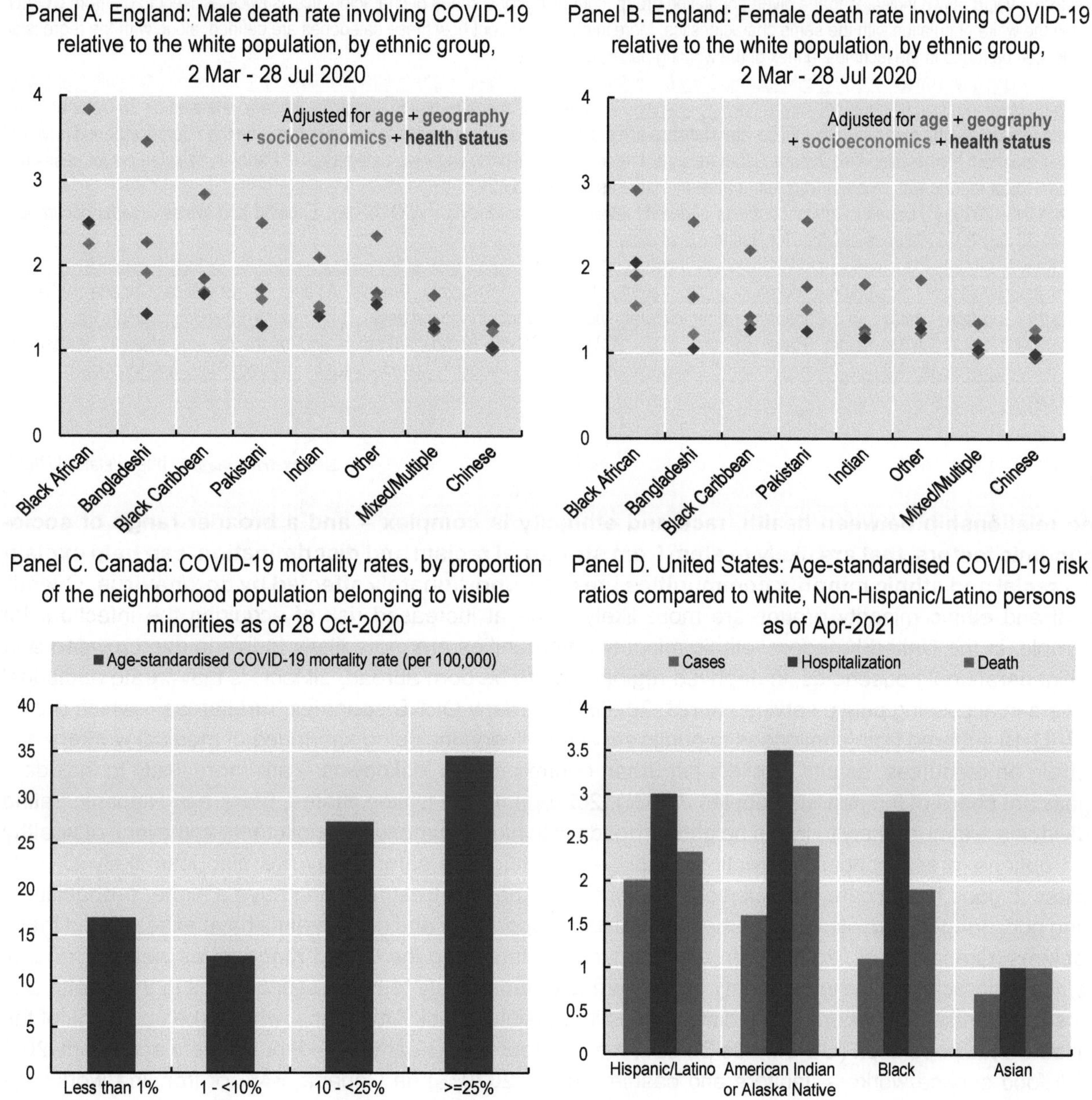

Note: In Panels A and B, Cox proportional hazards regression models are used to estimate how differences in the risk of death involving COVID-19 change when adjusting for a range of factors affecting both the risk of infection and the risk of death if infected, including age, geography (region of residence and population density), socio-economic characteristics (individual and household deprivation measures, based on income, employment, education, health and housing) and health status (self-reported health status and presence of pre-existing conditions). Both plots show the COVID-19 death rates for different racial and/or ethnic groups *relative* to the white population, adjusting for a range of characteristics. Therefore a value of two indicates that a given population group, controlling for a series of characteristics, is twice as likely to die from COVID-19 than the white population with the same characteristics. More information about how these categories are defined, along with the regression models, can be found in the technical annex of the working paper, located at https://www.ons.gov.uk/peoplepopulationandcommunity/birthsdeathsandmarriages/deaths/methodologies/coronaviruscovid19relateddeathsbyethnicgroupenglandandwalesmethodology#modelling-analysis. In Panel C, Canadian Vital Statistics Death data, released on 28 October 2020, are used to estimate the mortality rates; these vital statistics are provisional, as some deaths that occurred during the reference period have not yet been reported. Visible minorities include South Asian, Chinese, Black, Filipino, and Arab categories. In Panel D, calculations for cases use only the 61% of reports with race/ethnicity information available as of 3 April 2021.

Source: ONS (2020[25]), *Updating ethnic contrasts in deaths involving the coronavirus (COVID-19), England and Wales: deaths occurring 2 March to 28 July 2020* (database), Office for National Statistics, https://www.ons.gov.uk/peoplepopulationandcommunity/birthsdeathsandmarriages/deaths/articles/updatingethniccontrastsindeathsinvolvingthecoronaviruscovid19englandandwales/deathsoccurring2marchto28july2020#main-points (Panels A and B); Statistics Canada (2020[26]), *COVID-19 mortality rates in Canada's ethno-cultural neighbourhoods* (database), https://www150.statcan.gc.ca/n1/pub/45-28-0001/2020001/article/00079-eng.htm (Panel C); and CDC (2021[27]), *COVID-19 hospitalization and death by race/ethnicity* (database), https://www.cdc.gov/coronavirus/2019-ncov/covid-data/investigations-discovery/hospitalization-death-by-race-ethnicity.html#footnote01 (Panel D).

StatLink https://stat.link/7igkfx

The relationship between health, race and ethnicity is complex – and a broader range of socio-economic factors, that are likely to stem from structural racism and discrimination, can help explain why racial and ethnic minority communities are disproportionately affected by coronavirus. Overall, racial and ethnic minority groups are more likely to be at increased risk of acquiring the infection: for example, in the United Kingdom, ethnic minority communities are more likely to live in overcrowded and multigenerational households, in deprived regions and to be born abroad, all factors that create additional barriers in accessing public services (ONS, 2020[28]). In many OECD countries, rural areas – which during COVID-19 suffered from challenges to public service delivery, including shortages of medical workers and a strain on resources, as city dwellers left urban centres during lockdowns – are more likely to include a significant share of Indigenous peoples (OECD, 2020[29]). In the United States, Black and Hispanic/Latino individuals are more likely to live in neighbourhoods with higher exposure to pollutants and a lack of healthy food options, green spaces, recreational facilities, lighting and safety; they are also less likely to have access to good health care, are subject to racial bias in medical treatment and have a higher probability of being poor; longer-term systemic barriers in housing, opportunity and other realms have exacerbated these problems (Graham et al., 2020[30]). In both the United States and the United Kingdom as well as Canada, members of racial and ethnic minority groups are also more likely to hold essential jobs in the health and transportation sectors where social distancing is impossible: Black Americans, who make up 13.4% of the United States population (US Census Bureau, n.d.[31]), represent nearly 30% of bus drivers and nearly 20% of all food service workers, janitors and cashiers (Ray, 2020[32]); in Canada, 34% of frontline workers – including those employed as nurse aides, orderlies and patient service associates – identified as a member of a visible minority[8] in 2016 (compared with 21% in other sectors) (Statistics Canada, 2020[33]). Similarly, Black and Asian men in the United Kingdom are more likely to work in occupations that have a higher risk of COVID-19 death (Figure 6.5). Once they become infected, some racial and ethnic groups are also more likely to be at increased risk of poorer outcomes due to a range of prevalent co-morbidities such as asthma, diabetes and cardiovascular disease, partly due to the same structural factors listed above leading to the higher risk of infection (ONS, 2020[28]; Graham et al., 2020[30]). In the United States, the much higher hospitalisation and death risks of American Indians or Alaska Natives compared to white people (Figure 6.4, Panel D) partly reflect health disparities that have affected Native communities for decades (Lakhani, 2021[34]; Hlavinka, 2020[35]).[9]

Figure 6.5. Ethnic minority groups in England and Wales are more likely to work in jobs with higher COVID-19 death rates

Proportion of ethnic groups within high-risk occupations, and COVID-19 age-standardised death rates per 100 000 population (shown in parentheses), in England and Wales, 9 Mar - 25 May 2020

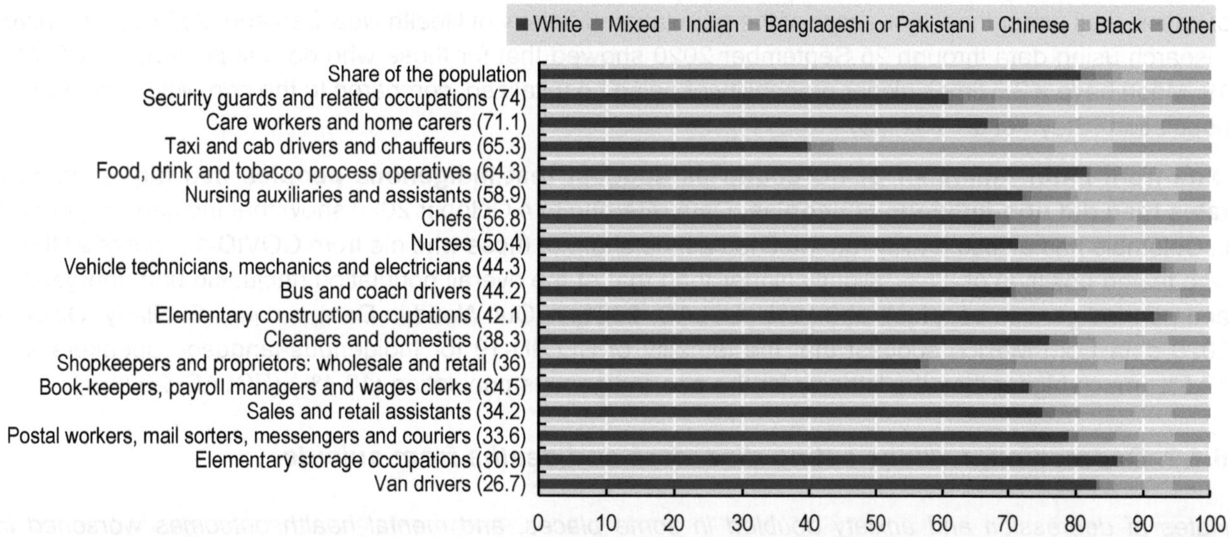

Note: The horizontal bars show the proportion of different ethnic groups within each high risk occupation. Data in parentheses refer to the age-standardised COVID-19 death rate, per 100 000 population, for each occupation type. The overall age-standardised mortality rate involving COVID-19 for the working-age population during this period was 19.1 deaths per 100 000 men and 9.7 deaths per 100 000 women.

Source: ONS (2020[28]), *Why have Black and South Asian people been hit hardest by COVID-19?* (database), Office for National Statistics, https://www.ons.gov.uk/peoplepopulationandcommunity/healthandsocialcare/conditionsanddiseases/articles/whyhaveblackandsouthasianpeoplebeenhithardestbycovid19/2020-12-14.

StatLink https://stat.link/1byse9

The health impact of COVID-19 on Indigenous communities, whose situation is not directly comparable across countries, has taken different turns depending on the context. Data up to February 2021 indicate that Indigenous communities in Australia experienced lower case rates and lower death rates than the general population: out of 909 deaths and 29 135 cases recorded in the whole country, there have been no deaths, 150 cases and only 20 hospitalisations among Indigenous Australians (Australian Government Department of Health, 2021[36]).[10] This pattern, which completely reversed the detrimental death toll of past pandemics like the 2009 H1N1 flu among Indigenous Australians, has been credited to multiple factors, including the government giving way to Indigenous leadership; increased training in Aboriginal-controlled health services; remote communities shutting down access to their territories as early as March 2020; Indigenous-tailored media messaging; and the promotion of consistent, culturally appropriate health literacy (Keck, 2020[37]; AIHW, 2021[38]). In Canada, First Nations, Inuit and Métis communities slowed the spread of cases during the first wave of the pandemic through self-imposed border closures and community-based responses such as public health campaigns grounded in the local context of the various nations. In July 2020, the prevalence of COVID-19 among Indigenous people in Canada was less than one-quarter that of non-Indigenous Canadians, with a third of the fatalities and a 30% higher recovery rate (Richardson and Crawford, 2020[39]). However, newly reported cases in Canada's First Nations communities rose rapidly during the second wave. During the week of 8-14 November 2020, there were a total of 558 new cases in First Nations communities (Government of Canada, 2020[40]) – close to four times the total number of Indigenous people infected during the first wave (Alhmidi, 2020[41]) – compared to an estimated 32 000 in Canada as a whole (based on a 7-day average of 4 560 new cases per day) (Dong, Du and Gardner, 2020[42]). While the share of cases for First Nations (1.7%) was lower than their population share (4.9%, as of 2016 (OECD, 2020[43])), it has nonetheless grown since the first wave of the pandemic.[11] In New Zealand, rapid measures imposed by the government also helped to contain the spread of COVID-19. With initial clusters concentrated in areas such as Southland and Canterbury, which have small Māori populations, Pākehā (i.e. non-Māori groups) tended to be over-represented among cases (Cook et al., 2020[44]). Up through February 2021, Māori represented only 8.4% of cases, well under their 16% share of the population (Ministry of Health New Zealand, 2021[45]). However research using data through 25 September 2020 showed that for those who do test positive for COVID-19, Māori have a 2.5 times higher probability of being hospitalized, compared to the non-Māori non-Pacific population (Steyn et al., 2021[46]).

Data from Latin American OECD countries suggest that Indigenous peoples had higher fatality rates than did non-Indigenous peoples. Data referring to 4 October 2020 show that Indigenous peoples in Colombia had a case fatality rate (defined as the share of those who die from COVID-19, out of all those who tested positive) of 3.5%, slightly higher than that of the overall population (including both Indigenous and non-Indigenous peoples), at 3.12% (ECLAC, 2021[47]; Our World in Data, n.d.[48]). Similarly, October 2020 data from Mexico suggest that the lethality of COVID-19 for Indigenous-language speakers was 17.5%, much higher than the lethality for the non-Indigenous population (10.4%) (ECLAC, 2021[47]).

6.1.2. Depression, anxiety, eating disorders and deaths from suicide

Rates of depression and anxiety doubled in some places, and mental health outcomes worsened in particular for women, parents of school-age children, young people, those with more precarious financial and employment situations, racial and ethnic minorities, and LGBTI+ youth

Women have higher reported rates of anxiety and depression than men, and these gaps have widened over the course of the pandemic. Data from 16 OECD countries collected from April through December 2020 show that women are more likely to be at risk of depression (29.4%) and anxiety (23.9%) than men (26% and 23.7%, respectively) (Figure 6.6, Panel A), using the PHQ-4 scale.[12] For seven of the eight European countries for which broadly comparable pre-COVID data are available,[13] the gender gaps in risks for depression have widened (Figure 6.6, Panel B). A study conducted during the first wave of the pandemic in the United Kingdom also found that working women experienced some of the largest deteriorations in mental health (OECD, 2021[49]). A longitudinal study of 1 301 Canadian women, from 20 May – 15 July 2020, found that anxiety and depression rose for all women, compared to baseline years, with larger increases for women experiencing negative income shocks, those who had trouble balancing home schooling and work responsibilities, and those with difficulty accessing childcare (Racine et al., 2021[50]) (see Box 6.2 for additional evidence of gender inequalities in mental health in Canada). A meta-analysis of 18 studies found that maternal depression and anxiety rose during the pandemic, and that older mothers were more likely to have higher clinically significant symptoms of depression and anxiety (Racine et al., 2021[51]).

Figure 6.6. Women have higher rates of depression and anxiety than men, and gender gaps in depression have widened since the start of the pandemic

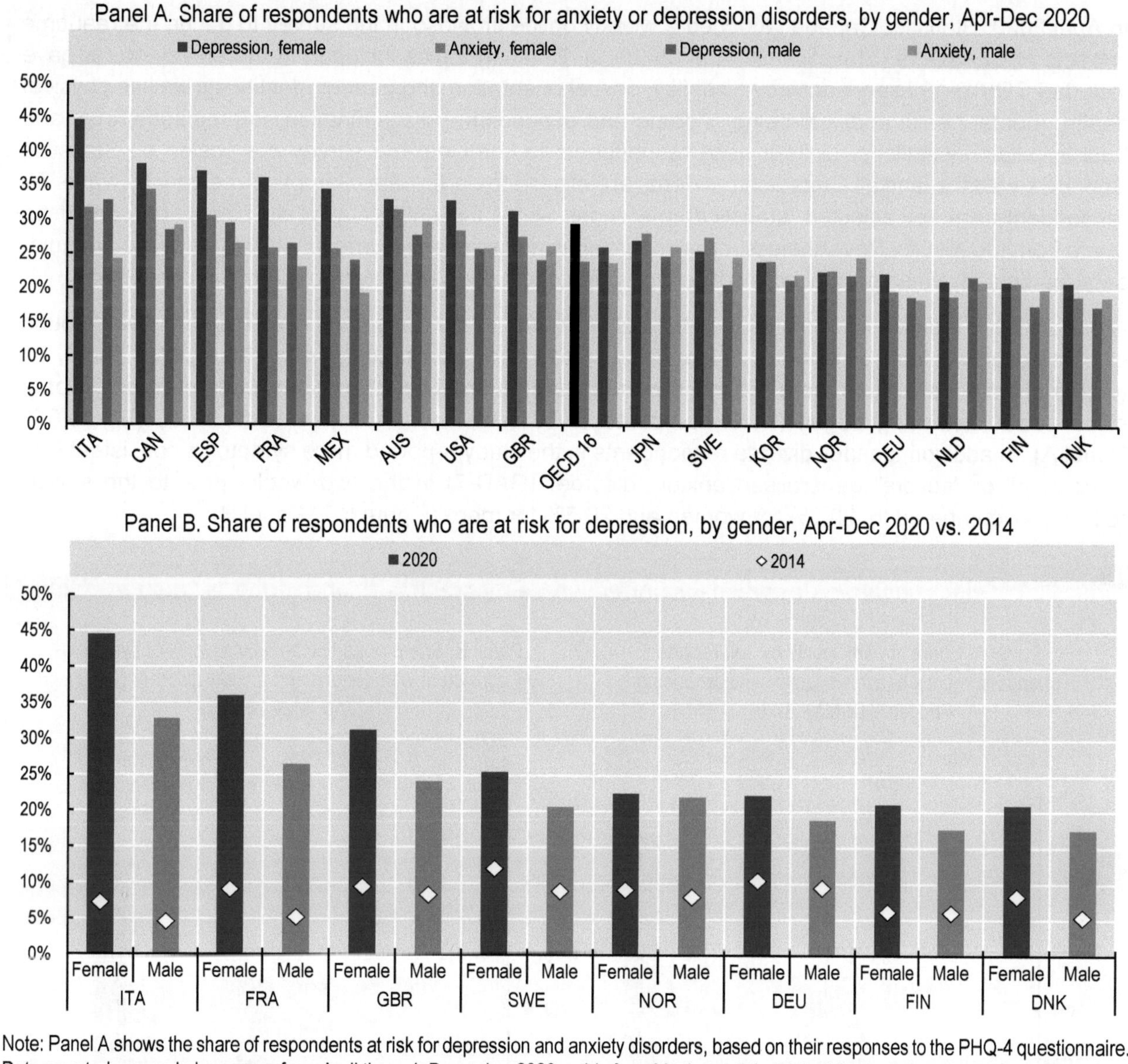

Note: Panel A shows the share of respondents at risk for depression and anxiety disorders, based on their responses to the PHQ-4 questionnaire. Data reported are pooled averages from April through December 2020, aside from Mexico and the United States, where they are averages from April through September 2020. The OECD average includes only the 16 countries shown. Panel B shows the share of respondents at risk of depression, based on responses to the PHQ-2 questionnaire, in 2020 and 2014. Data from 2020 come from a different data source than do data from 2014; although both use the same mental health diagnostic tool (PHQ-2), caution should be taken when interpreting exact numerical increases in any individual country. Baseline data come from the European Health Interview Survey (EHIS) wave 2.

Source: OECD calculations based on Imperial College London YouGov (2020[52]), *COVID-19 behaviour tracker data hub* (database), https://github.com/YouGov-Data/covid-19-tracker; and OECD calculations based on European Health Interview Survey (EHIS) wave 2 data (n.d.[53]), https://ec.europa.eu/eurostat/statistics-explained/index.php?title=Glossary:European_health_interview_survey_(EHIS).

StatLink https://stat.link/4swi0g

Box 6.2. Innovation: Statistics Canada's crowdsourced surveys to collect data on COVID-19

In April 2020, Statistics Canada launched a weekly online crowdsourcing survey to gauge the real-time impacts of COVID-19 (Statistics Canada, 2020[54]). Rotating topics included in the survey so far have included COVID-19 experiences by disability, sexual orientation and gender identity, as well as physical health, mental health and well-being, income and expenditure, discrimination, interpersonal trust and trust in public institutions. Links inviting respondents to complete the survey are posted on Statistics Canada's website, and all Canadian residents are eligible to participate. Sample sizes vary by wave. As respondents are self-selected, statistical inferences about the entire Canadian population cannot be made from the results. Nevertheless, crowdsourcing is a cost-effective and timely way to collect granular data, particularly when normal data collection operations have been interrupted by the pandemic.

Around 46 000 residents completed the *Impacts of COVID-19 on Canadians – Your mental health* round of data collection from 24 April to 11 May 2020. Canadians participating in the study who identify as gender diverse were much more likely to report that their mental health is "somewhat" or "much" worse since social distancing began (71%, compared to 57% for women and 47% for men) (Figure 6.7, Panel A). In addition, gender-diverse respondents in the study reported more symptoms consistent with "moderate" or "severe" generalised anxiety disorder (GAD-7) in the two weeks prior to the survey (61.8%, as compared to 29.3% for women and 20.5% for men) (Figure 6.7, Panel B).

Figure 6.7. Gender-diverse Canadians reported worse mental health and higher anxiety in 2020

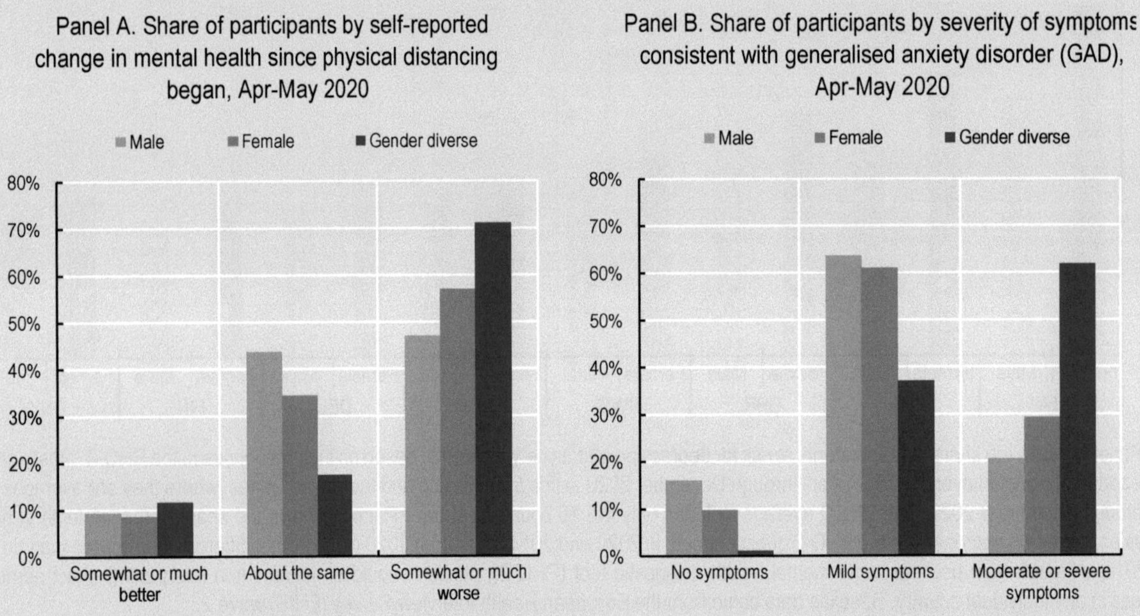

Note: Respondents are categorised as gender diverse if they do not report their gender as exclusively male or female (i.e. includes those who are unsure of their gender, who identify as both male and female, or who identify as neither). Note that outcomes for "male" and "female" respondents include both cisgender (current gender and sex assigned at birth) and transgender individuals.
Source: Statistics Canada (2020[55]), *Gender differences in mental health during the COVID-19 pandemic* (database), https://www150.statcan.gc.ca/n1/pub/45-28-0001/2020001/article/00047-eng.htm.

StatLink https://stat.link/prhdqo

Young people's mental health has been particularly affected during the pandemic, against a backdrop of school closures, labour market shocks and disruption to mental health services in schools and workplaces (Figure 3.9) (OECD, 2021[56]). Before the pandemic, 35% of adolescents receiving mental health services in the United States received these services exclusively from the school system – especially those from low-income households and those belonging to racial and ethnic minority groups – therefore disruptions to these services are likely to disproportionately impact these groups (Ali et al., 2019[57]). March 2021 data from Belgium, France and the United States showed that the share of young people with anxiety and depression symptoms had more than doubled compared to pre-pandemic data (OECD, 2021[56]). Survey data from 12 OECD countries from April 2020 to December 2020 meanwhile indicate that anxiety and depression rates for 15-24 year-olds are higher than older age cohorts (41.2% depression and 38.9% anxiety, compared to 27.9% and 26.0% for 25-64 year-olds, and 14.9% and 14.7% for those aged 65 and over) (Figure 6.8, Panels A and B). Similarly, data from 8 OECD countries throughout 2020 and 2021 show that full-time students had levels of depression and anxiety similar to those among the unemployed (Figure 6.8, Panels C and D): in 2020, 39.6% of full-time students in 8 OECD countries reported symptoms of depression and 35.0% symptoms of anxiety, compared to 39.4% and 37.2%, respectively, among the unemployed. Full-time students are likely to be younger, thus it is difficult to disentangle whether being a student or being younger is the factor driving their lower mental health.

In addition to elevated depression and anxiety, eating disorders have been on the rise for young people during the pandemic (Spettigue et al., 2021[58]; Touyz, Lacey and Hay, 2020[59])**.** In March 2021, the United Kingdom National Health Service noted that child and adolescent eating disorder referrals almost doubled in in the year since the start of the pandemic (Solmi, Downs and Nicholls, 2021[60]). According to the CMME (clinique des maladies mentales et de l'encéphale) clinic in Paris's Sainte-Anne hospital, cases of bulimia, overeating and anorexia have increased significantly since the start of the pandemic and subsequent lockdowns, while the French Anorexia Bulimia Federation's national (FFAB) hotline saw a 30% increase in calls in 2020 compared to previous years. Young people aged 18-21, primarily women, are most affected by eating disorders (Raybaud, 2021[61]).

LGBTI+ individuals, especially youth, reported poor mental health outcomes during the pandemic, especially those confined in homes where they may not be accepted. Surveys in the United States and United Kingdom found that those identifying as a sexual minority or LGBTI+ were more likely to report symptoms of depression (OECD, 2021[56]). Another study of LGBTI+ respondents in the United Kingdom, running from 27 April to 13 July, found that depression and stress were present in almost 70% of the population, with 17% reporting some form of discrimination since the start of the pandemic because of their sexual orientation (Kneale and Bécares, 2020[62]). One reason for these elevated levels of mental distress is that young LGBTI+ people may be forced to quarantine with family members who do not accept them. A study of 632 LGBTI+ youth aged 16 to 35 in Portugal, from 17 April to 4 May 2020, found that 59% of respondents felt uncomfortable within their family, 30% felt very uncomfortable living with their parents during confinement, and 35% reported feeling "suffocated" because they could not express their true identity with their family (Durães e Lusa, 2020[63]). Data from the mental health hotline opened by the Colombian Ministry of Health and Social Protection in April 2020 showed that a higher percentage of transgender callers (14%) reported problems with interpersonal relationships as compared to cisgender women (4.5%) or men (4.8%) (El Heraldo, 2021[64]).

Figure 6.8. Young people, full-time students and the unemployed experienced the highest rates of anxiety and depression symptoms throughout 2020 and 2021

Share of respondents who are at risk for anxiety or depression disorders, Apr 2020 - Jun 2021

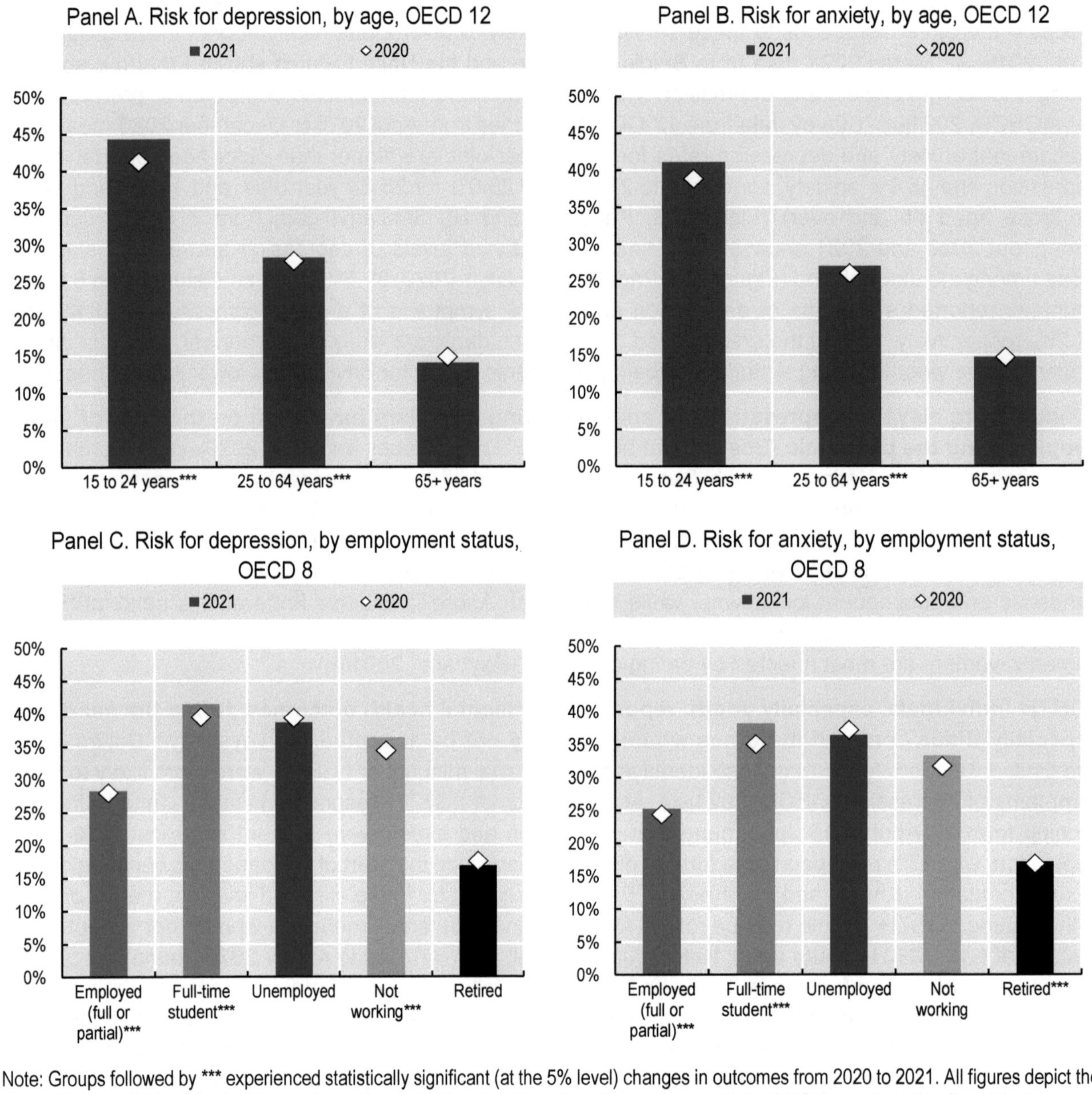

Note: Groups followed by *** experienced statistically significant (at the 5% level) changes in outcomes from 2020 to 2021. All figures depict the share of respondents at risk for depression and anxiety disorders, based on their responses to the PHQ-4 questionnaire. Panel A shows age breakdowns for the 12 OECD countries with complete data from April 2020 to June 2021: Australia, Canada, Denmark, France, Germany, Italy, Japan, Korea, Norway, Spain, Sweden and the United Kingdom. Panels C and D show employment status breakdowns for eight OECD countries with complete data: Canada, France, Germany, Italy, Japan, Korea, Spain and the United Kingdom.

Source: OECD calculations based on Imperial College London YouGov (2020[52]), *COVID-19 behaviour tracker data hub* (database), https://github.com/YouGov-Data/covid-19-tracker.

StatLink https://stat.link/se4j6f

Symptoms of depression and anxiety are also more common among the unemployed and those experiencing financial difficulties (OECD, 2021[49]). Survey data from the United Kingdom, collected between 27 January and 7 March 2021, showed that 40% of unemployed individuals reported depression, compared to only half that level among those employed or self-employed (19%) (ONS, 2021[65]). In the United States, survey data collected from the COVID Impact Survey in June 2020 reveal that households with income of less than USD 30 000 were among the groups that reported the highest rates of hopelessness (45% compared to 25% for households making more than USD 125 000) and depression (46%, compared to 33%) (Wozniak et al., 2020[66]; COVID Impact Survey, 2020[67]). Another United States-based study from 19-24 March 2020 found that 33% of lower-income Americans experienced high distress, compared to 17% of people in upper-income households (Keeter, 2020[68]).[14] An online national survey in Japan, administered in two waves (16-18 April 2020 and 15-17 May 2020) to 2 000 total respondents, found that the unemployed had higher rates of depression (measured using PHQ-9)[15] and anxiety (using GAD-7)[16] than did permanent employees: 31.2% vs. 18.9% at risk of depression, and 25.4% vs. 11.7% at risk of anxiety, respectively. Part-time temporary workers reported better mental health outcomes than the unemployed, but still significantly below those of permanent employees (20.6% at risk for depression, and 12.6% at risk of anxiety). Similarly, rates of depression and anxiety were more than twice as large for households whose finances were worse off following the start of the pandemic, compared to those whose finances were unchanged or improved (Ueda et al., 2020[69]).

Children from lower-income families also report low mental health outcomes. According to the Tulsa SEED study in the United States, low-income parents and their children have struggled with mental health since the pandemic began. One in four parents experienced depressive symptoms, which were often tied to food insecurity: parents who were food insecure were twice as likely to report feeling depressed as parents who were food secure. Similarly, 47% of parents said their child experienced increased emotional or behavioural problems since the pandemic began (Tulsa SEED Study Team, 2020[70]). A study from the United States Center for Translational Neuroscience reveals similar trends (Center for Translational Neuroscience, 2020[71]).[17]

An additional concern is the toll that COVID-19 is taking on the mental health of frontline health-care workers (United Nations, 2020[72]; OECD, 2021[49]). Frontline workers are facing the stress and anxiety of working long hours, the death of many patients – often without the presence of family members – and fear of contracting the virus themselves and/or infecting family members. In April 2020, a survey of 578 Canadian health-care workers revealed that 47% reported a need for psychological support; with regards to their current work situation, 67% felt anxious, 49% unsafe, 40% overwhelmed, 29% helpless, 28% sleep deprived and 28% discouraged (Potloc, 2020[73]). A 2021 study by McKinsey & Company of 400 frontline nurses found that 22% reported a desire to leave their current position; among these, 60% said their desire to quit their job had increased since the start of the pandemic (Berlin et al., 2021[74]). Even before the pandemic arrived, physicians around the world had higher suicide rates, alcoholism and general substance abuse rates than the general population (Schernhammer and Colditz, 2004[75]; Kaliszewski, 2021[76]).[18] There are also growing concerns about high suicide rates among health workers, including doctors and nurses treating COVID-19 patients, in some of the worst-hit areas (Rahman and Plummer, 2020[77]; MacBride, 2020[78]). Unpaid adult caregivers are also at risk for worse mental health outcomes, increased substance abuse and higher levels of suicidal ideation (Czeisler et al., 2020[79]).

Although there are few data, migrants' mental health seems to have declined more than non-migrants' during the pandemic. In Germany, those with a migration background experienced a sharper increase in symptoms of anxiety in April 2020 vis-à-vis pre-pandemic years, compared to those without a migration background (Figure 6.9, Panel A). In a nationally representative survey conducted in July and November 2020 in Australia, the share of those saying that they had been "unhappy" or "very unhappy" over the past year rose from 16% in 2018-19 to 23% for respondents born abroad with a non-English speaking background, compared to a decline in unhappiness for those born in Australia from 22% to 20% (The Scandlon Foundation, 2021[80]).

Figure 6.9. Everyone's mental health suffered during the pandemic, but some groups experienced worse deteriorations than others

Selected measures of COVID-19-related mental health outcomes throughout 2020, by immigration status and population group

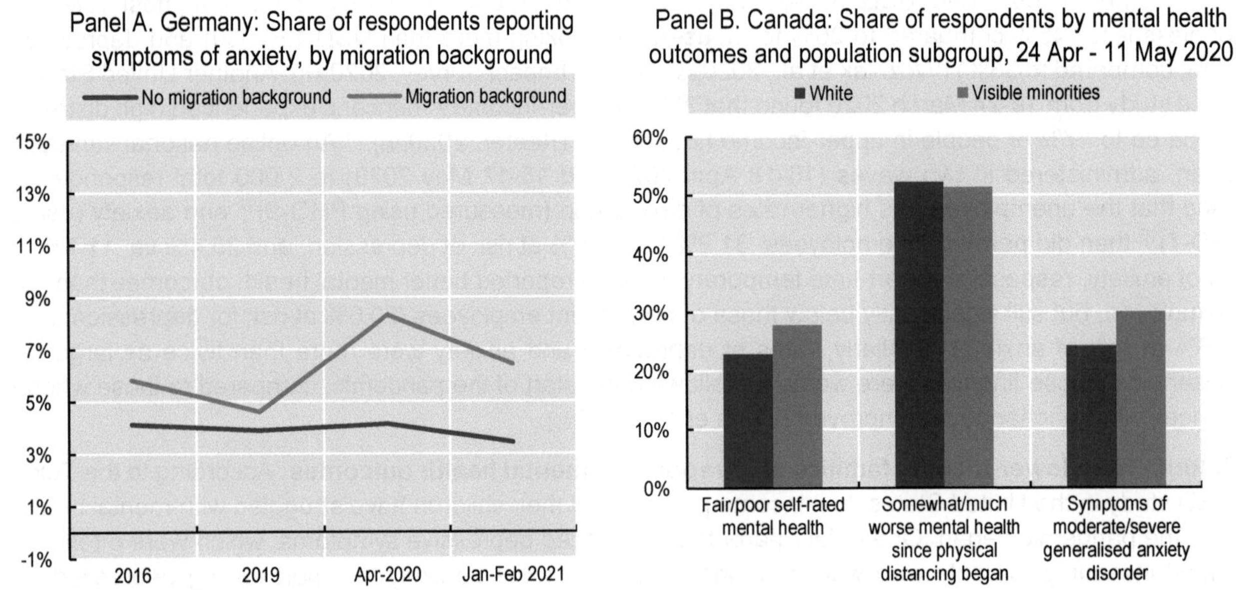

Note: In Panel A, the two-item Generalised Anxiety Disorder (GAD-2) scale was used to obtain information about symptoms of anxiety. In Panel B, visible minority groups include South Asian, Chinese, Black, Filipino, Latin American, Arab, Southeast Asian, West Asian, Korean, Japanese, visible minority not included elsewhere, and multiple visible minority categories; Indigenous peoples are not included. Outcomes are compared to the white (non-Indigeneous) population). Anxiety was measured using the GAD-7 scale; those with a score of 10 or higher are considered to have moderate to severe symptoms of generalised anxiety disorder in the two weeks prior to completing the survey.
Source: Kühne et al. (2020[81]), "The need for household panel surveys in times of crisis: The case of SOEP-CoV", *Survey Research Methods*, Vol. 14/2, pp. 195-203, https://doi.org/10.18148/srm/2020.v14i2.7748 (refer to Box 3.1 for methodological details) (Panel A); Statistics Canada (2020[82]), *The mental health of population groups designated as visible minorities in Canada during the COVID-19 pandemic* (database), https://www150.statcan.gc.ca/n1/pub/45-28-0001/2020001/article/00077-eng.htm (Panel B).

StatLink https://stat.link/9zx4a3

Mental health deteriorated for almost everyone in 2020, but gaps in mental health outcomes between racial and ethnic groups were large and in some cases increased over time. In Canada, similar proportions of visible minority[19] and white (non-Indigenous) participants reported that their mental health had worsened since the beginning of physical distancing in a survey in May and April 2020 (Statistics Canada, 2020[82]) (refer to Box 6.2 for survey methodology). However, a larger share of visible minority participants rated their mental health as fair or poor and exhibited symptoms of generalised anxiety disorder in the previous two weeks (Figure 6.9, Panel B). Moreover, 38% of Indigenous respondents, as compared to 23% of non-Indigenous respondents in the same survey, reported fair or poor mental health, and 48% of Indigenous women compared to 31% of Indigenous men experienced symptoms of anxiety (Statistics Canada, 2020[83]).[20] In the United Kingdom, self-reported mental health (based on the GHQ-12 score,[21] and after adjusting for a range of socio-economic and demographic conditions including social support) deteriorated across most groups during the first lockdown (April 2020 versus 2019), but the decline was most noticeable in the Indian group compared to those of white British or Other white ethnicity (ONS, 2020[84]).[22] In a different United Kingdom survey (the COVID-19 Social Study, a large longitudinal study but without a probability sample), 23.6% of respondents with an ethnic minority background reported thoughts of suicide or self-harm between 1 March and 20 April, as compared to 17.1% among white respondents (Iob, Steptoe and Fancourt, 2020[85]). Data from the United States Census Bureau Household

Pulse survey suggest gaps in mental health outcomes between different racial and ethnic groups were small in 2019, but widened in 2020 as overall levels of anxiety and depression increased rapidly during the pandemic (Figure 6.10). On average, more than 40% of Black and Hispanic/Latino Americans showed symptoms of anxiety and/or depressive disorder between April 2020 and May 2021, compared to 35% of white and 31% of Asian adults. However, additional nationally representative survey evidence indicates that, despite experiencing far greater material hardship during the pandemic (Chapter 5), levels of hope and optimism for the future among Hispanic/Latino and Black individuals remained more resilient.[23] This mirrors the lower prevalence of deaths by suicide, acute alcohol abuse and drug overdose ("deaths of despair") among these communities, compared to white communities, in the years preceding the pandemic (Graham et al., 2020[30]): the gap between Black and white respondents holds for all income levels, but is largest when comparing low-income Black and white adults.[24]

Figure 6.10. In the United States, Black and Hispanic/Latino Americans reported worse mental health outcomes throughout the pandemic

Share of adults reporting symptoms of anxiety and/or depressive disorder, by ethnicity and race, 2019-21

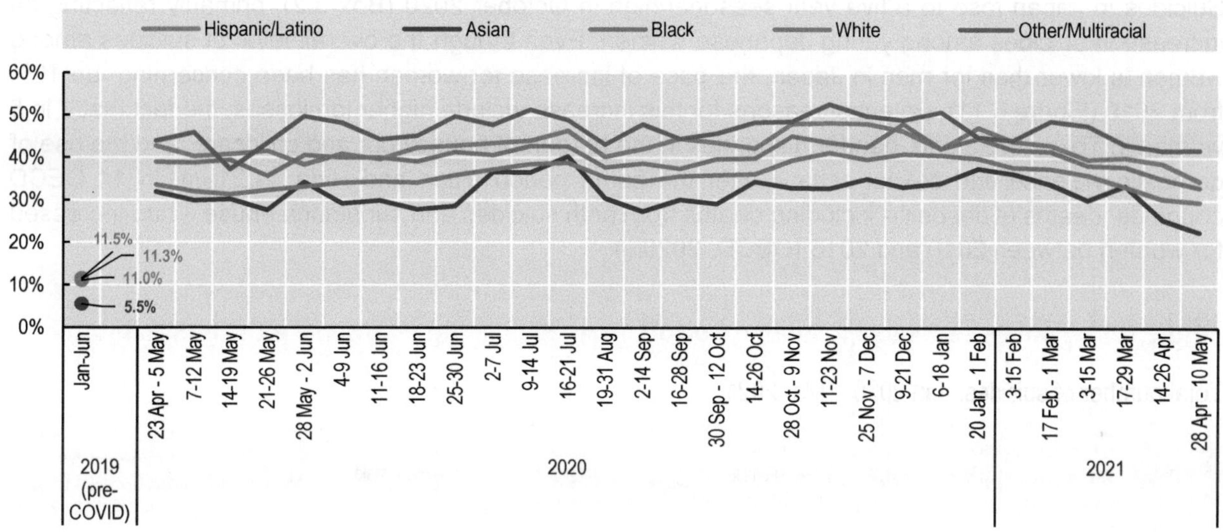

Note: Pre-pandemic data are January-June 2019 averages. Data before and during the pandemic use the two-item Patient Health Questionnaire (PHQ-2) and the two-item Generalised Anxiety Disorder (GAD-2) scale to obtain information on the frequency of anxiety and depression symptoms. The results may not be directly comparable as the two-week reference period in 2019 was modified to one week in 2020-2021. Results for the Other/Multiracial category are not available in 2019.
Source: 2019 data: NCHS (2020[86]), *National Health Interview Survey Early Release Program* (database), National Center for Health Statistics, https://www.cdc.gov/nchs/data/nhis/earlyrelease/ERmentalhealthbyrace-508.pdf; 2020-2021 data: United States Census Bureau (n.d.[87]), *Measuring household experiences during the coronavirus pandemic* (database), https://www.census.gov/householdpulsedata (refer to Box 3.1 for methodological details).

StatLink https://stat.link/gn49tx

Suicides among young people have not risen as feared, but intentional self-harm among some population groups is on the rise

Despite the rapid rise in mental health difficulties among young adults, prompting early fears of an increase in youth suicide rates in the United States, **later evidence showed no significant increases in 2020** (Bartlett, 2021[88]). In other countries, however, some studies have found evidence of increases in suicides or self-harm hospitalisations, especially among other segments of the population (see Box 6.3 for evidence from Japan). A study in England from 23 March to 17 May 2020, in Oxford and Derby hospitals, found that COVID-19 and lockdown restrictions contributed to self-harm, especially for women (Hawton et al., 2021[89]). Data from private health-care claims in the United States showed that claims for intentional self-harm as a percentage of all medical claim lines for those aged 13-18 nearly doubled from April 2019 to April 2020 (FAIR Health, 2021[90]).

Box 6.3. Spotlight: Rising suicide rates in Japan in the second and third quarter of 2020, mainly among women

Suicides in Japan rose to a five-year seasonal high in October 2020 (Box 3.2), primarily reflecting an increase in suicides among young Japanese women. Even though the overall level of suicides among women is lower than for men in Japan, the pace of increase for women has been concerning: up 15% from 2019 (Figure 6.11). Potential reasons for this increase include higher job losses, the fact that 1 in 5 women in Tokyo live alone, gender disparities in the burden of housework and childcare, and the rise of domestic violence and sexual assault over the same period (Rich and Hida, 2021[91]). In 14 OECD countries, deaths of despair – including deaths from both suicides and substance abuse – had increased for women between 2010 and 2016 (OECD, 2020[4]).

Figure 6.11. Female suicides in Japan rose 15% from 2019, a higher increase than for men

Total number of suicides, Jan 2020 – Mar 2021

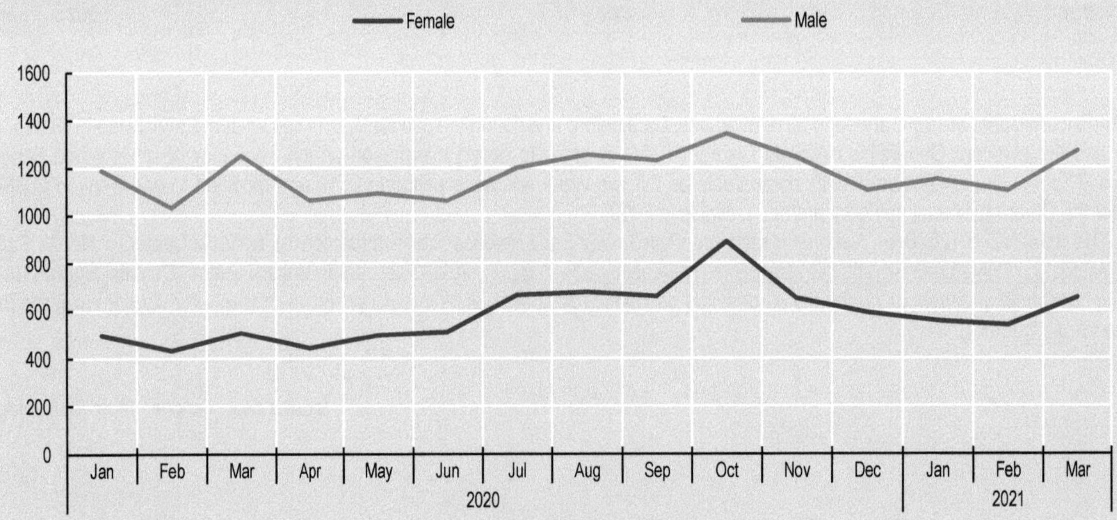

Source: Japanese National Police Agency (2021[92]), 令和２年中における自殺の状況, https://www.npa.go.jp/safetylife/seianki/jisatsu/R03/R02_jisatuno_joukyou.pdf.

StatLink https://stat.link/uev6q5

6.2. Subjective well-being

As compared to mental health, life satisfaction remained surprisingly resilient for many over the course of 2020 but declined for some groups

Although average measures of subjective well-being in OECD countries remained relatively stable from 2019 to 2020 (Chapter 3)**, some population groups were more adversely impacted by the pandemic than others** (Figure 6.12). Women (especially women who have children in the home), those living in a home with children under the age of 18, young people, and those working part-time experienced some of the largest declines in life satisfaction from 2019 to 2020. These declines in life satisfaction are more or less mirrored in negative affect balance.[25] In addition, life satisfaction in 2020 declined for the unemployed. Conversely, while the large changes in negative affect balance for the unemployed are visually striking (and counterintuitive), they are not statistically significant. They likely stem from the fact that overall unemployment rates increased in many countries in 2020, changing drastically the composition of the unemployed (Helliwell et al., 2021[93]).[26]

In 2020, women experienced slightly larger declines in both life satisfaction and negative affect balance relative to men (Figure 6.12). According to the Global Attitude Survey from the Pew Research Center, 68.8% of women in Germany, France and the United States reported in November-December of 2020 that their life had changed a great deal/fair amount as a result of the COVID-19 outbreak, while only 59.3% of men did (Devlin and Kent, 2021[94]).[27] According to data from the Gallup World Poll, life satisfaction for women fell by 0.06 points on a 0-10 scale, on average in the OECD, compared to 0.03 points for men; negative affect balance deteriorated by 1.4 percentage points, compared to 0.7pp for men. While these average falls are small, they mirror women's higher risk of job losses (Adams-Prassl et al., 2020[95]; Alon et al., 2020[96]) and domestic violence during lockdown periods (Leslie and Wilson, 2021[97]; Armbruster and Klotzbücher, 2020[98]), as well as higher childcare burdens stemming from school and day-care closures (Adams-Prassl et al., 2020[95]).

Regardless of gender, life satisfaction for parents of school-age children fell during 2020, and this effect was stronger in areas that underwent more school closures (Huebener et al., 2020[99]) (Figure 6.13). In fact, changes in life satisfaction were significant only for countries where school closures exceeded the OECD average (Figure 6.13, Panel A), with deteriorations for those with school-age children and significant improvements for partnered people with no children in the home. In countries with lower than OECD average school closures in 2020, none of the household groupings experienced significant changes in life satisfaction (Figure 6.13, Panel B). However, while parents saw their life satisfaction fall more than those without children (or with children over age 18), parents of school-age children still have higher levels of life satisfaction than single people with no children (6.8 vs. 6.51 in 2020, respectively). Those in partnerships – either married or in a consensual union – have higher life satisfaction than single people, regardless of whether they have children: 6.8 and 6.79 for those in partnerships with and without children, compared to 6.58 and 6.51 for single people with and without children, respectively (Figure 6.12).

Overall, across OECD countries, subjective well-being is higher among people in employment, relative to the unemployed, and this gap widened for life satisfaction in 2020. Average life satisfaction among the full-time employed fell from 6.88 to 6.85 in 2020, while for the unemployed it fell from 6.04 to 5.88 (Figure 6.12). For negative affect balance, the gap between the employed and the unemployed narrowed somewhat, but in 2020 the share of unemployed experiencing a negative affect balance was still very high at 21% (compared to 12% for the full-time employed). A much smaller gap exists between those in full-time and part-time employment, where full-time employees are slightly better off.[28] However, while full-time employees experienced little change in their subjective well-being, on average, from 2019 to 2020, part-time workers recorded some of the largest deteriorations of any group, across both measures.

Figure 6.12. Though measures of subjective well-being were fairly resilient overall, some groups experienced larger deteriorations than others

Selected measures of subjective well-being, by population group, 2019-20

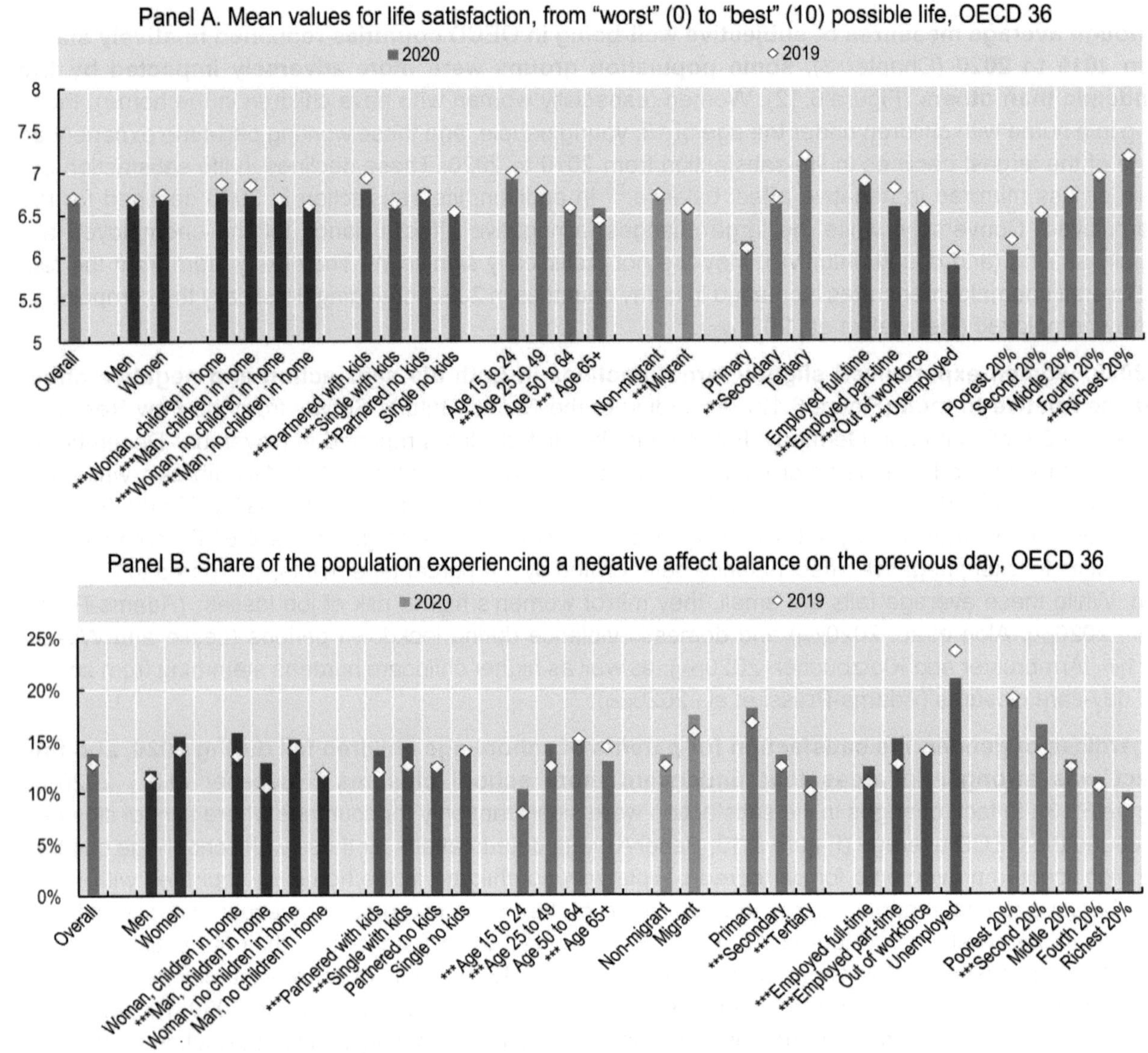

Note: In Panel A, life satisfaction is measured on a scale from 0 "not at all satisfied" to 10 "completely satisfied". In Panel B, a negative affect balance is recorded when a respondent reports more negative (anger, sadness or worry) than positive (well-rested, enjoyment, laughing or smiling a lot) feelings or states in the previous day. In both panels, the OECD average excludes Luxembourg (no data in 2020) and the Czech Republic (no data in 2019). Groups preceded by *** experienced statistically significant (at the 5% level) changes in outcomes from 2019 to 2020. Refer to the Reader's Guide for a complete list of Gallup World Poll data collection dates in 2020, and to Box 3.4 for additional information about the data collection methodology. "Women and men with children in the home" are respondents who report having at least one child under the age of 18 living in the household. "Women and men with no children" are defined as those who do not have any children under the age of 18 living in the household. Therefore, these indicators do not account for parents of adult children, or children who live outside of the household. "Partnered" is defined as being either married or in a consensual union. "Single" encompasses those who are not married, are not in a consensual union, are divorced, and/or are widowed. "Poorest 20%" refers to those in the bottom quintile of household income (income quintiles are defined by Gallup). See the Reader's Guide for a definition of educational categories.

Source: OECD calculations based on the *Gallup World Poll* (n.d.[100]) (database), https://www.gallup.com/178667/gallup-world-poll-work.aspx.

StatLink https://stat.link/u1f2xl

Declines in life satisfaction for low-income earners and those with low levels of education are not statistically significant (Figure 6.12). **This suggests that measures of subjective well-being are perhaps reflecting both the negative impacts of the pandemic** (health risks, job and income loss, social isolation, school closures, etc.) **as well as the buffering role that government policies played in protecting people's material conditions** (job retention schemes, more generous unemployment packages, etc.) and some positives for those who kept their jobs but saw changes in their working or living arrangements (e.g. more time to spend with family among those furloughed, on short-time working hours, or no longer commuting to work – see Chapters 5 and 7). In the case of life satisfaction, this has netted out as few large changes in life satisfaction at the national average level among OECD countries (see Figure 3.11), but significant falls (and some gains) for specific population groups.

Figure 6.13. Parents of school-age children experienced larger drops in life satisfaction in countries that had more days of school closures

Mean values for life satisfaction, from "worst" (0) to "best" (10) possible life", 2019-20

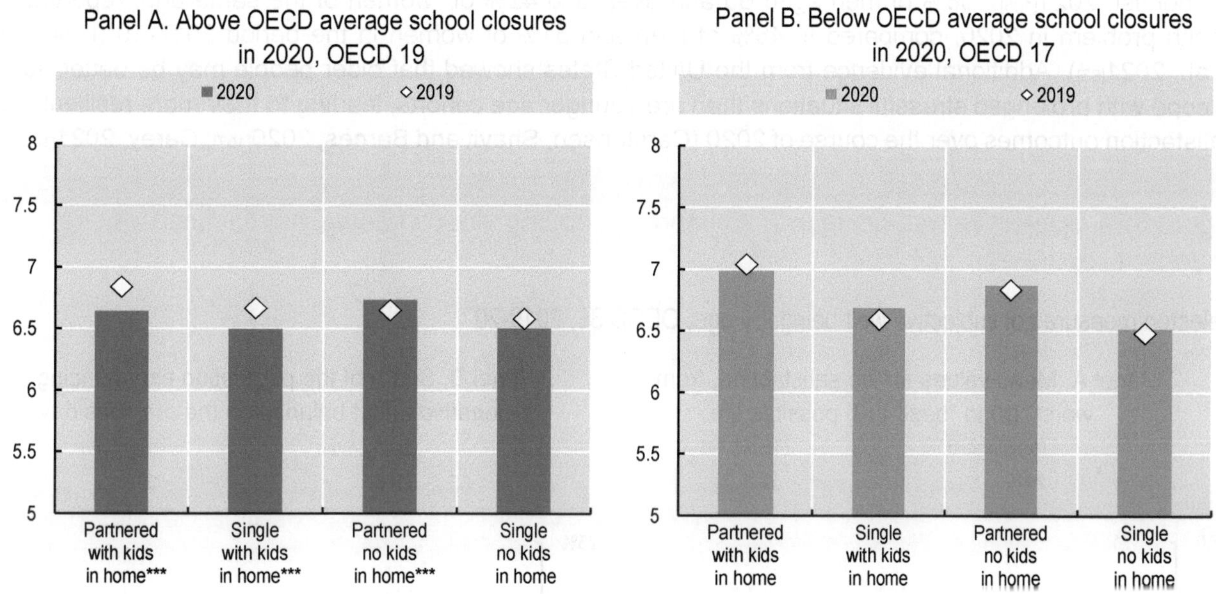

Note: Panel A displays life satisfaction averages by household type for countries where days of school closures exceeded the OECD 36 average during the Gallup fieldwork period (the OECD 19 average includes Canada, Chile, Colombia, Costa Rica, Finland, Ireland, Israel, Italy, Lithuania, Latvia, Mexico, the Netherlands, Norway, Portugal, Slovenia, Spain, Sweden, Turkey and the United States). Panel B shows outcomes for countries with below OECD average school closures (the OECD 17 average includes Australia, Austria, Belgium, Denmark, Estonia, France, Germany, Greece, Hungary, Iceland, Japan, Korea, New Zealand, Poland, the Slovak Republic, Switzerland and the United Kingdom). Luxembourg (no data in 2020) and the Czech Republic (no data in 2019) are not included in either group. School closure data (not pictured in the graphs, but used to categorise country groupings) come from the Oxford COVID-19 Government Response Tracker. Groups followed by *** experienced statistically significant (at the 5% level) changes in outcomes from 2019 to 2020. "Partnered" is defined as being either married or in a consensual union. "Single" encompasses those who are not married, are not in a consensual union, are divorced, and/or are widowed. A household is defined as having kids if the respondents indicate that at least one child under the age of 18 lives in the household. Therefore partnered or single people with children who do not live at home, or whose children are over the age of 18, are categorised as "no kids" for the purposes of this figure. Refer to the Reader's Guide for a complete list of Gallup World Poll data collection dates in 2020, and to Box 3.4 for additional information about the data collection methodology.

Source: OECD calculations based on the *Gallup World Poll* (n.d.[100]) (database), https://www.gallup.com/178667/gallup-world-poll-work.aspx; OECD calculations based on Hale et.al (2021[101]), "A global panel database of pandemic policies (Oxford COVID-19 Government Response Tracker)", *Nature Human Behaviour*, Vol. 5/4, pp. 529-538, http://dx.doi.org/10.1038/s41562-021-01079-8.

StatLink https://stat.link/90bp8k

The life satisfaction of young people fell more than any other age group in 2020, while there is some evidence that life satisfaction among those aged 65 or above improved (Figure 6.14). Data from both national statistics offices and international surveys in 2020 suggest that as young people have been especially hard hit by the pandemic – their schooling interrupted, their career prospects dimmed and their social lives dramatically diminished – their life satisfaction has fallen more than other age cohorts (Helliwell, Schellenberg and Fonberg, 2020[102]). Data from the United Kingdom Office for National Statistics show that the youngest age cohort had the lowest levels of life satisfaction from April-May 2020 (ONS, 2020[103]), while evidence from France shows that the steep drop in young people's life satisfaction occurred in early 2021, rather than 2020 (CEPREMAP/INSEE, n.d.[104]). Data from 26 countries from April to June, collected by Imperial College London YouGov (2020[52]), show that, across most countries, younger people were least satisfied with their life, while middle-aged and older cohorts reported better outcomes (SDSN Secretariat, 2020[105]).

The finding that life satisfaction improved for older people in 2020 is still not well understood. One theory posits that older people feel relatively healthier in the context of a global pandemic: those who were lucky enough to avoid contracting COVID-19 feel more grateful for their baseline health levels (The Economist, 2021[106]). 36% of men aged 60 and over, and 42% of women of the same age, reported a health problem in 2020, compared to 46% of men and 51% of women in the period 2017-19 (Helliwell et al., 2021[93]). Additional evidence from the United States showed that older people may be better able to cope with prolonged stressful situations than are younger age cohorts, leading to their more resilient life satisfaction outcomes over the course of 2020 (Carstensen, Shavit and Barnes, 2020[107]; Carey, 2021[108]).

Figure 6.14. Subjective well-being in 2020 improved among elderly people, but declined among younger people

Selected measures of subjective well-being, by age, OECD 36, 2019-20

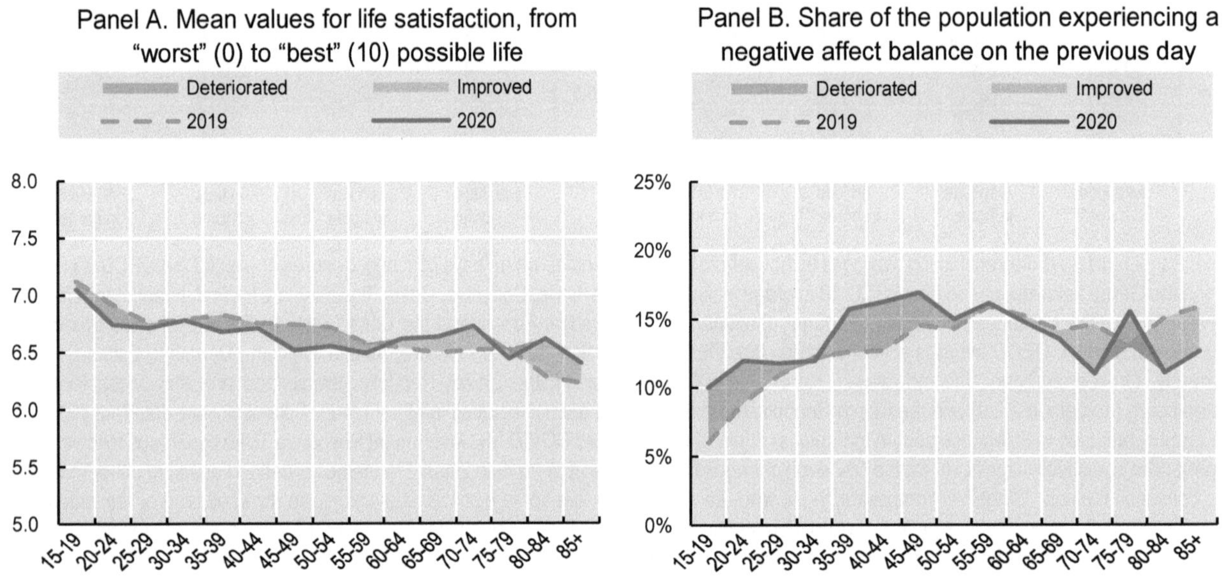

Note: In Panels A and B, the OECD average excludes Luxembourg (no data in 2020) and the Czech Republic (no data in 2019). The figure shows subjective well-being outcomes throughout the life course, in 5-year periods. Life course outcomes for 2020 are contrasted to those from 2019. Refer to the Reader's Guide for a complete list of Gallup World Poll data collection dates in 2020, and to Box 3.4 for additional information about the data collection methodology.
Source: OECD calculations based on the *Gallup World Poll* (n.d.[100]) (database), https://www.gallup.com/178667/gallup-world-poll-work.aspx.

StatLink https://stat.link/astrh9

Box 6.4. Spotlight: Evidence from four OECD countries shows declines in life satisfaction for some

French data show that women had lower levels of life satisfaction than men throughout 2019-21. When life satisfaction reached its 2020 peak (coinciding with the June/July deconfinement in the country) women's levels more or less equalled men's. However, the steep decline in life satisfaction in October/November 2020 – the beginning of strict second-wave lockdowns – was worse for women than men (Figure 6.15, Panel A).

Figure 6.15. Country-specific evidence for life satisfaction declines for women, racial and ethnic minorities, and low income earners

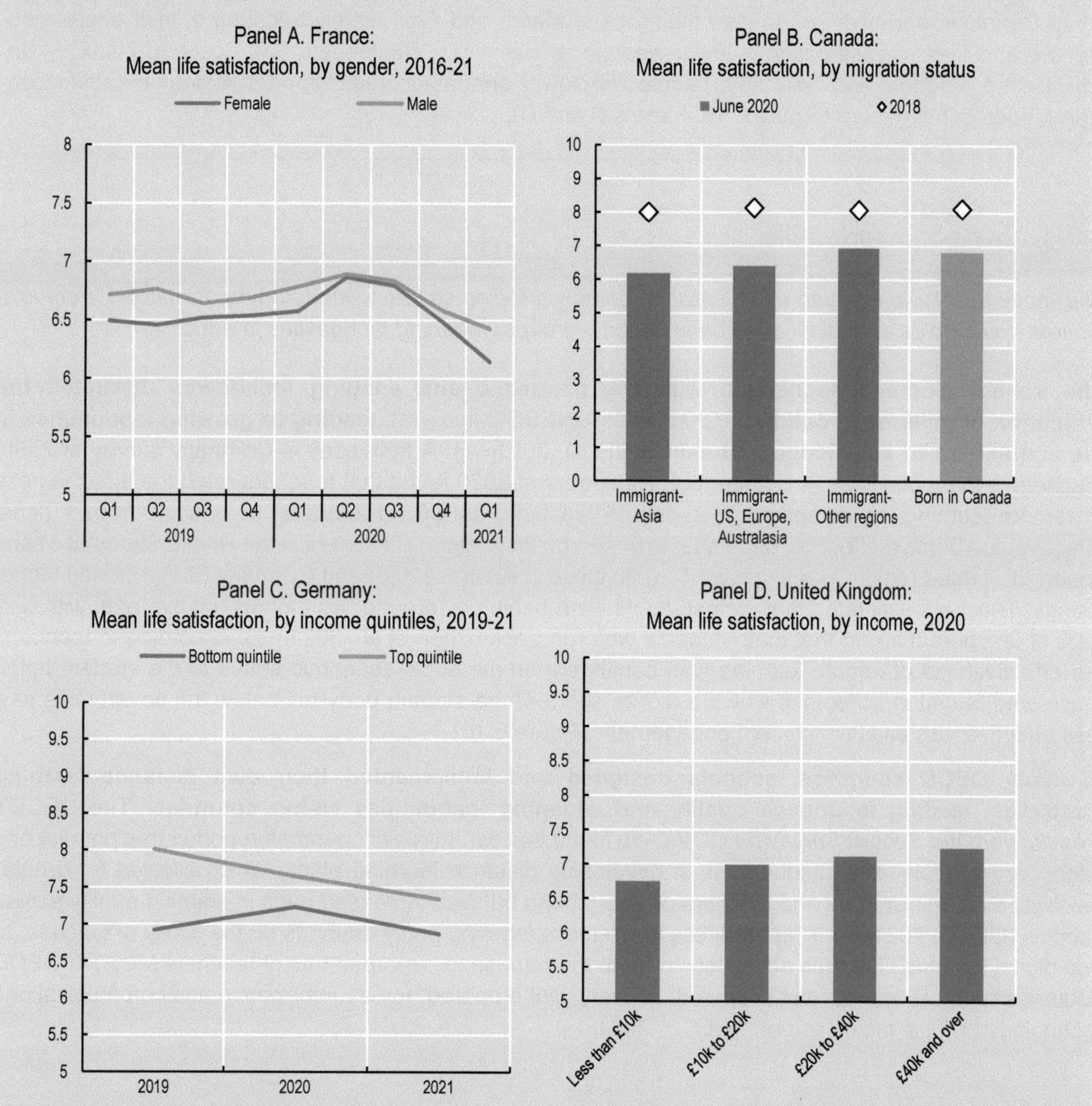

Note: All four panels show average life satisfaction on a scale from 0 "not at all satisfied" to 10 "completely satisfied".

Source: CEPREMAP/INSEE (n.d.[104]), *Le bien-être en France* (database), http://www.cepremap.fr/Duree.html (Panel A); Helliwell, Schellenberg and Fonberg (2020[102]), "Life satisfaction in Canada before and during the COVID-19 pandemic", *Analytical Studies Branch Research Paper Series*, No. 457, Statistics Canada, https://www150.statcan.gc.ca/n1/en/pub/11f0019m/11f0019m2020020-eng.pdf?st=s6m4rNgZ (Panel B); Kühne et al. (2020[81]), "The need for household panel surveys in times of crisis: The case of SOEP-CoV", *Survey Research Methods*, Vol. 14/2, pp. 195-203, https://doi.org/10.18148/srm/2020.v14i2.7748 (Panel C); and ONS (n.d.[109]), *Personal and economic well-being in Great Britain: September 2020* (database), Office for National Statistics, https://www.ons.gov.uk/peoplepopulationandcommunity/wellbeing/datasets/incomegroupsplitestimatesonpersonalandeconomicwellbeingacrosstime (Panel D).

StatLink https://stat.link/sfn4l6

In Canada, between 2019 and 2020, life satisfaction declined more among migrants from Asia, the United States, Europe and Australasia than it did among individuals born in Canada (Figure 6.15, Panel B). Both economic and social factors may account for this outcome. Recent migrants were more likely than Canadian-born workers to lose their jobs in March and April mainly because of their shorter job tenure and over-representation in lower-wage jobs (Helliwell, Schellenberg and Fonberg, 2020[102]). In the United Kingdom and Germany, people with lower annual incomes reported lower life satisfaction than those earning more (Figure 6.15, Panels C and D).

6.3. Knowledge and skills

The move to remote learning has disproportionately affected children with learning disabilities, from low-income households and racial and ethnic minority groups, widening inequalities in education

The school closures associated with the pandemic and ensuing lockdowns disrupted the education of millions of children (Chapter 3) (UNESCO, n.d.[110]), **leading to growing inequalities in the acquisition of knowledge and skills** (OECD, 2021[111]). A McKinsey & Company survey of 2 549 teachers in eight countries in October and November of 2020 found that teachers rated the effectiveness of remote learning, as compared to in-person teaching, as 4.8 on average, on a scale from 1 (least effective) to 10 (most effective, and equal to in-person instruction). Teachers in the United States (3.5) and Japan (3.3) rated remote learning lowest, while those in Australia (6.6) and Germany (6.1) reported higher ratings. Teachers estimated that their students were behind by around two months, on average, with only 12% of teachers thinking that their students were on track (Chen et al., 2021[112]). According to teachers, the effectiveness of remote learning was contingent on the socio-economic status of the student body: those who taught in schools in which a higher share of the student body fell below the poverty line saw less effectiveness and less student engagement (Figure 6.16).

In many OECD countries, schools designed and implemented their own distance learning strategies, leading to uneven quality and widening inequalities within countries. The OECD's *Results from the Special Survey on COVID-19* found that two-thirds of countries reported that primary and secondary schools were autonomous in developing distance learning plans, which allowed for greater flexibility by administrators and teachers on-the-ground but also increased gaps in learning quality across schools (OECD, 2021[113]). Preparedness for distance learning partly depends on the ability of teachers to use digital learning platforms effectively; prior to the pandemic, less than half of teachers (43%) in OECD countries reported feeling "well prepared" or "very well prepared" to use information and communications technology (ICT) in the classroom (OECD, 2021[113]).

Figure 6.16. The efficacy of remote learning is lower in schools in which a higher share of the student body lives in households below the poverty line

Panel A. Effectiveness of remote learning from 1 (least effective) to 10 (most effective), by the share of the student body living below the poverty line, Oct-Nov 2020

Panel B. Share of students engaged with remote learning by the share of the student body living below the poverty line, Oct-Nov 2020

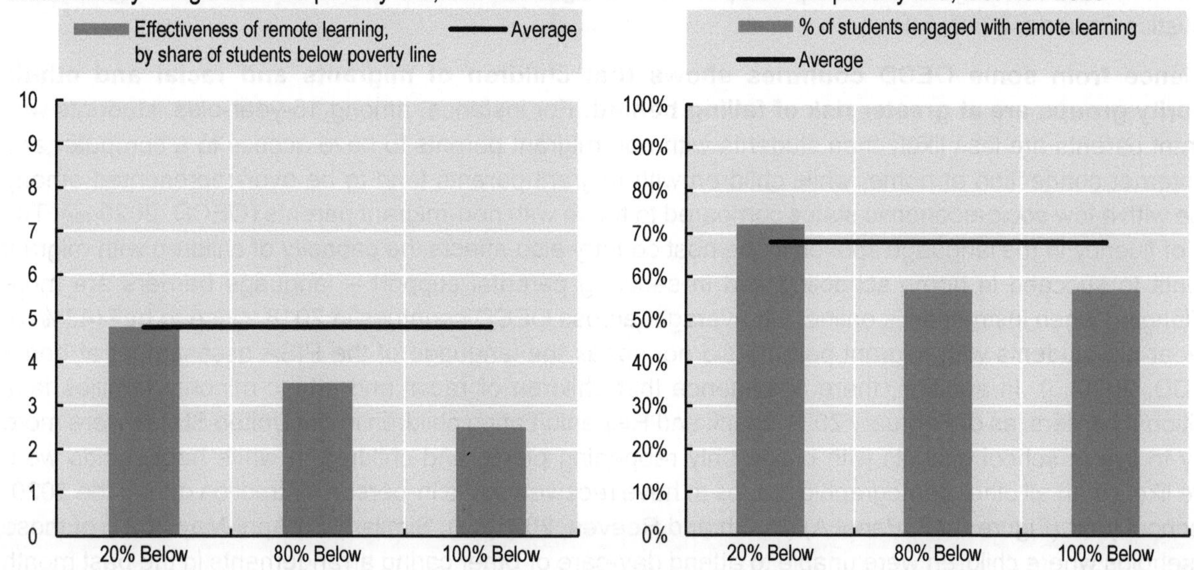

Note: Panel A shows the average effectiveness that teachers assigned to remote learning, where 1 is least effective and 10 is most effective (equal to in-person instruction), by the type of school: schools in which 20% of the student body live in households below the poverty line; 80% below, and 100% below. Panel B shows the share of students engaged with remote learning for each school type. The survey was administered to 2 549 teachers in eight countries: Australia (146 participants), Canada (350), China (350), France (278), Germany (274), Japan (350), the United Kingdom (351) and the United States (450). Data collection ran from 28 October to 17 November 2020.

Source: Chen, L. et al. (2021[112]), *Teacher survey: Learning loss is global--and significant*, McKinsey & Company, https://www.mckinsey.com/industries/public-and-social-sector/our-insights/teacher-survey-learning-loss-is-global-and-significant?cid=other-eml-alt-mip-mck&hdpid=1a57cf47-eae2-400f-b9f0-fd8edddbbfb6&hctky=2909643&hlkid=b53175decdec48bbb6888bd21b5a168b.

StatLink https://stat.link/6ztcmr

Findings from a number of national studies also show that children whose parents have lower income and/or educational levels experienced greater barriers to remote learning. Pre-pandemic evidence showed that children's academic performance is influenced by their parent's education level; this implies that school closures will likely widen existing learning gaps (OECD, 2021[114]). Students who do not have learning support from parents will be more at risk of falling behind their classmates whose parents are better equipped to help them (Di Pietro et al., 2020[115]). Preliminary findings from a study in the United Kingdom show that children from better-off families spent 30% more time on home learning than did students from disadvantaged backgrounds (Andrew et al., 2020[116]). A study in France found that working-class families allocated slightly more time to home learning, but that families from higher socio-economic backgrounds were able to provide higher quality supplemental instruction and that they experienced a lower decline in the parent-student relationship during the lockdown (Hélary, 2020[117]). In the Netherlands, a study of the 2020 eight-week school closure found that it led to 0.08 standard deviations of learning loss (equivalent to one-fifth of a school year), on average, but losses were 60% higher for low-income students (Engzell, Frey and Verhagen, 2021[118]). A United States study administered from May to July 2020 among children from low-income families in Tulsa – aged three to the end of fourth grade – and teachers found that only 29% of teachers reported that "nearly all" students participated in distance learning activities, one in five parents reported that their child never communicated with their teacher, and two in five children spent an hour per day or less on distance learning. Most parents (65%) noted challenges with distance learning, including: children needing more support than the parent(s) can provide (30%); lack of or inconsistent Internet access (16%); lessons and instructions too hard (14%); no dedicated space for schoolwork (13%); and lack of a device to connect to distance learning (10%) (Tulsa SEED Study Team, 2020[70]).[29] A study from Statistics Canada found that lower income households had less access to Internet-enabled devices, and were more likely to use mobile devices to connect to the Internet; these devices have more limited functionality than desktop computers, making them less suitable for remote learning activities (Statistics Canada, 2020[119]).

Evidence from some OECD countries shows that children of migrants and racial and ethnic minority groups are at greater risk of falling behind. For instance, among 15-year-olds, students with migrant parents are less likely than students with non-migrant parents to have access to a computer and an Internet connection at home, while children with migrant parents tend to be over-represented among those with a low socio-economic status compared to those with non-migrant parents (OECD, 2020[19]). The lack of fluency in the language spoken in the host country also affects the capacity of children with migrant parents to succeed in home schooling and in securing parental support – language barriers are more challenging when instruction is online. On average, across OECD countries in 2018, close to half (48%) of 15-year-old students with migrant parents did not speak the language of the PISA assessment at home (OECD, 2020[19]). In addition, there is evidence that children of racial and ethnic minority families face additional barriers: as of February 2021, Black and Hispanic/Latino children in the United States were more likely to live in school districts with online-only reopening plans, and children in white households were more likely than all other demographic groups to have received some in-person instruction during the 2020-21 school year (Figure 6.17, Panel A) (Smith and Reeves, 2021[120]). Similarly, in April-May 2021, of those households where children were unable to attend day-care or other caring arrangements in the past month due to COVID-19, white adults were more likely to cut their work hours compared to members of different racial and ethnic groups, but were less likely to lose their job (Figure 6.17, Panel B). Further, nearly half of Black children in the United States are raised by solo mothers, compared to 17% of all other children, making parental support during home schooling more difficult relative to work obligations (Smith and Reeves, 2021[120]).

Conversely, the shift to online parent-teacher conferences has facilitated inclusion of parents whose work schedules typically conflict with such meetings (OECD, 2021[111]). Results from a survey of 34 OECD countries in January and February 2021 showed that governments have provided school systems with guidelines for keeping communication channels with parents open during COVID-19 learning disruptions. The most commonly used methods include e-school platforms, phone calls to students and/or parents, emails to students and/or parents, regular conversations with parents, video conference technology and text/WhatsApp messaging (OECD, 2021[111]). Pre-pandemic evidence from the OECD's 2018 PISA study showed that parents with children in more socio-economically advantaged schools were more likely to discuss their child's academic progress with teachers, compared to more disadvantaged schools where teachers were more likely to take the initiative. The most commonly cited reason for parents to not participate in school activities was the need to work (34%), followed by inconvenient meeting times (33%) (OECD, 2019[121]).

Figure 6.17. In the United States, education and childcare arrangements during COVID-19 differ along racial and ethnic lines

Education- and child-care related outcomes for households with children in the United States, by race/ethnicity, Apr-May 2021

Panel A. Share of households in which children received in-person instruction from a teacher at their school during the 2020-21 school year, by race/ethnicity

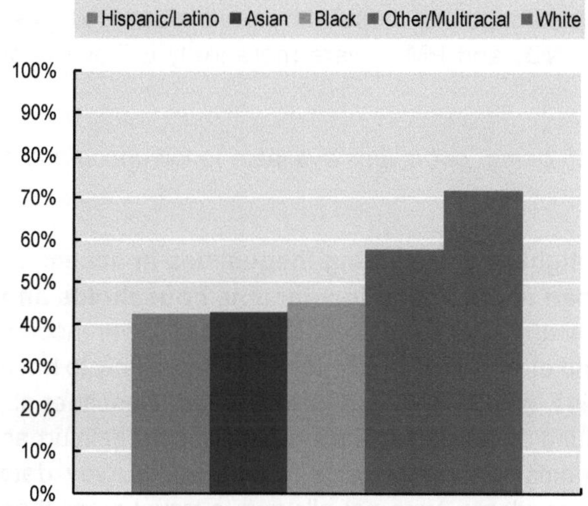

Panel B. Share of households in which children were unable to attend daycare because of COVID-19 in the past month (7% of all households with children), and in which in order to care for the children, an adult..., by race/ethnicity

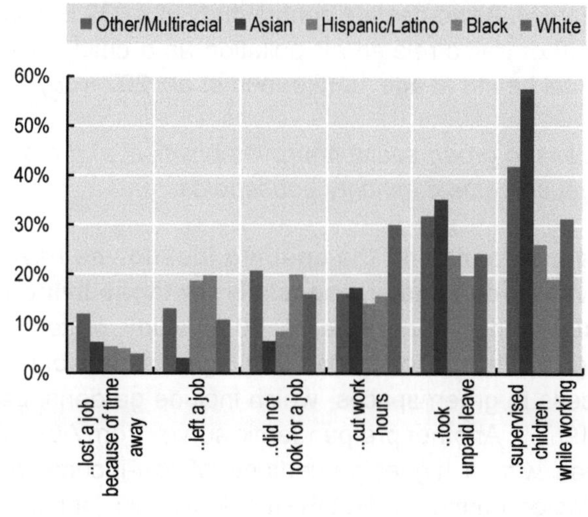

Source: United States Census Bureau (n.d.[87]), *Measuring household experiences during the coronavirus pandemic* (database), https://www.census.gov/householdpulsedata (refer to Box 3.1 for methodological details).

StatLink https://stat.link/ij4fgp

6.4. Environmental quality

6.4.1. Air pollution and access to green space

Confinement regulations have affected air pollution, leaving some groups more vulnerable to its negative impacts

Research suggests that prolonged exposure to air pollution exacerbates COVID-19 symptoms (Chapter 3)**, and that socio-economically disadvantaged households are often more exposed to air pollution** (Brunekreef, 2021[122]; Kerr, Goldberg and Anenberg, 2021[123]), which – coupled with a higher probability of having underlying health conditions, and a greater likelihood of inability to work from home – worsens their COVID-19 outcomes. Pre-COVID studies in England and the Netherlands showed that PM_{10} and NO_2 concentrations are higher in more deprived areas, as well as in ethnic minority neighbourhoods. However, while it is often assumed that poorer areas have worse air pollution, within Western Europe this is not always the case: some of the most polluted regions are among the wealthiest (examples include Lombardy and Emilia Romagna in northern Italy, and Flemish Brabant and Wallonia Brabant in Belgium) (Brunekreef, 2021[122]). While some studies in Europe may bring mixed results, research in North America shows that areas with a high concentration of low-economic status communities tend to have higher concentrations of air pollutants (Hajat, Hsia and O'Neill, 2015[124]).

Because of the pandemic, people are spending more time than ever indoors, which increases the risks of indoor air pollution from extended cooking time, gas stove usage and occupant density (Chapter 3). Occupants of lower socio-economic households are more likely to live in over-crowded dwellings with poor ventilation, exacerbating these risks (Ferguson et al., 2020[125]). These households also tend to have more smokers; the risk of second-hand smoke, especially for children, will be higher during COVID-19 due to increased time spent indoors (Brunekreef, 2021[122]).

Reductions in traffic pollutants may be especially important for children living in urban areas. Confinement measures led to short-term drops in traffic-related pollutants: NO_2 levels decreased 30-50% during European lockdowns, although $PM_{2.5}$ levels decreased only slightly (5 to 20%) (Brunekreef, 2021[122]). A two-decade cohort study of 2 039 British children found that those who were exposed to higher levels of traffic-related air pollution as a child, especially NO_2 and PM_{10}, were more likely to have poor mental health at age 18 (Reuben et al., 2021[126]).[30]

Access to green space improves physical and mental well-being, but is less available to low-income and racial and ethnic minority households

The pandemic and the ensuing lockdowns have highlighted pre-existing inequalities in access to private green space, especially for those living in urban areas and in low-income households and racial/ethnic minorities. A 2019 study of ten cities in the United States found that lower-income neighbourhoods, and those with higher shares of racial and ethnic minority groups, were less likely to have access to green spaces, which include gardens, balconies, small parks and nearby trees (Nesbitt et al., 2019[127]). Another pre-pandemic survey from Australia found that green space availability is lower in urban areas with a higher percentage of low-income households (Astell-Burt et al., 2014[128]). Survey data collected during the first French lockdown (during which residents were not allowed to travel more than 1 kilometre from their home) showed, perhaps unsurprisingly, that those living in urban areas were less likely to access green areas (Recchi et al., 2020[129]). Data collected in England during the pandemic found that those living in poverty were almost three times less likely to have access to either shared or private outdoor space (Natural England, 2020[130]; ONS, 2020[131]), and that Black people were four times as likely as white to have no access to outdoor space at home (including private or shared gardens, a patio or balcony) (Figure 6.18, Panel A). However, this same study found more equality in access to public spaces: people living in the most deprived areas have greater access to public parks within a five minutes' walk (at 34%) than do those living in the least deprived areas (18%) (ONS, 2020[131]).

The benefits of outdoor play for young children are well established (Burns and Gottschalk, 2020[132]; Brussoni, 2019[133]) **and outdoor activity has been disrupted due to confinement regulations in many OECD countries.** An online study of around 1 500 Canadian parents in April 2020 found that only 4.8% of children (5-11 years-old) and 0.6% of youth (12 to 17) were getting the recommended amount of physical activity time outdoors per day, compared to 12.7% of 5 to 17 year-olds before the pandemic. Children whose parents encouraged physical activity were more likely to play outdoors, as were children living in detached houses (rather than apartments) and those with pet dogs (Moore et al., 2020[134]). A study of 5-13 year-olds in the United States from 25 April to 16 May 2020 found that 36% of parents reported their child had engaged in much less physical activity over the past 7 days, as compared to February 2020 (before the start of the pandemic); only 11% stated their child had increased their amount of physical activity. However, for those engaging in exercise, the likelihood of exercising at home, in the garage or on sidewalks and roads in their neighbourhood increased from pre-COVID time periods (Dunton, Do and Wang, 2020[135]). Pre-pandemic research in the United States has shown that the majority of youth from low-income families engage in physical activity through after-school programmes: during lockdowns, children who do not have access to safe outdoor areas to exercise will be more adversely affected (Romero, 2005[136]). A study of 1 500 15-year-old children in England found that 60% reported having spent less time outdoors since the start of the pandemic (Figure 6.18, Panel B). Certain groups were more affected than others: 71% of children from ethnic minority backgrounds said they spent less time outdoors, compared to 57% of white children, as did 73% of children from low-income households, compared to 57% of children from higher-income households (Natural England, 2020[137]).

Figure 6.18. In England, access to green space was unequal before the pandemic, and children's use of outdoor space has fallen during the pandemic

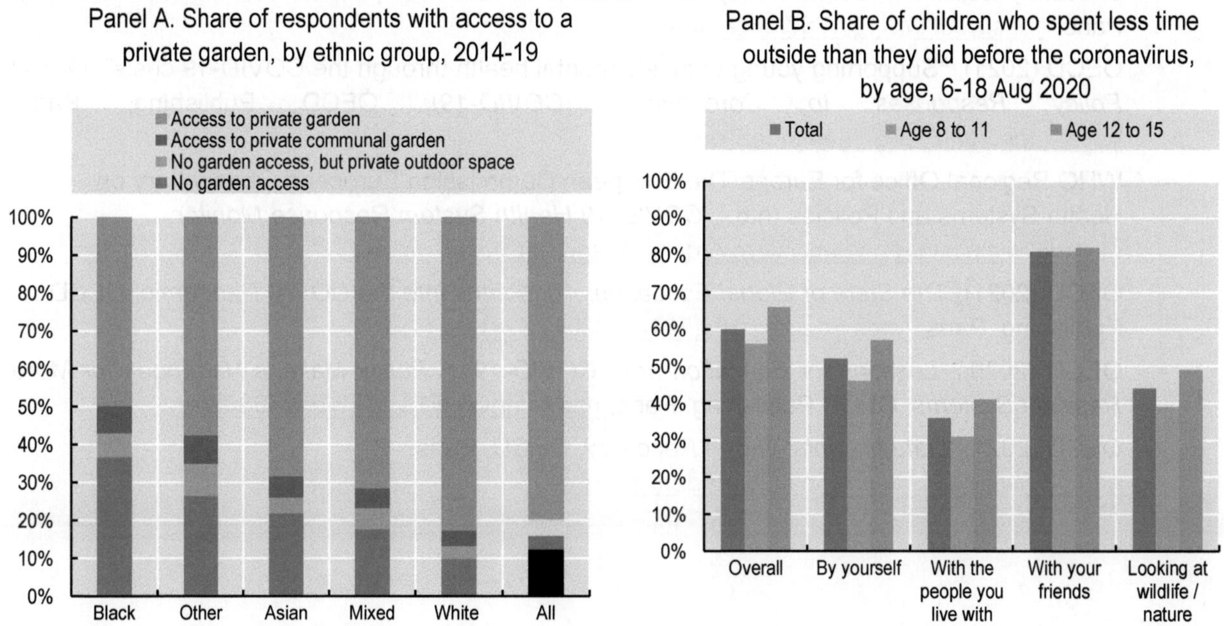

Note: Panel A shows the share of people with access to a private garden by ethnic group in England. Data come from the Natural England – Monitor of Engagement with Natural Environment Survey and refer to the years 2014-2019. Panel B depicts the share of children, by age, who report having spent less time outside since the start of COVID-19. Data come from the People and Nature Survey for England. The survey ran from 6-18 August 2020 and includes data from 1 501 respondents.

Source: ONS (2020[131]), *One in eight British households has no garden* (database), Office for National Statistics, https://www.ons.gov.uk/economy/environmentalaccounts/articles/oneineightbritishhouseholdshasnogarden/2020-05-14; and Natural England (2020[137]), *The people and nature survey for England: Children's survey (experimental statistics)* (database), Office for National Statistics, https://www.gov.uk/government/statistics/the-people-and-nature-survey-for-england-child-data-wave-1-experimental-statistics/the-people-and-nature-survey-for-england-childrens-survey-experimental-statistics#childrens-time-outside-during-the-pandemic.

StatLink https://stat.link/inv0kc

Box 6.5. Further reading

- OECD (forthcoming), *Health at a Glance 2021: OECD Indicators*, OECD Publishing, Paris
- OECD (2021), "Tackling the mental health impact of the COVID-19 crisis: An integrated, whole-of-society response," *OECD Policy Responses to Coronavirus (COVID-19),* OECD Publishing, Paris, https://doi.org/10.1787/0ccafa0b-en
- OECD (2021), "Supporting young people's mental health through the COVID-19 crisis", *OECD Policy Responses to Coronavirus (COVID-19),* OECD Publishing, Paris, https://doi.org/10.1787/84e143e5-en
- WHO Regional Office for Europe/The European Commission/European Observatory on Health Systems and Policies (n.d.), *COVID-19 Health System Response Monitor*, https://www.covid19healthsystem.org/mainpage.aspx
- OECD (2021), *The State of Global Education: 18 Months into the COVID Pandemic*, OECD Publishing, Paris, https://doi.org/10.1787/1a23bb23-en
- OECD (2020]), *Lessons for Education from COVID-19: A Policy Maker's Handbook for More Resilient Systems*, OECD Publishing, Paris, https://doi.org/10.1787/0a530888-en
- OECD (2021), *Data Insights: Green Recovery*, OECD, Paris, http://www.oecd.org/coronavirus/en/data-insights

References

Abdallah, S. and S. Shah (2012), *Well-being Patterns Uncovered: An analysis of UK data*, New Economics Foundation, https://neweconomics.org/2012/11/well-patterns-uncovered. [142]

ABS (2016), *Australian Demographic Statistics, Jun 2016*, Australian Demographic Statistics, https://www.abs.gov.au/AUSSTATS/abs@.nsf/7d12b0f6763c78caca257061001cc588/2d2860dfa430d432ca2580eb001335bb!OpenDocument (accessed on 21 June 2021). [144]

Adams-Prassl, A. et al. (2020), "Inequality in the impact of the coronavirus shock: Evidence from real time surveys", *IZA Discussion Paper* 13183, https://www.iza.org/publications/dp/13183/inequality-in-the-impact-of-the-coronavirus-shock-evidence-from-real-time-surveys. [95]

AIHW (2021), *The first year of COVID-19 in Australia: direct and indirect health effects, Summary - Australian Institute of Health and Welfare*, Australian Institute of Health and Welfare, https://www.aihw.gov.au/reports/burden-of-disease/the-first-year-of-covid-19-in-australia/summary. [38]

Alhmidi, M. (2020), "Feds need better data on COVID-19 in Indigenous communities, Marc Miller says", *CBC News*, https://www.cbc.ca/news/canada/saskatchewan/federal-government-covid-19-data-indigenous-communities-1.5811043. [41]

Ali, M. et al. (2019), "Utilization of mental health services in educational setting by adolescents in the United States", *Journal of School Health*, Vol. 89/5, pp. 393-401, http://dx.doi.org/10.1111/josh.12753. [57]

Alon, T. et al. (2020), "The impact of COVID-19 on gender equality", *NBER Working Paper Series*, No. 26947, National Bureau of Economics, https://www.nber.org/system/files/working_papers/w26947/w26947.pdf. [96]

Andrew, A. et al. (2020), *Learning during the lockdown: Real-time data on children's experiences during home learning*, Institute for Fiscal Studies, http://dx.doi.org/10.1920/BN.IFS.2020.BN0288. [116]

Arias, E., B. Tejada-Vera and F. Ahmad (2021), "Provisional life expectancy estimates for January through June, 2020", *Vital Statistics Rapid Release*, Vol. 10, https://www.cdc.gov/nchs/data/vsrr/VSRR10-508.pdf (accessed on 3 March 2021). [23]

Armbruster, S. and V. Klotzbücher (2020), "COVID-19, social distancing, and mental health in Germany", *Albert-Ludwigs-Universität Freiburg, Wilfried-Guth-Stiftungsprofessur für Ordnungs- und Wettbewerbspolitik, Freiburg i. Br.* Diskussionsbeiträge, 2020-04, http://hdl.handle.net/10419/218885. [98]

Astell-Burt, T. et al. (2014), "Do low-income neighbourhoods have the least green space? A cross-sectional study of Australia's most populous cities", *BMC Public Health*, Vol. 14/1, pp. 1-11, http://dx.doi.org/10.1186/1471-2458-14-292. [128]

Australian Government Department of Health (2021), "Communicable Diseases Intelligence 2021 - Aboriginal and Torres Strait Islander Epidemiology Report on COVID-19, 28 February 2021", *Communicable Diseases Intelligence*, No. 45, http://dx.doi.org/10.33321/cdi.2021.45.27. [36]

Australian Institute of Health and Welfare (2019), *Profile of Indigenous Australians*, Australia's Welfare 2019, https://www.aihw.gov.au/reports/australias-welfare/profile-of-indigenous-australians. [143]

Bartlett, T. (2021), "The pandemic suicide crisis is unsupported by the data", *The Atlantic*, https://www.theatlantic.com/health/archive/2021/04/pandemic-suicide-crisis-unsupported-data/618660/. [88]

Berlin, G. et al. (2021), *The US nursing workforce in 2021*, McKinsey & Company, https://www.mckinsey.com/industries/healthcare-systems-and-services/our-insights/nursing-in-2021-retaining-the-healthcare-workforce-when-we-need-it-most. [74]

Brunekreef, B. (2021), *Air Pollution and COVID-19*, Policy Department for Economic, Scientific and Quality of Life Policies, https://www.europarl.europa.eu/RegData/etudes/STUD/2021/658216/IPOL_STU(2021)658216_EN.pdf. [122]

Brussoni, M. (2019), "Why outdoor play?", *Encyclopedia on Early Childhood Development*, https://www.child-encyclopedia.com/outdoor-play. [133]

Burns, T. and F. Gottschalk (eds.) (2020), *Education in the Digital Age: Healthy and Happy Children*, Educational Research and Innovation, OECD Publishing, Paris, https://dx.doi.org/10.1787/1209166a-en. [132]

Carey, B. (2021), "Why older people managed to stay happier through the pandemic", *The New York Times*, https://www.nytimes.com/2021/03/12/health/covid-pandemic-happiness-age.html. [108]

Carstensen, L., Y. Shavit and J. Barnes (2020), "Age Advantages in Emotional Experience Persist Even Under Threat From the COVID-19 Pandemic", *Psychological Science*, Vol. 31/11, pp. 1374-1385, http://dx.doi.org/10.1177/0956797620967261. [107]

CDC (2021), *COVID-19 hospitalization and death by race/ethnicity (database)*, https://www.cdc.gov/coronavirus/2019-ncov/covid-data/investigations-discovery/hospitalization-death-by-race-ethnicity.html#footnote01 (accessed on 11 February 2021). [27]

Center for Translational Neuroscience (2020), "Flattening the other curve: Trends for young children's mental health are good for some but concerning for others", *Medium*, https://medium.com/rapid-ec-project/flattening-the-other-curve-7be1e574b340. [71]

CEPREMAP/INSEE (n.d.), *Le bien-être en France*, http://www.cepremap.fr/Duree.html (accessed on 15 June 2021). [104]

Chen, L. et al. (2021), *Teacher Survey: Learning loss is global — and significant*, McKinsey & Company, https://www.mckinsey.com/industries/public-and-social-sector/our-insights/teacher-survey-learning-loss-is-global-and-significant?cid=other-eml-alt-mip-mck&hdpid=1a57cf47-eae2-400f-b9f0-fd8edddbbfb6&hctky=2909643&hlkid=b53175decdec48bbb6888bd21b5a168b (accessed on 10 June 2021). [112]

Chetty, R. et al. (2016), "The association between income and life expectancy in the United States, 2001-2014", *JAMA - Journal of the American Medical Association*, Vol. 315/16, pp. 1750-1766, http://dx.doi.org/10.1001/jama.2016.4226. [6]

Chinnappan, S. (2021), *Long COVID: The impact on women and ongoing research*, Society for Women's Health Research, https://swhr.org/long-covid-the-impact-on-women-and-ongoing-research/. [2]

Cook, D. et al. (2020), "He kāhui waiora: Living standards framework and he ara waiora COVID-19: Impacts on wellbeing", *Discussion Papers*, No. 20/02, The New Zealand Treasury, https://www.treasury.govt.nz/publications/dp/dp-20-02. [44]

COVID Impact Survey (2020), *Social, economic, health impacts persist as Americans grapple with convergence of pandemic and civil unrest*, https://www.covid-impact.org/blog/social-economic-health-impacts-persist-as-americans-grapple-with-convergence-of-pandemic-and-civil-unrest. [67]

Czeisler, M. et al. (2020), "Mental health, substance use, and suicidal ideation during the COVID-19 pandemic — United States, June 24–30, 2020", *Morbidity and Mortality Weekly Report*, Vol. 69/32, pp. 1049-1057, http://dx.doi.org/10.15585/mmwr.mm6932a1. [79]

Department of Finance Canada (2021), *Budget 2021: A recovery plan for jobs, growth, and resilience, Annex 4: Gender, diversity, and quality of life statement*, https://www.budget.gc.ca/2021/report-rapport/anx4-en.html. [145]

Devlin, K. and N. Kent (2021), *As pandemic continues, more in US and Europe feel major impact on their lives*, Pew Research Center, https://www.pewresearch.org/global/2021/02/03/as-pandemic-continues-more-in-u-s-and-europe-feel-major-impact-on-their-lives/. [94]

Di Pietro, G. et al. (2020), *The Likely Impact of COVID-19 on Education: Reflections based on the existing literature and recent international datasets*, Publications Office of the European Union, Luxembourg, http://dx.doi.org/10.2760/126686. [115]

Dong, E., H. Du and L. Gardner (2020), "An interactive web-based dashboard to track COVID-19 in real time", *The Lancet Infectious Diseases*, Vol. 20/5, pp. 533-534, http://dx.doi.org/10.1016/S1473-3099(20)30120-1. [42]

Drefahl, S. et al. (2020), "A population-based cohort study of socio-demographic risk factors for COVID-19 deaths in Sweden", *Nature Communications*, Vol. 11/1, pp. 1-7, http://dx.doi.org/10.1038/s41467-020-18926-3. [8]

Dunton, G., B. Do and S. Wang (2020), "Early effects of the COVID-19 pandemic on physical activity and sedentary behavior in children living in the U.S", *BMC Public Health*, Vol. 20/1351, http://dx.doi.org/10.1186/s12889-020-09429-3. [135]

Durães e Lusa, M. (2020), "O confinamento em família foi "sufocante" para 35% dos jovens LGBT+", *Público*, https://www.publico.pt/2020/05/18/p3/noticia/confinamento-familia-sufocante-35-jovens-lgbt-1917027. [63]

ECLAC (2021), *The Impact of COVID-19 on Indigenous Peoples in Latin America (Abya Yala): Between invisibility and collective resistance*, United Nations Economic Commission for Latin America and the Caribbean, https://www.cepal.org/en/publications/46698-impact-covid-19-indigenous-peoples-latin-america-abya-yala-between-invisibility. [47]

Eichenbaum, M., S. Rebelo and M. Trabandt (2020), "Inequality in Life and Death", https://www.kellogg.northwestern.edu/faculty/rebelo/htm/inequality.pdf. [16]

El Heraldo (2021), "Línea de atención en salud mental recibió más de 18 mil llamadas en pandemia", *El Heraldo*, https://www.elheraldo.co/colombia/linea-de-atencion-en-salud-mental-recibio-mas-de-18-mil-llamadas-en-un-ano-de-pandemia. [64]

Engzell, P., A. Frey and M. Verhagen (2021), "Learning loss due to school closures during the COVID-19 pandemic", *Proceedings of the National Academy of Sciences of the United States of America*, Vol. 118/17, p. e2022376118, http://dx.doi.org/10.1073/PNAS.2022376118. [118]

Eurostat (n.d.), *European health interview survey (EHIS) (database)*, https://ec.europa.eu/eurostat/statistics-explained/index.php?title=Glossary:European_health_interview_survey_(EHIS) (accessed on 16 June 2021). [53]

FAIR Health (2021), "The impact of COVID-19 on pediatric mental health: A study of private healthcare claims", *FAIR Health White Paper*, https://s3.amazonaws.com/media2.fairhealth.org/whitepaper/asset/The%20Impact%20of%20COVID-19%20on%20Pediatric%20Mental%20Health%20-%20A%20Study%20of%20Private%20Healthcare%20Claims%20-%20A%20FAIR%20Health%20White%20Paper.pdf. [90]

Ferguson, L. et al. (2020), "Exposure to indoor air pollution across socio-economic groups in high-income countries: A scoping review of the literature and a modelling methodology", *Environment International*, Vol. 143, http://dx.doi.org/10.1016/j.envint.2020.105748. [125]

Finch, W. and M. Hernández Finch (2020), "Poverty and COVID-19: Rates of incidence and deaths in the United States during the first 10 weeks of the pandemic", *Frontiers in Sociology*, Vol. 5/47, http://dx.doi.org/10.3389/FSOC.2020.00047. [15]

Gallup (n.d.), *Gallup World Poll*, https://www.gallup.com/analytics/318875/global-research.aspx (accessed on 18 June 2021). [100]

Goldberg, D. and P. Williams (1988), *A User's Guide to the General Health Questionnaire*, NFER-Nelson, Windsor. [139]

Government of Canada (2020), *Government of Canada COVID-19 update for Indigenous Peoples and communities*, https://www.canada.ca/en/indigenous-services-canada/news/2020/11/government-of-canada-covid-19-update-for-indigenous-peoples-and-communities1.html. [40]

Graham, C. et al. (2020), *Well-being and mental health amid COVID-19: Differences in resilience across minorities and whites*, The Brookings Institution, https://www.brookings.edu/research/well-being-and-mental-health-amid-covid-19-differences-in-resilience-across-minorities-and-whites/. [30]

Hajat, A., C. Hsia and M. O'Neill (2015), "Socioeconomic disparities and air pollution exposure: A global review", *Current environmental health reports*, Vol. 2/4, pp. 440-450, http://dx.doi.org/10.1007/s40572-015-0069-5. [124]

Hale, T. et al. (2021), "A global panel database of pandemic policies (Oxford COVID-19 Government Response Tracker)", *Nature Human Behaviour*, Vol. 5/4, pp. 529-538, http://dx.doi.org/10.1038/s41562-021-01079-8 (accessed on 11 June 2021). [101]

Hawton, K. et al. (2021), “Self-harm and the COVID-19 pandemic: A study of factors contributing to self-harm during lockdown restrictions”, *Journal of Psychiatric Research*, Vol. 137, pp. 437-443, http://dx.doi.org/10.1016/j.jpsychires.2021.03.028. [89]

Hélary, L. (2020), “École à la maison: Des inégalités de pédagogie selon les familles”, *Ouest France*, https://www.ouest-france.fr/education/enseignement/ecole-la-maison-des-inegalites-de-pedagogie-selon-les-familles-6830947. [117]

Helliwell, J. et al. (2021), *World Happiness Report 2021*, Sustainable Development Solutions Network, https://worldhappiness.report/ed/2021/. [93]

Helliwell, J., G. Schellenberg and J. Fonberg (2020), “Life satisfaction in Canada before and during the COVID-19 pandemic”, *Analytical Studies Branch Research Paper Series*, No. 457, Statistics Canada, https://www150.statcan.gc.ca/n1/en/pub/11f0019m/11f0019m2020020-eng.pdf?st=s6m4rNgZ (accessed on 11 February 2021). [102]

Hlavinka, E. (2020), “Navajo Country: COVID-19 cases trend down, but need still high”, *MedPageToday*, https://www.medpagetoday.com/infectiousdisease/covid19/88041. [35]

Huebener, M. et al. (2020), “Parental well-being in times of COVID-19 in Germany”, *IZA Discussion Paper*, No. 13556, https://www.iza.org/de/publications/dp/13556/parental-well-being-in-times-of-covid-19-in-germany. [99]

Imperial College London YouGov (2020), *Covid-19 behaviour tracker data hub*, https://github.com/YouGov-Data/covid-19-tracker (accessed on 21 July 2021). [52]

Iob, E., A. Steptoe and D. Fancourt (2020), “Abuse, self-harm and suicidal ideation in the UK during the COVID-19 pandemic”, *The British Journal of Psychiatry*, Vol. 217/4, pp. 543-546, http://dx.doi.org/10.1192/BJP.2020.130. [85]

Japanese National Police Agency (2021), *令和２年中における自殺の状況*, https://www.npa.go.jp/safetylife/seianki/jisatsu/R03/R02_jisatuno_joukyou.pdf (accessed on 10 June 2021). [92]

Kaliszewski, M. (2021), *Substance Abuse in Doctors - Statistics and treatment options*, American Addiction Centers, https://americanaddictioncenters.org/medical-professionals/substance-abuse-among-doctors-key-statistics. [76]

Keck, M. (2020), “COVID-19 rates among Indigenous Australians are low thanks to an “extraordinary” Aboriginal-led response”, *Global Citizen*, https://www.globalcitizen.org/en/content/covid-19-rates-indigenous-australians/. [37]

Keeter, S. (2020), “People financially affected by COVID-19 outbreak are experiencing more psychological distress than others”, *Pewresearch.org*, https://www.pewresearch.org/fact-tank/2020/03/30/people-financially-affected-by-covid-19-outbreak-are-experiencing-more-psychological-distress-than-others/. [68]

Kelland, K. (2021), “Women in 40s, 50s who survive COVID more likely to suffer persistent problems: UK studies”, *Reuters*, https://www.reuters.com/article/us-health-coronavirus-longcovid-women-idUSKBN2BG1SO. [1]

Kerr, G., D. Goldberg and S. Anenberg (2021), “COVID-19 pandemic reveals persistent disparities in nitrogen dioxide pollution”, *Proceedings of the National Academy of Sciences*, Vol. 118/30, p. e2022409118, http://dx.doi.org/10.1073/PNAS.2022409118. [123]

Kneale, D. and L. Bécares (2020), "The mental health and experiences of discrimination of LGBTQ+ people during the COVID-19 pandemic: Initial findings from the Queerantine Study", *medRxiv*, http://dx.doi.org/10.1101/2020.08.03.20167403. [62]

Kroenke, K. et al. (2009), "An ultra-brief screening scale for anxiety and depression: the PHQ-4", *Psychosomatics*, Vol. 50/6, pp. 613-621, http://dx.doi.org/10.1176/APPI.PSY.50.6.613. [140]

Kühne, S. et al. (2020), "The need for household panel surveys in times of crisis: The case of SOEP-CoV", *Survey Research Methods*, Vol. 14/2, pp. 195-203, https://doi.org/10.18148/srm/2020.v14i2.7748 (accessed on 19 May 2021). [81]

Lakhani, N. (2021), "Exclusive: Indigenous Americans dying from COVID at twice the rate of white Americans", *The Guardian*, https://www.theguardian.com/us-news/2021/feb/04/native-americans-coronavirus-covid-death-rate. [34]

Leslie, E. and R. Wilson (2021), "Sheltering in place and domestic violence: Evidence from calls for service during COVID-19", *Journal of Public Economics*, http://dx.doi.org/10.2139/ssrn.3600646. [97]

Lu, D. (2021), "Which groups are still dying of Covid in the U.S.?", *The New York Times*, https://www.nytimes.com/interactive/2021/06/10/us/covid-death-patterns.html?action=click&module=Top%20Stories&pgtype=Homepage. [3]

MacBride, K. (2020), "With COVID-19, healthcare workers are even more vulnerable to suicide", *Healthline*, https://www.healthline.com/health/mental-health/healthcare-workers-suicide-covid-19#1. [78]

Marmot, M. et al. (2010), *Fair society healthy lives (The Marmot Review)*, Institute of Health Equity, https://www.instituteofhealthequity.org/resources-reports/fair-society-healthy-lives-the-marmot-review. [5]

McFarling, U. (2020), "Fearing deportation, many immigrants at higher risk of Covid-19 are afraid to seek testing or care", *StatNews*, https://www.statnews.com/2020/04/15/fearing-deportation-many-immigrants-at-higher-risk-of-covid-19-are-afraid-to-seek-testing-or-care/. [21]

Ministry of Health New Zealand (2021), *COVID-19: Case demographics*, https://www.health.govt.nz/our-work/diseases-and-conditions/covid-19-novel-coronavirus/covid-19-data-and-statistics/covid-19-case-demographics. [45]

Moore, S. et al. (2020), "Impact of the COVID-19 virus outbreak on movement and play behaviours of Canadian children and youth: A national survey", *International Journal of Behavioral Nutrition and Physical Activity*, Vol. 17/1, pp. 1-11, http://dx.doi.org/10.1186/s12966-020-00987-8. [134]

Morgan, D. et al. (2020), "Excess mortality: Measuring the direct and indirect impact of COVID-19", *OECD Health Working Papers*, No. 122, OECD Publishing, Paris, https://dx.doi.org/10.1787/c5dc0c50-en. [150]

Natural England (2020), *The people and nature survey for England: Adult data Y1Q1 (April - June 2020) (experimental statistics)*, Natural England, https://www.gov.uk/government/statistics/the-people-and-nature-survey-for-england-adult-data-y1q1-april-june-2020-experimental-statistics/the-people-and-nature-survey-for-england-adult-data-y1q1-april-june-2020-experimental-statistics (accessed on 24 February 2021). [130]

Natural England (2020), *The people and nature survey for England: Children's survey (experimental statistics)*, https://www.gov.uk/government/statistics/the-people-and-nature-survey-for-england-child-data-wave-1-experimental-statistics/the-people-and-nature-survey-for-england-childrens-survey-experimental-statistics#childrens-time-outside-during-the-pandemic (accessed on 10 June 2021). [137]

NCHS (2020), *National Health Interview Survey Early Release Program*, National Center for Health Statistics, https://www.cdc.gov/nchs/data/nhis/earlyrelease/ERmentalhealthbyrace-508.pdf (accessed on 11 February 2021). [86]

Nesbitt, L. et al. (2019), "Who has access to urban vegetation? A spatial analysis of distributional green equity in 10 US cities", *Landscape and Urban Planning*, Vol. 181, pp. 51-79, http://dx.doi.org/10.1016/J.LANDURBPLAN.2018.08.007. [127]

NPR (2020), "As pandemic deaths add up, racial disparities persist — And in some cases worsen", *National Public Radio*, https://www.npr.org/sections/health-shots/2020/09/23/914427907/as-pandemic-deaths-add-up-racial-disparities-persist-and-in-some-cases-worsen?t=1608509692531&t=1612899321921. [146]

OECD (2021), "Securing the recovery, ambition, and resilience for the well-being of children in the post-COVID-19 decade", *OECD Policy Responses to Coronavirus (COVID-19)*, OECD Publishing, Paris, https://doi.org/10.1787/0f02237a-en. [114]

OECD (2021), "Supporting young people's mental health through the COVID-19 crisis", *OECD Policy Responses to Coronavirus (COVID-19)*, OECD Publishing, Paris, https://doi.org/10.1787/84e143e5-en. [56]

OECD (2021), "Tackling the mental health impact of the COVID-19 crisis: An integrated, whole-of-society response", *OECD Policy Responses to Coronavirus (COVID-19)*, OECD Publishing, Paris, https://doi.org/10.1787/0ccafa0b-en. [49]

OECD (2021), *The State of Global Education: 18 Months into the Pandemic*, OECD Publishing, Paris, https://doi.org/10.1787/1a23bb23-en. [113]

OECD (2021), *The State of School Education: One Year into the COVID Pandemic*, OECD Publishing, Paris, https://doi.org/10.1787/201dde84-en. [111]

OECD (2020), *How's Life? 2020: Measuring Well-being*, OECD Publishing, Paris, https://dx.doi.org/10.1787/9870c393-en. [4]

OECD (2020), *International Migration Outlook 2020*, OECD Publishing, Paris, https://dx.doi.org/10.1787/ec98f531-en. [147]

OECD (2020), *Linking Indigenous Communities with Regional Development in Canada*, OECD Rural Policy Reviews, OECD Publishing, Paris, https://dx.doi.org/10.1787/fa0f60c6-en. [43]

OECD (2020), "Policy implications of Coronavirus crisis for rural development", *OECD Policy Responses to Coronavirus (COVID-19)*, OECD Publishing, Paris, https://doi.org/10.1787/6b9d189a-en. [29]

OECD (2020), "What is the impact of the COVID-19 pandemic on immigrants and their children?", *OECD Policy Responses to Coronavirus (COVID-19)*, OECD Publishing, Paris, https://dx.doi.org/10.1787/e7cbb7de-en. [19]

OECD (2019), *PISA 2018 Results (volume III): What School Life Means for Students' Lives*, PISA, OECD Publishing, Paris, https://dx.doi.org/10.1787/acd78851-en. [121]

OECD (2017), *Health at a Glance 2017: OECD Indicators*, OECD Publishing, Paris, https://dx.doi.org/10.1787/health_glance-2017-en. [7]

OECD (n.d.), *COVID-19 Health Indicators (database)*, https://stats.oecd.org/index.aspx?queryid=104676# (accessed on 19 September 2021). [12]

ONS (2021), *Coronavirus and depression in adults, Great Britain: January to March 2021*, Office for National Statistics, https://www.ons.gov.uk/peoplepopulationandcommunity/wellbeing/articles/coronavirusanddepressioninadultsgreatbritain/januarytomarch2021. [65]

ONS (2021), *Prevalence of ongoing symptoms following coronavirus (COVID-19) infection in the UK*, Office for National Statistics, https://www.ons.gov.uk/peoplepopulationandcommunity/healthandsocialcare/conditionsanddiseases/bulletins/prevalenceofongoingsymptomsfollowingcoronaviruscovid19infectionintheuk/4june2021 (accessed on 21 June 2021). [14]

ONS (2021), *Technical article: Updated estimates of the prevalence of post-acute symptoms among people with coronavirus (COVID-19) in the UK*, Office for National Statistics, https://www.ons.gov.uk/peoplepopulationandcommunity/healthandsocialcare/conditionsanddiseases/articles/technicalarticleupdatedestimatesoftheprevalenceofpostacutesymptomsamongpeoplewithcoronaviruscovid19intheuk/26april2020to1august2021. [13]

ONS (2020), *Coronavirus and the social impacts on different ethnic groups in the UK: 2020*, Office for National Statistics, https://www.ons.gov.uk/peoplepopulationandcommunity/culturalidentity/ethnicity/articles/coronavirusandthesocialimpactsondifferentethnicgroupsintheuk/2020. [84]

ONS (2020), *Coronavirus and the social impacts on young people in Great Britain*, Office for National Statistics, https://www.ons.gov.uk/peoplepopulationandcommunity/birthsdeathsandmarriages/ageing/articles/coronavirusandthesocialimpactsonyoungpeopleingreatbritain/3aprilto10may2020#impacts-on-well-being (accessed on 21 June 2021). [103]

ONS (2020), *One in eight British households has no garden*, Office for National Statistics, https://www.ons.gov.uk/economy/environmentalaccounts/articles/oneineightbritishhouseholdshasnogarden/2020-05-14 (accessed on 24 February 2021). [131]

ONS (2020), *Updating ethnic contrasts in deaths involving the coronavirus (COVID-19), England and Wales: deaths occurring 2 March to 28 July 2020*, Office for National Statistics, https://www.ons.gov.uk/peoplepopulationandcommunity/birthsdeathsandmarriages/deaths/articles/updatingethniccontrastsindeathsinvolvingthecoronaviruscovid19englandandwales/deathsoccurring2marchto28july2020#main-points (accessed on 11 February 2021). [25]

ONS (2020), *Why have Black and South Asian people been hit hardest by COVID-19?*, Office for National Statistics, https://www.ons.gov.uk/peoplepopulationandcommunity/healthandsocialcare/conditionsanddiseases/articles/whyhaveblackandsouthasianpeoplebeenhithardestbycovid19/2020-12-14 (accessed on 11 February 2021). [28]

ONS (n.d.), *Personal and economic well-being in Great Britain: September 2020 (database)*, Office for National Statistics, https://www.ons.gov.uk/peoplepopulationandcommunity/wellbeing/datasets/incomegroupsplitestimatesonpersonalandeconomicwellbeingacrosstime (accessed on 15 December 2020). [109]

Our World in Data (n.d.), *Colombia: Coronavirus Pandemic Country Profile (database)*, https://ourworldindata.org/coronavirus/country/colombia (accessed on 22 September 2021). [48]

Potloc (2020), *Insights from the Canadian front lines of the COVID-19 pandemic*, Potloc, https://www.potloc.com/blog/en/potloc-study-canadian-health-workers-insights-front-lines-covid-19-pandemic. [73]

Racine, N. et al. (2021), "When the bough breaks: A systematic review and meta-analysis of mental health symptoms in mothers of young children during the COVID-19 pandemic", http://dx.doi.org/10.31234/OSF.IO/U8PNH. [51]

Racine, N. et al. (2021), "Maternal depressive and anxiety symptoms before and during the COVID-19 pandemic in Canada: a longitudinal analysis", *The Lancet Psychiatry*, Vol. 8/5, pp. 405-415, http://dx.doi.org/10.1016/S2215-0366(21)00074-2. [50]

Rahman, A. and V. Plummer (2020), "COVID-19 related suicide among hospital nurses: Case study evidence from worldwide media reports", *Psychiatry Research*, Vol. 291, p. 113272, http://dx.doi.org/10.1016/J.PSYCHRES.2020.113272. [77]

Rao, A. et al. (2021), "A disproportionate epidemic: COVID-19 cases and deaths among essential workers in Toronto, Canada", *medRxiv*, http://dx.doi.org/10.1101/2021.02.15.21251572. [18]

Raybaud, A. (2021), "Anorexie, boulimie… La crise sanitaire provoque une hausse inquiétante des troubles alimentaires chez les jeunes adultes", *Le Monde*, https://www.lemonde.fr/campus/article/2021/04/27/anorexie-boulimie-la-hausse-inquietante-des-troubles-alimentaires-chez-les-jeunes-adultes_6078198_4401467.html#xtor=AL-32280270. [61]

Ray, R. (2020), *Why are Blacks dying at higher rates from COVID-19?*, The Brookings Institution, https://www.brookings.edu/blog/fixgov/2020/04/09/why-are-blacks-dying-at-higher-rates-from-covid-19/. [32]

Recchi, E. et al. (2020), "Lockdown for all, hardship for some: Insights from the first wave of the CoCo project", *HAL*, https://halshs.archives-ouvertes.fr/halshs-03070206/document. [129]

Rentsch, C. et al. (2020), "Patterns of COVID-19 testing and mortality by race and ethnicity among United States veterans: A nationwide cohort study", *PLOS Medicine*, Vol. 17/9, http://dx.doi.org/10.1371/journal.pmed.1003379. [138]

Reuben, A. et al. (2021), "Association of air pollution exposure in childhood and adolescence with psychopathology at the transition to adulthood", *JAMA Network Open*, Vol. 4/4, http://dx.doi.org/10.1001/JAMANETWORKOPEN.2021.7508. [126]

Rho, H., H. Brown and S. Fremstad (2020), *A basic demographic profile of workers in frontline industries*, Center for Economic and Policy Research, Washington, D.C., https://cepr.net/wp-content/uploads/2020/04/2020-04-Frontline-Workers.pdf?__cf_chl_jschl_tk__=pmd_.7KR_H_gmypiRrI3OgamZtEQpg9w0Ec20tjZf0aMaoc-1631627106-0-gqNtZGzNAlCjcnBszQcI. [17]

Richard, L. et al. (2021), "Testing, infection and complication rates of COVID-19 among people with a recent history of homelessness in Ontario, Canada: A retrospective cohort study", *Canadian Medical Association Open Access Journal*, Vol. 9/1, pp. E1-E9, http://dx.doi.org/10.9778/CMAJO.20200287. [11]

Richardson, L. and A. Crawford (2020), "How Indigenous communities in Canada organized an exemplary public health response to COVID", *Scientific American*, https://www.scientificamerican.com/article/how-indigenous-communities-in-canada-organized-an-exemplary-public-health-response-to-covid/. [39]

Rich, M. and H. Hida (2021), "As pandemic took hold, suicide rose among Japanese women", *The New York Times*, https://www.nytimes.com/2021/02/22/world/asia/japan-women-suicide-coronavirus.html. [91]

Robert Koch Institut (2021), *Soziale Unterschiede in der COVID-19-Sterblichkeit während der zweiten Infektionswelle in Deutschland*, https://www.rki.de/DE/Content/GesundAZ/S/Sozialer_Status_Ungleichheit/Faktenblatt_COVID-19-Sterblichkeit.html. [9]

Romero, A. (2005), "Low-income neighborhood barriers and resources for adolescents' physical activity", *Journal of Adolescent Health*, Vol. 36/3, pp. 253-259, http://dx.doi.org/10.1016/j.jadohealth.2004.02.027. [136]

Schernhammer, E. and G. Colditz (2004), "Suicide rates among physicians: A quantitative and gender assessment (meta-analysis)", *The American Journal of Psychiatry*, Vol. 161/12, pp. 2295-2302, http://dx.doi.org/10.1176/APPI.AJP.161.12.2295. [75]

SDSN Secretariat (2020), *New report highlights the impact of COVID-19 on life satisfaction worldwide*, Sustainable Development Solutions Network, https://www.unsdsn.org/new-report-highlights-the-impact-of-covid-19-on-life-satisfaction-worldwide. [105]

Smith, E. and R. Reeves (2021), *Black moms facing the toughest childcare crunch: How policy can help*, The Brookings Institution, https://www.brookings.edu/blog/how-we-rise/2021/02/24/black-moms-facing-the-toughest-childcare-crunch-how-policy-can-help/?utm_campaign=Economic%20Studies&utm_medium=email&utm_content=113794600&utm_source=hs_email. [120]

Solmi, F., J. Downs and D. Nicholls (2021), "COVID-19 and eating disorders in young people", *The Lancet Child and Adolescent Health*, Vol. 5, pp. 316-318, https://doi.org/10.1016/S2352-4642(21)00094-8. [60]

Spettigue, W. et al. (2021), "The impact of COVID-19 on adolescents with eating disorders: a cohort study", *Journal of Eating Disorders*, Vol. 9/1, p. 65, http://dx.doi.org/10.1186/s40337-021-00419-3. [58]

Spitzer, R. et al. (2006), "A brief measure for assessing generalized anxiety disorder: The GAD-7", *Archives of internal medicine*, Vol. 166/10, pp. 1092-1097, http://dx.doi.org/10.1001/ARCHINTE.166.10.1092. [141]

Stantcheva, S. (2021), *Inequalities in the times of a pandemic*, https://www.economic-policy.org/wp-content/uploads/2021/04/9103_Inequalities-in-the-Times-of-a-Pandemic.pdf. [10]

Statistics Canada (2021), *COVID-19 deaths among immigrants: Evidence from the early months of the pandemic*, https://www150.statcan.gc.ca/n1/pub/45-28-0001/2021001/article/00017-eng.htm (accessed on 22 September 2021). [20]

Statistics Canada (2021), *Provisional death counts and excess mortality, January to December 2020*, Statistics Canada, https://www150.statcan.gc.ca/n1/daily-quotidien/210310/dq210310c-eng.htm. [148]

Statistics Canada (2020), *COVID-19 mortality rates in Canada's ethno-cultural neighbourhoods*, https://www150.statcan.gc.ca/n1/pub/45-28-0001/2020001/article/00079-eng.htm (accessed on 11 February 2021). [26]

Statistics Canada (2020), *Gender differences in mental health during the COVID-19 pandemic*, StatCan COVID-19, https://www150.statcan.gc.ca/n1/pub/45-28-0001/2020001/article/00047-eng.htm (accessed on 3 March 2021). [55]

Statistics Canada (2020), *Impacts of COVID-19 on Canadians: Data collection series*, https://www23.statcan.gc.ca/imdb/p2SV.pl?Function=getSurvey&SDDS=5323. [54]

Statistics Canada (2020), *Impacts of COVID-19 on immigrants and people designated as visible minorities*, Statistics Canada, https://www150.statcan.gc.ca/n1/pub/11-631-x/2020004/s6-eng.htm. [33]

Statistics Canada (2020), *Indigenous people and mental health during the COVID-19 pandemic*, https://www150.statcan.gc.ca/n1/pub/45-28-0001/2020001/article/00035-eng.htm. [83]

Statistics Canada (2020), *School closures and the online preparedness of children during the COVID-19 pandemic*, https://www150.statcan.gc.ca/n1/pub/11-626-x/11-626-x2020001-eng.htm. [119]

Statistics Canada (2020), *The mental health of population groups designated as visible minorities in Canada during the COVID-19 pandemic*, https://www150.statcan.gc.ca/n1/pub/45-28-0001/2020001/article/00077-eng.htm (accessed on 10 February 2021). [82]

Steyn, N. et al. (2021), "Māori and Pacific People in New Zealand have higher risk of hospitalisation for COVID-19", *medRxiv*, http://dx.doi.org/10.1101/2020.12.25.20248427. [46]

Sze, S. et al. (2020), "Ethnicity and clinical outcomes in COVID-19: A systematic review and meta-analysis", *EClinicalMedicine*, Vol. 29-30, http://dx.doi.org/10.1016/j.eclinm.2020.100630. [22]

Tavernise, S. and A. Goodnough (2021), "Covid causes sharp drop in U.S. life expectancy", *The New York Times*, https://www.nytimes.com/2021/02/18/us/covid-life-expectancy.html. [24]

The COVID Tracking Project (2020), *The COVID Racial Data Tracker*, https://covidtracking.com/race (accessed on 9 February 2021). [149]

The Economist (2021), "The pandemic has changed the shape of global happiness", *The Economist*, https://www.economist.com/international/2021/03/20/the-pandemic-has-changed-the-shape-of-global-happiness. [106]

The Scandlon Foundation (2021), *Mapping social cohesion: The Scanlon Foundation surveys*, https://scanloninstitute.org.au/sites/default/files/2021-02/SC2020%20Report%20Final.pdf (accessed on 15 September 2021). [80]

Touyz, S., H. Lacey and P. Hay (2020), "Eating disorders in the time of COVID-19", *Journal of Eating Disorders*, Vol. 8/1, pp. 1-3, http://dx.doi.org/10.1186/s40337-020-00295-3. [59]

Tulsa SEED Study Team (2020), "Parents, teachers, and distance learning during the COVID-19 pandemic: A snapshot from Tulsa", https://medium.com/@TulsaSEED/parents-teachers-and-distance-learning-during-the-covid-19-pandemic-a-snapshot-from-tulsa-ok-5b5fdb54ea18. [70]

Ueda, M. et al. (2020), "Mental health status of the general population in Japan during the COVID-19 pandemic", *Psychiatry and Clinical Neurosciences*, Vol. 74/9, pp. 505-506, http://dx.doi.org/10.1111/PCN.13105. [69]

UNESCO (n.d.), *Global Monitoring of School Closures, COVID-19 (database)*, United Nations Educational, Scientific and Cultural Organization, https://en.unesco.org/covid19/educationresponse (accessed on 5 October 2021). [110]

United Nations (2020), *COVID-19 and the need for action on mental health*, United Nations Policy Brief, https://www.un.org/sites/un2.un.org/files/un_policy_brief-covid_and_mental_health_final.pdf. [72]

US Census Bureau (n.d.), *Measuring household experiences during the coronavirus pandemic*, https://www.census.gov/householdpulsedata (accessed on 16 June 2021). [87]

US Census Bureau (n.d.), *US Census Bureau QuickFacts: United States (database)*, https://www.census.gov/quickfacts/fact/table/US/PST045219 (accessed on 22 September 2021). [31]

Wozniak, A. et al. (2020), *COVID Impact Survey*, National Opinion Research Center, https://www.covid-impact.org/ (accessed on 9 August 2021). [66]

Notes

[1] Excess death statistics are better able to capture the full effect of the pandemic on fatality rates. The quality of official statistics on COVID-19 deaths may vary across countries due to differences in how deaths are recorded and the quality of measurement. Furthermore, COVID-19 fatality data do not capture the indirect health impacts of the pandemic – such as delays in non-COVID related medical care due to the fact that hospitals are overrun with COVID patients. See Chapter 3 and Morgan et al. (2020[150]) for further discussion of excess mortality statistics.

[2] The two countries that follow a different pattern, in which the 0-44 age cohort has the highest excess death rate, are Iceland and Canada. In Iceland, this pattern is driven by its small population: there were 22, 17 and -21 excess deaths for the 0-44, 45-64, and 65+ age cohorts during this time period, respectively. The data for Canada are more puzzling, in that the trends are not driven by small population groups. Statistics Canada suggested that this might reflect the indirect consequences of the pandemic, including increases in opioid overdoses in some provinces. However, until more specific cause-of-death data are available it is too soon to say what precisely is driving this trend (Statistics Canada, 2021[148]). Furthermore, the higher excess death rates for younger age groups occurred during the summer and autumn, when COVID deaths were very low nationwide; therefore, it may be indirect or unrelated factors that are playing a role.

[3] Trend lines for those aged 0-44 are not depicted in Figure 6.2, but on whole point to lower excess mortality rates than the two older age cohorts. Overall death rates (i.e. deaths from all causes) for the youngest age cohort are much lower, meaning that small changes in a given week can lead to large spikes in the data. The erratic nature of the 0-44 trend line is an indication that the excess mortality statistic is picking up a number of things that are unrelated to COVID-19, as very few members of this age group died from the virus.

[4] Assessing to what extent COVID-19 has affected ethnic and racial minority populations is challenging for a number of reasons. Basic statistics on the number and characteristics of COVID-19 cases are registered by national health systems, based on administrative sources such as testing and hospitalisations. Not all OECD countries consistently record diversity information (or other key socio-economic variables) in case numbers, hospital records or death certificates, nor do they always transmit these data for the compilation of national health and mortality statistics. For example, information on race, ethnicity or migrant status on death certificates is not transferred to the federal level in Germany; is incompletely recorded in Scotland; and is not recorded at all in England, Wales and Northern Ireland. This implies that data from census records, death registrations and hospital statistics in the latter countries have to be linked to provide information about the impact of COVID-19 by race and/or ethnicity (ONS, 2020[25]; OECD, 2020[19]). Many states in the United States have been slow to implement this practice: in May 2020, 51% of cases and 88% of deaths could be attributed to people with an identified race (though states have been working to identify the race of deaths previously recorded without one); by September 2020, only 65% of new cases included an identified race/ethnicity code (The COVID Tracking Project, 2020[149]; NPR, 2020[146]). A year on, 39% of all cumulative cases recorded by April 2021 lacked this information (CDC, 2021[27]). Native Americans in the United States and First Nations, Inuit and Métis communities in Canada, many of whom operate their own health systems, are also not officially required to report COVID-19 data. What is more, numbers of confirmed cases by ethnicity or origin are impacted by the ability of each country to reach the most vulnerable groups; rates of testing among military veterans in the United States up to July 2020 have been found to be lower for Hispanic/Latino and Black communities compared to whites, for instance (Rentsch et al., 2020[138]). Hence, relative COVID-19 related risks among groups, especially those of younger ages less likely to show symptoms, are likely to be underestimated. Moreover, many population surveys, especially the non-official and experimental ones launched throughout 2020 to capture the pandemic's psychosocial impact in real-time, often either do not contain questions on identity, or have such small sample sizes that any statements would be misleading. For this reason, this chapter uses only surveys with more than 500 observations for each aspect of diversity.

[5] Consistent with OECD practice (e.g. in the *International Migration Outlook* (2020[147])), this report uses the words "migrants", "immigrants" and "foreign-born" synonymously. Unless mentioned otherwise, this includes all persons born abroad, regardless of their migration category, legal status or nationality. Likewise, unless mentioned otherwise, native-born or "non-migrant" include all persons born in the country, regardless of the country of birth of their parents.

[6] The study included data from 18 728 893 patients from 50 studies in the United Kingdom and the United States.

[7] The term "visible minority" is used here because it is the official demographic category defined by the Canadian Employment Equity Act, and it is used by Statistics Canada in their surveys. The Employment Equity Act defines visible minorities as "persons, other than Aboriginal peoples, who are non-Caucasian in race or non-white in colour". The visible minority population consists mainly of South Asian, Chinese, Black, Filipino, Latin American, Arab, Southeast Asian, West Asian, Korean and Japanese people. The question of appropriate terminology is currently being reviewed in Canada, in the context of a task force on modernizing the Employment Equity Act (Department of Finance Canada, 2021[145]).

[8] See endnote 7 (above).

[9] For instance, in 2018 one in four positions at the Indian Health Service facilities were vacant, one in three households on the Navajo reservation lacked running water, while American Indians, especially in rural areas, have higher risks of many chronic health conditions, including diabetes (three times higher than for white Americans in the United States) and obesity (50% higher).

[10] As of 2016, Indigenous Australians represented around 3.3% of the Australian population (around 798 365, out of a total population of 24.1 million) (Australian Institute of Health and Welfare, 2019[143]) (ABS, 2016[144]); as of February 2021, they represent only 0.5% of total COVID-19 cases in Australia (Australian Government Department of Health, 2021[36]).

[11] Since First Nations communities are not officially required to consistently report COVID-19 data, these only present cases of Indigenous peoples residing on reserves, and are likely to be even higher among Indigenous people living off-reserve.

[12] The full Patient Health Questionnaire (PHQ) contains 59 questions, with modules focusing on mood, anxiety, alcohol, eating and somatoform disorders. The PHQ-4 screening tool is a short, four-question survey administered to respondents to gauge their mental condition, and to identify the presence and severity of depression and anxiety. PHQ-4 pulls two depression-related questions from the PHQ-9/8 (itself called the PHQ-2), and two anxiety-related questions from the Generalised Anxiety Disorder (GAD-7) questionnaire (itself called the GAD-2). Thus, the PHQ-4 is a combination of PHQ-2 and GAD-2. All question items are added together to provide a total score of mental distress: 0-2 normal, 3-5 moderate, 9-12 severe. A total score greater than or equal to 2 for the first two questions, pulled from the GAD-7, indicates that the respondent is at risk for anxiety. A total score greater than or equal to 2 for the final two questions, pulled from the PHQ-8, indicates that the respondent is at risk for depression (Kroenke et al., 2009[140]). The self-reported values from the PHQ surveys have been validated in separate studies comparing survey outcomes with actual diagnostic interviews with mental health professionals.

[13] The source of the baseline data is different from the source of the pandemic-era data, therefore caution should be exercised in interpreting any individual country trajectory; however, both data sources use the same instrument (PHQ-2) to assess the risk of depression, therefore the overall trend of increasing gender gaps is likely to be true.

[14] Pew Research Center conducted this study in the United States to understand people's assessments of their personal financial situation during the current period of economic slowdown and high unemployment rates caused by the coronavirus outbreak. For this analysis, Pew surveyed 13 200 United States adults in August 2020. Everyone who took part was a member of Pew Research Center's American Trends Panel (ATP), an online survey panel that is recruited through national, random sampling of residential addresses; this way nearly all United States adults have a chance of selection. The survey is weighted to be representative of the United States adult population by gender, race, ethnicity, partisan affiliation, education and other categories.

[15] The PHQ-8 and PHQ-9 questionnaires are a common shortened version of the full PHQ survey (see endnote 4 above for more information). PHQ-9 is a nine-question survey designed to detect the presence and severity of depression disorders. The PHQ-8 questionnaire is the same but removes the final question regarding suicidal ideation.

[16] The Generalised Anxiety Disorder Questionnaire (GAD) identifies the risk of anxiety. Similar to the PHQ, data are self-reported and validated against clinical diagnostic interviews (Spitzer et al., 2006[141]).

[17] The Rapid Assessment of Pandemic Impact on Development Early Childhood Household Survey Project is a weekly survey of United States households with children aged five and under launched on 6 April 2020. Since then, the study has been gathering weekly data about child and adult emotional well-being, financial and work circumstances, availability of health care, and access to childcare/early childhood education. These analyses are based on responses collected from 4 586 caregivers between 6 April 2020 and 11 June 2020. These caregivers represent a range of voices: 12.6% are Black, 17.5% are Hispanic/Latino and 9.4% live at or below 1.5 times the federal poverty line. Proportions are calculated based on the item-level response rates, not out of the total sample size. The data for these analyses are *not* weighted.

[18] Schernhammer and Colditz (2004[75]) conducted a meta-analysis of studies investigating physician suicide covering Australia, Denmark, Estonia, Finland, Germany, Great Britain, Iceland, South Africa (white population only), Sweden and the United States.

[19] See endnote 7 (above). Outcomes for visible minorities are compared to those of the white, non-Indigenous, population.

[20] For context, in the 2017 Canadian Aboriginal Peoples Survey, 16% of the Indigenous adult population (First Nations people living off reserve, Métis and Inuit) reported fair or poor mental health.

[21] The twelve items of the General Health Questionnaire (GHQ-12) are added together to provide a total score from 0 to 36, where higher values indicate worse mental health (Goldberg and Williams, 1988[139]). The questionnaire contains four subscales, focussing on somatic symptoms, anxiety and insomnia, social dysfunction and severe depression. 6 of the questions are positively phrased, while 6 are negatively phrased.

[22] These patterns seem to have been driven by increased or persistent loss of sleep over worry, which was the only question within the GHQ-12 that showed any significant variation across ethnic groups, after adjusting for age. Indeed, Indians reported greater difficulty with sleep over worry during this time (36% versus 23% for white British and 18% of Other white respondents). While 35% of those from the Black, African, Caribbean or Black British ethnic group also said they lost sleep, the change in mental health for these groups were not as marked, though definite statements are difficult to make due to large confidence intervals.

[23] The study by Graham et al. (2020[30]) compares outcomes for low-income and high-income groups by ethnicity but does not include other socio-economic controls.

[24] A nationally representative survey fielded by the Social Policy Institute at Washington University in St. Louis from 27 April to 12 May found that, after controlling for socio-economic and demographic variables such as age, gender, income, education and place of residence, Black and Hispanic/Latino respondents scored higher on life satisfaction, optimism for the future and a self-reported mental health question compared to whites, with the largest racial differences between those of low income.

[25] Negative affect balance is measured as the share of the population reporting more negative feelings (anger, sadness, worry) than positive feelings (enjoyment, laughing or smiling a lot, feeling well-rested) the day prior.

[26] While the composition of all the different labour market categories changed markedly in 2020, it is only unemployment that shows such large counterintuitive movements in negative affect balance from 2019 to 2020. This may also reflect the small sample size of the unemployed, compared to other labour market groups. According to the Gallup World Poll data, 5.8% of respondents in 33 OECD countries were unemployed in 2020, compared to 13.1% who were working part-time, 35.5% who were out of work and 45.7% who were employed full-time. The smaller sample size my lead to more noise in the data, meaning that though there appears to be more movement the changes are insignificant.

[27] This study analyses public opinion in the United States and three European countries: France, Germany and the United Kingdom. Data are from nationally representative telephone surveys of 4 069 adults from 10 November to 23 December 2020 in the three countries.

[28] Analysis of United Kingdom data has shown the importance of whether part-time work is voluntary (i.e. individuals who work part-time out of choice) or involuntary (i.e. individuals who want to work more hours, but were unable to find a full-time job). Specifically, those working part-time voluntarily have higher subjective well-being than full-time workers, while those working part-time involuntarily experience lower levels of subjective well-being than full-time workers (Abdallah and Shah, 2012[142]).

[29] The Tulsa School Experiences and Early Development (SEED) Study, initiated in 2016, is following a diverse sample of children from low-income families from age 3 through 4th grade to understand the effects of attending pre-K programmes on children's learning and development. The Tulsa SEED Study surveyed both parents (N=586) and teachers (N=118) in a 6-week period between May and July 2020. Participants in this pair of COVID-19 surveys were the parents (90% mothers) and the first-grade teachers of the SEED study children. These children have been followed since ages 3–4, when they experienced a range of public preschool arrangements in the Tulsa Public School (TPS) district. Of the families still enrolled in the study by 1st grade, 43% responded to this special COVID-19 survey (85% of whom are still enrolled in the TPS district). COVID-19 survey respondents resembled the TPS population with respect to family income, child race/ethnicity and child special needs status, but were slightly more likely to be dual language learners.

[30] Poor mental health is measured via a "psychopathology factor", a composite measure that synthesises symptoms associated with ten psychiatric disorders, including alcohol dependence, ADHD and generalised anxiety disorder.

7 Inclusion, community relations and COVID-19

While the COVID-19 pandemic has affected the way almost everyone connects with each other, spends their time, relates to society and experiences safety, some groups have suffered more than others. Those with financial difficulties, the unemployed, women and people without university education felt particularly lonely in 2020, as did younger people and those living alone. Apart from the youngest age group, these characteristics were already risk factors for well-being pre-COVID, but absolute gaps widened for vulnerable groups since then. Similar patterns can be observed for feeling left out of society. Both men and women experienced an increase in the burden of unpaid domestic work and care for children (or other family members), but most of this additional burden still fell on women. Women have also been affected by increases in domestic violence.

7.1. Social connections

Loneliness has hit everyone, but particularly vulnerable groups

A year of multiple lockdown rounds, social distancing and restrictions on travel and gatherings has made nearly everyone more lonely, but some groups more so than others. In European OECD countries, nearly 1 in 5 people overall felt lonely most or all of the time in February-March 2021, up from 1 in 7 in April-May a year earlier (see Chapter 4). A closer look at different subgroups reveals that people with financial difficulties, the unemployed, younger people, those with up to secondary education, women, people living alone as well as single parents were disproportionally affected (Figure 7.1).

Figure 7.1. People in precarious financial and work situations, the young and those living without a partner felt loneliest in the first year of the pandemic

Share of people feeling lonely most or all of the time in the past two weeks, by population group, OECD 22, Apr-Jun 2020 - Feb-Mar 2021

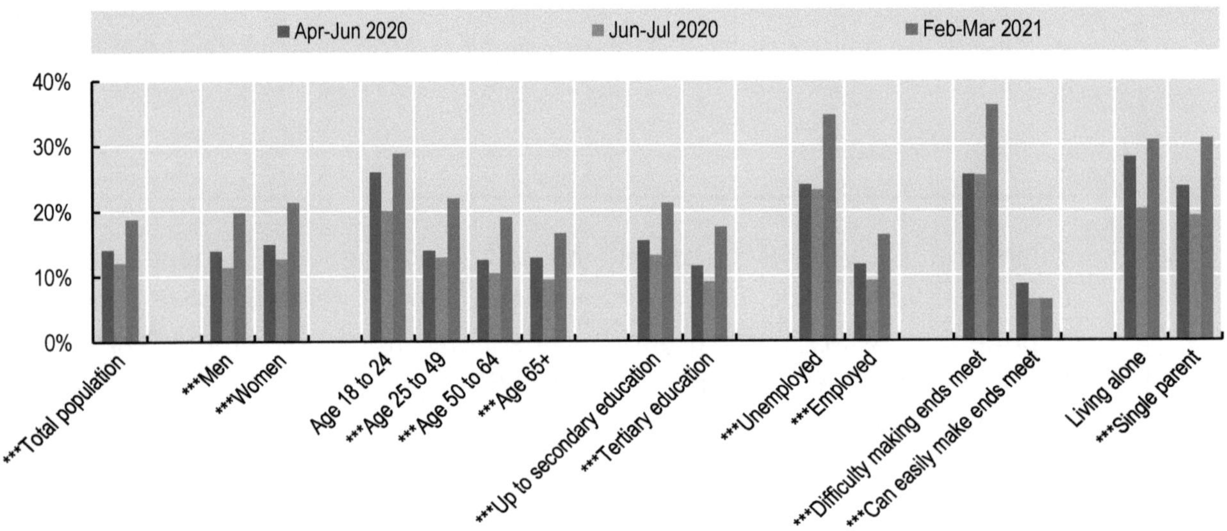

Note: The OECD average includes Austria, Belgium, the Czech Republic, Denmark, Estonia, Finland, France, Germany, Greece, Hungary, Ireland, Italy, Latvia, Lithuania, Luxembourg, the Netherlands, Poland, Portugal, Slovenia, the Slovak Republic, Spain and Sweden. Categories preceded by *** saw statistically significant (at the 5% level) changes from April-June 2020 to February-March 2021. Difficulty making ends meet is captured by the question: "A household may have different sources of income and more than one household member may contribute to it. Thinking of your household's total monthly income: is your household able to make ends meet?". "With difficulty" refers to respondents answering with difficulty or with great difficulty, while "easily" refers to respondents answering fairly easily, easily or very easily. Refer to Box 2.1 for methodological details on the Living, working and COVID-19 survey.
Source: OECD calculations based on Eurofound (n.d.[1]), *Living, working and COVID-19 e-survey* (database), http://eurofound.link/covid19data.

StatLink https://stat.link/52feh7

The risk factors for loneliness were nearly identical before and during the pandemic. In 2016, people in European OECD countries who were struggling financially, without a job, living alone, lower educated or female were already more likely to be lonely (Figure 7.2, Panel A). In addition, single parents, people living in urban areas, and those with a disability or diagnosed mental health condition felt most lonely pre-COVID and throughout 2020 (Eurofound, 2020[2]; Loneliness New Zealand Charitable Trust, 2020[3]; ANUPoll, 2020[4]; ONS, 2020[5]; Kühne et al., 2020[6]; NZ Social Wellbeing Agency, 2020[7]). However, two patterns stand out about the impact of COVID-19. First, while between 2016 and 2020 *relative* loneliness inequalities by ability to make ends meet, employment status, educational attainment or gender narrowed (because every population group, including those previously protected, experienced increases in loneliness), these inequalities remain very substantial (Figure 7.2, Panel B). For instance, in the first year of the pandemic a person living in a European OECD country who had difficulty making ends meet was more than three times more likely to feel lonely compared to a person who could easily meet household expenses; similarly, someone with up to a secondary education was 1.3 times more likely to be lonely than a peer with a tertiary degree.

Figure 7.2. Gaps in loneliness between population groups have narrowed since 2016 as overall levels increased for everyone but remain substantial

Loneliness, by population group, OECD 22, 2016, average over 3 survey waves in Apr-Jun 2020, Jun-Jul 2020, Feb-Mar 2021

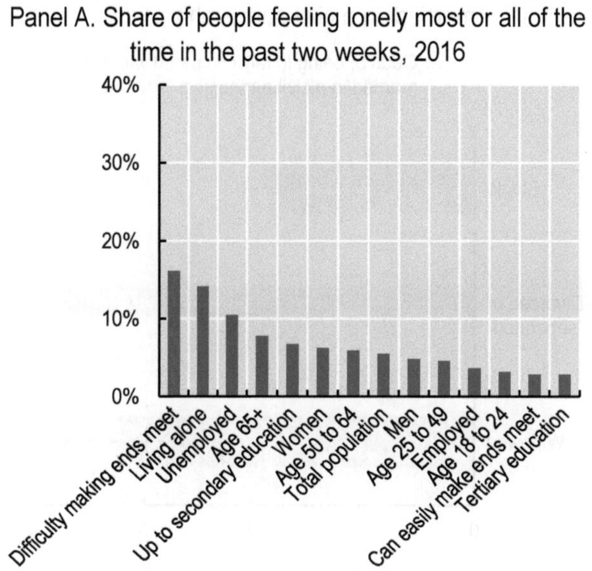

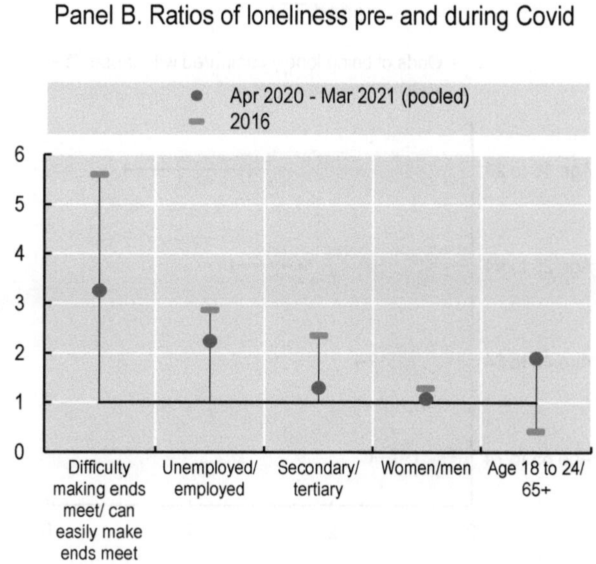

Note: The OECD average includes Austria, Belgium, the Czech Republic, Denmark, Estonia, Finland, France, Germany, Greece, Hungary, Ireland, Italy, Latvia, Lithuania, Luxembourg, the Netherlands, Poland, Portugal, Slovenia, the Slovak Republic, Spain and Sweden. See the note of Figure 7.1 for the definition of difficulty making ends meet. In Panel B, ratios with values above 1 indicate worse outcomes for the population subgroups listed first, values below 1 indicate worse outcomes for the population subgroups listed second. While the 2020-2021 and 2016 data are not directly comparable due to differences in sampling between the Living, working and COVID-19 e-survey and the European Quality of Life Survey (although the question asked is the same), the ratios provide a useful point of comparison over time. Refer to Box 2.1 for methodological details on the Living, working and COVID-19 e-survey.

Source: OECD calculations based on Eurofound (2018[8]), *European Quality of Life Survey 2016*, https://www.eurofound.europa.eu/publications/report/2017/fourth-european-quality-of-life-survey-overview-report; and Eurofound (n.d.[1]), *Living, working and COVID-19 e-survey* (database), http://eurofound.link/covid19data.

StatLink https://stat.link/38wlnt

Second, younger people have been particularly hit by loneliness during the pandemic. Before COVID-19, some evidence supported the idea of loneliness increasing with age, while other sources pointed to loneliness being more prevalent among younger cohorts.[1] Conversely, in 2020 young people consistently emerged as the age group feeling the most lonely during the pandemic (Figure 7.2). Official statistics from New Zealand and Great Britain confirm this pattern: in the former, 57% of New Zealanders aged 18–24-years felt lonely at least a little of the time during the past four weeks in March 2021, compared to 34% of those aged 65 years and older (StatsNZ, 2021[9]). In the latter, the 16-24 and 25-44 years age cohorts had 4.2 and 3 times the odds of being lonely in the past week between October 2020 - February 2021, compared to people aged 74 years or over (Figure 7.2, Panel A). In February 2021, loneliness prevalence among students in England was more than triple that of the general population (ONS, 2021[10]). Marital status and household size, which vary by age, are also important drivers of loneliness: in Great Britain, those living alone had almost 1.6 times the odds of feeling lonely compared to people in two-person households, and all categories of unmarried people were more lonely than those married or living in a civil partnership (Figure 7.2, Panel B).

Figure 7.3. In Great Britain, younger and unmarried people were more likely to experience loneliness during lockdown

Odds of reporting feeling lonely in the last 7 days, among people in Great Britain who said their well-being was affected by the coronavirus, Oct 2020 - Feb 2021

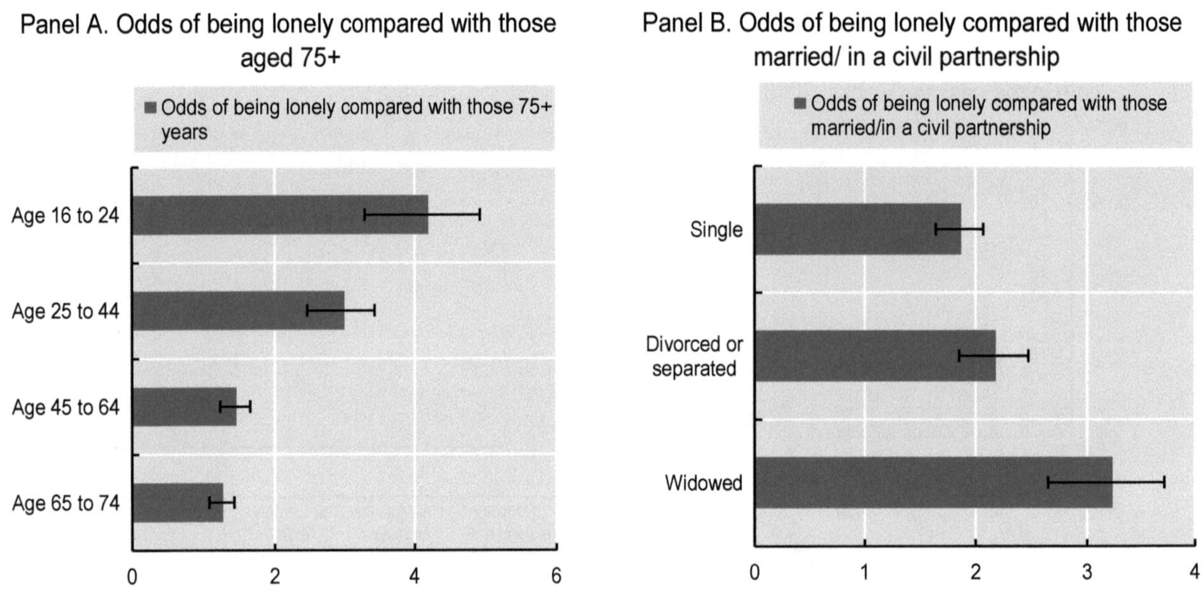

Note: In Panel A, odds ratios compare the likelihood of reporting lockdown loneliness for someone in a specified age group compared with those aged 75 years or over, while controlling for other possible influences. In Panel B, odds ratios compare the likelihood of reporting lockdown loneliness for someone in a specified living arrangement compared with those in married/civil partnership, while controlling for other possible influences. Lockdown loneliness is defined as those who said their well-being had been affected by the coronavirus through feeling lonely in the last seven days. The error bars show the degree of confidence of the estimates.
Source: ONS (2021[11]), *Mapping loneliness during the coronavirus pandemic*, https://www.ons.gov.uk/peoplepopulationandcommunity/wellbeing/articles/mappinglonelinessduringthecoronaviruspandemic/2021-04-07.

StatLink https://stat.link/x3hrfp

Box 7.1. Spotlight: Differences between loneliness and social isolation during the pandemic

Loneliness and social isolation are two related but different aspects of social connectedness. Generally speaking, social isolation refers to the amount of social contact a person has in terms of the number and frequency of contacts. Loneliness, in contrast, occurs when social relationships are perceived by a person to be less in quantity, and especially in quality, than desired (Social Wellbeing Agency, 2020[12]; OECD, 2021[13]). This implies that someone can feel lonely despite regular contact with family and friends, and that a person can be isolated without necessarily feeling lonely. While isolation is not a requirement for feeling lonely, being socially isolated does increase the likelihood of being lonely.

German data on self-reported social isolation from 2017 and at two time points during the COVID-19 pandemic show that, as with the loneliness trends described in this chapter, social isolation has progressively increased for all population groups since the start of 2020 (Figure 7.4). Many of the risk factors for perceived social isolation – low income, being female, being younger, having a lower education – were similar to those identified for loneliness in the broader European context.

Figure 7.4. In Germany, income, gender and younger age were associated with feeling socially isolated pre-outbreak, and remained so during the pandemic

Share of people in Germany feeling socially isolated, by population group, 2017, Apr-Jun 2020, Jan-Feb 2021

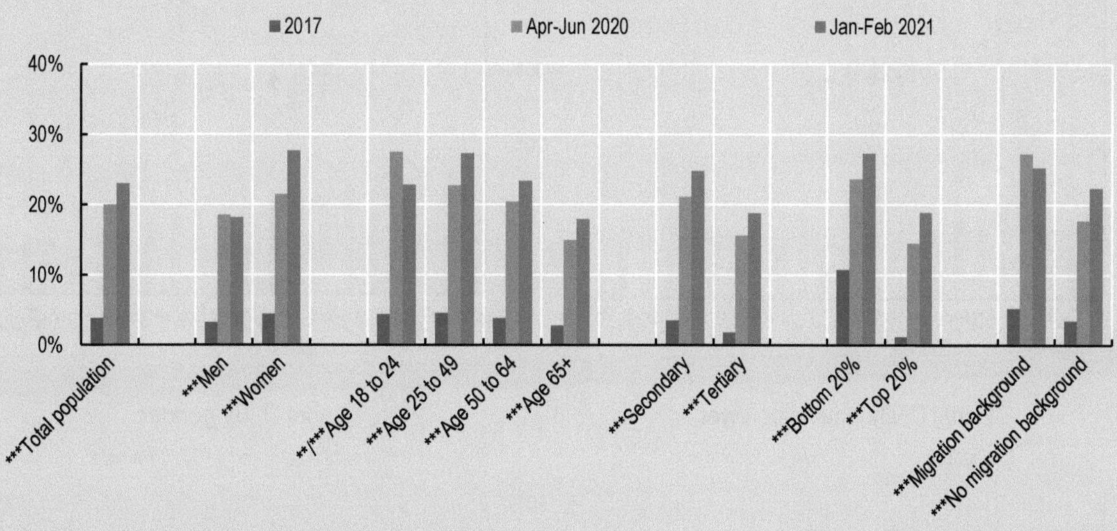

Note: Socially isolated is defined as respondents who say they feel very often or often socially isolated. Migration background is defined as respondents or either of their parents being born in a country other than Germany. ** denotes categories with between 100 and 300 observations in April-June 2020 and January-February 2021. More than 500 observations per category are available for all other categories. Categories preceded by *** saw statistically significant (at the 5% level) changes from 2017-2021. Funded by the German Federal Ministry of Education and Research (BMBF). The data can be accessed via the research data centre of the SOEP. Refer to Box 3.1 for methodological details.
Source: Kühne et al. (2020[6]), "The need for household panel surveys in times of crisis: The case of SOEP-CoV", *Survey Research Methods*, Vol. 14/2, pp. 195-203, https://doi.org/10.18148/srm/2020.v14i2.7748.

StatLink https://stat.link/c4kv32

Socio-economic risk factors for loneliness are similar across OECD countries. In all European OECD members covered by the Eurofound Living, working and COVID-19 e-survey, a larger share of people with difficulty making ends meet, of the unemployed and of those with secondary or lower education felt lonely between April - June 2020, compared to those who are better-off financially, employed or more highly educated (Figure 7.5, Panels A-C). The same was true for women compared to men in most countries, though gaps are much smaller than those relating to socio-economic status and only significant for Hungary and Ireland (Figure 7.5, Panel D). In Great Britain, 9% of people who earn up to GBP 10 000 were lonely between March 2020 - April 2021 compared to 3.3% of those with a yearly income of GBP 40 000 or above (Figure 7.6). Further, local authority areas with higher unemployment (in October 2019 - September 2020) had higher proportions of lonely residents between October 2020 - February 2021 (ONS, 2021[11]).[2] In Germany, gender gaps in loneliness progressively widened over the course of the pandemic: in 2017, the prevalence of loneliness among women was around 3 percentage points higher than among men. This gap rose to 6.5 percentage points in April-June 2020, and to close to 10 percentage points in January-February 2021. Similar patterns can be observed for social isolation (Figure 7.7).

Figure 7.5. Socio-economic risk factors for loneliness during COVID-19 are similar across European OECD countries

Share of people feeling lonely all or most of the time in the past two weeks, OECD 22, average over 3 survey waves in Apr-Jun 2020, Jun-Jul 2020, Feb-Mar 2021

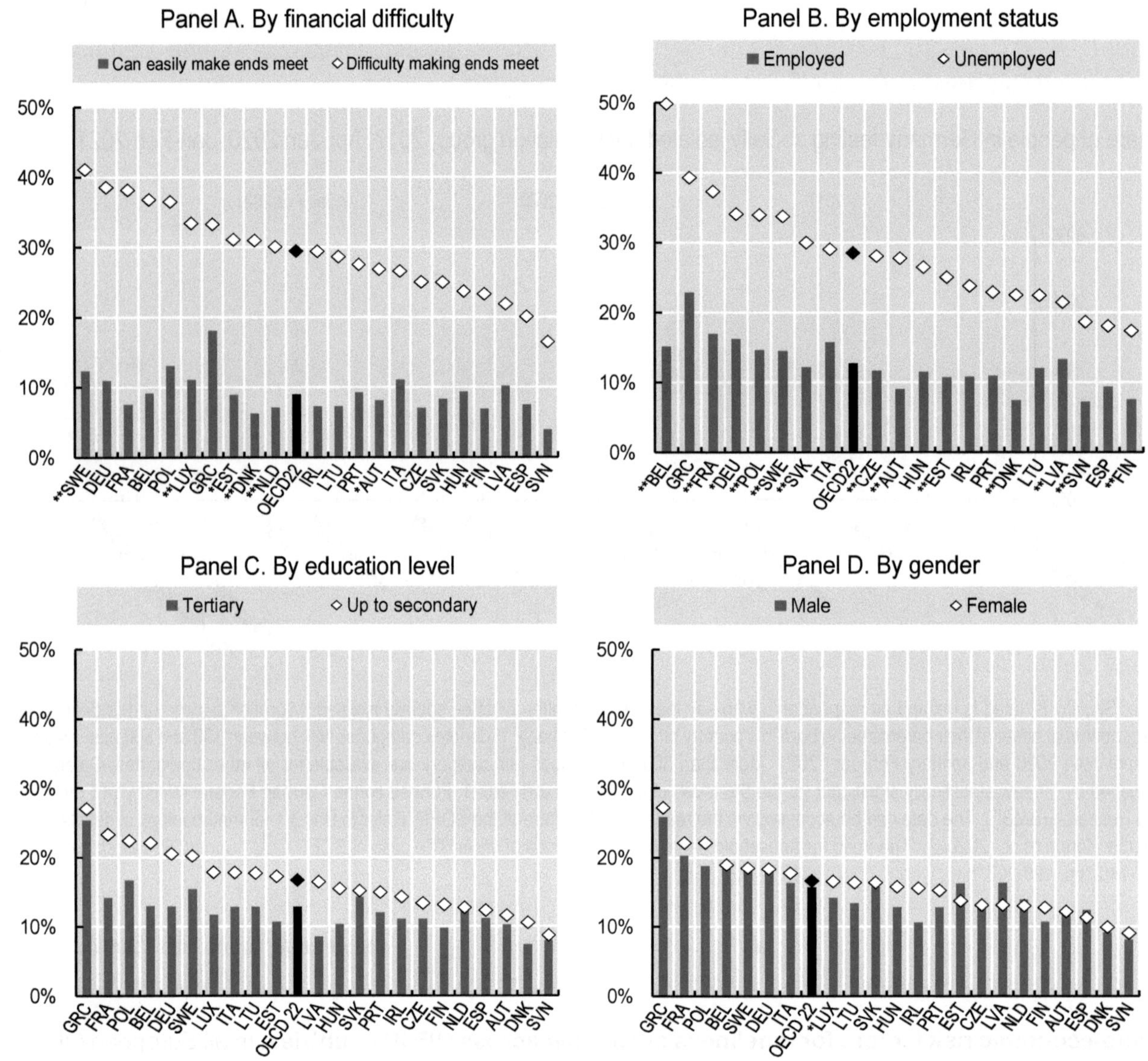

Note: In all panels, the OECD 22 average includes Austria, Belgium, the Czech Republic, Denmark, Estonia, Finland, France, Germany, Greece, Hungary, Ireland, Italy, Latvia, Lithuania, Luxembourg, the Netherlands, Poland, Portugal, the Slovak Republic, Slovenia, Spain and Sweden. Data are not reported for countries where fewer than 100 observations are available. ** denotes countries with between 100 and 300 observations per category; * denotes countries with between 301 and 500 observations per category. More than 500 observations per category are available for all other countries. Refer to Box 2.1 for methodological details on the Living, working and COVID-19 survey. In Panel A, see the note of Figure 7.1 for the definition of difficulty making ends meet. Differences between groups are significant (at the 5% level) for all countries, including OECD 22. In Panel B, differences between groups are significant (at the 5% level) for all countries, including OECD 22, except for Latvia and the Netherlands. In Panel C, differences between groups are significant (at the 5% level) for Belgium, Estonia, France, Germany, Hungary, Italy, Latvia, Lithuania, OECD 22, Poland and Portugal. In Panel D, differences between groups are significant (at the 5% level) for Hungary and Ireland.

Source: OECD calculations based on Eurofound (n.d.[1]), *Living, working and COVID-19 e-survey* (database), http://eurofound.link/covid19data.

StatLink https://stat.link/a29w34

Figure 7.6. In Great Britain, loneliness in the first year of COVID-19 was worse for lower-income groups

Share of people in Great Britain feeling often or always lonely, by annual personal income, Mar 2020 - Apr 2021

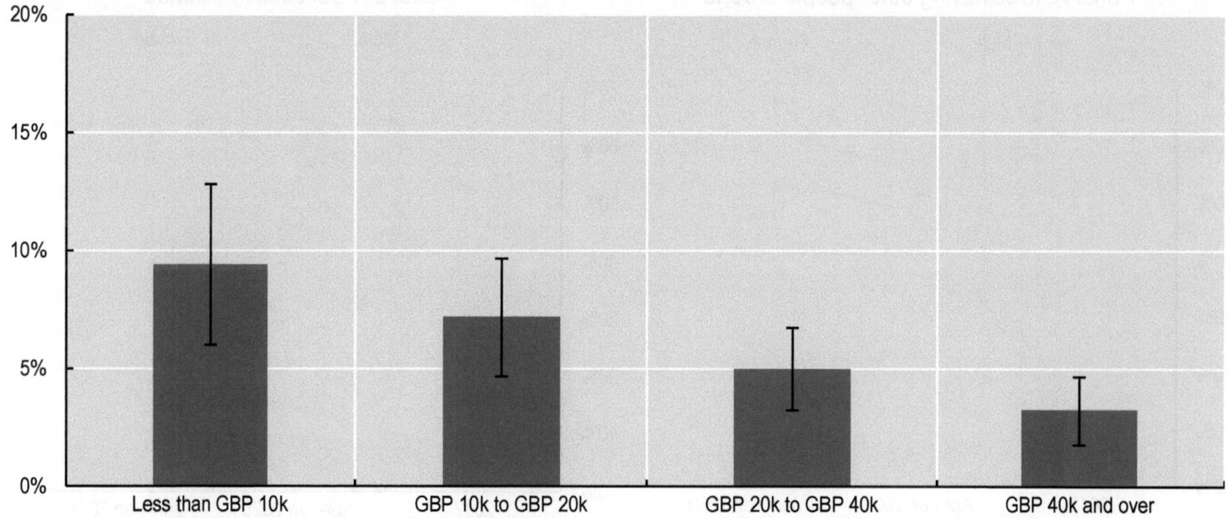

Note: Chronic loneliness is defined as adults aged 16 years or over that were asked how often they felt lonely and responded with often or always. Income refers to total annual income of individuals from all sources, gross of tax. The error bars show the lower and upper intervals of the estimates.
Source: ONS (2020[14]), *Personal and economic well-being in Great Britain: January 2021*, https://www.ons.gov.uk/peoplepopulationandcommunity/wellbeing/datasets/incomegroupsplitestimatesonpersonalandeconomicwellbeingacrosstime.

StatLink https://stat.link/eivc01

Very little COVID-19 specific data by race, ethnicity or migration status currently exist with regard to social connections. In the United Kingdom, a quarter of people from the white Irish and Indian ethnic groups reported either continuing to feel lonely often or experiencing an increase in feelings of loneliness between 2019 - April 2020 (ONS, 2020[15]). In comparison, only 18% of white British, 11% of Black, African, Caribbean or Black British, and 10% of Chinese and other Asian ethnic groups said the same, after controlling for a range of other factors.[3] In Germany, rates of loneliness have risen in the first year of the pandemic for those both with and without a migration background; but, by early 2021 gaps flipped compared to 2017, with those with a migration background feeling less lonely than those without (Figure 7.8).[4] However, people with a migration background were still more likely to say that they feel socially isolated (Figure 7.4).

Figure 7.7. In Germany, gender gaps in loneliness and social isolation widened

Share of people in Germany saying they very often or often miss having people around or feel socially isolated, by gender, 2017, Apr-Jun 2020, Jan-Feb 2021

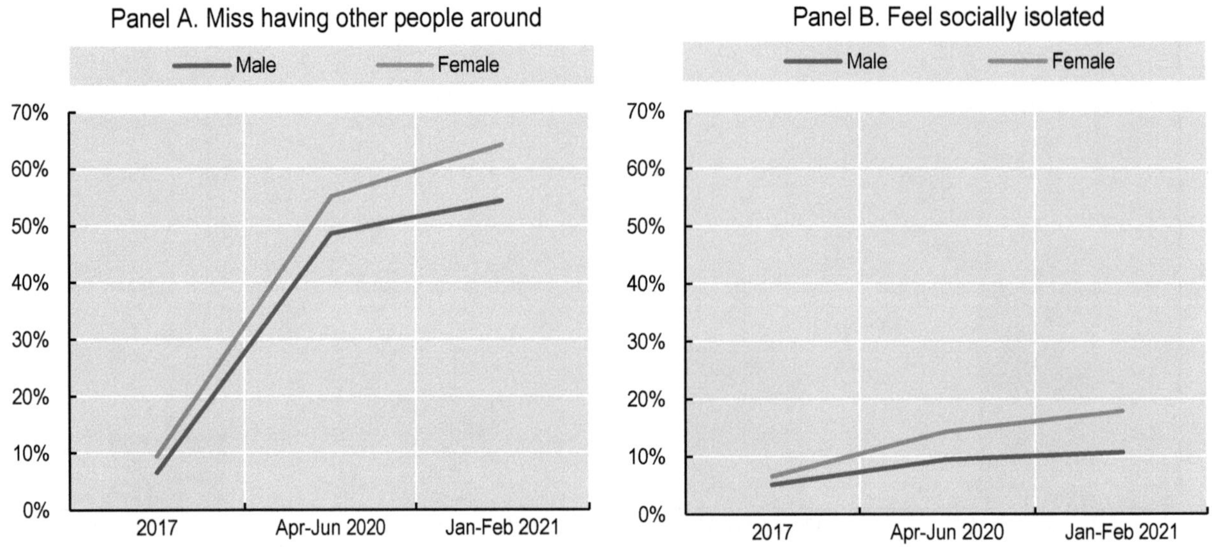

Note: Funded by the German Federal Ministry of Education and Research (BMBF). The data can be accessed via the research data centre of the SOEP. Refer to Box 3.1 for methodological details.
Source: Kühne et al. (2020[6]), "The need for household panel surveys in times of crisis: The case of SOEP-CoV", *Survey Research Methods*, Vol. 14/2, pp. 195-203, https://doi.org/10.18148/srm/2020.v14i2.7748.

StatLink https://stat.link/dtbz4p

Figure 7.8. In Germany, people with a migration background felt comparatively less lonely

Share of people in Germany saying they often or very often miss having other people around, by migration background, 2017, Apr-Jun 2020, Jan-Feb 2021

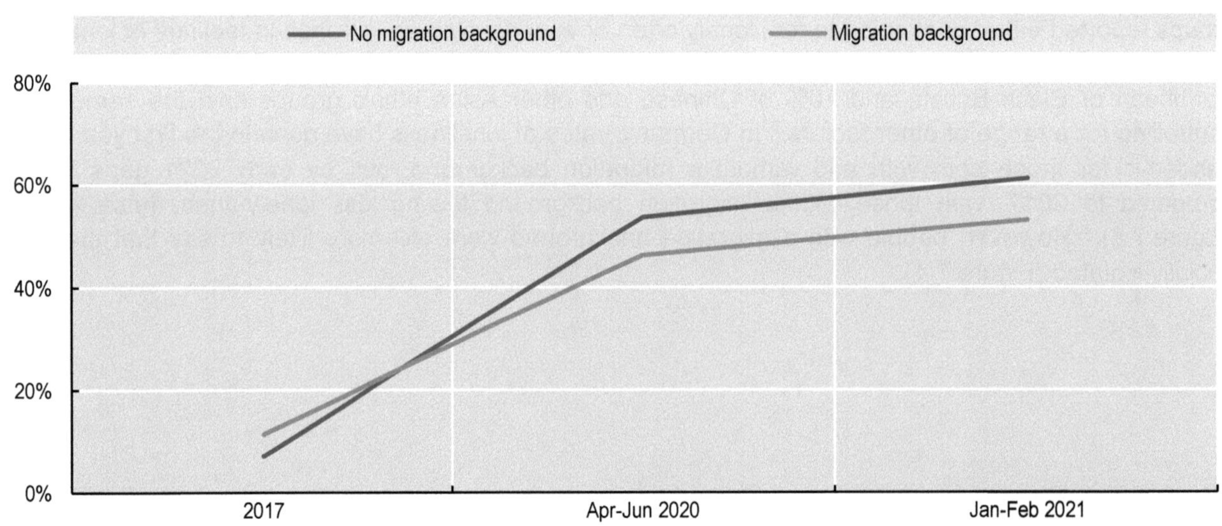

Note: Migration background refers to respondents/parents being born outside Germany. Funded by the German Federal Ministry of Education and Research (BMBF). The data can be accessed via the research data centre of the SOEP. Refer to Box 3.1 for methodological details.
Source: Kühne et al. (2020[6]), "The need for household panel surveys in times of crisis: The case of SOEP-CoV", *Survey Research Methods*, Vol. 14/2, pp. 195-203, https://doi.org/10.18148/srm/2020.v14i2.7748.

StatLink https://stat.link/jh61kp

7.2. Work-life balance

Changed working conditions have brought benefits and challenges to different groups…

Working conditions in 2020 (including both telework and contact restrictions for those at a work location outside the home) have worn most people out, but especially those struggling financially, people with young children and women. In April-June 2020, 22% of workers in 22 European OECD countries said they had always or most of the time felt too tired after work to do some household chores in the previous two weeks, while by February-March 2021 this share had risen to 29.5% (see Chapter 4). A closer look at different population groups shows that the prevalence of exhaustion was higher than the population average for people struggling to make ends meet, single parents, people living with children, those aged 18-49, women, and people with up to secondary education (Figure 7.9). People with difficulty making ends meet were particularly affected: more than a third in April-June 2020 and almost half by February-March 2021 reported being too tired after work to finish household chores.

Figure 7.9. All employed people have felt more exhausted as the pandemic dragged on, but particularly those with difficulty making ends meet

Share of employed people reporting feeling too tired after work to do necessary household chores, by population group, OECD 22, average over 3 survey waves in Apr-Jun 2020, Jun-Jul 2020, Feb-Mar 2021

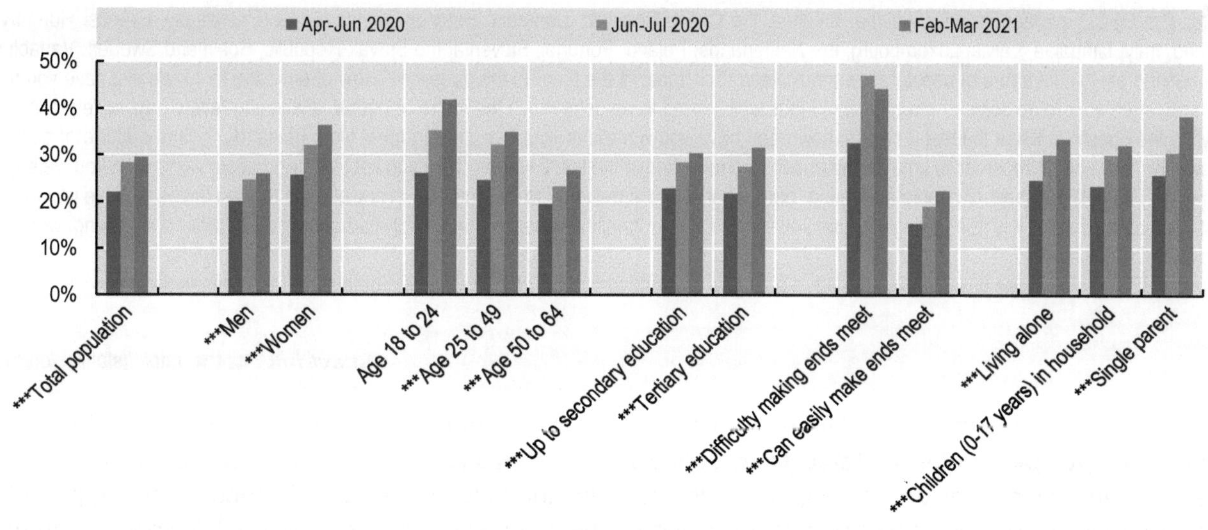

Note: The OECD average includes Austria, Belgium, the Czech Republic, Denmark, Estonia, Finland, France, Germany, Greece, Hungary, Ireland, Italy, Latvia, Lithuania, Luxembourg, the Netherlands, Poland, Portugal, the Slovak Republic, Slovenia, Spain and Sweden. Categories preceded by *** saw statistically significant (at the 5% level) changes from April-June 2020 to February-March 2021. See the note of Figure 7.1 for the definition of difficulty making ends meet. Refer to Box 2.1 for methodological details on the Living, working and COVID-19 survey.
Source: OECD calculations based on Eurofound (n.d.[1]), *Living, working and COVID-19 e-survey* (database), http://eurofound.link/covid19data.

StatLink https://stat.link/725hny

Those working from home felt less exhausted at the end of the day, but work was more likely to seep into their regular lives. Between June 2020 - March 2021, workers in 22 European OECD countries who were working exclusively from home were almost 4 percentage points less likely to feel too tired at the end of the day to do necessary household chores, and less likely to feel that their job prevented them from spending time with family. However they were also nearly 12 percentage points more likely to work in their free time to meet work demands, and 4 percentage points more likely to keep worrying about their job when not working (Figure 7.10).

Figure 7.10. Those working at home were less tired and could spend more time with their family, but were more likely to work after hours and to worry about their jobs

Share of employed people experiencing work-life balance challenges, by work location, OECD 22, average over 2 survey waves in Jun-Jul 2020, Feb-Mar 2021

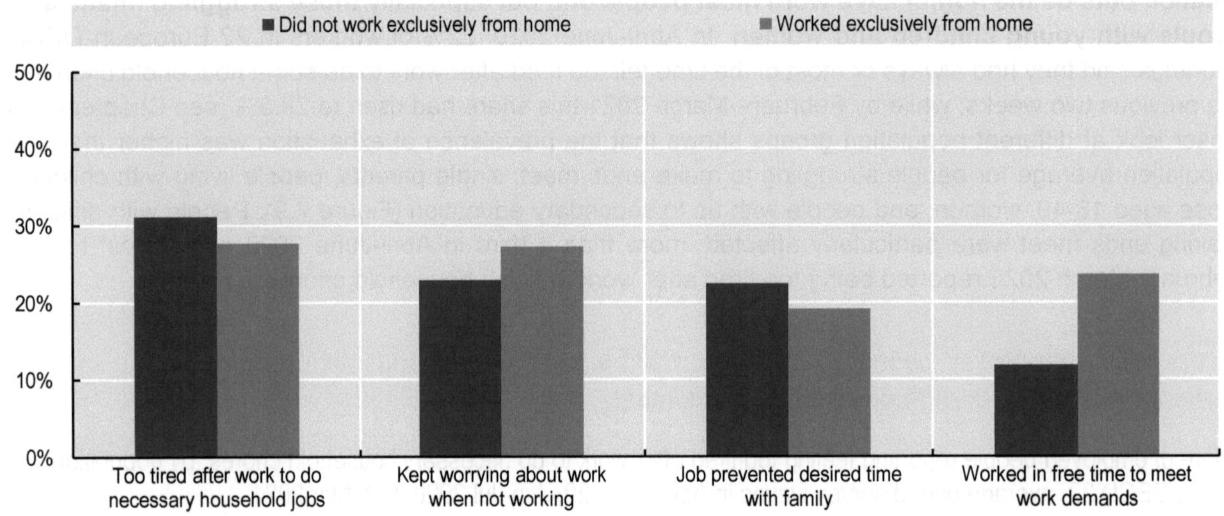

Note: The OECD average includes Austria, Belgium, the Czech Republic, Denmark, Estonia, France, Finland, Germany, Greece, Hungary, Ireland, Italy, Lithuania, Latvia, Luxembourg, the Netherlands, Poland, Portugal, Slovenia, the Slovak Republic, Spain and Sweden. Variables are defined as: (1) the share of people answering "always" or "most of the time" to the question: "How often in the last 2 weeks, have you felt too tired after work to do some of the household jobs which need to be done?"; (2) the share of people answering "every day" or "every other day" to the question: "Over the last 2 weeks, how often have you worked in your free time to meet work demands?"; (3) the share of people answering "always" or "most of the time" to the question: "How often in the last 2 weeks, have you kept worrying about work when you were not working?"; and (4) the share of people answering "always" or "most of the time" to the question: "How often in the last 2 weeks, have you found that your job prevented you from giving the time you wanted to your family?" Refer to Box 2.1 for methodological details on the Living, working and COVID-19 e-survey.

Source: OECD calculations based on Eurofound (n.d.[1]), *Living, working and COVID-19 e-survey* (database), http://eurofound.link/covid19data.

StatLink https://stat.link/c6io15

Focusing on different types of teleworkers, parents experienced more flexibility and family time, while younger people felt isolated from colleagues and prone to "workaholism" (see Box 5.5). On the one hand, there is evidence that, due to the combination of teleworking and school closures, parents were more likely than non-parents to report being unable to meet deadlines, and that teleworking parents with children up to 18 years found it more difficult to get their work done without interruptions compared to parents without minor children (Parker, Menasce Horowitz and Minkin, 2020[16]). But, across the EU 27 members in June-July 2020, teleworkers with children under age 12 were also less likely to report that their job prevented them from spending time with family than those working at other locations (Eurofound, 2020[2]). Teleworking experiences have also differed by age. According to a survey conducted in 9 countries by the Capgemini Research Institute in September-October 2020, 61% of employees aged 31-40 (compared to just over half of all surveyed employees) felt burnt out as a result of working remotely, while "workaholism" was found to be more common among younger workers living alone (Capgemini Research Institute, 2020[17]). Younger workers have also been less likely to feel motivated to do their work since the pandemic started, and more likely to feel isolated at work (see Box 5.5).

...but many people would like to continue working from home to some degree

Overall, preferences for working remotely in the future are substantial. Almost half of all employed people in 22 European OECD countries (45.8%) would like to work from home at least several days a week after COVID-19 subsides (see Chapters 2 and 4), a feeling that is shared across all socio-demographic subgroups interviewed between June 2020 - March 2021 (Figure 7.11). Preferences for telework are highest among those with children or in the age range more likely to have children (aged 25-49), among women, the well-educated and those who can easily make ends meet (who are likely to be in jobs that allow for remote work and to have larger living spaces to turn into a home office – see Chapter 5). But even among people with up to secondary education and those struggling to make ends meet, more than a third would prefer working from home at least a few times a week.

Figure 7.11. Preferences for remote work are highest for those with child-caring responsibilities, women and the better educated

Share of employed people who, if they had the choice, would like to work from home daily or several times a week if there were no restrictions due to COVID-19, by population group, OECD 22, average over 2 survey waves in Jun-Jul 2020, Feb-Mar 2021

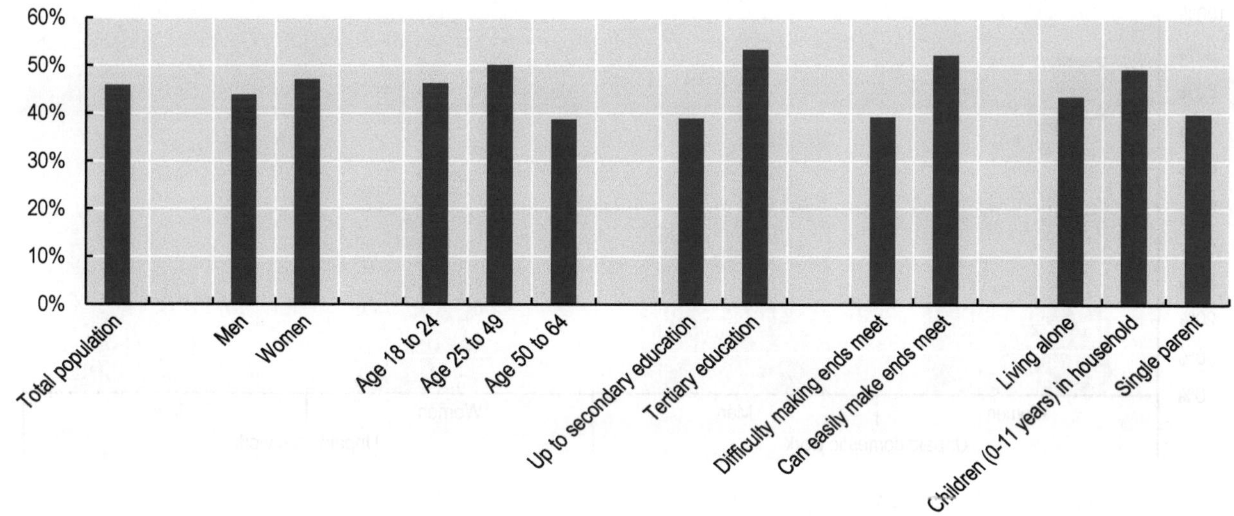

Note: The OECD 22 average includes Austria, Belgium, the Czech Republic, Denmark, Estonia, Finland, France, Germany, Greece, Hungary, Ireland, Italy, Latvia, Lithuania, Luxembourg, the Netherlands, Poland, Portugal, the Slovak Republic, Slovenia, Spain and Sweden. See the note of Figure 7.1 for the definition of difficulty making ends meet. Refer to Box 2.1 for methodological details on the Living, working and COVID-19 survey.
Source: OECD calculations based on Eurofound (n.d.[11]), *Living, working and COVID-19 e-survey* (database), http://eurofound.link/covid19data.

StatLink https://stat.link/bfwsiq

Women still spend more time on care and housework than men

With more people at home due to pandemic-related measures, household chores and care have multiplied in some countries – and the majority of this work falls on the shoulders of women. Evidence from UN Women Rapid Gender Assessment Surveys conducted in April 2020 in Chile, Mexico and Turkey suggest that both women and men reported an increase in time spent on unpaid domestic work and care work since COVID-19 struck, with stronger rises for women (Figure 7.12). In Australia, more than one in three women (38%) and one in three men (33%) surveyed in June-July 2020 reported an increase in unpaid time spent caring for others. However, women were twice as likely as men to report performing most of the unpaid domestic work, and more than three times as likely to perform most of the unpaid caring responsibilities in their household (ABS, 2020[18]). The Future of Business Survey, a collaboration between the OECD, the World Bank and Facebook that documented the experience of over 150 000 business leaders from over 50 countries between May - October 2020, also found that 31% of female business leaders reported spending more time on domestic tasks since the pandemic began, compared to 25% of male business leaders. The gap widened when considering only business leaders with a spouse: in October 2020, 23% of female business leaders with a partner spent more than six hours per day on domestic tasks, compared to only 12% of male business leaders with a partner. The most cited domestic responsibilities were home-schooling (25% female to 19% male), household chores (41% to 27%) and caring for dependents (31% to 24%) (Facebook; OECD;The World Bank, 2020[19]).

Figure 7.12. In Chile, Mexico and Turkey, being at home more at the outset of the pandemic has meant more work for everyone, especially women

Share of people who reported an increase in time spent on at least one unpaid domestic and care work activity since COVID-19, by gender, Apr-2020

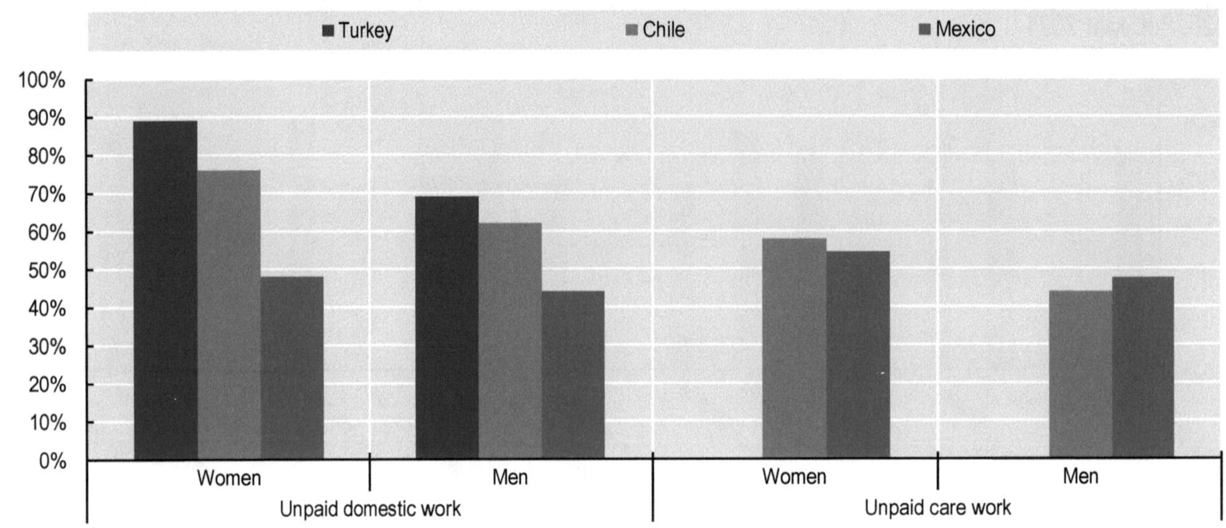

Source: UN Women (n.d.[20]), Covid-19 Data Monitor (database), https://data.unwomen.org/COVID19.

StatLink https://stat.link/khw6qb

Figure 7.13. After a temporary reduction in March-April 2020, the gender gap in unpaid work in Great Britain reverted to pre-pandemic levels six months later

Minutes per day spent on paid and unpaid work for adults aged 18 years or over, by gender, 2014-15 for the United Kingdom, Mar-Apr 2020 and Sep-Oct 2020 for Great Britain

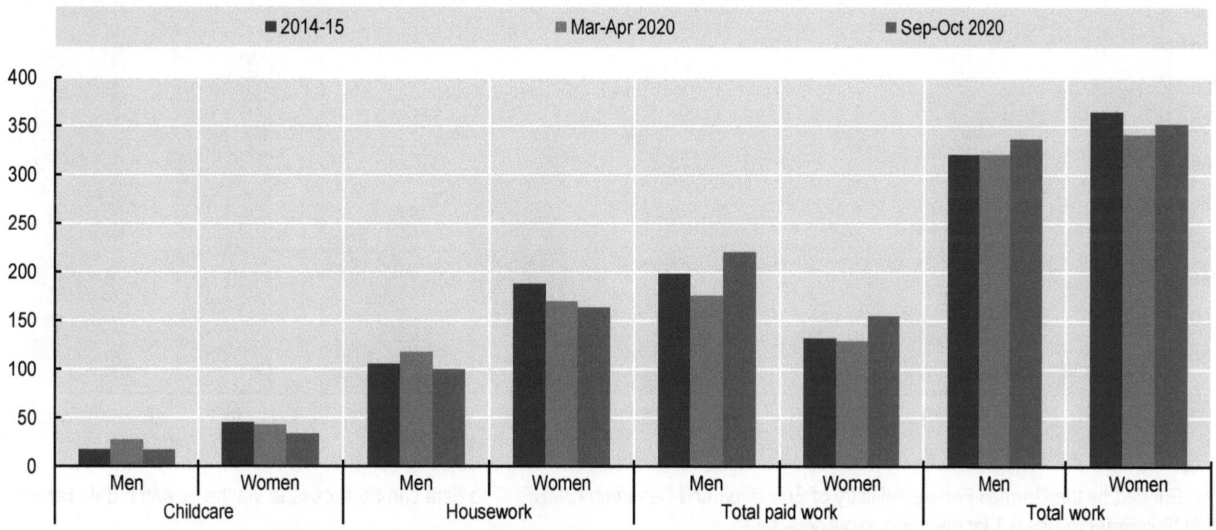

Note: Only times that people identify as their main activity at any given point are shown. Refer to Box 7.2 for methodological details.
Source: ONS (2021[21]), *A "new normal"? How people spent their time after the March 2020 coronavirus lockdown*, https://www.ons.gov.uk/peoplepopulationandcommunity/healthandsocialcare/conditionsanddiseases/articles/anewnormalhowpeoplespenttheirtimeafterthemarch2020coronaviruslockdown/2020-12-09.

StatLink https://stat.link/7ieyfa

In other countries, men stepped up their share of unpaid work in return for being more affected by reduced paid working hours – though this seems to be a temporary phenomenon and the increase was still not enough to match women's contribution. During the first national lockdown in the United Kingdom in March-April 2020, the gap in unpaid work between men and women initially declined slightly compared to 2014-15 (it still remained large, at 1 hour and 7 minutes a day). However, as people returned to work and schools reopened in September-October 2020, so did older gender patterns: men reduced their daily contribution to household tasks by three times the amount of women (18 and 6 minutes, respectively) compared to six months earlier (Figure 7.13). In Germany, by January-February 2021, men increased their daily time spent on housework by 15 minutes (compared to 12 minutes for women). Nevertheless, women still performed the majority of unpaid work, increased their time spent on childcare more than men (12 vs 9 minutes), and worked half an hour more if both unpaid and paid work are considered (Figure 7.14). In addition, existing gender gaps in dissatisfaction with family time, sleep and leisure time have increased in Germany over this same period (Figure 7.15). In June 2021, women in Columbia were more likely than men to feel consistently overburdened by domestic chores (25.2% vs 12.8%) (DANE, n.d.[22]).

Figure 7.14. In Germany, women continue to work more than men if unpaid work is taken into account

Minutes per day spent on paid and unpaid work in Germany, by gender, 2019, Apr-Jun 2020, Jan-Feb 2021

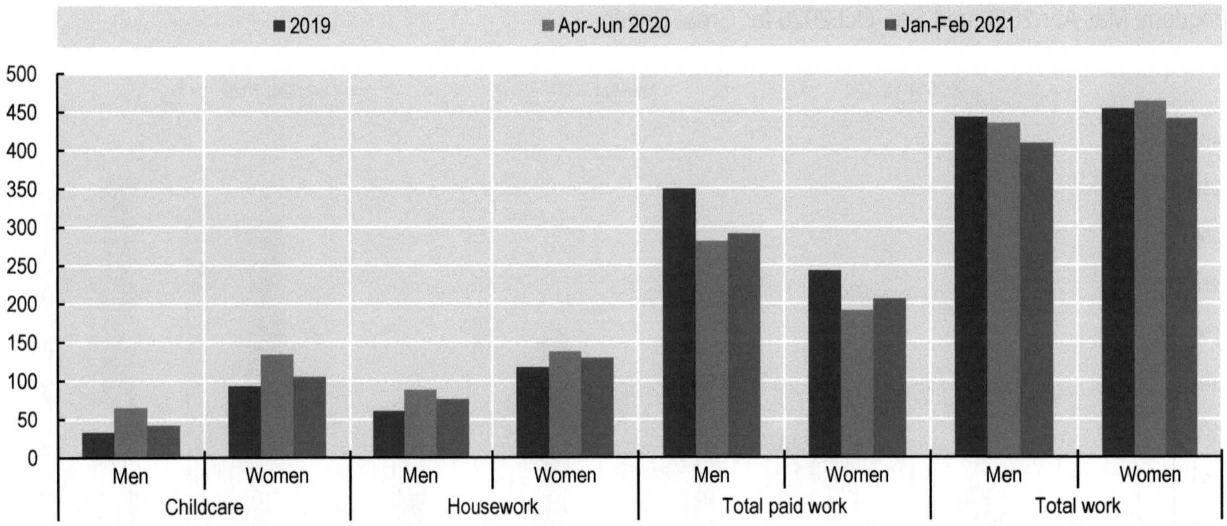

Note: Funded by the German Federal Ministry of Education and Research (BMBF). The data can be accessed via the research data centre of the SOEP. Refer to Box 3.1 for methodological details.
Source: Kühne et al. (2020[6]), "The need for household panel surveys in times of crisis: The case of SOEP-CoV", *Survey Research Methods*, Vol. 14/2, pp. 195-203, https://doi.org/10.18148/srm/2020.v14i2.7748.

StatLink https://stat.link/7gap6c

Figure 7.15. Gender gaps in dissatisfaction with how time is spent have widened in Germany compared to 2019

Share of people in Germany dissatisfied with their time use in selected areas, by gender, 2019, Jan-Feb 2021

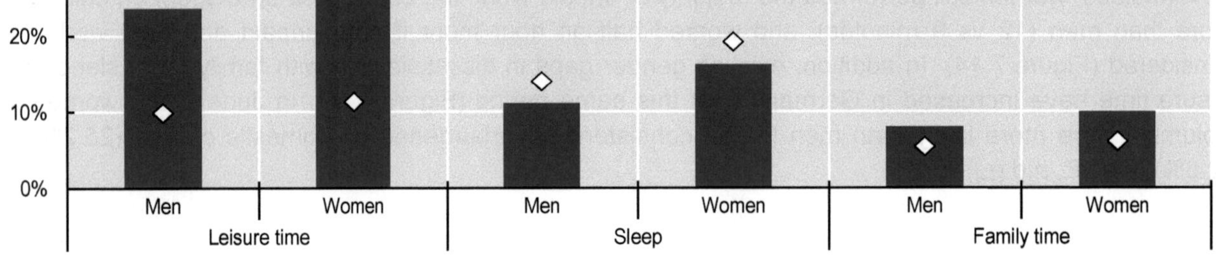

Note: People who answered 4 or less on a scale of 0 (not at all satisfied) to 10 (completely satisfied) for each of the areas of time use are defined as dissatisfied. Funded by the German Federal Ministry of Education and Research (BMBF). The data can be accessed via the research data centre of the SOEP. Refer to Box 3.1 for methodological details.
Source: Kühne et al. (2020[6]), "The need for household panel surveys in times of crisis: The case of SOEP-CoV", *Survey Research Methods*, Vol. 14/2, pp. 195-203, https://doi.org/10.18148/srm/2020.v14i2.7748.

StatLink https://stat.link/e4ah7z

Working parents, most of all working mothers, have struggled with care work. In the United States, 52% of employed parents with children younger than 12 reported difficulties in meeting their childcare responsibilities in October 2020, up from 38% in March 2020. In addition, 36% of teleworking mothers reported having heavy childcare duties, as compared to 16% of teleworking fathers (Pew Research Center, 2020[23]).[5] An earlier study from the United States, relying on data from the Current Population Survey up to May 2020, found that school closures and stay-at-home orders particularly affected working mothers (forcing them to take leave) but had no immediate impact on fathers' leave or leave of women without school-age children (Heggeness, 2020[24]).

Some evidence also suggests that the contributions of men to unpaid work could be overestimated. In Canada, when asked in June 2020, men were much more likely than women to report that they shared parental tasks equally with their partner (Figure 7.16). This pattern is consistent with previous studies (Pew Research Center, 2015[25]). Indeed, research shows that men tend to overestimate the time they spend on unpaid family work, particularly when this information is collected using stylized questions (i.e. respondents answer questions about their activities retrospectively) instead of time-use diaries (i.e. respondents record their activities over a period of time in a diary) (Kan, 2008[26]; UN, 2005[27]).

Figure 7.16. In Canada, men's and women's perceptions of how parental tasks are divided differ

Share of men and women in Canada reporting that they perceive a task to be equally shared by both parents, Jun-2020

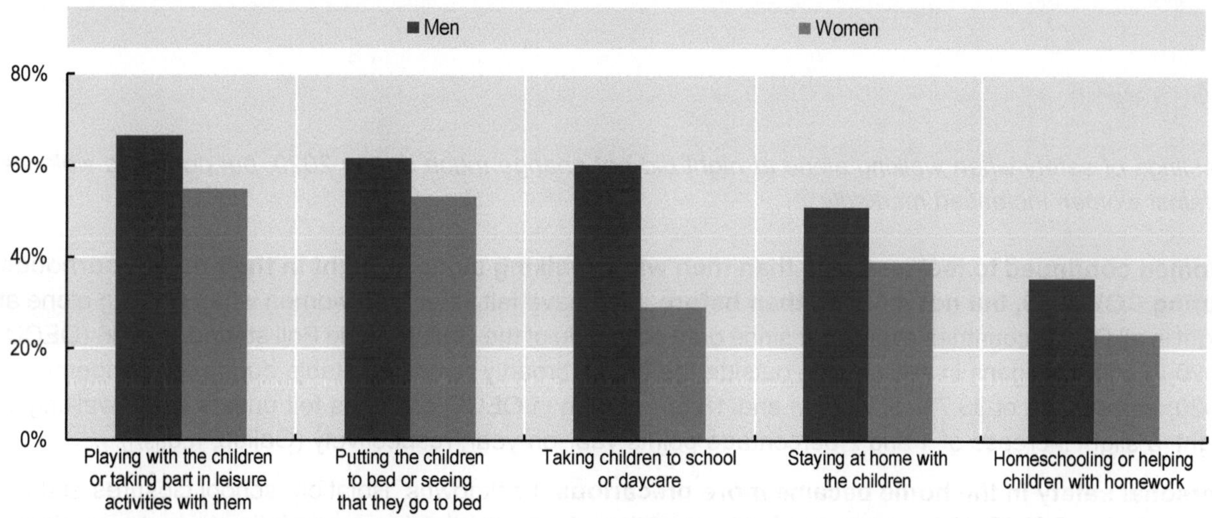

Note: The analysis is limited to respondents who were living with a spouse or partner at the time of the survey.
Source: Statistics Canada (2020[28]), *Caring for their children: Impacts of COVID-19 on parents*, https://www150.statcan.gc.ca/n1/pub/45-28-0001/2020001/article/00091-eng.htm.

StatLink https://stat.link/k2iv5x

Box 7.2. Innovation: Online time-use surveys in times of a pandemic

Several OECD countries have moved towards online collection of time-use data during the pandemic.

United Kingdom: 2020 online time-use study

Under COVID-19 restrictions in Great Britain, the Office of National Statistics (ONS) carried out a special online time-use survey for adults aged 18 years or over between 28 March - 26 April 2020, with a second wave conducted six months later, between 5 September - 11 October 2020 (ONS, 2020[29]; ONS, 2021[21]). As part of trying to understand the impact of the COVID-19 pandemic and associated restrictions on household behaviour more broadly, respondents were asked to record the average minutes per day and week spent on various activities (e.g. travelling and transport, working from and away from home, total paid work, unpaid childcare and other unpaid work, study, keeping fit, personal care, entertainment and socialising).

Australia: Australia's Time-Use Survey

The Australian Bureau of Statistics (ABS) launched an online time-use survey in 2021 to collect information about how Australians balance their time between work, family, leisure, caring and other activities (ABS, 2021[30]). The survey collects general information on everyone in the household and includes questions about employment, childcare and health, asking each household member who is aged 15 or over to complete a time-use diary and record all activities over a two-day period.

7.3. Safety

Feelings of safety when walking alone at night did not change much during 2020, but domestic violence against women increased markedly

Women continued to feel less safe than men when walking alone at night in their neighbourhoods during COVID-19, but not more so than before. Men have felt safer than women when walking alone at night in all OECD countries every year since data collection of the Gallup World Poll started in 2006 (OECD, 2020[31]). Gender gaps in feeling safe outside the house broadly remained stable during the pandemic: in 2020, an average of 33.7% of women and 18.5% of men in OECD countries felt unsafe when walking at night, a slight increase of 1 and 2 percentage points year-on-year, respectively (Gallup, n.d.[32]).

Personal safety in the home became more precarious. Lockdowns, isolation, school closures and job losses during COVID-19 have created fertile conditions for domestic abuse, and intimate partner violence against women and girls worldwide has intensified since the pandemic outbreak (OECD, 2020[33]).[6] Population surveys and official crime statistics both suggest a rise of domestic violence: for instance, according to an online survey by the Australian Institute of Criminology, close to 1 in 4 Australian women experienced domestic violence in the three months prior to May 2020, with many of them identifying the pandemic as the onset of their experience (Figure 7.17). One in 10 women (as well as 1 in 17 men) in Canada were very or extremely concerned about the possibility of violence in the home in April-May 2020 (Statistics Canada, 2020[34]). In England and Wales, police records indicate a 7% increase in the total number of offences related to domestic abuse from March to June 2020 year-on-year (Figure 7.18), and the number of domestic abuse killings of women in the United Kingdom was the highest of any 21-day period in the past decade during the first three weeks of the first national lockdown in March-April 2020 (Home Office, 2020[35]).

Demand for victim support services also suggests the rise of domestic violence. In the United Kingdom, the National Domestic Abuse Helpline registered a 65% increase in calls and contacts logged between April and June 2020 compared to the year's first three months. Victim Support handled 12% more domestic abuse in the first week that lockdown restrictions were eased in mid-May compared to the previous week, reflecting the difficulties victims faced in safely seeking support during confinement (ONS, 2020[36]). Similarly, Canada's Assaulted Women's Helpline handled 77% more calls from March to December 2020 compared to the average annual number of contacts, while in Mexico City, there were 58% more requests to the Línea Mujeres helpline from January to September 2020 than in the same period for 2019 (Data-Pop Alliance, 2020[37]; AWHL, n.d.[38]). Calls to national helplines for victims of domestic violence also markedly increased in Italy (by 73% during the first lockdown from March to mid-April 2020 compared to the same period in 2019) and France (by around 400% between prior to the first lockdown in March and the end of April 2020) (Istat, 2020[39]; Republique Francaise, 2020[40]).

Figure 7.17. More than 20% of all Australian women cohabiting with a partner experienced emotionally abusive, harassing or controlling behaviours in May-June 2020

Share of women in Australia who reported experiencing different types of domestic violence in the last three months, May-Jun 2020

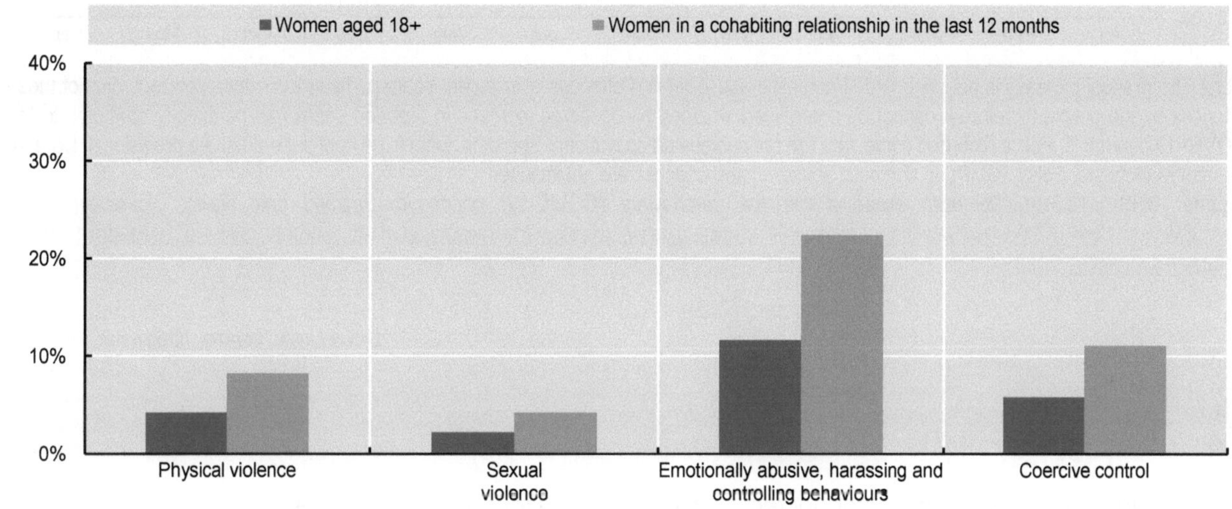

Note: The survey was conducted by i-Link Research Solutions between 6 May and 1 June 2020. Domestic violence is defined here as physical violence, sexual violence and emotionally abusive, harassing or controlling behaviour involving intimate partners.
Source: Australian Institute of Criminology (2020[41]), *The prevalence of domestic violence among women during the COVID-19 pandemic*, https://www.aic.gov.au/sites/default/files/2020-07/sb28_prevalence_of_domestic_violence_among_women_during_covid-19_pandemic.pdf.

StatLink https://stat.link/seirf0

Figure 7.18. Domestic abuse offences in England and Wales were on the rise in the first half of 2020

Number of offences (excluding fraud) in England and Wales (excluding GMP) flagged as domestic abuse-related, Jan 2018 - Jun 2020

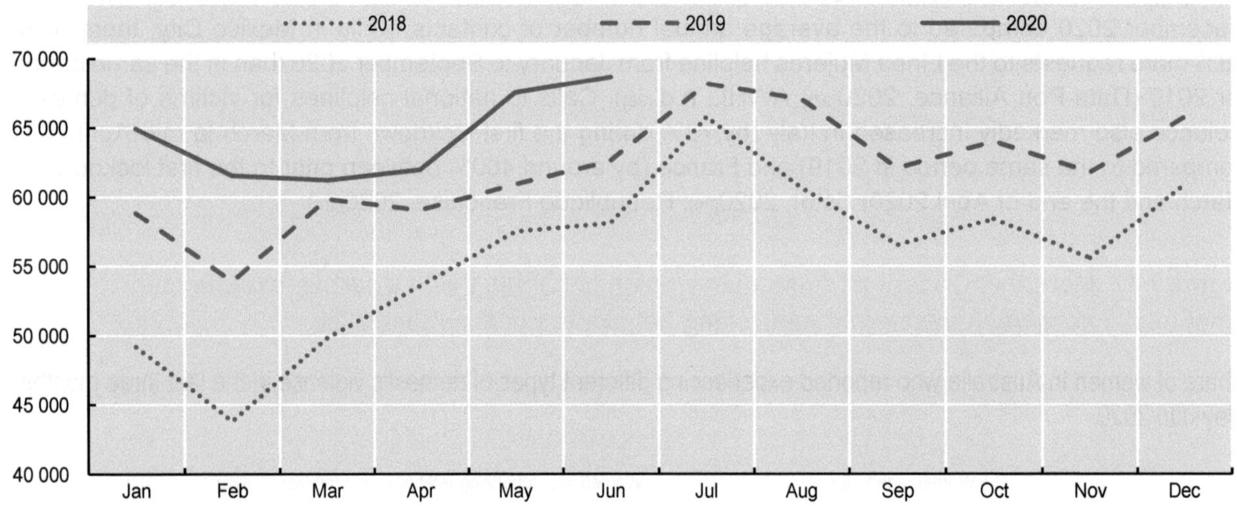

Note: The gradual increase in police-recorded domestic abuse-related offences over recent years partly reflects improved recording of these offences by the police; therefore it cannot be determined whether the observed increase in reported cases can be directly attributed to the COVID-19 pandemic. Police-recorded crime data are not designated as National Statistics. Data from April-June 2020 are provisional. Data for Greater Manchester Police (GMP) on domestic abuse-related offences are not included.
Source: ONS (2020[42]), *Domestic abuse during the coronavirus (COVID-19) pandemic, England and Wales: November 2020*, https://www.ons.gov.uk/peoplepopulationandcommunity/crimeandjustice/articles/domesticabuseduringthecoronaviruscovid19pandemicenglandandwales/november2020.

StatLink https://stat.link/s7ptlk

7.4. Civic engagement

Vulnerable groups feel more disconnected from community life during COVID-19

Many people feel disconnected from communal life and unable to shape the society they live in. In June-July 2020, when economies were temporarily re-opening, 18.6% of respondents in European OECD countries agreed with the statement that they felt left out of their societies. Six months later, this share had risen to 27.5% (see Chapter 4). This feeling was particularly acute among those with difficulty making ends meet, the unemployed, the lower educated (all of whom were already more likely to feel left out in 2016) as well as younger people up to age 24 (Figure 7.19). This pattern holds at both the OECD average and individual country level (Figure 7.20).

Figure 7.19. The unemployed, those with financial difficulties or less than university education and younger people were all more likely to feel left out of society in the first year of the pandemic

Share of people agreeing or strongly agreeing with the statement "I feel left out of society", by population group, OECD 22, 2016, Jun-Jul 2020, Feb-Mar 2021

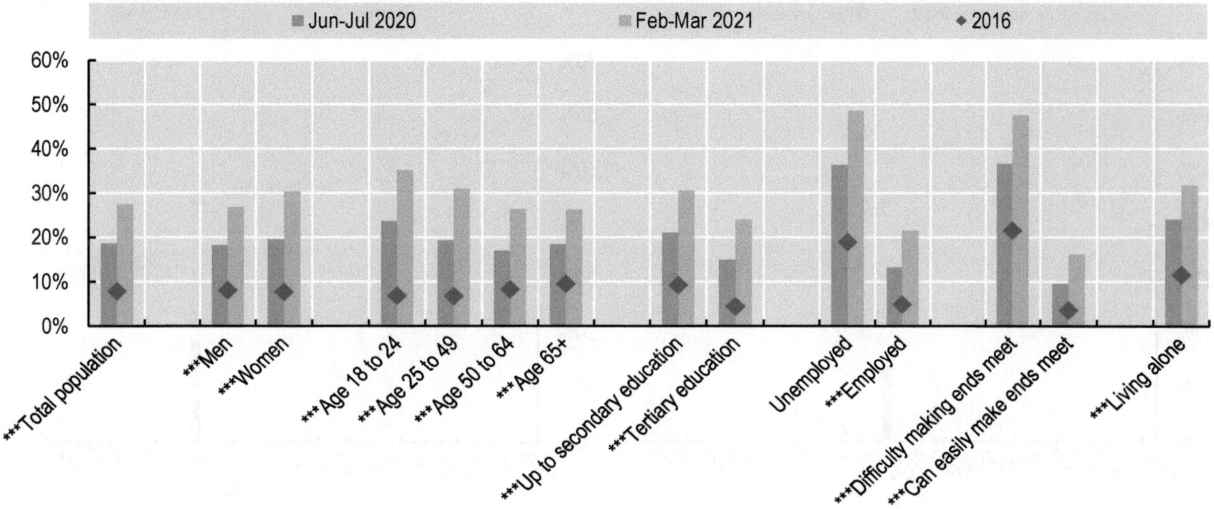

Note: The OECD average includes Austria, Belgium, the Czech Republic, Denmark, Estonia, Finland, France, Germany, Greece, Hungary, Ireland, Italy, Latvia, Lithuania, Luxembourg, the Netherlands, Poland, Portugal, the Slovak Republic, Slovenia, Spain and Sweden. Categories preceded by *** saw statistically significant (at the 5% level) changes from June-July 2020 to February-March 2021. See the note of Figure 7.1 for the definition of difficulty making ends meet, and Box 2.1 for methodological details on the Living, working and COVID-19 e-survey. The 2020-2021 and 2016 data points are not directly comparable due to differences in sampling between the Living, working and COVID-19 e-survey and the European Quality of Life Survey (although the question asked is the same).

Source: OECD calculations based on Eurofound (2018[8]), *European Quality of Life Survey 2016*, https://www.eurofound.europa.eu/publications/report/2017/fourth-european-quality-of-life-survey-overview-report; and Eurofound (n.d.[1]), *Living, working and COVID-19 e-survey* (database), http://eurofound.link/covid19data.

StatLink https://stat.link/0hivrw

Figure 7.20. Inequalities in feeling left out of society are similar across European OECD countries

Share of people agreeing or strongly agreeing with the statement "I feel left out of society", by financial difficulty, employment status, education and gender, average over 2 survey waves in Jun-Jul 2020, Feb-Mar 2021

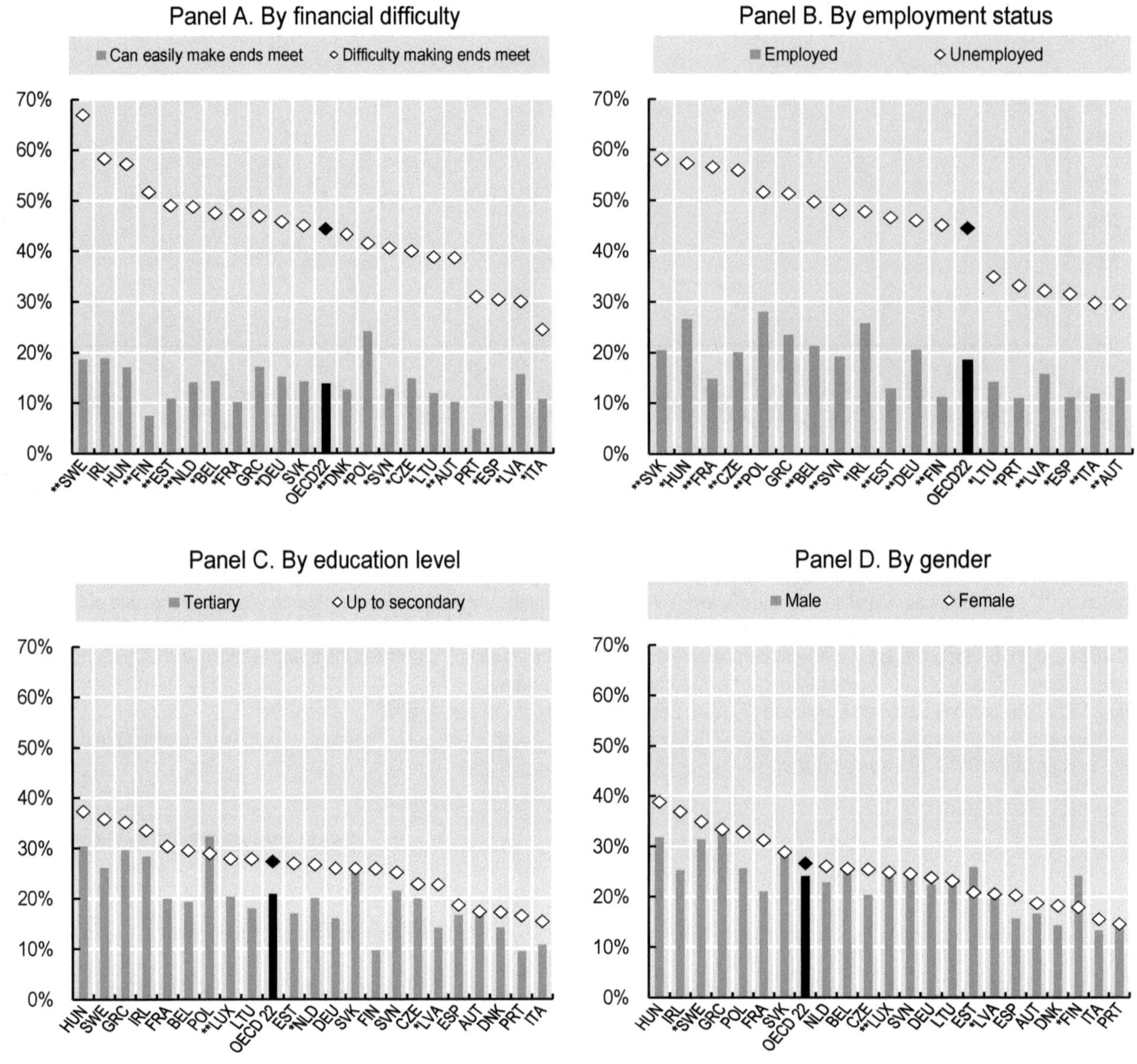

Note: In all panels, the OECD average includes Austria, Belgium, the Czech Republic, Denmark, Estonia, Finland, France, Germany, Greece, Hungary, Ireland, Italy, Latvia, Lithuania, Luxembourg, the Netherlands, Poland, Portugal, the Slovak Republic, Slovenia, Spain and Sweden. Data are not reported for countries where fewer than 100 observations are available. ** denotes countries with between 100 and 300 observations per category; * denotes countries with between 301 and 500 observations per category. More than 500 observations per category are available for all other countries. See Box 2.1 for methodological details on the Living, working and COVID-19 survey. In Panel A, see the note of Figure 7.1 for the definition of difficulty making ends meet. Differences between groups are significant (at the 5% level) for all countries, including OECD 22. In Panel B, differences between groups are significant (at the 5% level) for all countries, including OECD 22, except for the Netherlands. In Panel C, differences between groups are significant (at the 5% level) for all countries, including OECD 22, except for Austria, the Czech Republic, Denmark, Ireland, Italy, Latvia, Luxembourg, Poland, the Slovak Republic, Slovenia and Spain. In Panel D, differences between groups are significant (at the 5% level) for the Czech Republic, Finland, France, Hungary, Ireland and OECD 22.

Source: OECD calculations based on Eurofound (n.d.[1]), *Living, working and COVID-19 e-survey* (database), http://eurofound.link/covid19data.

StatLink https://stat.link/p15xhl

Box 7.3. Further reading

- OECD (2021), "Towards gender-inclusive recovery", *OECD Policy Responses to Coronavirus (COVID-19)*, OECD Publishing, Paris, https://doi.org/10.1787/ab597807-en
- OECD (2021), "All the lonely people: Education and loneliness", *Trends Shaping Education Spotlights*, No. 23, OECD Publishing, Paris, https://doi.org/10.1787/23ac0e25-en
- OECD (2020), *Taking Public Action to End Violence at Home: Summary of Conference Proceedings*, OECD Publishing, Paris, https://doi.org/10.1787/cbff411b-en
- Eurofound (2020), *Living, working and COVID-19*, COVID-19 series, Publications Office of the European Union, Luxembourg, https://www.eurofound.europa.eu/publications/report/2020/living-working-and-covid-19

References

ABS (2021), *Australia's Time Use Survey*, https://www.abs.gov.au/tus#Anchor1. [30]

ABS (2020), *Household Impacts of COVID-19 Survey*, https://www.abs.gov.au/statistics/people/people-and-communities/household-impacts-covid-19-survey/6-10-july-2020#unpaid-caring-responsibilities-and-domestic-work. [18]

ANUPoll (2020), *Tracking outcomes during the COVID-19 pandemic (August 2020)*, Australian National University, https://csrm.cass.anu.edu.au/sites/default/files/docs/2020/9/Tracking_wellbeing_outcomes_during_the_COVID-19_pandemic_February_to_August_2020.pdf. [4]

Australian Institute of Criminology (2020), *The prevalence of domestic violence among women during the COVID-19 pandemic*, https://www.aic.gov.au/sites/default/files/2020-07/sb28_prevalence_of_domestic_violence_among_women_during_covid-19_pandemic.pdf. [41]

AWHL (n.d.), *Assaulted Women's Helpline*, https://www.awhl.org/ (accessed on 18 June 2021). [38]

Capgemini Research Institute (2020), *The Future of Work: From remote to hybrid*, https://www.capgemini.com/it-it/research/the-future-of-work/. [17]

DANE (n.d.), *Encuesta Pulso Social (database)*, Departamento Administrativo Nacional de Estadística, https://www.dane.gov.co/index.php/estadisticas-por-tema/encuesta-pulso-social (accessed on 21 September 2021). [22]

Data-Pop Alliance (2020), *Using Data to Shed Light on the Shadow Pandemic of Domestic Violence in Mexico*, https://datapopalliance.org/using-data-to-shed-light-on-the-shadow-pandemic-of-domestic-violence-in-mexico/. [37]

Eurofound (2020), *Living, working and COVID-19*, Publications Office of the European Union, Luxembourg, https://www.eurofound.europa.eu/publications/report/2020/living-working-and-covid-19. [2]

Eurofound (2018), *European Quality of Life Survey 2016*, Publications Office of the European Union, Luxembourg, https://www.eurofound.europa.eu/publications/report/2017/fourth-european-quality-of-life-survey-overview-report. [8]

Eurofound (n.d.), *Living, working and COVID-19 dataset*, https://www.eurofound.europa.eu/data/covid-19 (accessed on 21 August 2021). [1]

Eurostat (n.d.), *Database - EU Survey on Income and Living Conditions*, https://ec.europa.eu/eurostat/web/income-and-living-conditions/data/database (accessed on 20 May 2021). [45]

Facebook; OECD;The World Bank (2020), *Global State of Small Business Report: Reflections on six waves of data collection*, https://dataforgood.fb.com/wp-content/uploads/2020/12/State-of-Small-Business-Wave-VI-Report.pdf. [19]

Gallup (n.d.), *Gallup World Poll (database)*, https://www.gallup.com/178667/gallup-world-poll-work.aspx (accessed on 18 June 2021). [32]

Heggeness, M. (2020), "Estimating the immediate impact of the COVID-19 shock on parental attachment to the labor market and the double bind of mothers", *Review of Economics of the Household*, Vol. 18/4, http://dx.doi.org/10.1007/s11150-020-09514-x. [24]

Home Office (2020), *Home Office preparedness for Covid-19 (Coronavirus): domestic abuse and risks of harm within the home Contents*, https://publications.parliament.uk/pa/cm5801/cmselect/cmhaff/321/32105.htm#footnote-109. [35]

Istat (2020), *Gender-based violence in the time of COVID-19: calls to the 1522 helpline*, https://www.istat.it/en/archivio/245001. [39]

John, N. et al. (2020), "Lessons Never Learned: Crisis and gender-based violence", *Developing World Bioethics*, Vol. 20/2, http://dx.doi.org/10.1111/dewb.12261. [44]

Kan, M. (2008), *Measuring Housework Participation: The Gap Between "Stylised" Questionnaire Estimates and Diary-Based Estimates*, https://www.researchgate.net/publication/225682128_Measuring_Housework_Participation_The_Gap_Between_Stylised_Questionnaire_Estimates_and_Diary-Based_Estimates. [26]

Kühne, S. et al. (2020), "The need for household panel surveys in times of crisis: The case of soep-cov", *Survey Research Methods*, Vol. 14/2, pp. 195-203. [6]

Kuhnt, A. and S. Krapf (2020), "Partnership Living Arrangements of Immigrants and Natives in Germany", *Frontiers in Sociology*, Vol. 5, http://dx.doi.org/10.3389/fsoc.2020.538977. [43]

Loneliness New Zealand Charitable Trust (2020), *Prolonged loneliness in New Zealand before, during, and after lockdown*, Loneliness NZ, https://loneliness.org.nz/wp-content/uploads/2020/07/Prolonged-loneliness-in-New-Zealand-1-Aug-2020.pdf. [3]

NZ Social Wellbeing Agency (2020), *Short Report: Social Isolation, loneliness and COVID-19*, https://swa.govt.nz/assets/Publications/reports/Short-Report-V3.pdf. [7]

OECD (2021), "All the lonely people: Education and loneliness", *Trends Shaping Education Spotlights*, No. 23, OECD Publishing, Paris, https://doi.org/10.1787/23ac0e25-en. [13]

OECD (2020), *How's Life? 2020 - Measuring Well-being*, OECD Publishing, Paris, https://doi.org/10.1787/9870c393-en. [31]

OECD (2020), *Taking Public Action to End Violence at Home: Summary of Conference Proceedings*, OECD Publishing, Paris, https://dx.doi.org/10.1787/cbff411b-en. [33]

ONS (2021), *A "new normal"? How people spent their time after the March 2020 coronavirus lockdown*, https://www.ons.gov.uk/peoplepopulationandcommunity/healthandsocialcare/conditionsanddiseases/articles/anewnormalhowpeoplespenttheirtimeafterthemarch2020coronaviruslockdown/2020-12-09. [21]

ONS (2021), *Coronavirus and higher education students: England, 19 February to 1 March 2021*, https://www.ons.gov.uk/peoplepopulationandcommunity/healthandsocialcare/healthandwellbeing/bulletins/coronavirusandhighereducationstudents/19februaryto1march2021. [10]

ONS (2021), *Mapping loneliness during the coronavirus pandemic*, https://www.ons.gov.uk/peoplepopulationandcommunity/wellbeing/articles/mappinglonelinessduringthecoronaviruspandemic/2021-04-07. [11]

ONS (2020), *Coronavirus and how people spent their time under lockdown: 28 March to 26 April 2020*, https://www.ons.gov.uk/economy/nationalaccounts/satelliteaccounts/bulletins/coronavirusandhowpeoplespenttheirtimeunderrestrictions/28marchto26april2020. [29]

ONS (2020), *Coronavirus and loneliness, Great Britain: 3 April to 3 May 2020*, https://www.ons.gov.uk/peoplepopulationandcommunity/wellbeing/bulletins/coronavirusandlonelinessgreatbritain/3aprilto3may2020. [5]

ONS (2020), *Coronavirus and the social impacts on different ethnic groups in the UK: 2020*, https://www.ons.gov.uk/peoplepopulationandcommunity/culturalidentity/ethnicity/articles/coronavirusandthesocialimpactsondifferentethnicgroupsintheuk/2020. [15]

ONS (2020), *Domestic abuse during the coronavirus (COVID-19) pandemic, England and Wales: November 2020*, https://www.ons.gov.uk/peoplepopulationandcommunity/crimeandjustice/articles/domesticabuseduringthecoronaviruscovid19pandemicenglandandwales/november2020. [42]

ONS (2020), *Domestic abuse in England and Wales overview: November 2020*, https://www.ons.gov.uk/peoplepopulationandcommunity/crimeandjustice/bulletins/domesticabuseinenglandandwalesoverview/november2020. [36]

ONS (2020), *Personal and economic well-being in Great Britain: September 2020, Opinions and Lifestyle Survey (COVID-19 module), 20 March to 26 July 2020, Estimates for Income Groups*, https://www.ons.gov.uk/peoplepopulationandcommunity/wellbeing/datasets/incomegroupsplitestimatesonpersonalandeconomicwellbeingacrosstime. [14]

ONS (2018), "Loneliness - What characteristics and circumstances are associated with feeling lonely?", https://www.ons.gov.uk/peoplepopulationandcommunity/wellbeing/articles/lonelinesswhatcharacteristicsandcircumstancesareassociatedwithfeelinglonely/2018-04-10. [47]

Parker, K., J. Menasce Horowitz and R. Minkin (2020), *How the Coronavirus outbreak has – and hasn't – changed the way americans work*, Pew Research Center, https://www.pewresearch.org/social-trends/2020/12/09/how-the-coronavirus-outbreak-has-and-hasnt-changed-the-way-americans-work/. [16]

Pew Research Center (2020), *A rising share of working parents in the U.S. say it's been difficult to handle child care during the pandemic*, https://www.pewresearch.org/fact-tank/2021/01/26/a-rising-share-of-working-parents-in-the-u-s-say-its-been-difficult-to-handle-child-care-during-the-pandemic/. [23]

Pew Research Center (2015), *Raising Kids and Running a Household: How Working Parents Share the Load*, https://www.pewresearch.org/wp-content/uploads/sites/3/2015/11/2015-11-04_working-parents_FINAL.pdf. [25]

Republique Francaise (2020), *Violences conjugales : l'effet "révélateur" du confinement*, https://www.vie-publique.fr/en-bref/275691-violences-conjugales-le-confinement-revelateur. [40]

Social Wellbeing Agency (2020), *Short Report: Social Isolation, loneliness and COVID-19*, https://swa.govt.nz/assets/Publications/reports/Short-Report-V3.pdf. [12]

Statistics Canada (2020), *Canadian Perspectives Survey Series 1: Impacts of COVID-19*, https://www150.statcan.gc.ca/n1/daily-quotidien/200408/dq200408c-eng.htm. [34]

Statistics Canada (2020), *Caring for their children: Impacts of COVID-19 on parents*, https://www150.statcan.gc.ca/n1/pub/45-28-0001/2020001/article/00091-eng.htm. [28]

StatsNZ (2021), *Wellbeing statistics: A year in review (June 2020 to March 2021 quarter)*, https://www.stats.govt.nz/reports/wellbeing-statistics-a-year-in-review-june-2020-to-march-2021-quarter#worse. [9]

StatsNZ (n.d.), *Wellbeing data for New Zealanders - Loneliness*, https://wellbeingindicators.stats.govt.nz/en/loneliness/ (accessed on 26 February 2021). [46]

UN (2005), *Guide to Producing Statistics on Time Use: Measuring Paid and Unpaid Work.*, https://unstats.un.org/unsd/publication/SeriesF/SeriesF_93E.pdf. [27]

UN Women (n.d.), *Covid 19 and gender monitor*, https://data.unwomen.org/COVID19 (accessed on 31 April 2021). [20]

Notes

[1] For instance, 2018 data from the European Union Statistics on Income and Living Conditions (EU-SILC) as well as 2016 data from the European Quality of Life Survey showed that older age groups were more lonely than those 18-24 year old (Eurofound, 2018[8]) (Eurostat, n.d.[45]). However, in the United Kingdom, younger adults aged 16 to 24 already reported feeling lonely more often than those in older age groups in 2016-17 (ONS, 2018[47]), as was the case for young people aged 15-24 in New Zealand in 2018 (StatsNZ, n.d.[46]). Further research on the impact of question wording on responses to questions about loneliness, as well as on whether people adapt their frame of reference with age will be needed to understand these patterns better.

[2] Higher unemployment in a local area was also linked to greater average anxiety in that area as well as poorer life satisfaction, with the link between high levels of unemployment and poorer life satisfaction becoming stronger during the pandemic.

[3] These include the respondent's age, gender, whether living alone, changes in help and support received since the start of the coronavirus pandemic, and having a health condition.

[4] This might be partly due to the fact that persons with a migration background are less likely to live alone (Kuhnt and Krapf, 2020[43]).

[5] This study is based on 2 029 U.S. adults who have children younger than 18, were working part time or full time, and had either one or more than one job. Data were collected as part of the online survey Center's American Trends Panel conducted from 13-19 October 2020.

[6] Evidence from previous disease outbreaks also highlights a strong relationship between gender-based violence and crisis situations. For instance, the Ebola outbreak in sub-Saharan Africa during 2015-16 significantly increased the risk of sexual exploitation for women and children (John et al., 2020[44]).

8 Economic capital and COVID-19

The impact of the pandemic on economic capital, which includes both produced (man-made) and financial assets, has differed across sectors and types of assets. Total investment in OECD countries has significantly declined due to high uncertainty in the economy. In particular, private sector investment has fallen, while investment in intellectual assets (as a share of the total) has increased slightly. Both household savings and household financial net worth have increased, while the impact of the crisis on household debt has been limited. These averages, however, mask divergent trends, with both wealth and savings increasing faster among the wealthy. In one-third of the 23 OECD countries with data, corporate debt either reached or exceeded levels observed during the Global Financial Crisis. Government financial net worth declined and gross government debt increased due to unprecedented public spending on pandemic support programmes.

The global economy plunged into recession following the outbreak of the COVID-19 pandemic as most economic activities were impaired by the lockdown. Over the past century, the depth of the current recession has been exceeded only by World War Two and the Great Depression (World Bank, 2021[1]). Across OECD countries, GDP growth rates shrank on average by 10.4% in the second quarter of 2020 although growth rebounded sharply in the third quarter of 2020 and reverted to its pre-pandemic level in the first quarter of 2021 (Figure 8.1). This unprecedented crisis is having a large impact not only on current well-being, but also on the future, due to disruptions to investment in the resources that sustain well-being over time – including stocks of economic capital. In addition, economic sustainability is at risk when debt (incurred by governments, the corporate sector or households) rises. Although the COVID-19 pandemic has had severe impacts on short-term economic production, the impact on economic capital has differed across economic sectors and types of assets. In 2021, global economy recovered, but the recovery remains uneven across countries, sectors and demographic groups in terms of output and employment (OECD, 2021[2]).

Figure 8.1. The fall in GDP among OECD countries during the pandemic was well in excess of that recorded during the financial crisis

Gross domestic product, growth rate based on seasonally adjusted volume data, percentage change from previous quarter, OECD

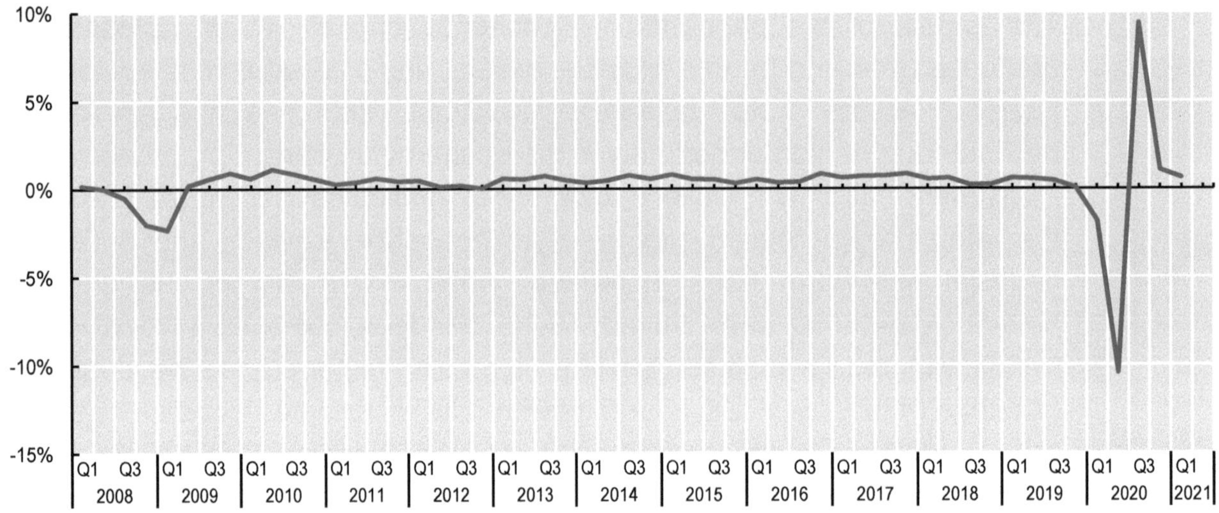

Source: OECD (n.d.[3]), *National Accounts Statistics, Quarterly National Accounts* (database), https://stats.oecd.org/Index.aspx?DataSetCode=QNA.

StatLink https://stat.link/w41gf5

Uncertainty remains high after peaking at the onset of the COVID-19 pandemic. Across 29 OECD countries, the World Uncertainty Index (WUI) from the IMF – an index derived by counting the occurrences of the word "uncertainty" in Economist Intelligence Unit country reports (Ahir, Bloom and Furceri, 2020[4]) – was 0.49 in the first quarter of 2020, an all-time high since the index was started in 1952. This measure of uncertainty decreased in the fourth quarter of 2020, yet remained around 60% above its average level during the 1996-2010 period. The expectations of businesses and consumers about future economic performance also stayed low throughout 2020. Across OECD countries, confidence indices among both businesses and consumers, as measured by opinion surveys, were mostly below 100 during 2020, indicating continuing pessimism about future performance (OECD, 2021[5]; OECD, 2021[6]). This pessimism risks weighing heavily on investment decisions, with long-term consequences for GDP growth and people's well-being. At the same time, the ambitious recovery packages being designed and implemented in most OECD countries include a strong focus on investments in digital, energy and transport infrastructure, and on the replacement of energy intensive durable goods with more climate-friendly alternatives. Achieving the medium-term goal of net zero emissions of greenhouse gases will require an overhaul of the stock of economic capital, spurring investment growth in the future.

8.1. Investment in economic assets

Gross fixed capital formation fell sharply during the pandemic in all OECD countries, although with different intensity across different types of assets

The level of investment in fixed capital declined sharply throughout the OECD area as economic activities were disrupted and uncertainty reigned during the first wave of the pandemic. In the second quarter of 2020, gross fixed capital formation (GFCF) across OECD countries fell by close to 12%, on average (Figure 8.2, Panel A). This compares to a growth rate of 1.9% in the second quarter in 2019. As many OECD countries exited the first wave of the pandemic in the third quarter of 2020, GFCF rebounded strongly, but this rebound was only temporary and was followed by a further fall as the health crisis deepened further towards the end of 2020 (Figure 8.2, Panel B).

The contraction in GFCF extended to most types of assets, although with different intensity.[1] Across 28 OECD countries,[2] GFCF in all different types of assets contracted in the second quarter of 2020 compared to the same period of 2019, with smaller declines for cultivated biological resources (-0.6 percentage points) and intellectual property products (-16.2) and much larger ones for: dwellings (-30.6 percentage points), other buildings and structures (-34.1), and machinery and equipment (-38.2) (OECD, 2021[7]). As a consequence, the share of investment in machinery in total GFCF across 32 OECD countries declined by 3.1 percentage points in the second quarter of 2020 relative to the previous year, while that of buildings increased by 1.7 percentage points (Figure 8.3) and that of intellectual property assets (across 31 countries) increased by 1.0 percentage points, although edging down more recently (Figure 8.4, Panel A and Panel B).

High uncertainty has contributed to the volatility of investment in the first year of the pandemic, and this volatility weighed heavily on business decisions. The share of business investment in GDP across the 27 EU members declined by 0.6 percentage points in 2020 relative to the previous year, while that of government and households increased by 0.3 and 0.1 percentage points, respectively (Eurostat, 2021[8]). In the United Kingdom, the business sector (i.e. private and public corporations) reduced its total investment by 11.9% between the fourth quarter of 2020 and the first quarter of 2021, the second-largest fall on record after the 22.5% fall recorded in the second quarter of 2020. Lower investment in transport equipment contributed the most to the fall in business investment, followed by ICT and other machinery and equipment. Evidence suggests that uncertainty in the UK business sector was already rising pre-pandemic, but reached new heights in 2020: text analysis of comments from two official business sector surveys run by the UK Office of National Statistics showed a continuous increase in references to uncertainty and to delaying or cancelling investments since the third quarter of 2018, peaking in the second quarter of 2020 (Figure 8.5).

The pandemic hit small and medium-sized businesses harder than large businesses, due to their difficulties in mobilising liquidity and accessing finance as their revenues declined (OECD, 2021[9]). Evidence from 41 SME surveys across OECD countries, conducted by business associations, think tanks, chambers of commerce or banks since February 2020, shows that more than half of SMEs reported severe losses in revenues; one-third of them feared being out of business without further support within one month, and up to 50% within three months (OECD, 2020[10]). A survey on the business impacts of COVID-19 conducted by the Australian Bureau of Statistics in August 2020 reported that 35% of small businesses (employing fewer than 20 people) expected that it would be difficult or very difficult to meet their financial commitments over the next three months; this compared to 33% among medium-sized business (below 200 people) and 18% among large business (200 people and above) (ABS, 2020[11]).

Figure 8.2. Gross fixed capital formation fell in almost all OECD countries in the second quarter of 2020

Gross fixed capital formation, growth rate based on seasonally adjusted volume data, percentage change from the previous quarter

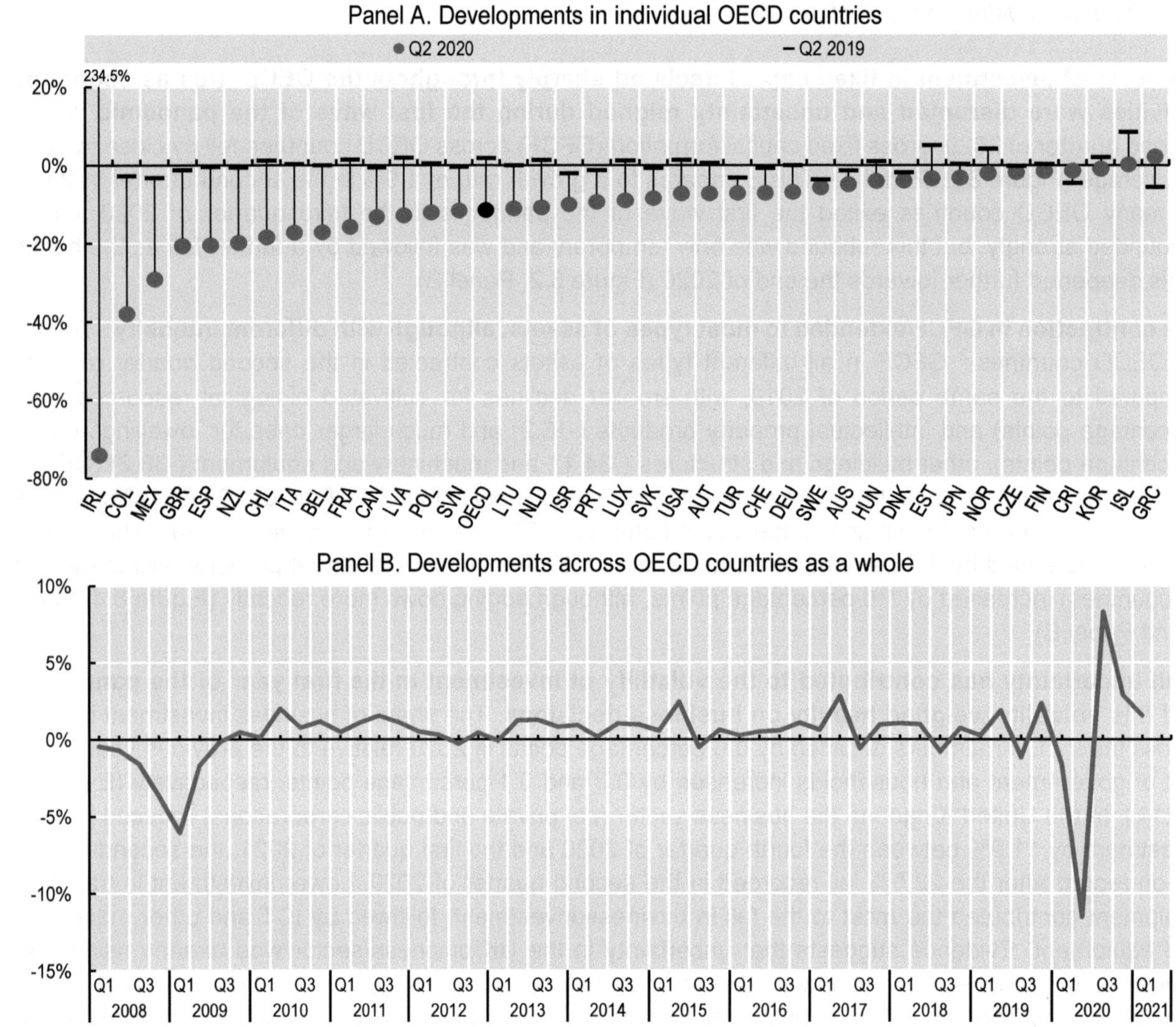

Source: OECD (n.d.[3]), *National Accounts Statistics, Quarterly National Accounts* (database), https://stats.oecd.org/Index.aspx?DataSetCode=QNA.

StatLink https://stat.link/jr6twq

Figure 8.3. The share of tangible assets to total investment declined in most OECD countries

Investment in building and machinery, as a share of total gross fixed capital formation

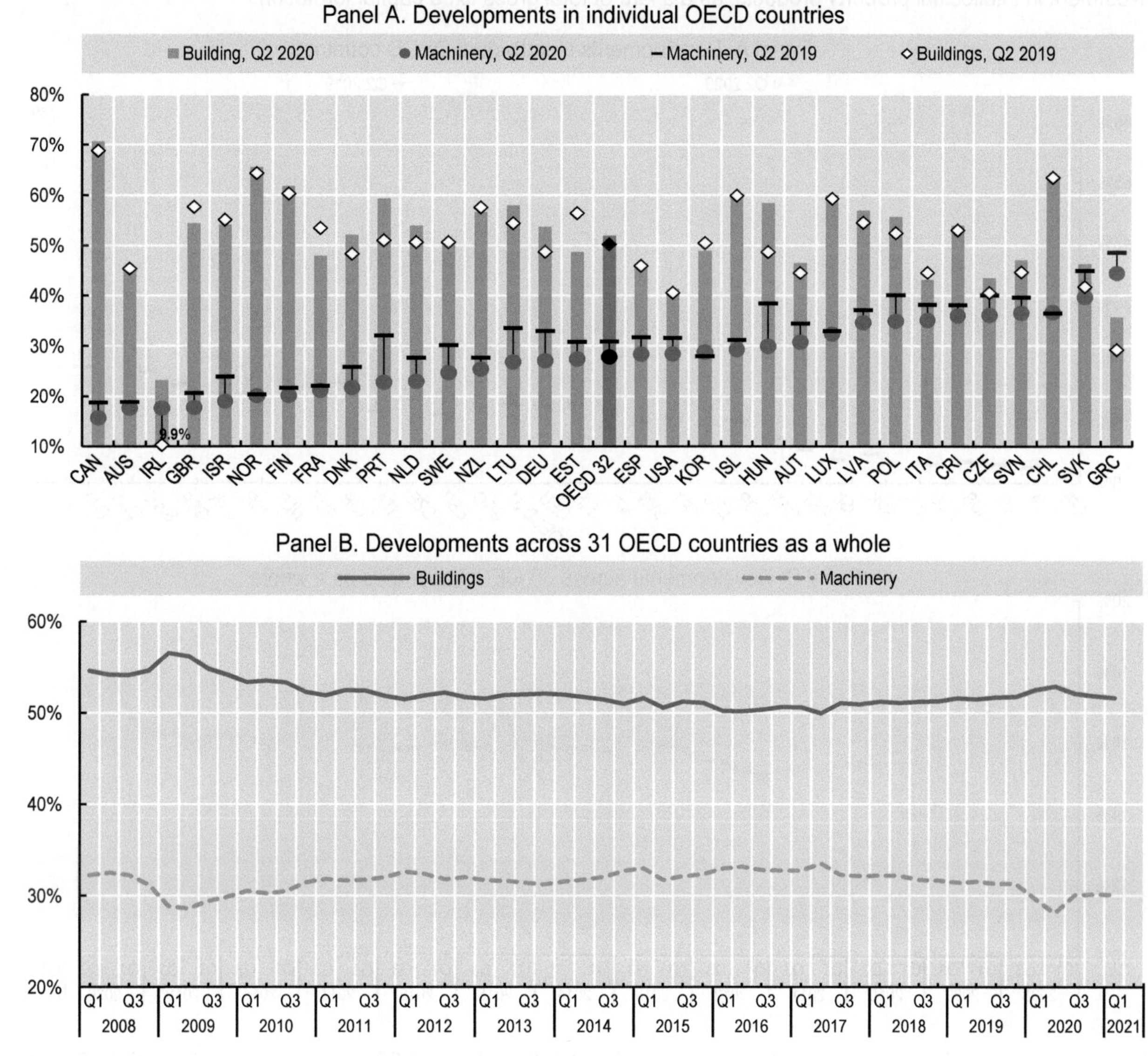

Note: Data are expressed in current prices and are seasonally adjusted. In the figure, building assets include both dwellings and other buildings and structures. In Panel A, the OECD average excludes Belgium, Colombia, Japan, Mexico, Switzerland and Turkey due to a lack of data. In Panel B, the OECD average excludes Ireland, in addition to all the countries excluded from Panel A, due to a lack of data over the period reviewed.

Source: OECD (n.d.[3]), *National Accounts Statistics, Quarterly National Accounts* (database), https://stats.oecd.org/Index.aspx?DataSetCode=QNA.

StatLink https://stat.link/ai2obu

Figure 8.4. The share of intellectual assets in total investment rose slightly in most OECD countries in the early phase of the lockdown

Investment in intellectual property products, as a share of total gross fixed capital formation

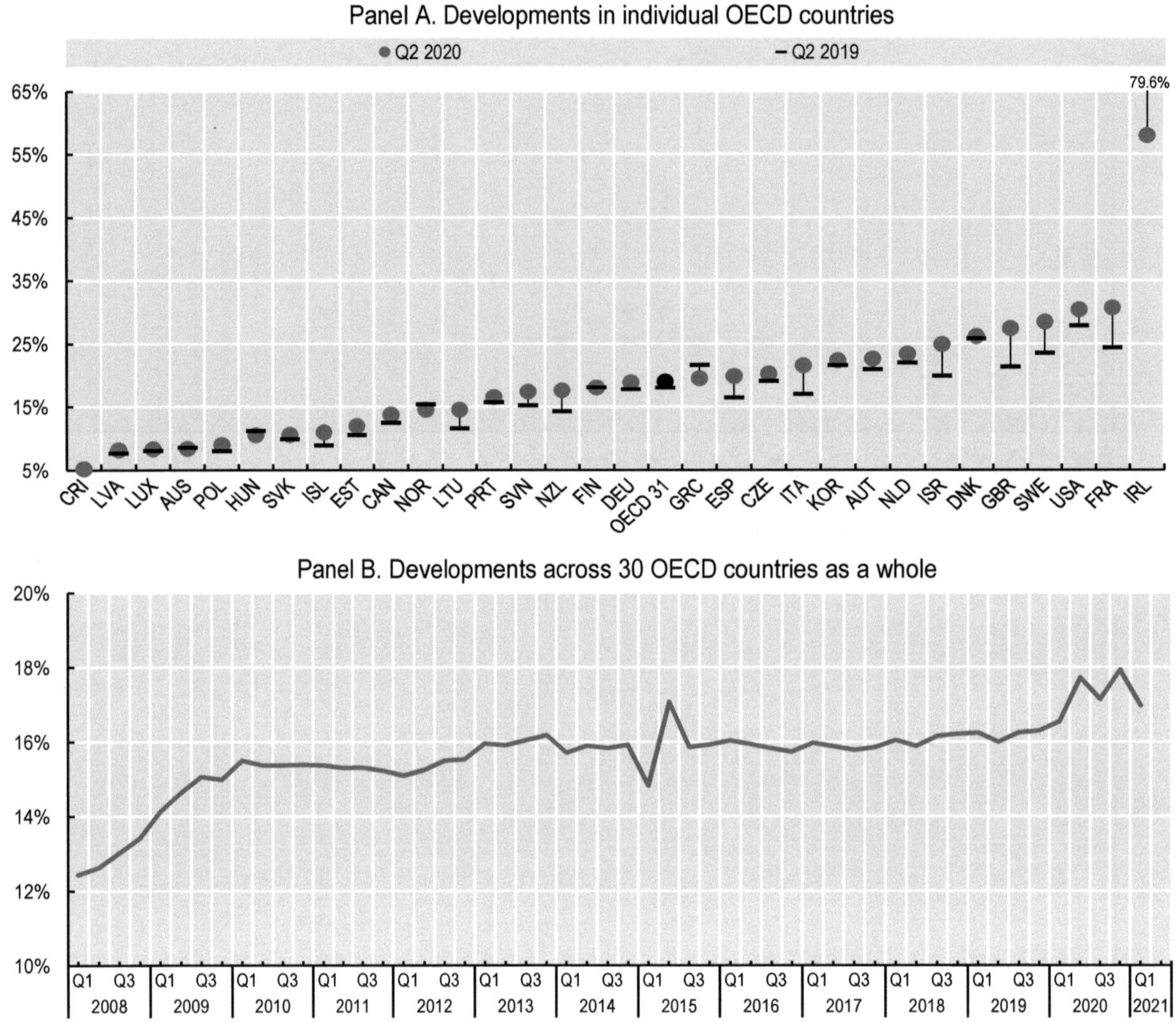

Note: Data are expressed in current prices and are seasonally adjusted. In Panel A, the OECD average excludes Belgium, Chile, Colombia, Japan, Mexico, Switzerland and Turkey due to a lack of data. In Panel B, the OECD average excludes Ireland, in addition to those excluded from Panel A, due to a lack of data over the period reviewed.

Source: OECD (n.d.[3]), *National Accounts Statistics, Quarterly National Accounts* (database), https://stats.oecd.org/Index.aspx?DataSetCode=QNA.

StatLink https://stat.link/b0mg1t

Box 8.1. Innovation: Text analysis of business surveys in the United Kingdom

The Office of National Statistics (ONS) in the United Kingdom collects the comments left by businesses responding to both the Quarterly Acquisitions and Disposals of Capital Assets Survey (QCAS) and the Quarterly Stocks Survey (QSS). Text analysis summarises the most commonly cited words, in the context of popular phrases and themes. The analysis shown in Figure 8.5 tracks the frequency of common phrases and key words over time. Results of this analysis suggest that the percentage of comments referring to investments being delayed or cancelled peaked (at 30.6% and 3.1%, respectively) in the second quarter of 2020. References to business investment being delayed or cancelled subsequently fell back in the second half of 2020, but remained higher than at the end of 2019.

Table 8.1. Comments in UK surveys on business investment plans by theme in late 2020

Number of comments, Q4 2020; themes may not be mutually exclusive

QCAS		QSS	
Theme	Number of comments (%)	Theme	Number of comments
COVID	700 (29.0%)	COVID	389 (15.5%)
ICT Investment	165 (6.8%)	Stockpiling	233 (8.7%)
Brexit	81 (3.4%)	Brexit	282 (10.5%)
Lockdown	116 (4.8%)	Increasing Stock Levels	653 (24.3%)
Investment Delayed	576 (23.8%)	Decreasing Stock Levels	495 (18.4%)
Investment Cancelled	61 (2.6%)		

Source: ONS (2021[12]), *Quarterly Stocks Survey (QSS) and Capital Assets Survey (QCAS) textual data analysis* (database), Office for National Statistics, https://www.ons.gov.uk/economy/grossdomesticproductgdp/datasets/quarterlystockssurveyqssandcapitalassetssurveyqcastextualdataanalysis

Figure 8.5. Many UK businesses made references to delaying or cancelling their investments

Share of comments, Q4 2017 - Q4 2020

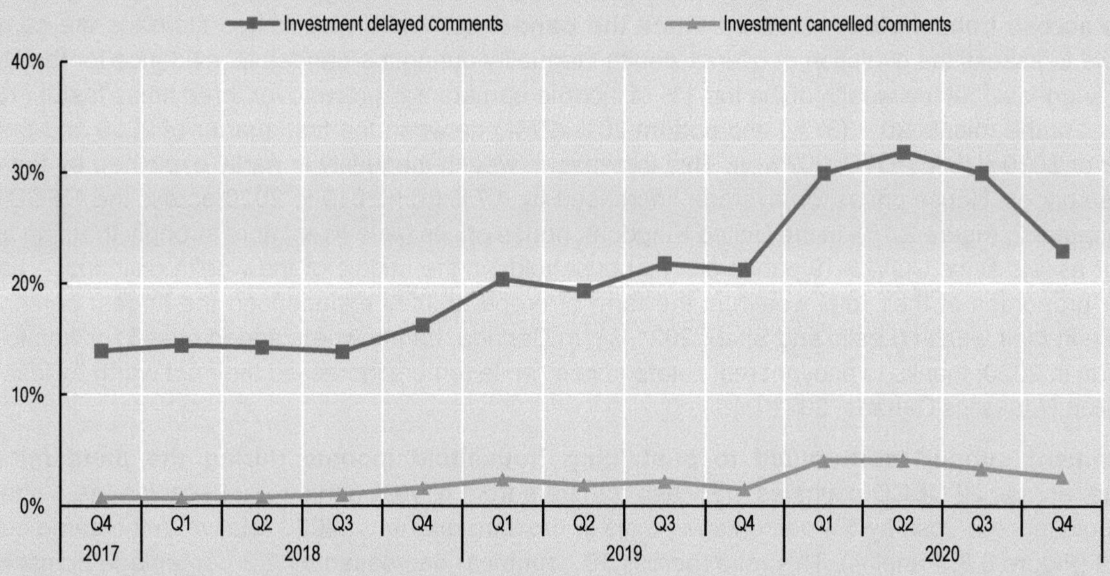

Note: Data are sourced from comments left by businesses participating in the two surveys cited below. These summarise the most commonly cited words that businesses responded with, in the context of popular phrases and themes. For some single words, to prevent business disclosure, a common phrase has been derived based on variations of instances in which the top word appeared.
Source: ONS (2021[12]), *Quarterly Stocks Survey (QSS) and Capital Assets Survey (QCAS) textual data analysis* (database), Office for National Statistics, https://www.ons.gov.uk/economy/grossdomesticproductgdp/datasets/quarterlystockssurveyqssandcapitalassetssurveyqcastextualdataanalysis.

StatLink https://stat.link/qi6ax7

8.2. Financial net worth

Average financial net worth of households increased during 2020 while that of governments fell

Household financial net worth rose in 2020, as savings rates increased sharply and consumption expenditure fell. Across 23 OECD countries, household financial assets exceeded financial liabilities by 282% of Household Gross Disposable Income (GDI) in the fourth quarter of 2020 (Figure 8.6). This represents an average increase of 15.8 percentage points relative to the same quarter in 2019. High saving rates (i.e. the ratio of household gross savings to their gross disposable income plus the change in pension entitlements) contributed to this rise. Across 23 OECD countries, the saving rates of households jumped by 12.3 percentage points in the second quarter of 2020 relative to the second quarter of 2019, while household expenditure decreased by 14.4% (Figure 8.7, Panel A). By the third quarter of 2020, consumption expenditure was beginning to recover and savings rates to decline, but both remained far from pre-pandemic levels (Figure 8.7, Panel B).

Growth in average savings rates masked different experiences among different households. A Bank of England survey in the United Kingdom conducted between August and September 2020 found that high and middle-income households were more likely to increase their savings, while low-income, unemployed and furloughed households were more likely to deplete their savings (ONS, 2021[13]). For example, the share of high-income households who reported that they saved more than in the past (42%) was almost two times larger than the share among low-income employed households (22%). In the United States, a Pew Research Center survey conducted in January of 2021 indicated that 32% of high-income households and 22% of middle-income households reported they saved more since the COVID-19 outbreak began, whereas only 16% of low-income households did (Pew Research Center, 2021[14]).

Looking beyond household financial net worth, some evidence suggests that inequality in (total) wealth across households increased since the pandemic. While very limited statistics are currently available to assess the evolution of overall wealth inequality during the pandemic, evidence for the Unites States suggests that the wealth of the top 1% of income earners has grown over three times faster (135%) than that of the middle 20% (37%) and bottom 20% (27%) between the first quarter of 2009 and the last quarter of 2020 (USAFACTS, 2021[15]). This increase in wealth inequality is partly explained by the rises in house prices. House prices, on average, increased by 4.7% from 2019 to 2020 across the OECD area (see Chapter 2, Figure 2.15). In the United Kingdom, house prices have risen more strongly than the prices of other assets since COVID-19 pandemic; as households in the middle of the wealth distribution have a greater proportion of their total wealth in the form of property, they experienced the largest percentage increase in their wealth (Leslie and Shah, 2021[16]). In Canada, homeowners added over $1 trillion to their net worth in 2020, thanks to buoyant real estate prices, while renters increased their net worth by less than $90 billion (Statistics Canada, 2021[17]).

Government support contributed to sustaining household income during the pandemic. On average, across 22 OECD countries, net cash transfers from governments to households, as a share of household income, rose by 5.4 percentage points in the third quarter of 2020 relative to the same quarter of 2019 (Figure 8.8, Panel A). This ratio (across 20 countries) decreased by 2.2 percentage points in the first quarter of 2021, while still remaining higher than pre-pandemic levels (Figure 8.8, Panel B).

Figure 8.6. Household financial net worth across 23 OECD countries increased slightly

Financial net worth of households, as a share of gross disposable income

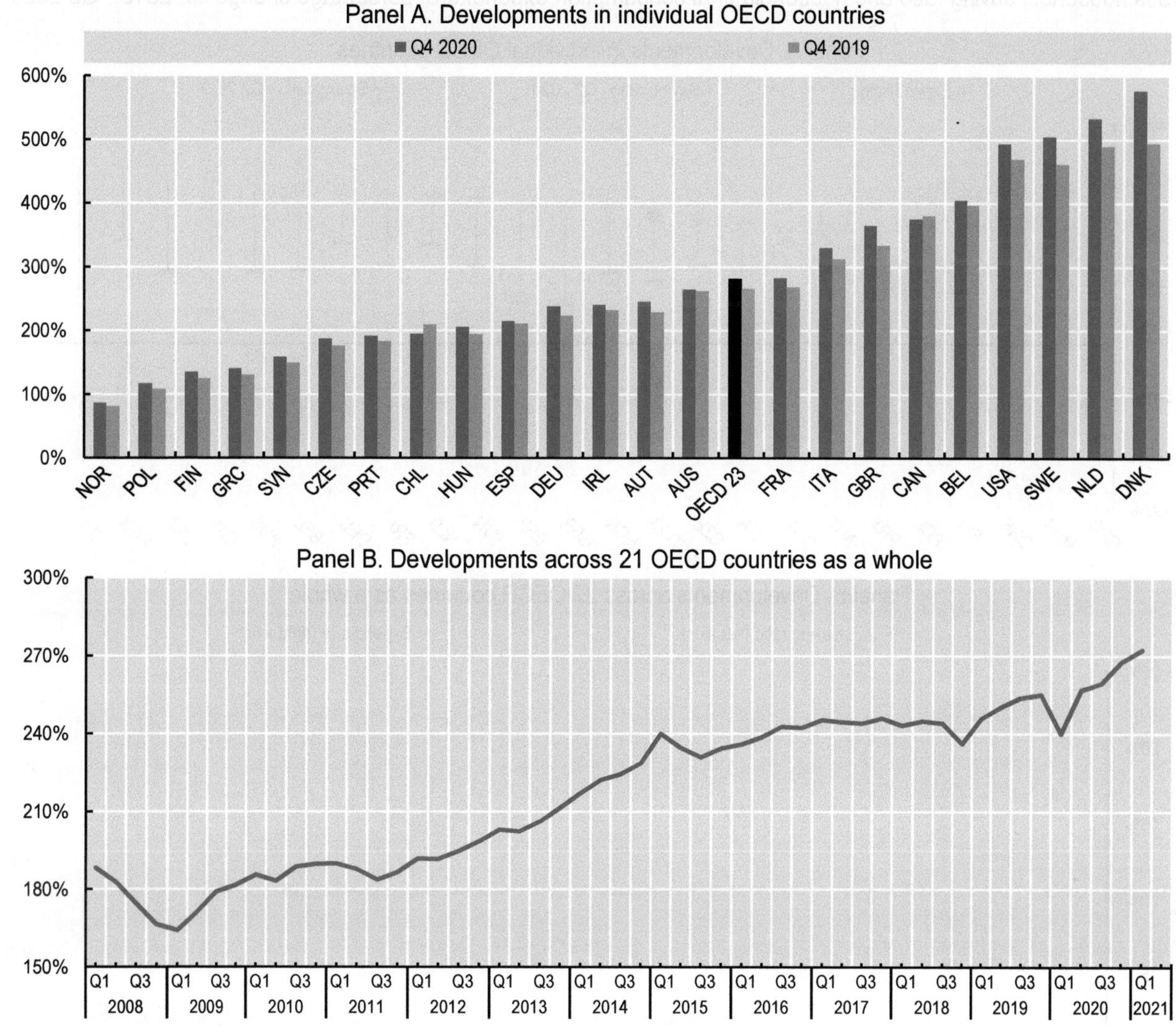

Note: Data are not seasonally adjusted. In Panel A, the OECD average includes only those 23 countries shown. In Panel B, the OECD average excludes Denmark and France, in addition to those excluded from Panel A, due to a lack of data over the period reviewed.
Source: OECD (n.d.[18]), *National Accounts Statistics, Household Dashboard* (database), http://stats.oecd.org/Index.aspx?DataSetCode=HH_DASH.

StatLink https://stat.link/80dqs1

Figure 8.7. Households in 23 OECD countries increased their saving rates and reduced their consumption expenditure

Gross household saving ratio and household final consumption expenditure, percentage change Q2 2019 - Q2 2020

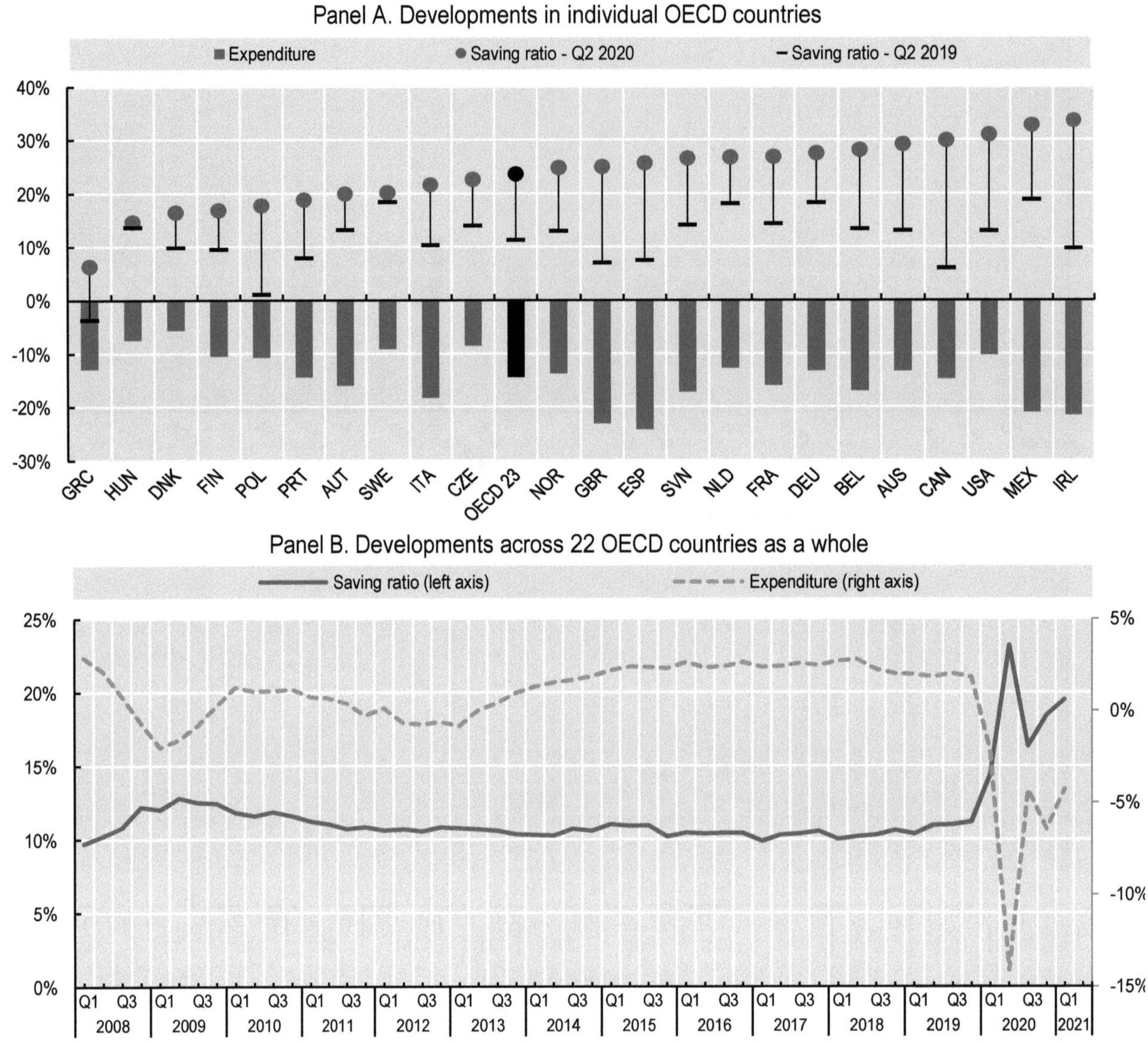

Note: Gross household saving is defined as household gross disposable income plus the change in pension entitlements less household final consumption expenditure. The household gross savings rate is calculated as the ratio of household gross savings to household gross disposable income plus the change in pension entitlements. Household consumption expenditure is the percentage change from the same quarter of the previous year based on seasonally adjusted volume data. In Panel A, the OECD average includes only those 23 countries shown. In Panel B, the OECD average excludes Mexico, in addition to those countries excluded from Panel A, due to a lack of Q1 2021 data.
Source: OECD (n.d.[18]), *National Accounts Statistics, Household Dashboard* (database), http://stats.oecd.org/Index.aspx?DataSetCode=HH_DASH.

StatLink https://stat.link/3xkmyd

Figure 8.8. Government supported household income in order to reduce the shock of the pandemic

Net cash transfers, ratio of households gross disposable income to gross primary income

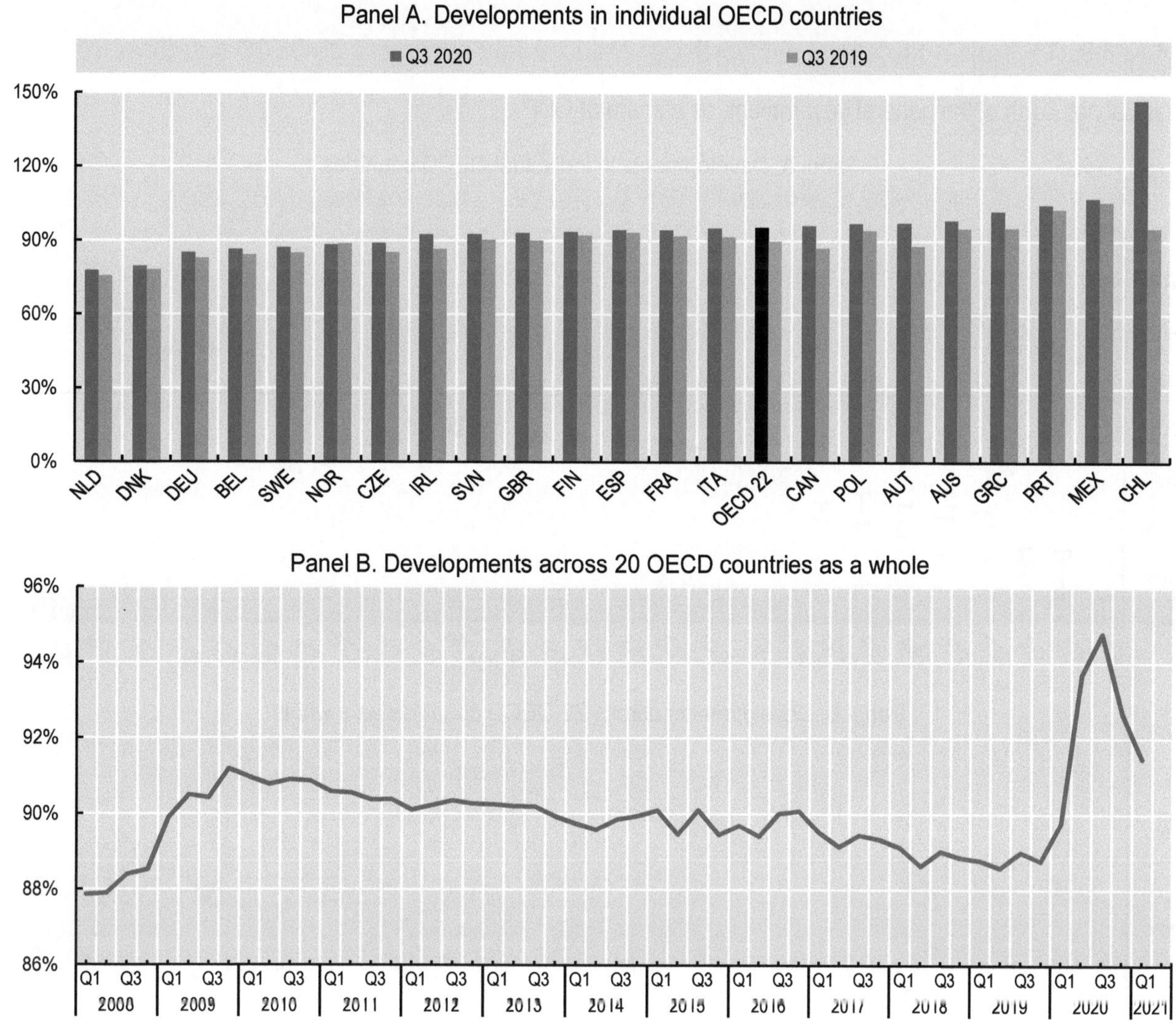

Note: This ratio shows the impact of government transfers on the income of households. The indicator is calculated as the ratio of gross disposable income to gross primary income. Household gross disposable income is derived from primary income by taking into account net current transfers – for example, the payment of taxes on income and wealth and social contributions, and the receipt of social benefits from government. It does not include in-kind transfers, such as those related to health care and education provided free or at economically insignificant prices by government. The taxes deducted from income do not include consumption taxes (such as value-added taxes). In Panel A, the OECD average includes only those 22 countries shown. In Panel B, France and Mexico are excluded, in addition to the countries excluded from Panel A, due to a lack of Q1 2021 data.

Source: OECD (n.d.[18]), *National Accounts Statistics, Household Dashboard* (database), http://stats.oecd.org/Index.aspx?DataSetCode=HH_DASH.

StatLink https://stat.link/f7ku3o

The unprecedented support provided by government to households and businesses in the first year of the pandemic translated into a large decline in government financial net worth. In the second quarter of 2020, the financial net worth of general government as a share of GDP was 6.3 percentage points lower than in the same quarter of 2019 (Figure 8.9, Panel A). Among 26 OECD countries, only Norway experienced an increase in government net financial worth (by 37.9 percentage points), while in

Chile, Korea, Sweden and Luxembourg it remained broadly stable. Overall, the OECD average decline in the financial net worth of the government sector during the first year of the pandemic has been steep, but has not yet reached the lows experienced in 2011-14 (Figure 8.9, Panel B).

Figure 8.9. Government financial net worth declined steeply in most of 26 OECD countries

Financial net worth of the general government, as a share of GDP

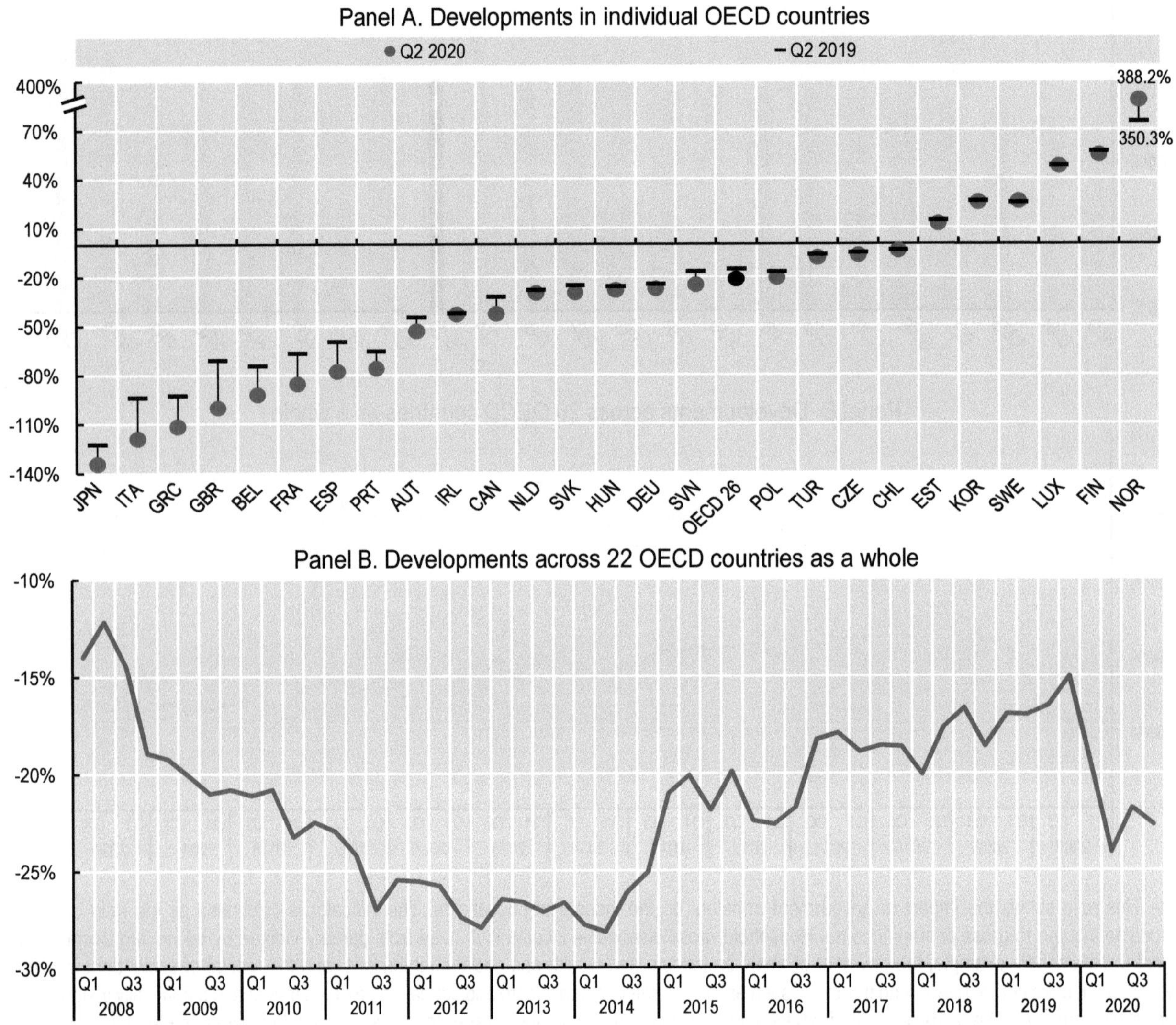

Note: Data are not seasonally adjusted. In Panel A, the OECD average includes only those 26 countries shown. In Panel B, the OECD average excludes Hungary, Korea, Poland and Turkey, in addition to those countries excluded from Panel A, due to a lack of data over the period reviewed.

Source: OECD (n.d.[19]), *National Accounts Statistics, Quarterly Sector Accounts, Non-consolidated financial balance sheets by economic sector* (database), https://stats.oecd.org/Index.aspx?DataSetCode=QASA_TABLE720R.

StatLink https://stat.link/r6f7yo

8.3. Debt

Government support during the pandemic has helped to keep household debt levels stable, while corporate debt remains high

The pandemic had limited impacts on average household debt so far in 2020, thanks to increased household savings and government income support. In the third quarter of 2020, across 23 OECD countries, the ratio of total outstanding debt of households as a percentage of their disposable income was 121.3% on average, little changed from the same quarter in 2019 (Figure 8.10, Panel A) and well below the 2011 peak (Figure 8.10, Panel B). Nevertheless, the debt burden of low-income households seem to have increase during the pandemic. According to a survey by the Resolution Foundation in the United Kingdom, 54% of adults in households from the lowest income quintile borrowed more to cover daily costs such as food and housing in March-June of 2020 than in the corresponding period of the previous year (Francis-Devine, 2021[20]). Different developments are visible when looking at different types of debt. Total unsecured debt in the United Kingdom declined sharply between March and November of 2020, while mortgage debt decreased by less (Francis-Devine, 2021[20]). In the United States, credit card balances declined substantially, by about USD 76 billion in the second quarter of 2020, while mortgage debt increased slightly (Congressional Research Service, 2020[21]).

The large decline in government financial net worth described in the previous section is mirrored by the sharp rise in government (gross) debt. The share of government gross debt to GDP in the fourth quarter of 2020 was 95.5% on average across 27 OECD countries (Figure 8.11). Between the fourth quarter of 2019 and the corresponding quarter of 2020, all OECD countries recorded rises in their government debt. On average, this share increased by 14.4 percentage points, and by a further 1.6 percentage points in the first quarter of 2021. This reflected expansionary fiscal policies targeted towards reducing the economic impact of the pandemic. Many governments implemented measures to support business cash-flow (e.g. extending deadlines for tax filing, deferring tax payments and granting tax exemptions) and household income and employment (e.g. cash benefits; broadening the coverage of unemployment benefits to self-employed workers; furlough and short-time work schemes) (OECD, 2020[22]). In 2020, the gross borrowings of OECD governments from the market hit the record high of USD 18 trillion, equal to almost 29% of GDP, and are projected to reach USD 19.1 trillion in 2021, remaining at the same share of GDP as in 2020 (OECD, 2021[23]).

Corporate debt remained high during the pandemic, signalling significant financial vulnerabilities. Although central banks continue to support financial markets through a variety of programmes, substantial risks remain (OECD, 2021[24]). A slow economic recovery or an early phasing out of support schemes could trigger additional debt delinquencies and defaults, with higher non-performing loans putting pressures on lenders (OECD, 2021[24]). In the third quarter of 2020, the debt service ratio (DSR)[3] of the private non-financial sector increased by 0.2 percentage points on average across 23 OECD countries (to 16.6%) compared to the same quarter in 2019 (Figure 8.12). The corporate debt burden either reached or exceeded levels last observed during the 2008 Global Financial Crisis in over one-third of OECD countries. This escalating debt burden is raising pressure on small firms, many of whom struggle to repay these loans and face an uncertain future. Higher levels of corporate debt also threaten to choke off the recovery by constraining firms' ability to invest in tangible and intangible assets and to innovate (OECD, 2021[25]).

Figure 8.10. Average household debt across 23 OECD countries remained relatively stable in the first three quarters of 2020

Household indebtedness, as a share of gross household disposable income

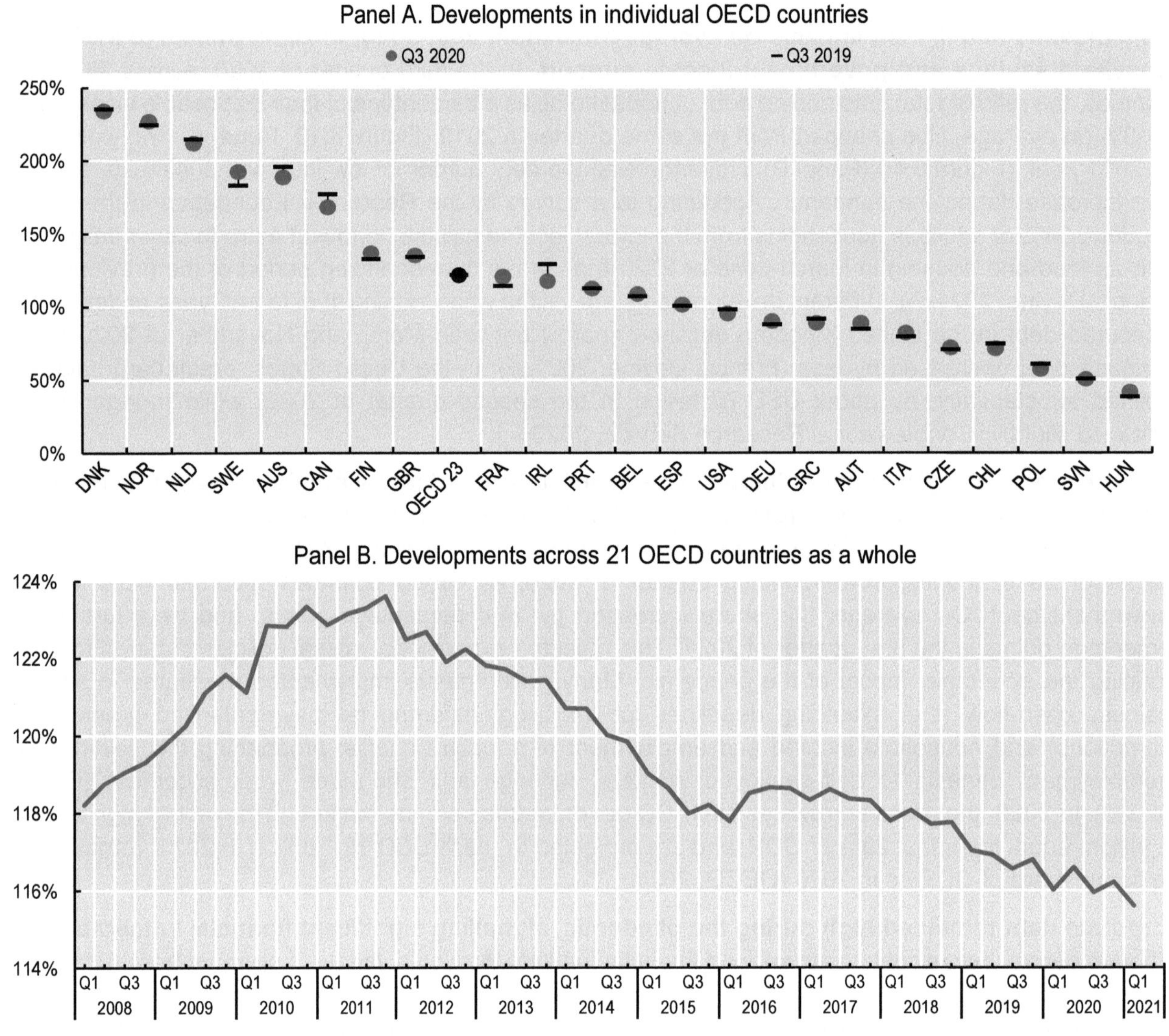

Note: Data are not seasonally adjusted. In Panel A, the OECD average includes only those 23 countries shown. In Panel B, the OECD average excludes Denmark and France, in addition to those countries excluded from Panel A, due to a lack of data over the period reviewed.
Source: OECD (n.d.[18]), *National Accounts Statistics, Household Dashboard* (database), http://stats.oecd.org/Index.aspx?DataSetCode=HH_DASH.

StatLink https://stat.link/76i2rf

Figure 8.11. Government debt increased in all 27 OECD countries

Government gross debt, as a share of GDP

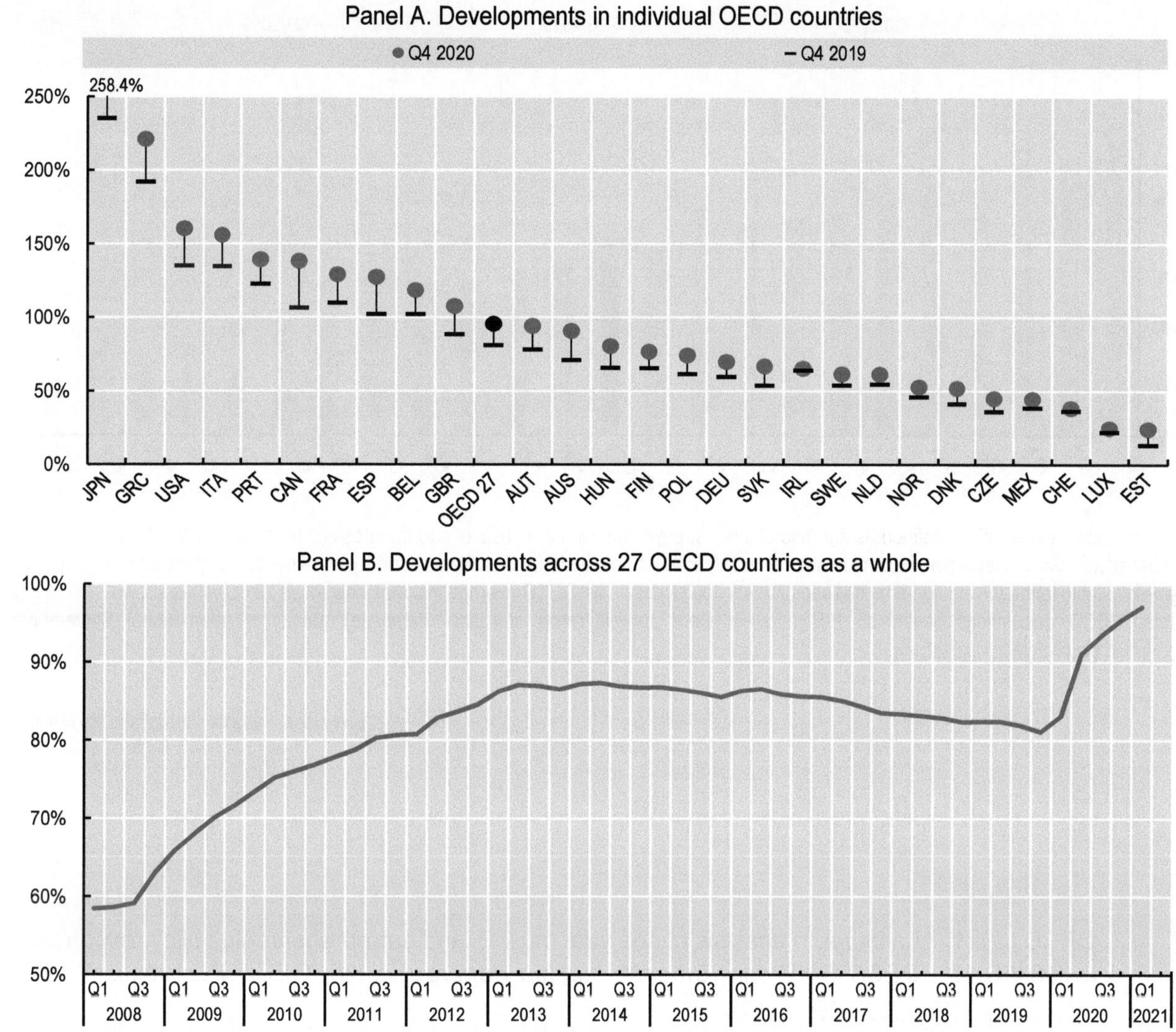

Note: Data are not seasonally adjusted. In both panels, the OECD average includes only those 27 countries shown in Panel A.
Source: OECD (n.d.[26]), *National Accounts Statistics, Quarterly Public Sector Debt, Public sector debt, consolidated, nominal value* (database), https://stats.oecd.org/Index.aspx?DataSetCode=QASA_TABLE7PSD.

StatLink https://stat.link/4tajrs

Figure 8.12. Debt burden of the private non-financial sector rose in half of 23 OECD countries

Debt service ratio of the private non-financial sector

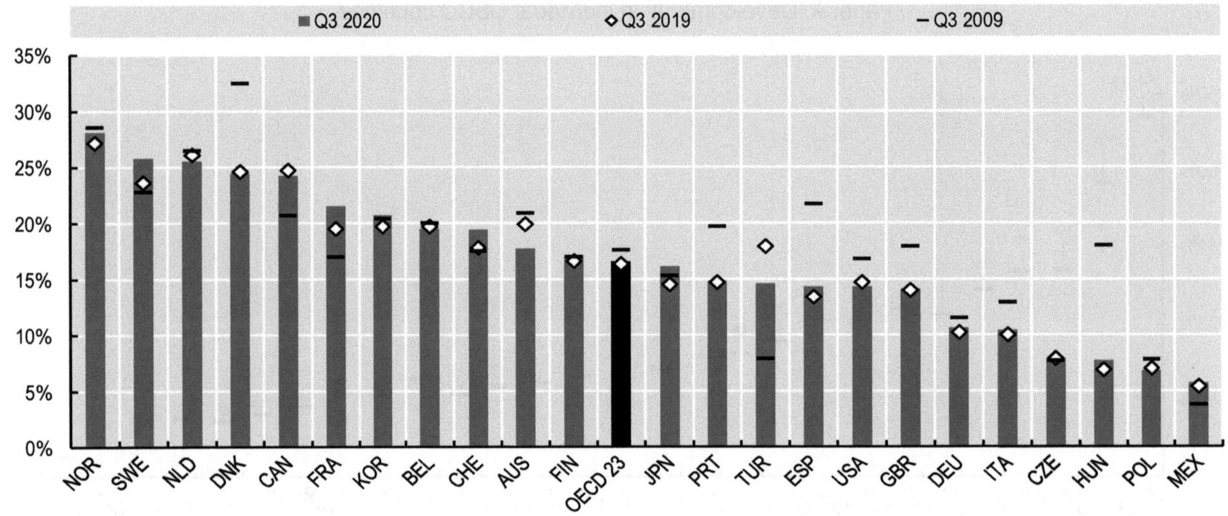

Note: The debt service ratio is defined as the ratio of interest payments plus amortisations to the gross disposable income of the private non-financial sector. Gross disposable income is augmented by interest payments (and dividends paid by non-financial corporations) to reflect the income available to the private non-financial sector to service its debt. The OECD average includes only those 23 countries shown.
Source: OECD calculations based on BIS (n.d.[27]), *Debt service ratios statistics* (database), Bank for International Settlements, https://www.bis.org/statistics/dsr.html.

StatLink https://stat.link/4ay0o5

Box 8.2. Further reading

- OECD (2021), "An in-depth analysis of one year of SME and entrepreneurship policy responses to COVID-19", *OECD SME and Entrepreneurship Papers*, No. 25, OECD Publishing, Paris, https://doi.org/10.1787/6407deee-en
- OECD (2021), *OECD Economic Outlook, Interim Report March 2021*, OECD Publishing, Paris, https://dx.doi.org/10.1787/34bfd999-en
- OECD (2021), *OECD Economic Outlook, Interim Report September 2021: Keeping the Recovery on Track*, OECD Publishing, Paris, https://doi.org/10.1787/490d4832-en
- OECD (2021), *OECD Sovereign Borrowing Outlook 2021*, OECD Publishing, Paris, https://doi.org/10.1787/48828791-en
- OECD (2020), *OECD Economic Outlook, Volume 2020, Issue 2*, OECD Publishing, Paris, https://doi.org/10.1787/39a88ab1-en
- OECD (2020), "Tax and fiscal policy in response to the Coronavirus crisis: Strengthening confidence and resilience", *OECD Policy Responses to Coronavirus (COVID-19)*, OECD Publishing, Paris, https://doi.org/10.1787/60f640a8-en

References

ABS (2020), *Business Impacts of COVID-19*, Australian Bureau of Statistics, https://www.abs.gov.au/statistics/economy/business-indicators/business-conditions-and-sentiments/aug-2020. [11]

Ahir, H., N. Bloom and D. Furceri (2020), *60 Years of uncertainty*, IMF Finance & Development, https://www.imf.org/external/pubs/ft/fandd/2020/03/imf-launches-world-uncertainty-index-wui-furceri.htm. [4]

BIS (2019), *BIS Statistical Bulletin*, Bank for International Settlements, http://www.bis.org/statistics/relcal.htm. [28]

BIS (n.d.), *Debt service ratios statistics (database)*, Bank for International Settlements, https://www.bis.org/statistics/dsr.htm (accessed on 12 August 2021). [27]

Congressional Research Service (2020), *COVID-19: Household Debt During the Pandemic*, https://crsreports.congress.gov. [21]

Eurostat (2021), *Investment by institutional sectors (database)*, https://ec.europa.eu/eurostat/databrowser/view/tec00132/default/table?lang=en (accessed on 29 September 2021). [8]

Francis-Devine, B. (2021), *Coronavirus: Impact on household debt and savings*, House of Commons Library, https://commonslibrary.parliament.uk/research-briefings/cbp-9060/. [20]

Leslie, J. and K. Shah (2021), *The impact of the coronavirus crisis on UK household wealth*, Resolution Foundation, https://www.resolutionfoundation.org/app/uploads/2021/07/Wealth-gap-year.pdf. [16]

OECD (2021), "An in-depth analysis of one year of SME and entrepreneurship policy responses to COVID-19: Lessons learned for the path to recovery", *OECD SME and Entrepreneurship Papers*, No. 25, OECD Publishing, Paris, https://doi.org/10.1787/6407deee-en. [25]

OECD (2021), *Business confidence index*, https://data.oecd.org/leadind/business-confidence-index-bci.htm#indicator-chart (accessed on 25 June 2021). [5]

OECD (2021), *Consumer confidence index*, https://data.oecd.org/leadind/consumer-confidence-index-cci.htm#indicator-chart (accessed on 25 June 2021). [6]

OECD (2021), *National Accounts, Quarterly National Accounts (database)*, https://stats.oecd.org/Index.aspx?DataSetCode=QNA (accessed on 29 September 2021). [7]

OECD (2021), *OECD Economic Outlook, Interim Report March 2021*, OECD Publishing, Paris, https://dx.doi.org/10.1787/34bfd999-en. [24]

OECD (2021), *OECD Economic Outlook, Interim Report September 2021: Keeping the Recovery on Track*, OECD Publishing, Paris, https://doi.org/10.1787/490d4832-en. [2]

OECD (2021), *OECD SME and Entrepreneurship Outlook 2021*, OECD Publishing, Paris, https://doi.org/10.1787/97a5bbfe-en. [9]

OECD (2021), *OECD Sovereign Borrowing Outlook 2021*, OECD Publishing, Paris, https://dx.doi.org/10.1787/48828791-en. [23]

OECD (2020), "Coronavirus (COVID-19): SME policy responses", *OECD Policy Responses to Coronavirus (COVID-19)*, OECD Publishing, Paris, https://doi.org/10.1787/04440101-en. [10]

OECD (2020), "Tax and fiscal policy in response to the Coronavirus crisis: Strengthening confidence and resilience", *OECD Policy Responses to Coronavirus (COVID-19)*, OECD Publishing, Paris, https://doi.org/10.1787/60f640a8-en. [22]

OECD (n.d.), *National Accounts Statistics, Household Dashboard (database)*, http://stats.oecd.org/Index.aspx?DataSetCode=HH_DASH (accessed on 12 August 2021). [18]

OECD (n.d.), *National Accounts Statistics, Quarterly National Accounts (database)*, https://stats.oecd.org/Index.aspx?DataSetCode=QNA (accessed on 12 August 2021). [3]

OECD (n.d.), *National Accounts Statistics, Quarterly Public Sector Debt, Public Sector Debt, consolidated, nominal value (database)*, https://stats.oecd.org/Index.aspx?DataSetCode=QASA_TABLE7PSD (accessed on 12 August 2021). [26]

OECD (n.d.), *National Accounts Statistics, Quarterly Sector Account, Non-consolidated financial balance sheets by economic sector (database)*, https://stats.oecd.org/Index.aspx?DataSetCode=QASA_TABLE720R (accessed on 12 August 2021). [19]

ONS (2021), *Coronavirus and the Impact on UK households and businesses: 2020*, Office for National Statistics, https://www.ons.gov.uk/economy/nationalaccounts/uksectoraccounts/articles/coronavirusandtheimpactonukhouseholdsandbusinesses/2020. [13]

ONS (2021), *Quarterly Stocks Survey (QSS) and Capital Assets Survey (QCAS) textual data analysis*, Office for National Statistics, https://www.ons.gov.uk/economy/grossdomesticproductgdp/datasets/quarterlystockssurveyqssandcapitalassetssurveyqcastextualdataanalysis (accessed on 12 August 2021). [12]

Pew Research Center (2021), *A Year Into the Pandemic, Long-Term Financial Impact Weighs Heavily on Many Americans*, https://www.pewresearch.org/social-trends/2021/03/05/a-year-into-the-pandemic-long-term-financial-impact-weighs-heavily-on-many-americans/. [14]

Statistics Canada (2021), *National balance sheet and financial flow accounts, fourth quarter 2020*, https://www150.statcan.gc.ca/n1/daily-quotidien/210312/dq210312b-eng.htm. [17]

USAFACTS (2021), *American wealth is growing, even during the pandemic. So is wealth inequality*, https://usafacts.org/articles/us-wealth-distribution-and-inequality-recession-pandemic-2020/. [15]

World Bank (2021), *Global Economic Prospects, January 2021*, World Bank, New York, http://dx.doi.org/10.1596/978-1-4648-1612-3. [1]

Notes

[1] National Account data on Investment distinguish between five different asset types: i) dwellings (excluding land); ii) other buildings and structures (roads, bridges, airfields, dams, etc.); iii) machinery and equipment (such as ICT equipment, telecommunications equipment, etc.) including transport equipment (ships, trains, aircraft, etc.) and weapon systems; iv) cultivated biological resources (managed forests, livestock raised for milk production, etc.); and v) intellectual property products (such as R&D, mineral exploration, software and databases, literary and artistic originals, etc.).

[2] 28 OECD countries are Australia, Austria, Colombia, Costa Rica, the Czech Republic, Denmark, Estonia, Finland, France, Germany, Greece, Hungary, Ireland, Israel, Italy, Lithuania, Latvia, Luxembourg, the Netherlands, New Zealand, Norway, Poland, Portugal, the Slovak Republic, Slovenia, Spain, Sweden and the United Kingdom.

[3] The DSR reflects the share of income used to service debt, given interest rates, principal repayments and loan maturities. It provides a more comprehensive assessment of credit burdens than the credit-to-income ratio or simple measures of interest payments relative to income, because it takes both interest payments and amortisations into account (BIS, 2019[28]).

9 Human capital and COVID-19

Human capital is vital to long-term well-being, since it addresses the future health, knowledge, competencies and skills of society. The pandemic has adversely impacted current well-being, but it has also weakened the stocks of human capital that will shape future well-being and resilience. In OECD countries, COVID-19 has led to millions of potential years of life lost and exacerbated the dangers of certain health risk factors, including obesity and smoking. As more young people drop out of school due to learning disruptions from the pandemic, long-term educational attainment could fall. Record numbers of people are finding themselves unemployed, underemployed or marginally attached to the labour market – particularly those in the youngest age cohort – which could lead to scarring effects that persist well into the future. For young adults who began their careers in the midst of the Global Financial Crisis, the pandemic is set to compound their disadvantages.

The OECD defines human capital as the knowledge, skills, competencies and attributes embodied by individuals that coalesce to create personal, social and economic well-being at a societal level (OECD, 2013[1]; OECD, 2020[2]). While different institutions may have different ways of defining human capital, all definitions encompass outcome measures of knowledge, skills and health, all of which influence the total stock of human capital in a society at a given point in time, and the broad range of benefits that this stock could deliver in the future (OECD, 2013[1]). Human capital can be nurtured in many ways – be it through formal schooling, job training, parenting, social interactions, individual health choices and more – many of which are covered in this chapter, and some others were considered in previous chapters (see especially Chapters 3 and 4).

9.1. Health risks and premature deaths

Data from 81 countries show that, as of January 2021, more than 20 million years of life may have been lost due to COVID-19 since the start of the pandemic…

The COVID-19 pandemic has led to tens of millions of years of life lost across more than 80 countries worldwide (Pifarré i Arolas et al., 2021[3]). While excess mortality is a useful indicator to measure the short-term impact of COVID-19 on mortality rates (see Chapters 3 and 6), measures of premature mortality are useful in framing COVID's impact on human capital loss. Potential years of life lost (PYLL) is a measure of premature mortality that more heavily weighs deaths that occur at younger ages.[1] Although older age groups experienced higher mortality rates, especially in the early waves of the pandemic, younger age cohorts have suffered a substantial loss of potential years of life. In addition to the human tragedy of losing so many young lives, these losses deprive societies of the human resources and competencies that they will need to thrive in the future. A study focusing on countries with high incidence of COVID-19 concluded that years of life lost to the pandemic, using different thresholds per age group, exceeded four million by July 2020 (Oh et al., 2020[4]).[2] A further study covering over 81 countries, using country/age-specific thresholds, found that 20.5 million years of life had been lost to COVID-19 as of January 2021 (Pifarré i Arolas et al., 2021[3]); three-quarters of this loss occurred in the under-75 population.[3] In the United States, although only one-fifth of recorded COVID-19 deaths occurred in the under-65 population, this group accounted for almost half of the years of potential life lost (Wu, 2020[5]; Elledge, 2020[6]).[4]

The years of life lost to COVID-19 dwarf those from the seasonal flu, even when focusing on the oldest age cohorts who are most susceptible to severe outcomes from the flu (Figure 9.1). Annual data indicate that the years of life lost from the pandemic in 2020 were at least two to nine times higher than the average from seasonal influenza (Pifarré i Arolas et al., 2021[3]). Data from England and Wales illustrate this point: in a bad flu year, an average of 30 000 people die from the flu or pneumonia, for a total of around 250 000 years of life lost. As of March 2021, 146 000 had died from COVID-19 for a total of 1.5 million potential years of life lost, i.e. 4.9 and 6 times more, respectively (The Health Foundation, 2021[7]; Krelle and Tallack, 2021[8]). The gaps in life lost between COVID-19 and the flu are large for both women and men, though more so for men (Figure 9.1).

Figure 9.1. Years of life lost due to COVID-19 dwarf those from flu or pneumonia in England and Wales, even among the elderly

Potential years of life lost for COVID-19 (2020) and the flu or pneumonia (2018), by gender and age, in England and Wales

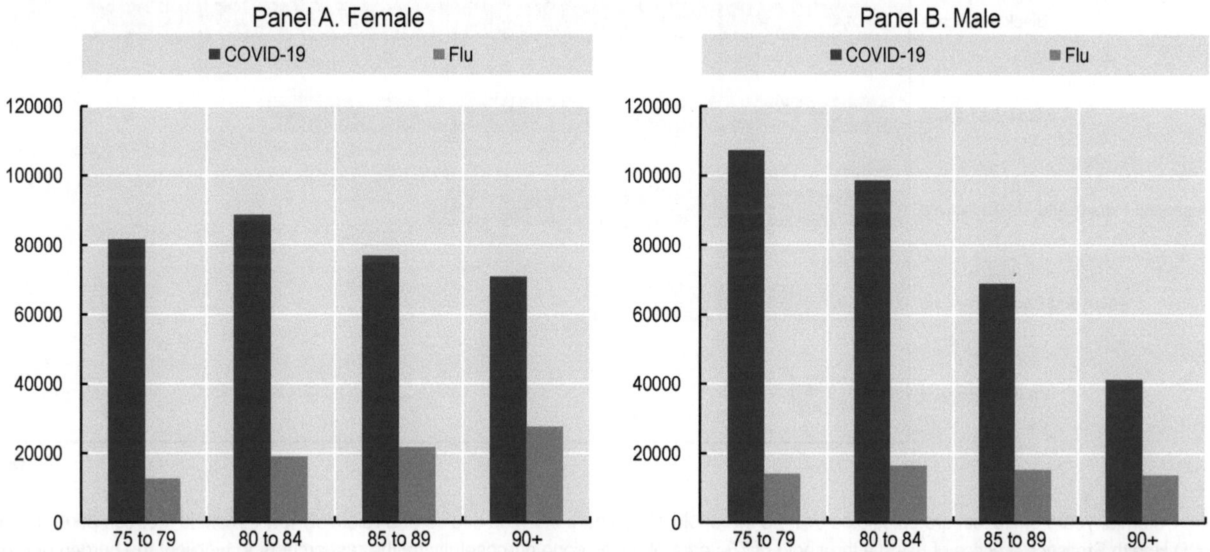

Note: Data refer to the population aged 75 or over. Flu and pneumonia data refer to the 2018 flu season. Actuarial life expectancy tables are used to calculated years of life lost for each age group.
Source: Krelle and Tallack (2021[8]), *One year on: Three myths about COVID-19 that the data proved wrong*, The Health Foundation, https://www.health.org.uk/publications/long-reads/one-year-on-three-myths-about-COVID-19-that-the-data-proved-wrong.

StatLink https://stat.link/0kxlti

…and these years of life lost are unequally distributed across the population

Men have lost more years of life than women (The Health Foundation, 2021[7]; Pifarré i Arolas et al., 2021[3]; Wu, 2020[5]) (Figure 9.1), despite having lower life expectancies on average than women, because men had higher fatality rates from the virus. However, as a measure based on mortality, PYLL does not take into account the long-term debilitating effects of an illness; measures such as disability-adjusted life years (DALYS) and quality-adjusted life-years (QALY) are therefore better able to provide the full picture of the COVID-19 disease burden (Pifarré i Arolas et al., 2021[3]). As women are more likely to suffer severe symptoms from long COVID (Torjesen, 2021[9]; Jackson, 2021[10]) (see also Box 6.1), data referring only to years of life lost do not provide the full gender picture.

Certain population groups have been more adversely affected than others, especially those with underlying medical conditions, those from low-income households and those belonging to racial and ethnic minority groups. Those with underlying health conditions, such as obesity, diabetes and heart disease, are more likely to die of COVID-19 were they to contract the virus, and hence have higher rates of years of life lost (Wu, 2020[5]). Data from England show that those living in the most deprived parts of England were twice as likely to die from COVID-19, and to die at younger ages, than those from wealthier areas (Krelle and Tallack, 2021[8]). In the United States, evidence referring to the spring of 2020 illustrates stark racial/ethnic inequalities (Figure 9.2). Black Americans lost around 127.6 years of life before age 65 per 100 000 population, compared to only 18.9 years per 100 000 population for white Americans (Bassett, Chen and Krieger, 2020[11]). The gaps in COVID-19 outcomes are widest at lower age groups: Black Americans aged 35-44 have seven to nine times higher mortality rates than white Americans (Resnick, 2020[12]).[5]

Figure 9.2. Striking racial/ethnic inequalities in years of life lost due to COVID-19 in the United States

Potential years of life lost to COVID-19 (under 65 years), per 100 000 population, 1 Feb – 20 May 2020

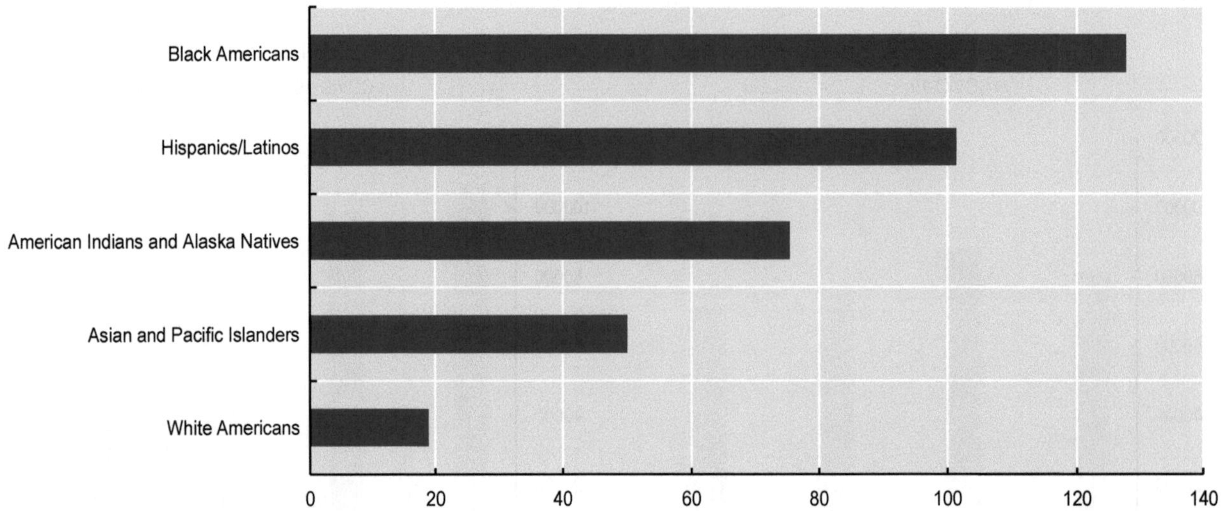

Note: Potential years of life lost are calculated using a threshold of 65-years-old. The choice of a relatively low threshold (i.e. compared to the OECD Health Statistics practice of using a threshold of 75-years-old) was done purposefully by the researchers to highlight the burden of lives lost on younger people and on those still in the labour market.
Source: Bassett, Chen and Krieger (2020[11]), "The unequal toll of COVID-19 mortality by age in the United States: Quantifying racial/ethnic disparities", HCPDS *Working Paper Series*, No. 3, Harvard Center for Population and Development Studies, https://cdn1.sph.harvard.edu/wp-content/uploads/sites/1266/2020/06/20_Bassett-Chen-Krieger_COVID-19_plus_age_working-paper_0612_Vol-19_No-3_with-cover.pdf.

StatLink https://stat.link/umfvwq

Despite initial disagreements, experts now agree that smoking is a risk factor for COVID-19

Public health officials warn that smoking may put individuals at risk of more severe COVID-19 symptoms (WHO, 2020[13]; Galiatsatos, 2020[14]; CDC, 2021[15]). Initial meta-analyses identified links between regular smoking or vaping and the severity of COVID-19, including in terms of rates of hospitalisation and death (WHO, 2020[16]; Galiatsatos, 2020[14]; HCSP, 2020[17]). These patient-based findings have been confirmed by population-based studies, such as the Zoe COVID-19 Symptom Study. This UK study used a mobile phone app to provide longitudinal data on over 2.4 million people, tracking their health and COVID-19 symptoms from 24 March to 23 April 2020. The study showed that regular smokers were at an increased risk of developing COVID-19 symptoms, including cough, fever and breathlessness (Hopkinson et al., 2020[18]).[6]

Smoking rates vary substantially across OECD countries, though they have been falling almost everywhere over the last 10 years (OECD, 2020[2]; OECD, 2019[19]). An average of 18% of adults across OECD countries smoked tobacco daily in 2017, down from an average of 23% in 2007 (OECD, 2019[19]). However, significant cross-country differences in tobacco usage remain: Greece, Turkey and Hungary have some of the highest rates, at 25% or over, while Costa Rica, Mexico and Iceland have rates below 10%. In general men are more likely to smoke than women, and those with lower levels of education are more likely to be smokers than those with higher educational attainment (OECD, 2019[19]); these groups have heightened risk profiles, and indeed experienced higher mortality rates from COVID-19 (Chapter 6).

While some people may have used the pandemic as an opportunity to quit smoking, some non-smokers also took up smoking, and tobacco use increased in some countries. Survey data collected by Ipsos Global Advisor in October/November 2020 showed that individuals in eight OECD countries were more likely to report having given up smoking than having started smoking since the pandemic began (Bailey et al., 2021[20]) (Figure 9.3, Panel D).[7] In some of the countries in which a relatively high share of respondents have reported stopping smoking (Mexico, Sweden), overall smoking rates were already relatively low; however, in others (Chile, Turkey) higher rates of quitting may be linked to higher smoking prevalence when the pandemic started (OECD, 2020[2]). Only four OECD countries included in the research – Chile, Turkey, Mexico and Israel – had a higher share of respondents indicating that they had taken up smoking since the start of the COVID-19 pandemic relative to those who reported quitting smoking. A cross-sectional study of 6 870 smokers in Australia, Canada, England and the United States found that while 46.7% considered quitting during the pandemic, the vast majority (70.2%) made no changes to their behaviour (Gravely et al., 2021[21]).

Evidence from individual countries shows that for those who already smoke, and did not quit in 2020, the pandemic led to an increase in tobacco consumption. A nationally representative survey in the United Kingdom conducted from 27 April to 24 May 2020 found that 25.5% of current smokers reported smoking more during the pandemic, compared to 51% who reported no change in smoking levels and 20% who reported smoking less: young women aged 16-29 were most likely to increase their smoking behaviours (Chen, 2020[22]). Data from Ireland found similar patterns for young women (Box 9.1). Consumption data from the United States show that the years-long decline in cigarette sales flattened in 2020 (Fakuade, 2020[23]), while calls to state "quitlines" – call centres that provide advice to those who want to quit smoking – fell 27% from 2019 to 2020 (North American Quitline Consortium, 2021[24]). Those who reported smoking more than usual had higher rates of anxiety, stress and isolation and poorer mental health in general (Chen, 2020[22]; The Lancet Respiratory Medicine, 2021[25]).

Obesity worsens individuals' COVID-19 outcomes, including death…

Those who are obese are at greater risk of more severe outcomes from COVID-19, including death. Unlike smoking, the evidence surrounding obesity and negative health outcomes from the virus has been clear-cut from the start. As a risk factor for COVID-19 mortality, obesity is second only to age (World Obesity Federation, 2021[26]). Studies from Brazil, China, France, Italy, Mexico, Spain, Sweden, the United States and the United Kingdom show that obesity increases the risk of having severe symptoms of COVID, including risks of hospitalisation, admission to intensive care units (ICUs), the need for ventilators and death (CDC, n.d.[27]; Public Health England, 2020[28]; Yang, Hu and Zhu, 2021[29]; Simonnet et al., 2020[30]; Popkin et al., 2020[31]; World Obesity Federation, 2021[26]). These findings hold even when controlling for demographic and socio-economic factors (Public Health England, 2020[28]) and can be distinguished from COVID-19 deaths stemming from other cardiometabolic conditions closely related to obesity, such as diabetes mellitus, hypertension and heart failure (O'Hearn et al., 2021[32]). It is not just those who are obese (i.e. with a BMI of 30 or above) who are at an increased risk: simply being overweight (with a BMI of 25 or above) also puts one at risk for worse COVID-19 outcomes (Kompaniyets et al., 2021[33]). Stigma and discrimination against the obese may play a role: stigma results in obese patients avoiding the healthcare system, which can exacerbate pre-existing conditions, hinder the prevention of chronic disease and delay COVID treatment (Wadman, 2020[34]; Public Health England, 2020[28]).

Among OECD countries, rates of overweight and obesity vary substantially and have been rising in the large majority of them over the last 10 years (OECD, 2019[19]). Of the 27 OECD countries with time-series data, none showed a decline in obesity rates from 2005 to 2017, though there is wide variation in prevalence – from 30% in the United States, Chile, Mexico, New Zealand and Australia to less than 5% in Japan and Korea (OECD, 2020[2]). Countries with higher obesity rates therefore have a higher share of the population at risk of severe COVID-19 complications and potentially face a higher burden on the health care system for a given rate of infection. A report by the World Obesity Federation concluded that countries with higher rates of overweight or obese adults had higher mortality rates from COVID-19, even when accounting for the age structure of the population, GDP per capita and the quality of COVID-19 data reporting (World Obesity Federation, 2021[26]; Boseley, 2021[35]).

...and the risk posed by obesity may have been exacerbated by weight put on during pandemic lockdowns and confinement

Survey data show that more respondents have gained weight, as opposed to lost weight, over the course of 2020 (Figure 9.3, Panel A). Ipsos survey data from late 2020 show that on average in 19 OECD countries, 31% of respondents had gained weight since the start of the pandemic, compared to only 18% who had lost weight (Bailey et al., 2021[20]). Women were more likely than men to gain weight, as were younger people (Figure 9.4, Panels A and B). Another international survey of 7 800 participants conducted online from April to May 2020 found that 27% of respondents had gained weight since lockdowns began, compared to 17% who had lost weight (Flanagan et al., 2021[36]).[8] Weight gains were largest for those who were already classified as obese (33%), likely driven by a reduction in exercise and time spent outside (O'Connor, 2020[37]). Survey data from individual countries support the finding that more people have gained rather than lost weight in 2020. In the United States, a survey by the American Psychological Association found that 42% experienced unwanted weight gain, versus 18% with unwanted weight loss. Women (45%), young adults aged 18-25 (52%), parents (51%) and essential workers (50%) were more likely to experience unwanted weight gain (APA, 2021[38]). An online poll in Canada found that 33% had gained weight compared to 15% who had lost weight (Alhmidi, 2020[39]); 55% of Israelis reported weight gain (I24news, 2020[40]); and in Italy, overweight boys experienced more weight gain compared to girls (Maltoni et al., 2021[41]) (see Box 9.1 for data from Ireland). While these numbers appear striking, baseline data provide a sense of how much they deviate from a normal, non-pandemic, year. Using data from the 2007 to 2010 National Health and Nutritional Examination Surveys, the US Center for Disease Control estimates that the average adult gains 1-2 pounds (0.45-0.91 kg) a year from early adulthood to middle-age, with the highest weight gain concentrated in the early 20s (Fryar CD, Gu Q and Ogden CL, 2012[42]; Ingraham, 2016[43]). By way of comparison, a longitudinal study of 269 participants in the United States from 1 February to 1 June 2020, which collected weight data from Bluetooth-connected scales, concluded that respondents gained 1.5 pounds (0.68 kg) per month, on average (Lin et al., 2021[44]).

Weight gain is in part driven by higher consumption of alcohol (Figure 9.3, Panel C) and **unhealthy foods** (see Box 9.1 for data from Ireland). People consume unhealthy "comfort" foods in response to stressful situations (Gapper, 2021[45]; O'Connor, 2020[37]). 26.8% of Canadians surveyed by Statistics Canada between 29 March and 3 April 2020 reported they had increased eating junk food or sweets, compared to 14.7% who reported eating less; the numbers were higher for younger people aged 15 to 49 (37.1% of them increased consumption) (Statistics Canada, 2020[46]). Alcohol is also used as a means to cope (Grossman, Benjamin-Neelon and Sonnenschein, 2020[47]). Data from Australia, Belgium, the United Kingdom and France found that women, parents of young children, those with higher income and/or those with worse mental health were more likely to increase their alcohol consumption during lockdown (OECD, 2021[48]) (see also Chapter 3). In mid-March, Nielsen (a US data and market measurement company) reported that sales of alcohol in the United States had increased 54% from the same week in the previous year (Grossman, Benjamin-Neelon and Sonnenschein, 2020[47]). A study of 1 540 Americans conducted by the RAND corporation showed that alcohol consumption increased by 14% from 29 April – 9 June 2019 (the baseline period) to 28 May – 16 June 2020 (Pollard, Tucker and Green, 2020[49]). Similarly, 14% of Canadians reported they had increased their alcohol consumption during the COVID crisis, with a stronger rise (20%) among younger people (aged 15-49) (Statistics Canada, 2020[46]).[9] Men were more likely to increase their consumption of alcohol than women (Figure 9.4, Panel A); a US survey found that 48% of fathers reported drinking more to cope with stress, compared to 29% of mothers (APA, 2021[38]).

Figure 9.3. In most OECD countries with data, more people adopted unhealthy, rather than healthy, behaviours since the start of the pandemic

Share of respondents who reported changes in health behaviour since the start of the pandemic, Oct-Nov 2020

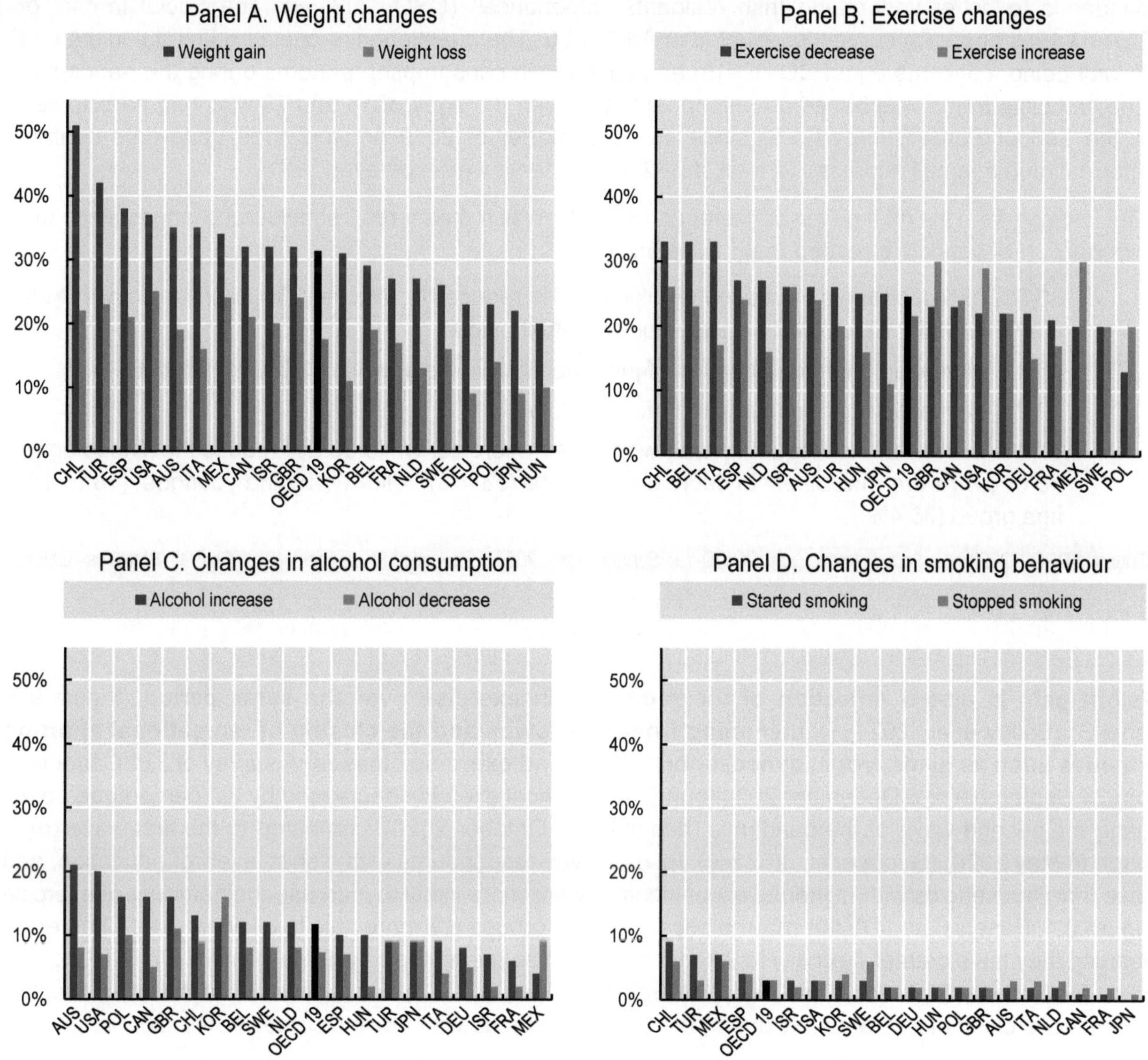

Note: The healthy behaviours considered refer to weight gain/loss; exercise increase/decrease; increase/decrease in alcohol consumption; and start/stop smoking. Data are rounded to the nearest percent. The OECD average includes only those 19 countries shown.
Source: Bailey et al. (2021[20]), *Diet and health under COVID-19*, Ipsos, https://www.ipsos.com/sites/default/files/ct/news/documents/2021-01/diet-and-health-under-covid-19.pdf.

StatLink https://stat.link/xuotd0

Box 9.1. Innovation: The Ireland Social Impact of COVID-19 Survey

The Irish Central Statistics Office (CSO) has implemented a series of surveys since the start of the pandemic to better understand Irish residents' experiences (CSO, 2021[50]). The Social Impact of COVID-19 is one such survey, conducted in April 2020. The questionnaire contained modules relating to well-being, concerns about COVID-19, and changes in consumption patterns during the pandemic. The sampling frame was based on respondents between the ages of 18 and 75 who had participated in the Labour Force Survey (LFS) since the first quarter of 2019 and provided up-to-date contact information (i.e. email address). In total, 1 362 respondents were surveyed.

Key findings from the changes in consumption module, which measures behavioural changes since the introduction of pandemic-related restrictions, include:

- 30.5% of respondents increased smoking, 8.6% reduced it. Women (34.7%) were more likely than men (26.2%) to have increased smoking behaviour.
- 45.4% increased their consumption of junk food and sweets, while 12.3% reduced it.
- 22.2% increased their consumption of alcohol, while 17.2% reduced it.
- 37.1% increased the frequency with which they exercise, while 33.2% reduced it. Those aged 70 or over were most likely to decrease exercise (53.4%), followed by the youngest (18 to 34) age group (36.4%).

Source: CSO (2020[51]), *Social Impact of COVID-19 Survey April 2020: Changes in consumption*, Central Statistics Office, https://www.cso.ie/en/releasesandpublications/ep/p-sic19/socialimpactofcovid-19surveyapril2020/changesinconsumption

Weight gain is also a reflection of the reduction in exercise over the same period (Figure 9.3, Panel B) (Bailey et al., 2021[20]), **stemming from lockdowns and the closing of recreational sporting activities such as gyms, yoga, dance, sports clubs and exercise classes.** A survey of 221 Canadians from 24 September to 8 December 2020 found that physical exercise decreased by 3.1 percentage points during the second wave of the pandemic (beginning in October 2020), compared to the first wave (mid-March to May 2020) (Gupta et al., 2021[52]). Ipsos survey respondents with higher levels of education, and those from households with higher levels of income, were more likely to increase their amount of exercise (Figure 9.4, Panels C and D); this may be because these groups are more able to telework (see Chapter 5), meaning they have greater flexibility to take time to exercise during the day. Data from the United Kingdom Office for National Statistics (ONS) Time Use Survey (see Box 7.2) also showed that those with higher incomes exercised more frequently during the week than those with lower incomes (ONS, 2020[53]).

Figure 9.4. On average in 19 OECD countries, changes in health behaviour were unequally distributed across the population

Share of respondents who reported changes in health behaviour since the start of the pandemic, by different characteristics, OECD 19, Oct-Nov 2020

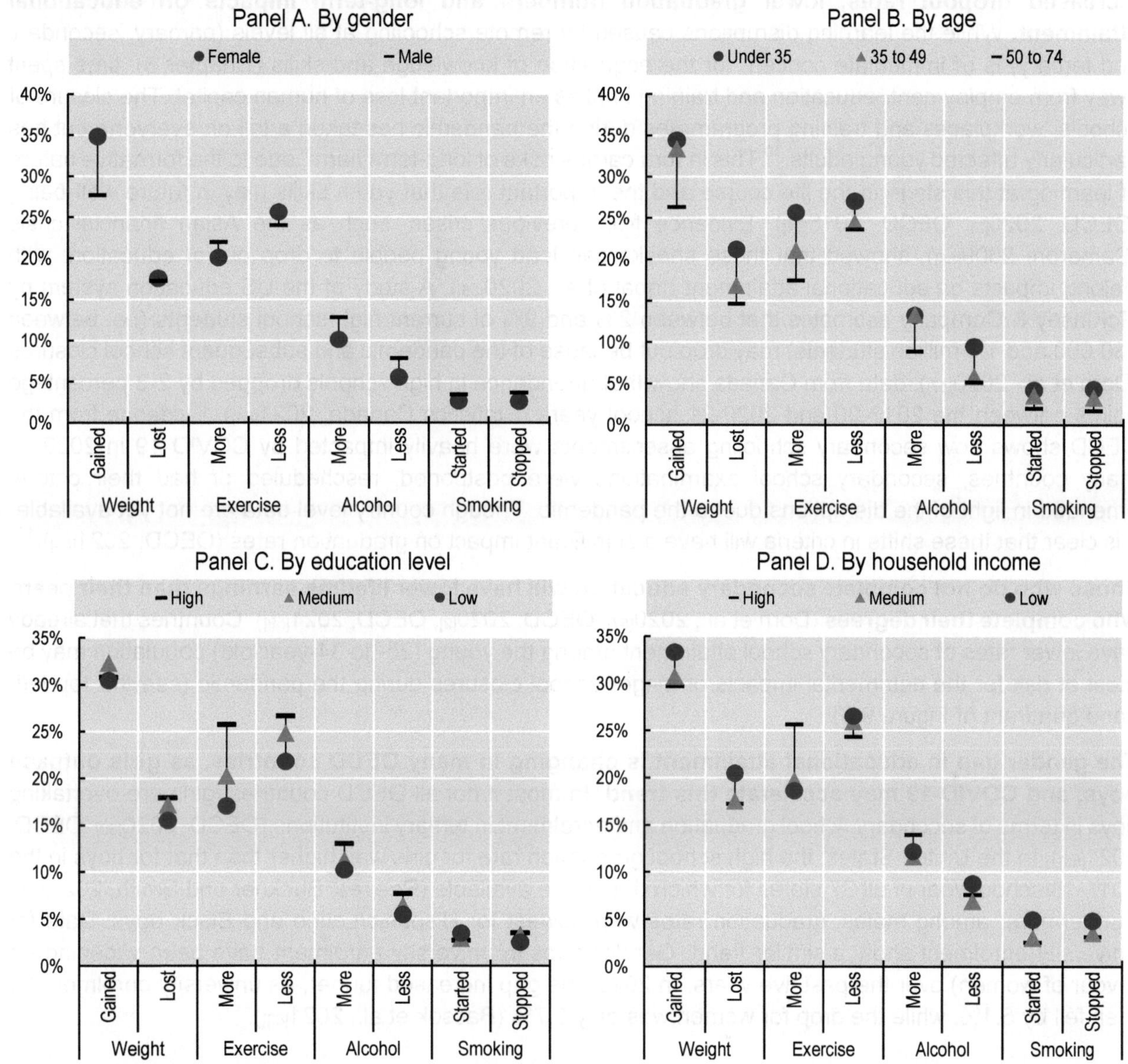

Note: Health behaviours include weight gain/loss; exercise more/less; more/less alcohol consumption; and start/stop smoking. The OECD average includes Australia, Belgium, Canada, Chile, France, Germany, Hungary, Israel, Italy, Japan, Korea, Mexico, the Netherlands, Poland, Spain, Sweden, Turkey, the United Kingdom and the United States. Data are rounded to the nearest percent.
Source: Bailey et al. (2021[20]), *Diet and health under COVID-19*, Ipsos, https://www.ipsos.com/sites/default/files/ct/news/documents/2021-01/diet-and-health-under-covid-19.pdf.

StatLink https://stat.link/7cu3p0

9.2. Knowledge and skills among youth and young adults

When extended over time, remote schooling may increase dropout rates and lower educational attainment

The pandemic and ensuing lockdowns have critically impacted schooling, leading to fears of increased dropout rates, lower graduation numbers and long-term impacts on educational attainment. While the learning disruptions caused by remote schooling at all levels (primary, secondary and tertiary) is of immediate concern for the acquisition of knowledge and skills (Chapter 3), time spent away from employment, education and training implies an important loss of human capital. The closure of schools, workplaces and training programmes during the pandemic has taken a toll on everyone but has particularly affected young adults.[10] This in turn carries risks of long-term harm, due to the formative nature of learning at this stage in the life course and the important role that youth skills play in future well-being (OECD, 2020[2]; OECD, 2015[54]). Evidence from previous crises, such as the Asian financial crisis (Cameron, 2009[55]), showed that these shocks can lead young people to drop out of education, with lifelong impacts on educational attainment (Iqbal et al., 2020[56]). A study of the US education system by McKinsey & Company estimates that between 2% and 9% of current high school students (i.e. between 230 000 and 1.1 million students) may drop out because of the pandemic and subsequent school closures (Dorn et al., 2020[57]); data from Canada show that attendance in high schools dropped by 2-3 percentage points between the 2019-20 and 2020-21 school years (Statistics Canada, 2021[58]). Evidence from the OECD shows how secondary schooling assessments were heavily impacted by COVID-19 in 2020: in many countries, secondary school examinations were postponed, rescheduled or had their criteria amended in light of the disruptions due to the pandemic. Though country level data are not yet available, it is clear that these shifts in criteria will have a significant impact on graduation rates (OECD, 2021[59]).[11]

Those who do not complete secondary education will have lower lifetime earnings than their peers who complete their degrees (Dorn et al., 2020[57]; OECD, 2020[2]; OECD, 2021[59]). Countries that already have lower rates of secondary school attainment among the young (25- to 34-year-old) population may be most at risk for the detrimental impacts of longer school closures during the pandemic (see the top left-hand quadrant of Figure 9.5).

The gender gap in educational attainment is changing in many OECD countries, as girls outpace boys, and COVID-19 may accelerate this trend. In most if not all OECD countries, girls are overtaking boys in terms of secondary school graduation and enrolment in tertiary institutions (OECD, 2020[60]; OECD, 2021[59]). In the United States, the high school graduation rate for girls was higher than that for boys in the 2017-18 school year in all 37 states for which data were available (Reeves, Buckner and Smith, 2021[61]). Furthermore, among males, graduation rates were lowest for Hispanic/Latino and Black boys. Data for university enrolment show a similar trend. Gender gaps in university enrolment have been widening (in favour of women) over the past five years. In 2020, the gap increased further, as university enrolment for men fell by 5.1%, while the drop for women was only 0.7% (Bassok et al., 2021[62]).

Figure 9.5. OECD countries with low educational attainment for young adults and more school closures due to COVID-19 may be most at risk of losing human capital

Share of instruction days when schools were fully or partially closed due to the pandemic (Mar 2020 – Jun 2021), and share of 25-34 year-olds with at least an upper secondary education (2020 or latest available)

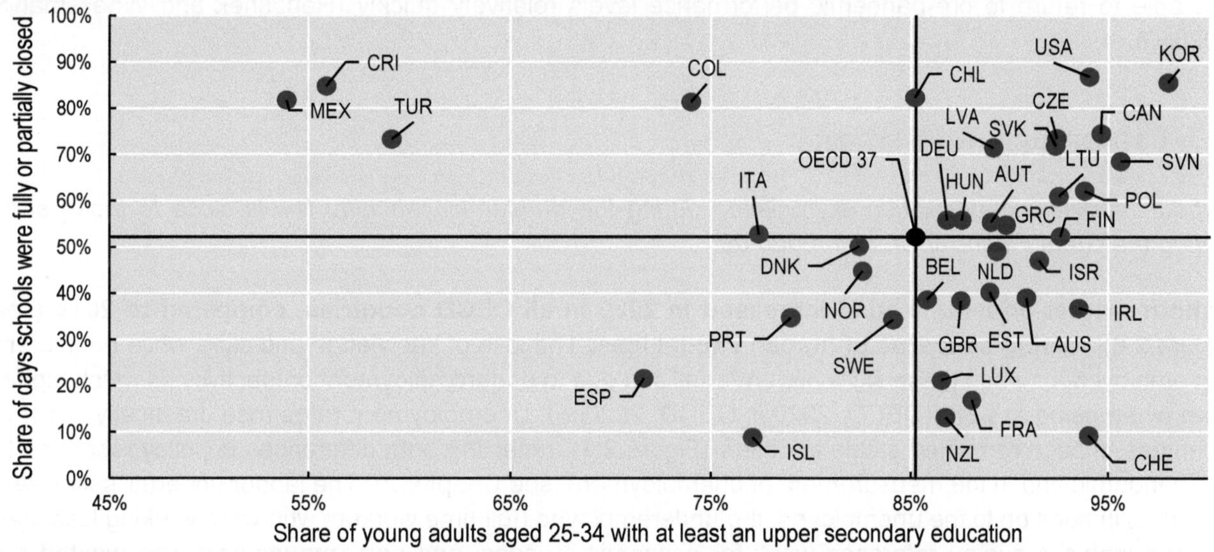

Note: Data on school closures refer to the share of days during which schools were fully or partially closed due to COVID-19, as a share of the total number of all instruction days (i.e., excluding school holidays, public holidays and weekends), as a pooled average from March 2020 to June 2021. "Fully closed" is defined as government-mandated closures of schools (pre-primary through upper secondary, ISCED levels 0 through 3) because of the COVID-19 pandemic. "Partially closed" refers to instances in which schools are closed in certain regions only, and/or are closed for some grade levels/age groups but not others, and/or are employing a hybrid (in-person combined with distance learning) approach. Educational attainment data refers to 2020 for all countries aside from Chile (2017), Denmark (2019) and Turkey (2019). The OECD average excludes Japan, which is missing educational attainment data.

Source: UNESCO (n.d.[63]), *Global Monitoring of School Closures, COVID-19* (database), United Nations Educational, Scientific and Cultural Organization, https://en.unesco.org/covid19/educationresponse; and OECD (n.d.[64]), *OECD Education Statistics* (database), https://doi.org/10.1787/edu-data-en.

StatLink https://stat.link/9nvkuh

For those who stay in school, learning losses may affect their ability to access higher education and lower lifetime earnings

For students who remain in education, the disruptions associated with remote schooling may lead to learning losses, especially for the most vulnerable (see Chapters 3 and 6). A wide evidence base shows that remote schooling leads to a reduction in instruction time (OECD, 2020[65]) and that children who do not have sufficient digital tools perform worse on schoolwork and standardised tests as compared to their better-equipped peers (The Pew Charitable Trusts, 2020[66]). The learning gap between high- and low-income groups has likely grown, as a consequence. Lacking quality equipment can make it more difficult for students to follow online schooling, making it more likely for them to be absent. Chronic absenteeism is associated with worse academic performance – increasing with the number of school days missed – and is a large risk factor for eventual dropout (OECD, 2019[67]; García and Weiss, 2020[68]).

Learning losses today foreshadow lost income and lower economic growth in the future. An OECD study estimates that students in primary and secondary education may experience 3% lower income over the course of their lifetime as a result of pandemic disruptions to learning, which in turn could translate to an annual loss of 1.5% of GDP for the rest of the 21st century. Students from disadvantaged backgrounds will be particularly at risk. It may be difficult to make up for these learning losses, even if school systems are able to return to pre-pandemic performance levels relatively quickly (Hanushek and Woessmann, 2020[69]).

9.3. Labour underutilisation

Labour market underutilisation skyrocketed during the pandemic, reaching levels close to those seen during the Great Financial Crisis in 2008-09…

Labour market underutilisation increased in 2020 in all OECD countries, compared to 2019 (see Figure 2.8), **raising concerns of human capital loss.** The loss of knowledge and skills while people are not employed, or when these skills are underutilised due to underemployment or inactivity, is much higher than when being at work (OECD, 2020[2]; OECD, 2020[70]). Unemployment rates rose drastically in some countries, though remained stable in others (Figure 2.7), reflecting both differences in policy response to the pandemic and in the measurement of unemployment (see Chapter 2). The labour underutilisation rate includes, in addition to the unemployed, the underemployed (full-time workers who were working less than usual during the survey reference week for economic reasons, and part-time workers who wanted but could not find full-time work) and the marginally attached (persons not in the labour force who did not actively seek work during the previous four weeks but who wish to and are available to work). On average in 32 OECD countries in 2020, labour underutilisation was more than twice as high as unemployment (17% and 7%, respectively), due to the large number of underemployed (6%) and marginally attached (4%) workers (Figure 9.6).

The rise in labour underutilisation from 2019 to 2020, for 32 OECD countries on average, was almost five times higher than the rise in unemployment over the same period. This is because, in contrast to trends in unemployment rates that differed across countries, the share of underemployed and marginally attached workers increased in all OECD countries in 2020 (with the exceptions of underemployment in Chile and marginally attached workers in Latvia) (Figure 9.7, Panels A and B). The large increase in labour market underutilisation underscores that the loss of knowledge and skills stemming from COVID may affect many more people than those who are conventionally counted as unemployed.

The increases in labour market underutilisation are large and reached levels comparable to those seen during the Great Financial Crisis in 2008-09 (Figure 9.8). Time-series data of 17 OECD countries show that the year-on-year increase in the OECD average labour market underutilisation was higher from 2019-20 (4.4 percentage points) than for all previous years aside from 2008-09 (5.3 percentage points).

Figure 9.6. Labour underutilisation increased in all OECD countries, reflecting higher numbers of people underemployed and marginally attached to the labour market

Labour market underutilisation, as a share of the total labour force, 2020

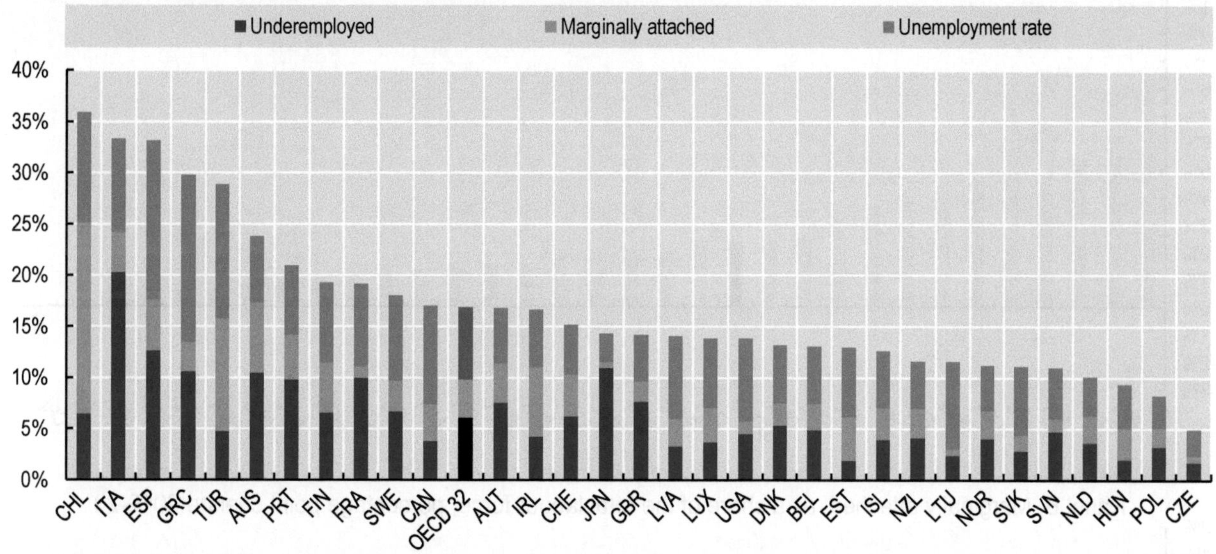

Note: The figure shows overall labour market underutilisation in 2020, decomposed into each component: the unemployed, the underemployed (full-time workers working less than usual during the survey reference week for economic reasons, and part-time workers who wanted but could not find full-time work) and the marginally attached (persons not in the labour force who did not actively seek work during the previous four weeks but who wish to and are available to work), expressed as a ratio of the total labour force. The OECD average excludes Colombia, Costa Rica, Germany (data are not available due to the introduction of the new German system of integrated household surveys since the beginning of 2020), Israel, Korea and Mexico (data are not available due to changes in survey collection during the year).
Source: OECD calculations based on OECD (n.d.[71]), *OECD Household Dashboard* (database), http://stats.oecd.org/Index.aspx?DataSetCode=HH_DASH.

StatLink https://stat.link/uiqewh

…and unemployment among the young is of particular concern

Across the OECD, the unemployment rate for young people has long been higher than for other age cohorts, and the pandemic has further widened this gap (Figure 9.9, Panel A) (Figure 5.7). Young adults were particularly affected by rising unemployment in the aftermath of the Great Financial Crisis and are again most at risk in the current pandemic (Figure 9.9). This is in part because they had yet to recover from the previous recession, and in part because they were more likely to work in service industry jobs that were the first to lay off workers during the first wave of the pandemic (Aaronson and Alba, 2020[72]). Young people aged 25-34 with an upper secondary education experienced a larger increase in unemployment from 2019 to 2020 (2 percentage points) than did young people with a tertiary degree (1 percentage point) (OECD, 2021[59]). Youth unemployment impacts not only short- to medium-term career prospects, but also lifelong earnings, access to training, skills improvement and mental health (Reuters, 2020[73]; Douine, 2020[74]; OECD, 2020[75]; OECD, 2020[70]).

Figure 9.7. Higher numbers of people underemployed and marginally attached to the labour market drove labour underutilisation increases in 2020 in all OECD countries

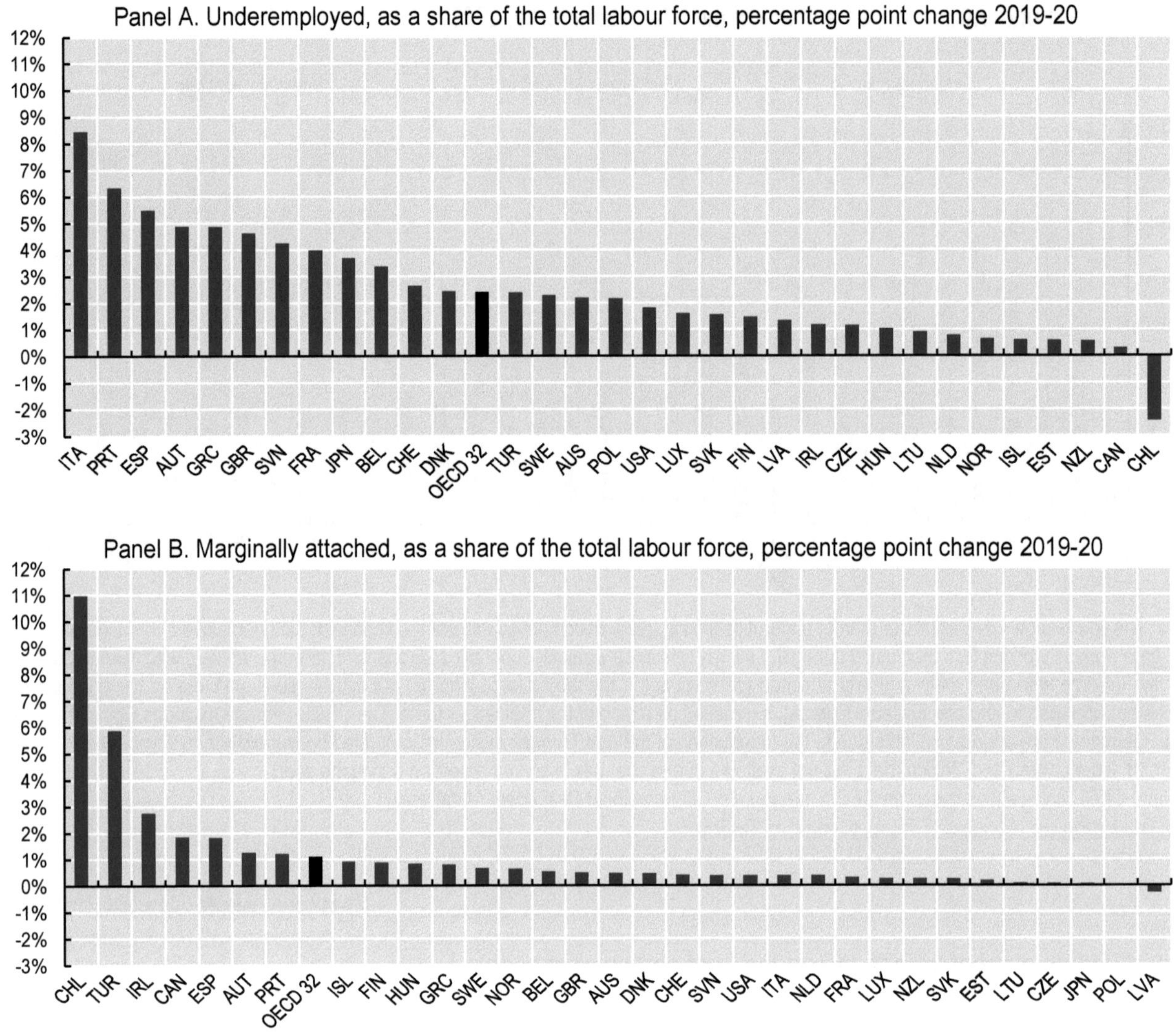

Note: Panel A shows the percentage point change in 2020 compared to 2019 for rates of underemployment (full-time workers working less than usual during the survey reference week for economic reasons, and part-time workers who wanted but could not find full-time work); Panel B shows the same for the marginally attached (persons not in the labour force who did not actively seek work during the previous four weeks but who wish to and are available to work), expressed as a ratio of the total labour force. Positive values mean the indicator has increased from the year prior, whereas negative values indicate the indicator has declined. In both panels, the OECD average excludes Colombia, Costa Rica, Germany (data are not available due to the introduction of the new German system of integrated household surveys since the beginning of 2020), Israel, Korea and Mexico (data are not available due to changes in survey collection during the year).
Source: OECD calculations based on OECD (n.d.[71]), *OECD Household Dashboard* (database), http://stats.oecd.org/Index.aspx?DataSetCode=HH_DASH.

StatLink https://stat.link/bw3r14

Figure 9.8. The sharp jump in labour market underutilisation in 2020 is close to that experienced during the Great Financial Crisis

As a percentage of the total labour force, OECD 17, 2007-20

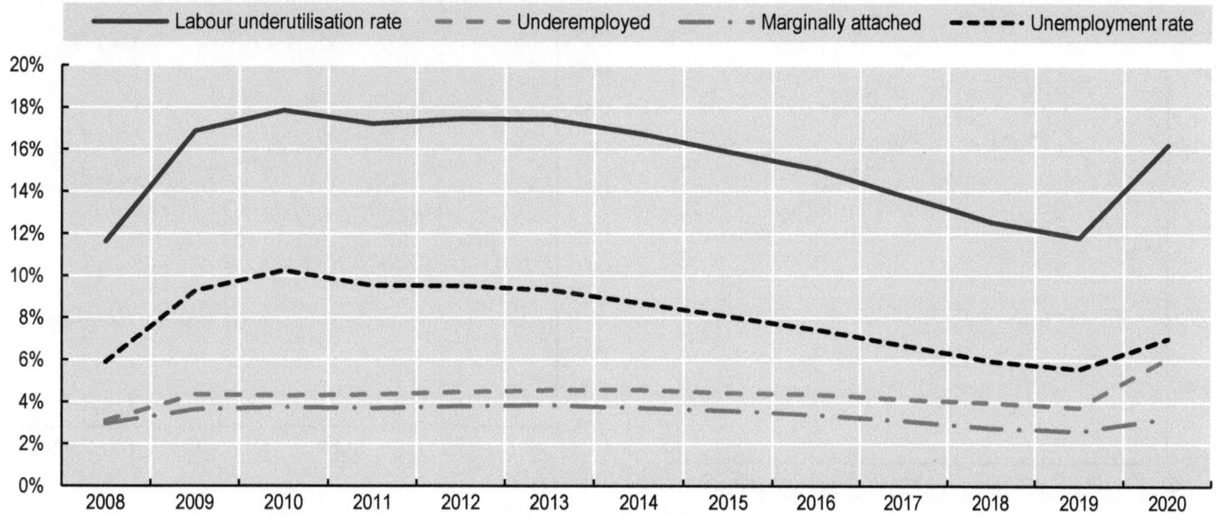

Note: The OECD average includes Australia, Austria, Canada, Spain, Estonia, Finland, the United Kingdom, Hungary, Iceland, Italy, Lithuania, Latvia, the Netherlands, Norway, New Zealand, Slovenia and the United States. Other OECD countries are omitted due to breaks in time series.
Source: OECD calculations based on OECD (n.d.[71]), *OECD Household Dashboard* (database), http://stats.oecd.org/Index.aspx?DataSetCode=HH_DASH.

StatLink https://stat.link/lyd3p4

While the number of young people not in education, employment or training (NEET) had been declining over the past few years, the pandemic reversed this trend (Figure 9.9, Panel B) (Figure 5.8). NEET rates are particularly high for migrants: across OECD countries, 19% of young migrants are NEET compared to 14% of native-born youths (OECD, 2021[59]). Traditionally, young people with lower educational attainment are more likely to be NEET than those with tertiary attainment; however in 2020 the share of NEETs with some amount of tertiary education rose sharply in many OECD countries (OECD, 2021[76]).[12] Quarterly data for some OECD countries showed large changes in early 2020: in Canada, the share of young people (aged 15 to 29) neither in employment nor in education or training increased from 12% in February to 18% in March 2020 and 24% in April 2020 (Brunet, 2020[77]).[13] However in the United Kingdom, NEET rates fell continuously throughout the pandemic, reaching historic lows by June 2021 (ONS, 2021[78]). This is likely due to young people choosing to stay in education, rather than enter the labour market during a period of instability (ONS, 2021[78]; Adcock, 2020[79]). OECD data show a similar pattern among youths aged 18-24 in Austria, France, Poland, Portugal and Slovenia (OECD, 2021[59]).

Figure 9.9. The pandemic has exacerbated poor labour market outcomes for younger age cohorts

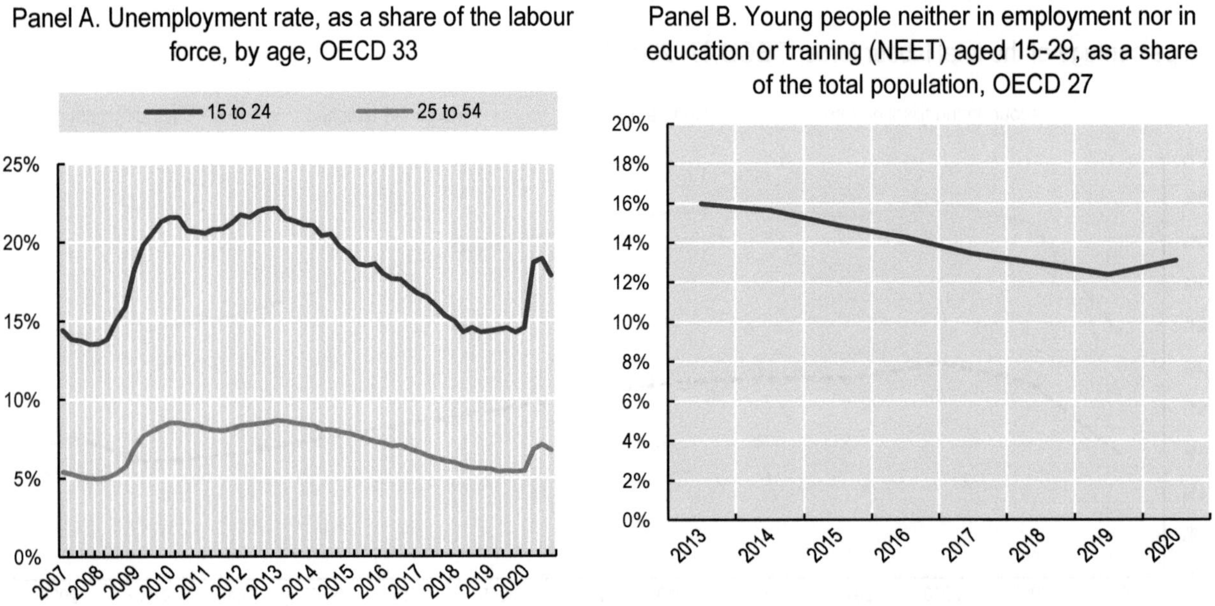

Note: In Panel A, the OECD average excludes Costa Rica, Germany, Mexico, Switzerland and the United Kingdom due to breaks in the time series. In Panel B, the OECD average includes Australia, Austria, Belgium, Canada, the Czech Republic, Estonia, Finland, France, Greece, Hungary, Iceland, Ireland, Israel, Italy, Latvia, Mexico, the Netherlands, New Zealand, Norway, Poland, Portugal, the Slovak Republic, Slovenia, Spain, Sweden, the United States and the United Kingdom.
Source: OECD (n.d.[80]), *Unemployment rate by age group* (database), https://doi.org/10.1787/997c8750-en; and OECD (n.d.[64]), *OECD Education Statistics* (database), https://doi.org/10.1787/edu-data-en.

StatLink https://stat.link/vke4wn

Box 9.2. Further reading

- OECD (forthcoming), *Health at a Glance 2021: OECD Indicators*, OECD Publishing, Paris
- OECD (2021), *Preventing Harmful Alcohol Use, OECD Health Policy Studies*, OECD Publishing, Paris, https://dx.doi.org/10.1787/6e4b4ffb-en
- OECD (2021), *Education at a Glance 2021: OECD Indicators,* OECD Publishing, Paris, https://dx.doi.org/10.1787/b35a14e5-en
- OECD (2020), *Education and COVID-19: Focusing on the long-term impact of school closures*, OECD Publishing, Paris, https://doi.org/10.1787/2cea926e-en
- OECD (2020), *OECD Employment Outlook 2020: Worker Security and the COVID-19 Crisis*, OECD Publishing, Paris, https://dx.doi.org/10.1787/1686c758-en

References

Aaronson, S. and F. Alba (2020), *Unemployment among young workers during COVID-19*, The Brookings Institution, https://www.brookings.edu/research/unemployment-among-young-workers-during-covid-19/. [72]

Adcock, J. (2020), *NEET Data: August 2021*, Youth Employment UK, https://www.youthemployment.org.uk/neet-data-august-2021/. [79]

Alhmidi, M. (2020), "Many Canadians gaining weight during COVID-19: Poll", *CTV News*, https://www.ctvnews.ca/health/many-canadians-gaining-weight-during-covid-19-poll-1.5202007. [39]

APA (2021), *One year on: Unhealthy weight gains, increased drinking reported by Americans coping with pandemic stress*, American Psychological Association, https://www.apa.org/news/press/releases/2021/03/one-year-pandemic-stress. [38]

Bailey, P. et al. (2021), *Diet and Health under COVID-19*, Ipsos, https://www.ipsos.com/sites/default/files/ct/news/documents/2021-01/diet-and-health-under-covid-19.pdf (accessed on 3 May 2021). [20]

Bassett, M., J. Chen and N. Krieger (2020), "The unequal toll of COVID-19 mortality by age in the United States: Quantifying racial/ethnic disparities", *HCPDS Working Paper Series*, No. 3, Harvard Center for Population and Development Studies, https://cdn1.sph.harvard.edu/wp-content/uploads/sites/1266/2020/06/20_Bassett-Chen-Krieger_COVID-19_plus_age_working-paper_0612_Vol-19_No-3_with-cover.pdf (accessed on 28 April 2021). [11]

Bassok, D. et al. (2021), *Coronavirus and Schools: Reflections on education one year into the pandemic*, The Brookings Institution, https://www.brookings.edu/blog/brown-center-chalkboard/2021/03/12/coronavirus-and-schools-reflections-on-education-one-year-into-the-pandemic/?utm_campaign=brookings-comm&utm_medium=email&utm_content=115585308&utm_source=hs_email. [62]

Boseley, S. (2021), "COVID deaths high in countries with more overweight people, says report", *The Guardian*, https://www.theguardian.com/world/2021/mar/03/covid-deaths-high-in-countries-with-more-overweight-people-says-report. [35]

Brunet, S. (2020), *Impact of the COVID-19 pandemic on the NEET (not in employment, education or training) indicator, March and April 2020*, Statistics Canada, https://www150.statcan.gc.ca/n1/en/pub/81-599-x/81-599-x2020001-eng.pdf?st=ssLobgbk. [77]

Cameron, L. (2009), "Can a public scholarship program successfully reduce school drop-outs in a time of economic crisis? Evidence from Indonesia", *Economics of Education Review*, Vol. 28/3, pp. 308-317, http://dx.doi.org/10.1016/j.econedurev.2007.09.013. [55]

CDC (2021), *Certain Medical Conditions and Risk for Severe COVID-19 Illness*, Centers for Disease Control and Prevention, https://www.cdc.gov/coronavirus/2019-ncov/need-extra-precautions/people-with-medical-conditions.html#smoking. [15]

CDC (n.d.), *Obesity, Race/ethnicity, and COVID-19*, Centers for Disease Control and Prevention, https://www.cdc.gov/obesity/data/obesity-and-covid-19.html. [27]

Chen, D. (2020), "The psychosocial impact of the COVID-19 pandemic on changes in smoking behavior: Evidence from a nationwide survey in the UK", *Tobacco Prevention and Cessation*, Vol. 6/October, pp. 1-5, http://dx.doi.org/10.18332/tpc/126976. [22]

CSO (2021), *Social Impact of COVID-19*, Central Statistics Office, https://www.cso.ie/en/methods/socialconditions/socialimpactofcovid-19/. [50]

CSO (2020), *Social Impact of COVID-19 Survey April 2020: Changes in consumption*, Central Statistics Office, https://www.cso.ie/en/releasesandpublications/ep/p-sic19/socialimpactofcovid-19surveyapril2020/changesinconsumption/ (accessed on 4 May 2021). [51]

Dorn, E. et al. (2020), *COVID-19 and student learning in the United States: The hurt could last a lifetime*, McKinsey & Company, https://www.mckinsey.com/industries/public-and-social-sector/our-insights/covid-19-and-student-learning-in-the-united-states-the-hurt-could-last-a-lifetime (accessed on 4 May 2021). [57]

Douine, H. (2020), "Les décrocheurs, premières victimes de la crise économique", *Le Figaro*, https://www.lefigaro.fr/economie/les-decrocheurs-premieres-victimes-de-la-crise-economique-20201202. [74]

Elledge, S. (2020), "2.5 million person-years of life have been lost due to COVID-19 in the United States", medRxiv, http://dx.doi.org/10.1101/2020.10.18.20214783. [6]

Fakuade, M. (2020), "How the COVID-19 pandemic got people smoking again", *Vox*, https://www.vox.com/the-goods/21561419/smoking-cigarettes-covid-19-pandemic-juul-health-boredom. [23]

Flanagan, E. et al. (2021), "The impact of COVID-19 stay-at-home orders on health behaviors in adults", *Obesity*, Vol. 29/2, pp. 438-445, http://dx.doi.org/10.1002/oby.23066. [36]

Fryar CD, Gu Q and Ogden CL (2012), "Anthropometric reference data for children and adults: United States, 2007-2010", *Vital Health Stat 11*, No. 252, National Center for Health Statistics, Washington, D.C., https://www.cdc.gov/nchs/data/series/sr_11/sr11_252.pdf. [42]

Galiatsatos, P. (2020), *Coronavirus: Smoking, vaping, wildfire smoke and air pollution*, Johns Hopkins Medicine, https://www.hopkinsmedicine.org/health/conditions-and-diseases/coronavirus/coronavirus-smoking-vaping-wildfire-smoke-and-air-pollution. [14]

Gapper, J. (2021), "Pandemic comfort food offers too much solace", *Financial Times*, https://www.ft.com/content/74497d5f-4bf4-4031-b424-b70a4547d23c?accessToken=zwAAAXnL70_okc90SX1fS_RAMdO0JLcKRUfSPA.MEUCIH4AVXychlq-IpnNXN_ZbIklnHTGXFUfk0DAuvgd5b_vAiEA_GiqfOP_gGlshu0pB-jsUwGqYGDsjhCPHfsACWih5R0&sharetype=gift?token=7f029a0b-262b-469a-8210-ba3c3aa4944c. [45]

García, E. and E. Weiss (2020), *COVID-19 and student performance, equity, and US education policy: Lessons from pre-pandemic research to inform relief, recovery, and rebuilding*, Economic Policy Institute, https://www.epi.org/publication/the-consequences-of-the-covid-19-pandemic-for-education-performance-and-equity-in-the-united-states-what-can-we-learn-from-pre-pandemic-research-to-inform-relief-recovery-and-rebuilding/. [68]

Gravely, S. et al. (2021), "Smokers' cognitive and behavioural reactions during the early phase of the COVID-19 pandemic: Findings from the 2020 ITC Four Country Smoking and Vaping Survey", *PLOS ONE*, Vol. 16/6, p. e0252427, http://dx.doi.org/10.1371/JOURNAL.PONE.0252427. [21]

Grossman, E., S. Benjamin-Neelon and S. Sonnenschein (2020), "Alcohol consumption during the COVID-19 pandemic: A cross-sectional survey of US adults", *International Journal of Environmental Research and Public Health*, Vol. 17/24, pp. 1-10, http://dx.doi.org/10.3390/ijerph17249189. [47]

Gupta, A. et al. (2021), "A cross-sectional survey of activities to support mental wellness during the COVID-19 pandemic", *Journal of Affective Disorders Reports*, Vol. 5, http://dx.doi.org/10.1016/J.JADR.2021.100167. [52]

Hanushek, E. and L. Woessmann (2020), "The economic impacts of learning losses", *OECD Education Working Papers*, No. 225, OECD Publishing, Paris, https://doi.org/10.1787/21908d74-en. [69]

HCSP (2020), *Notice Concerning the Link between Smoking and COVID-19*, Haut Conseil de la Santé Publique, https://www.hcsp.fr/explore.cgi/avisrapportsdomaine?clefr=891. [17]

Hopkinson, N. et al. (2020), "Current smoking and COVID-19 risk: Results from a population symptom app in over 2.4 million people", *Thorax*, Vol. 76/7, pp. 714-722, http://dx.doi.org/10.1136/thoraxjnl-2020-216422. [18]

I24news (2020), "Coronavirus lockdown caused 55% of Israelis to gain weight", *I24news*, https://www.i24news.tv/en/news/israel/1589287179-coronavirus-lockdown-caused-55-of-israelis-to-gain-weight. [40]

Ingraham, C. (2016), "Look at how much weight you're going to gain", *The Washington Post*, https://www.washingtonpost.com/news/wonk/wp/2016/01/29/the-age-when-you-gain-the-most-weight/. [43]

Iqbal, S. et al. (2020), *We should avoid flattening the curve in education – Possible scenarios for learning loss during the school lockdowns*, World Bank Blogs, https://blogs.worldbank.org/education/we-should-avoid-flattening-curve-education-possible-scenarios-learning-loss-during-school. [56]

Jackson, G. (2021), "Women are more susceptible to long COVID, but will we listen to them?", *The Guardian*, https://www.theguardian.com/lifeandstyle/2021/mar/25/women-coronavirus-long-covid-health. [10]

Kompaniyets, L. et al. (2021), "Body mass index and risk for COVID-19–related hospitalization, intensive care unit admission, invasive mechanical ventilation, and death — United States, March–December 2020", *Morbidity and Mortality Weekly Report*, Vol. 70/10, pp. 355-361, http://dx.doi.org/10.15585/mmwr.mm7010e4. [33]

Krelle, H. and C. Tallack (2021), *One year on: Three myths about COVID-19 that the data proved wrong*, The Health Foundation, https://www.health.org.uk/publications/long-reads/one-year-on-three-myths-about-COVID-19-that-the-data-proved-wrong (accessed on 28 April 2021). [8]

Lin, A. et al. (2021), "Body weight changes during pandemic-related shelter-in-place in a longitudinal cohort study", *JAMA Network Open*, Vol. 4/3, p. e212536, http://dx.doi.org/10.1001/JAMANETWORKOPEN.2021.2536. [44]

Maltoni, G. et al. (2021), "Adolescent males suffered from reduced physical activity and increased BMI during COVID-19 pandemic", *Nutrition, Metabolism and Cardiovascular Diseases*, Vol. 31/7, pp. 2181-2185, http://dx.doi.org/10.1016/j.numecd.2021.03.018. [41]

North American Quitline Consortium (2021), *Report on the Impact of the COVID-19 Pandemic on Smoking Cessation*, North American Quitline Consortium, Phoenix, AZ, http://dx.doi.org/10.7326/M20-7271. [24]

O'Hearn, M. et al. (2021), "Coronavirus disease 2019 hospitalizations attributable to cardiometabolic conditions in the United States: A comparative risk assessment analysis", *Journal of the American Heart Association*, Vol. 10/5, pp. 1-27, http://dx.doi.org/10.1161/JAHA.120.019259. [32]

O'Connor, A. (2020), "Weight gain and stress eating are downside of pandemic life", *The New York Times*, https://www.nytimes.com/2020/12/04/well/live/pandemic-weight-gain.html. [37]

OECD (2021), *Education at a Glance 2021: OECD Indicators*, OECD Publishing, Paris, https://dx.doi.org/10.1787/b35a14e5-en. [59]

OECD (2021), *OECD Employment Outlook 2021: Navigating the COVID-19 Crisis and Recovery*, OECD Publishing, Paris, https://dx.doi.org/10.1787/5a700c4b-en. [76]

OECD (2021), *Preventing Harmful Alcohol Use*, OECD Health Policy Studies, OECD Publishing, Paris, https://dx.doi.org/10.1787/6e4b4ffb-en. [48]

OECD (2021), *The State of Global Education: 18 Months into the Pandemic*, OECD Publishing, Paris, https://doi.org/10.1787/1a23bb23-en. [85]

OECD (2021), *The State of School Education: One Year into the COVID Pandemic*, OECD Publishing, Paris, https://doi.org/10.1787/201dde84-en. [82]

OECD (2020), *Education at a Glance 2020: OECD Indicators*, OECD Publishing, Paris, https://dx.doi.org/10.1787/69096873-en. [60]

OECD (2020), *How's Life? 2020: Measuring Well-being*, OECD Publishing, Paris, https://dx.doi.org/10.1787/9870c393-en. [2]

OECD (2020), *OECD Employment Outlook 2020: Worker Security and the COVID-19 Crisis*, OECD Publishing, Paris, https://dx.doi.org/10.1787/1686c758-en. [75]

OECD (2020), "Schooling disrupted, schooling rethought: How the COVID-19 pandemic is changing education", *OECD Policy Responses to Coronavirus (COVID-19)*, OECD Publishing, Paris, https://doi.org/10.1787/68b11faf-en. [65]

OECD (2020), "Youth and COVID-19: Response, recovery and resilience", *OECD Policy Responses to Coronavirus (COVID-19)*, OECD Publishing, Paris, https://doi.org/10.1787/c40e61c6-en. [70]

OECD (2019), *Health at a Glance 2019: OECD Indicators*, OECD Publishing, Paris, https://dx.doi.org/10.1787/4dd50c09-en. [19]

OECD (2019), *PISA 2018 Results (Volume III): What School Life Means for Students' Lives*, PISA, OECD Publishing, Paris, https://dx.doi.org/10.1787/acd78851-en. [67]

OECD (2015), *How's Life? 2015: Measuring Well-being*, OECD Publishing, Paris, https://dx.doi.org/10.1787/how_life-2015-en. [54]

OECD (2013), *How's Life? 2013: Measuring Well-being*, OECD Publishing, Paris, https://doi.org/10.1787/9789264201392-en. [1]

OECD (n.d.), *OECD Education Statistics (database)*, https://doi.org/10.1787/edu-data-en (accessed on 26 September 2021). [64]

OECD (n.d.), *OECD Household Dashboard (database)*, https://stats.oecd.org/Index.aspx?DataSetCode=HH_DASH (accessed on 29 April 2021). [71]

OECD (n.d.), *Unemployment rate by age group (database)*, https://doi.org/10.1787/997c8750-en (accessed on 2 June 2021). [80]

Oh, I. et al. (2020), "Years of life lost attributable to COVID-19 in high-incidence countries", *Journal of Korean Medical Science*, Vol. 35/32, p. e300, http://dx.doi.org/10.3346/jkms.2020.35.e300. [4]

ONS (2021), *Young people not in education, employment or training (NEET), UK: August 2021*, Office for National Statistics, https://www.ons.gov.uk/employmentandlabourmarket/peoplenotinwork/unemployment/bulletins/youngpeoplenotineducationemploymentortrainingneet/august2021. [78]

ONS (2020), *Coronavirus and how people spent their time under lockdown: 28 March to 26 April 2020*, Office for National Statistics, https://www.ons.gov.uk/economy/nationalaccounts/satelliteaccounts/bulletins/coronavirusandhowpeoplespenttheirtimeunderrestrictions/28marchto26april2020. [53]

Pifarré i Arolas, H. et al. (2021), "Years of life lost to COVID-19 in 81 countries", *Scientific Reports*, Vol. 11/3504, http://dx.doi.org/10.1038/s41598-021-83040-3. [3]

Pollard, M., J. Tucker and H. Green (2020), "Changes in adult alcohol use and consequences during the COVID-19 pandemic in the US", *JAMA network open*, Vol. 3/9, p. e2022942, http://dx.doi.org/10.1001/jamanetworkopen.2020.22942. [49]

Popkin, B. et al. (2020), "Individuals with obesity and COVID-19: A global perspective on the epidemiology and biological relationships", *Obesity Reviews*, Vol. 21/11, p. e13128, http://dx.doi.org/10.1111/obr.13128. [31]

Public Health England (2020), *Excess Weight and COVID-19: Insights from new evidence*, Public Health England, London, https://assets.publishing.service.gov.uk/government/uploads/system/uploads/attachment_data/file/907966/PHE_insight_Excess_weight_and_COVID-19__FINAL.pdf. [28]

Reeves, R., E. Buckner and E. Smith (2021), *The unreported gender gap in high school graduation rates*, The Brookings Institution, https://www.brookings.edu/blog/up-front/2021/01/12/the-unreported-gender-gap-in-high-school-graduation-rates/. [61]

Resnick, B. (2020), "New study calculates "years of potential life lost" from coronavirus", *Vox*, https://www.vox.com/science-and-health/2020/6/23/21299109/covid-19-pandemic-years-potential-life-lost. [12]

Reuters (2020), "Youth unemployment: A scourge of the COVID-19 economy", *Reuters*, https://www.reuters.com/article/uk-health-coronavirus-gen-z-economy-grap-idUKKBN28Y0MU. [73]

Simonnet, A. et al. (2020), "High prevalence of obesity in severe acute respiratory syndrome coronavirus-2 (SARS-CoV-2) requiring invasive mechanical ventilation", *Obesity*, Vol. 28/7, pp. 1195-1199, http://dx.doi.org/10.1002/oby.22831. [30]

Statistics Canada (2021), *Alcohol and cannabis use during the pandemic: Canadian Perspectives Survey Series 6*, The Daily, https://www150.statcan.gc.ca/n1/daily-quotidien/210304/dq210304a-eng.htm. [83]

Statistics Canada (2021), *Gendered impacts of the COVID-19 pandemic on the proportion of youth neither in employment nor education at the start of the school year*, Insights on Canadian Society, https://www150.statcan.gc.ca/n1/pub/75-006-x/2021001/article/00003-eng.htm. [58]

Statistics Canada (2021), *Labour Force Survey, May 2021*, The Daily, https://www150.statcan.gc.ca/n1/daily-quotidien/210604/dq210604a-eng.htm. [84]

Statistics Canada (2020), *Change in weekly habits as a result of COVID-19, March and April 2020*, https://www150.statcan.gc.ca/n1/daily-quotidien/200408/t002c-eng.htm. [46]

The Health Foundation (2021), *1.5 million potential years of life lost to COVID-19 in the UK, with each life cut short by 10 years on average*, The Health Foundation, https://www.health.org.uk/news-and-comment/news/1.5-million-potential-years-of-life-lost-to-covid-19. [7]

The Lancet Respiratory Medicine (2021), "COVID-19, smoking, and cancer: A dangerous liaison", *The Lancet Respiratory Medicine*, Vol. 9/9, p. 937, http://dx.doi.org/10.1016/S2213-2600(21)00373-8. [81]

The Lancet Respiratory Medicine (2021), "Pandemic fans the flames of smoking and health inequity", *The Lancet Respiratory Medicine*, Vol. 9/5, p. 435, http://dx.doi.org/10.1016/s2213-2600(21)00180-6. [25]

The Pew Charitable Trusts (2020), *What COVID-19 underscores about how broadband connectivity affects educational attainment*, https://www.pewtrusts.org/en/research-and-analysis/articles/2020/12/08/what-covid-19-underscores-about-how-broadband-connectivity-affects-educational-attainment. [66]

Torjesen, I. (2021), "COVID-19: Middle aged women face greater risk of debilitating long term symptoms", *BMJ*, Vol. 372, p. n829, http://dx.doi.org/10.1136/bmj.n829. [9]

UNESCO (n.d.), *Global Monitoring of School Closures, COVID-19 (database)*, United Nations Educational, Scientific and Cultural Organization, https://en.unesco.org/covid19/educationresponse (accessed on 12 July 2021). [63]

Wadman, M. (2020), "Why obesity worsens COVID-19", *Science*, Vol. 369/6509, pp. 1280-1281, http://dx.doi.org/10.1126/SCIENCE.369.6509.1280. [34]

WHO (2020), *Smoking and COVID-19*, World Health Organization, https://www.who.int/news-room/commentaries/detail/smoking-and-covid-19. [16]

WHO (2020), *Tobacco Use and COVID-19*, World Health Organization, https://www.who.int/news/item/11-05-2020-who-statement-tobacco-use-and-covid-19. [13]

World Obesity Federation (2021), *COVID-19 and Obesity: The 2021 Atlas*, World Obesity Federation, London, https://www.worldobesityday.org/assets/downloads/COVID-19_and_Obesity-The_2021_Atlas.pdf. [26]

Wu, K. (2020), "The coronavirus has claimed 2.5 million years of potential life in the US, study finds", *The New York Times*, https://www.nytimes.com/2020/10/21/health/coronavirus-statistics-deaths.html. [5]

Yang, J., J. Hu and C. Zhu (2021), "Obesity aggravates COVID-19: A systematic review and meta-analysis", *Journal of Medical Virology*, Vol. 93/1, pp. 257-261, http://dx.doi.org/10.1002/jmv.26237. [29]

Notes

[1] The OECD calculates Potential Years of Life Lost (PYLL) by summing up the deaths that occur at each age and multiplying this by the number of remaining years up to a selected threshold: 75 years. PYLL are standardised to allow for cross-country and cross-year comparisons (OECD, 2019[19]; OECD, 2015[54]). PYLL is a measure of *premature* mortality if the threshold is around 75-years-old or below. PYLL may be calculated somewhat differently across studies. Some studies use a different threshold year (65, 70, 80, etc.). Other statistical offices, such as the UK Office for National Statistics (ONS), use actuarial life expectancy tables to assign a threshold value for each year of death. For example, a man aged 80 in England or Wales has an expected life expectancy of an additional 8.2 years, meaning that if he were to die at age 80 his potential years lost would be 8.2 (Krelle and Tallack, 2021[8]).

[2] This study calculated Years of Life Lost (YLL) attributable to the virus in 30 countries with the highest rates of COVID-19 as of July 2020: Australia, Austria, Brazil, Belgium, Canada, China, Chile, Ecuador, France, Germany, India, Iran, Ireland, Israel, Italy, Japan, Korea, the Netherlands, Norway, Peru, Poland, Portugal, Romania, the Russian Federation, Sweden, Switzerland, Spain, Turkey, the United Kingdom and the United States. COVID-19 incidence and mortality data were collected from official statistics within each country. YLLs were calculated using life expectancy tables for Japanese females at one-year age intervals, who have the longest life expectancy globally. United Nations demography data were used to calculate YLL per 100 000 population (Oh et al., 2020[4]).

[3] The Pifarré i Arolas et al. (2021[3]) study uses country-specific life expectancy tables to calculate years of life lost for deaths at a given age (YLL). YLL is calculated as the difference between an individual's age at time of death from COVID-19 and their life expectancy at that age in their country.

[4] The Elledge (2020[6]) study uses actuarial life expectancy tables to set thresholds for each age.

[5] The disparity in outcomes may be in part a result of the higher poverty rates experienced by racial and ethnic minority groups, which can limit access to quality health care services.

[6] Lung cancer and COVID-19 share some symptoms – including cough, shortness of breath and lowered oxygen levels – leading to fears that the pandemic may result in delayed diagnoses of lung cancer (The Lancet Respiratory Medicine, 2021[81]).

[7] The Ipsos Global Advisor survey ran from 23 October to 6 November 2020 and collected data from 22 008 individuals across 30 countries: Argentina, Australia, Belgium, Brazil, Canada, Chile, China, France, Germany, Great Britain, Hong Kong, Hungary, India, Israel, Italy, Japan, Malaysia, Mexico, the Netherlands, Peru, Poland, the Russian Federation, Saudi Arabia, Singapore, South Africa, Spain, Sweden, Turkey, the United Kingdom and the United States. Only findings from OECD countries are used in this chapter. Surveys were conducted online via the Ipsos Online Panel system. Data are weighted to be nationally representative; however, Ipsos notes that the samples in certain countries, such as Brazil, may be more urban, educated and/or affluent than the general population (Bailey et al., 2021[20]).

[8] This survey was administered to 7 753 respondents between 3 April and 3 May 2020. Participants were invited to participate in the survey via paid advertisements on Facebook. Respondents from any country could participate; however, the researchers paid for advertisements to target participants from the United States, Australia, Canada, Ireland and the United Kingdom. The survey was also accessible via the research team's website, through email invites and word of mouth (Flanagan et al., 2021[36]).

[9] However a subsequent study from Statistics Canada, using data through January 2021, found that – of the Canadians aged 15 to 29 who consumed alcohol in the past month – 33% reported decreasing their consumption since the start of the pandemic, compared to only 18% of those aged 30-64 (Statistics Canada, 2021[83]). Therefore there is some variability in alcohol consumption rates by age, depending on the study and the time frame.

[10] In the early stages of the pandemic, education institutions of all levels shifted to remote learning in the majority of OECD countries. However, as the pandemic wore on, many OECD countries prioritised keeping primary schools open, while in a number of countries remote learning in secondary and tertiary institutions continued (see Chapter 3, as well as (OECD, 2021[85])).

[11] Graduation ratios (defined as the ratio of those who graduate from upper-secondary institutions compared to those who attended) for 2020 are not yet available in full. Early evidence suggests falls in some OECD countries, stability in others, and increases in graduation rates primarily stemming from vocational students (OECD, 2021[82]).

[12] One facet not captured by NEET or youth unemployment rates is the fall in student employment during the pandemic, which, in the case of Canada, had unequal gendered impacts: the employment rate for young women aged 15-24 attending school full-time declined by 10.6 percentage points from 2019 to 2021, compared to a 4.2 percentage point decline for men (Statistics Canada, 2021[84]).

[13] Statistics Canada notes that sharp increases in the NEET rates of the youngest age cohorts (aged 15 to 19) in the first two months of the pandemic may have been affected by measurement issues, such as young people reporting they were not in schooling due to remote learning, or changes to education delivery. However, the large increases among older age cohorts (20 to 24, and 25 to 29) were most likely due to increases in unemployment, rather than measurement issues (Brunet, 2020[77]).

10 Social capital and COVID-19

Social capital is about social norms, shared values and institutional arrangements that foster co-operation. Volunteering via official organisations, already on a downward trend, dropped in 2020, but signs of increased solidarity were also visible across the OECD, and charitable giving rose. Faster adoption of and adherence to containment measures in communities with higher interpersonal trust also led to fewer COVID-19 cases. The 2020 increase in trust in institutions in face of the common threat of COVID-19 started to wear off by early 2021. The pandemic forced governments to make difficult choices about temporarily restraining personal freedoms, to fast-track new regulations and cut back on impact assessments and active stakeholder engagement. Progress towards gender parity in politics, a proxy for the inclusiveness of institutions, continued but remains far from parity, including in COVID-19 task forces. More digital parliamentary practices have both positive and negative implications for female political participation.

10.1. Volunteering

The pandemic made volunteering via official organisations more difficult, but signs of mutual solidarity were visible throughout the OECD, and charitable giving increased

The way in which formal organisations co-ordinated volunteering in the past were impacted by the pandemic in multiple respects. For sanitary reasons, hospitals had to suspend many volunteer programmes, while religious, sports and recreation, as well as arts and cultural gatherings and events, were cancelled, with only some activity moving online. Community-led services (such as food banks) had to quickly implement social distancing and other health protection measures in the face of increasing demand for their services. In addition, increased care responsibilities due to COVID-19 restrictions are likely to have cut into people's available time for volunteering, particularly for women, parents with young children and elderly people.

As a consequence, formal volunteering fell across the OECD. In 2020, only 17% of people in OECD countries said they volunteered for an organisation in the past month, compared to 20% in 2019 (Figure 10.1, Panel A). Although volunteering increased in a small number of countries in Eastern Europe as well as in Iceland and Greece, more than half of OECD members recorded losses, including drops of more than 9 percentage points in Canada, Israel, Korea, Norway, the United Kingdom and the United States. Overall, this represents the lowest share of volunteers across the OECD in the past decade, accelerating the historical downward trend of voluntary engagement via formally established civil society organisations, neighbourhood clubs and charities (Figure 10.1, Panel B).[1] Available official data confirms this pattern: for instance, 21% of Australians said in March 2021 that they had volunteered for an organisation or group in the last 12 months, compared to 26% a year before (ABS, 2021[1]).[2] The loss of key social relationships and of a sense of purpose by giving up volunteering is likely to have had detrimental effects on social connectedness and the mental health particularly of elderly volunteers (What Works Wellbeing, 2020[2]). Indeed, a representative April 2020 survey in Australia revealed that volunteers over the age of 65, as well as women, were more likely to have stopped volunteering compared to the general population (Biddle and Gray, 2020[3]).

Informal support between people in OECD countries remained robust through the crisis. Almost half (44%) of people across all OECD countries reported having helped a stranger in the preceding month during 2020, a similar share as in 2019 (Gallup, n.d.[4]). And, a quarter of people across 14 OECD countries stated in September 2020 that they had provided assistance in the past week, such as running an errand or providing childcare for friends, neighbours or co-workers without expecting anything in return (Imperial College London YouGov, 2020[5]).

Figure 10.1. Volunteering via organisations, already on a long-term downward trend, was difficult to carry out during the pandemic

Share of people reporting to have volunteered for an organisation in the past month

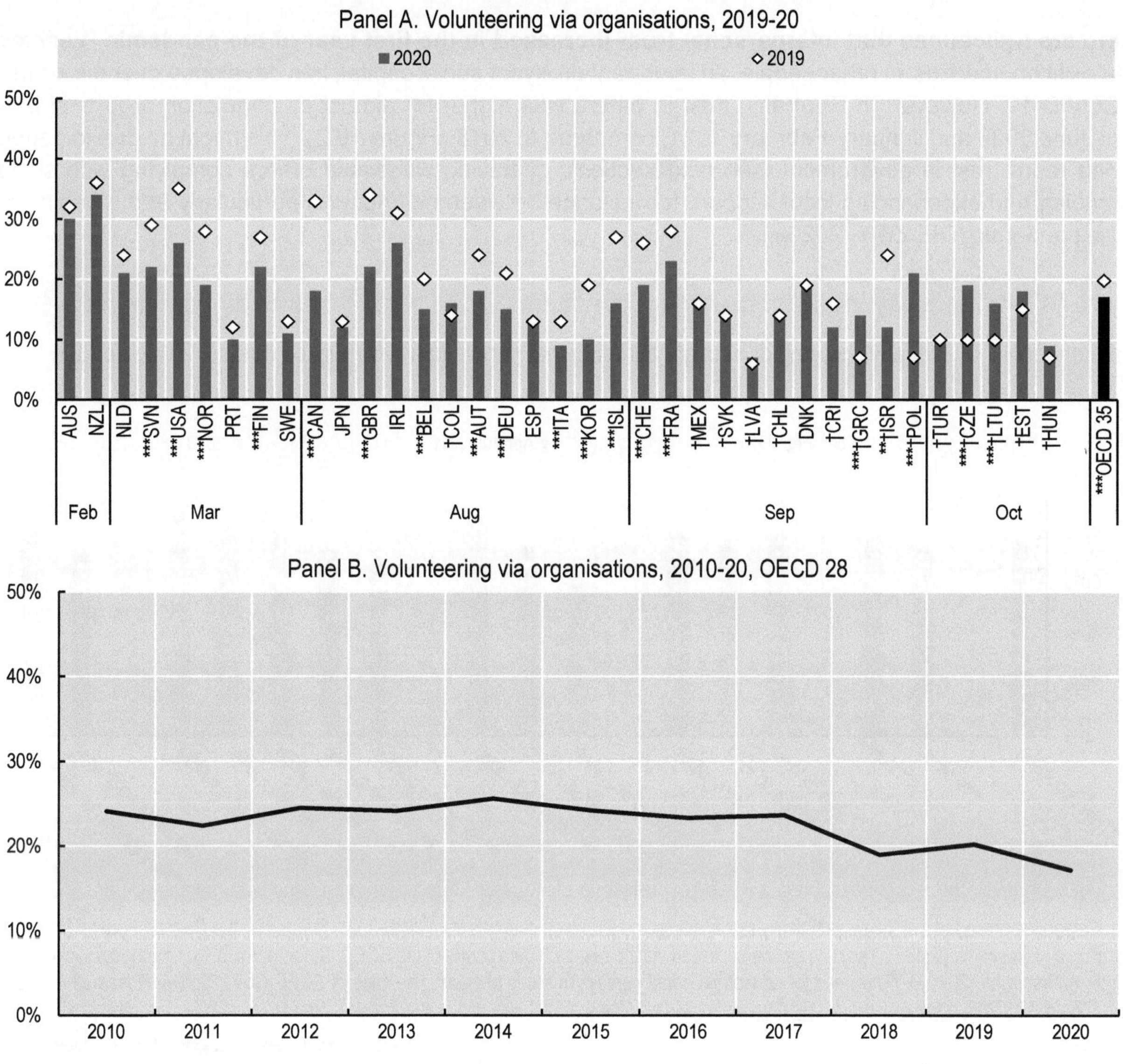

Note: In Panel A, † denotes countries in which the mode of data collection changed between 2019 and 2020 (generally, moving from face-to-face interviews to phone-based interviews). The OECD average excludes Luxembourg (no data in 2020), the Czech Republic and Iceland (no data in 2019). The 2019 value refers to 2018 for the Czech Republic and to 2017 for Iceland. Countries preceded by *** saw statistically significant (at the 5% level) changes from 2019-2020. Countries are ranked by fieldwork start date (earliest to latest) in 2020. Refer to the Reader's Guide for a complete list of Gallup World Poll data collection dates in 2020, and to Box 3.4 for additional information about the data collection methodology. In Panel B, the OECD average excludes Chile, the Czech Republic, Estonia, Greece, Iceland, Latvia, Luxembourg, Norway, Slovenia and the Slovak Republic due to missing data for at least one of the years. 2010 has been selected as the starting year (vs. 2006 when the Gallup World Poll was launched) to maximise country coverage.

Source: OECD calculations based on the *Gallup World Poll* (n.d.[4]) (database), https://www.gallup.com/178667/gallup-world-poll-work.aspx.

StatLink https://stat.link/8a0cns

10.2. Trust in others

Trust in others has increased in some countries, but many perceive their societies to be more divided since the onset of COVID-19

There are indications that interpersonal trust increased in the first year of the pandemic. Very few data exist on how trust in other people, an important proxy for social capital, has developed over the course of COVID-19. However, In Germany, trust in others was higher for almost all population groups in both April-June 2020 and January-February 2021, compared to 2018 (Figure 10.2). This might be due to people having more trust in government (see next section), or having witnessed others complying with social distancing and experiencing local support, for instance between neighbours, particularly at the beginning of the pandemic (DIE ZEIT, 2020[6]).[3]

Figure 10.2. In Germany, trust in others over the course of the pandemic was higher than in 2018

Share of people in Germany agreeing or strongly agreeing that people can generally be trusted, 2018, Apr-Jun 2020, Jan-Feb 2021

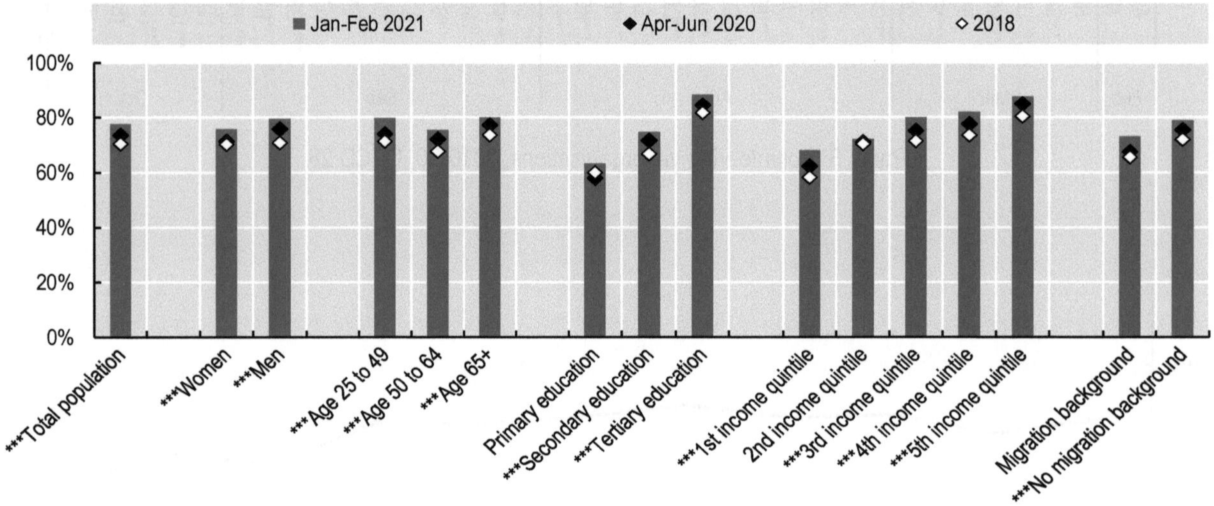

Note: Categories preceded by *** saw statistically significant (at the 5% level) changes from 2018-2021. Funded by the German Federal Ministry of Education and Research (BMBF). The data can be accessed via the research data centre of the SOEP. Refer to Box 3.1 for methodological details.
Source: Kühne et al. (2020[7]), "The need for household panel surveys in times of crisis: The case of SOEP-CoV", *Survey Research Methods*, Vol. 14/2, pp. 195-203, https://doi.org/10.18148/srm/2020.v14i2.7748.

StatLink https://stat.link/lm7h2j

It remains to be seen whether such effects will be long-lived. In New Zealand, levels of interpersonal trust increased in June 2020, but then returned to their 2018 baseline by September (Figure 10.7).[4] Previous pandemics, such as the 1918–19 Spanish flu, ended up having *negative* effects on interpersonal trust that persisted for at least a generation, while evidence from the Global Financial Crisis links regional income decline in Russia with decreasing trust in others (which did not revert to pre-crisis levels again despite economic recovery) (Aassve et al., 2020[8]; Ananyev and Guriev, 2019[9]). In addition, after being evenly split on whether the pandemic had brought people together in June-August 2020, the majority of adults in 12 OECD members found their country to be "more divided now than before the coronavirus outbreak" by February-May 2021 (Figure 10.3, Panels A and B). In all countries surveyed, those who think their country has done a bad job of dealing with the coronavirus outbreak were more likely to say that their country is more divided (Pew Research Center, 2020[10]). In addition, interpersonal trust and political preferences are related to perceptions of unity: across the surveyed OECD members, at least a third of respondents who said their country is more divided also reported that "most people cannot be trusted"; and in Europe, right-wing populist party supporters see more division since the pandemic began (Figure 10.3, Panel C).

Figure 10.3. By early 2021, between 53% and 88% of adults felt their countries were more divided than before COVID-19, a perception partly tied to interpersonal distrust and political preferences

Indicators of social cohesion, OECD 12, Jun-Aug 2020 - Feb-May 2021

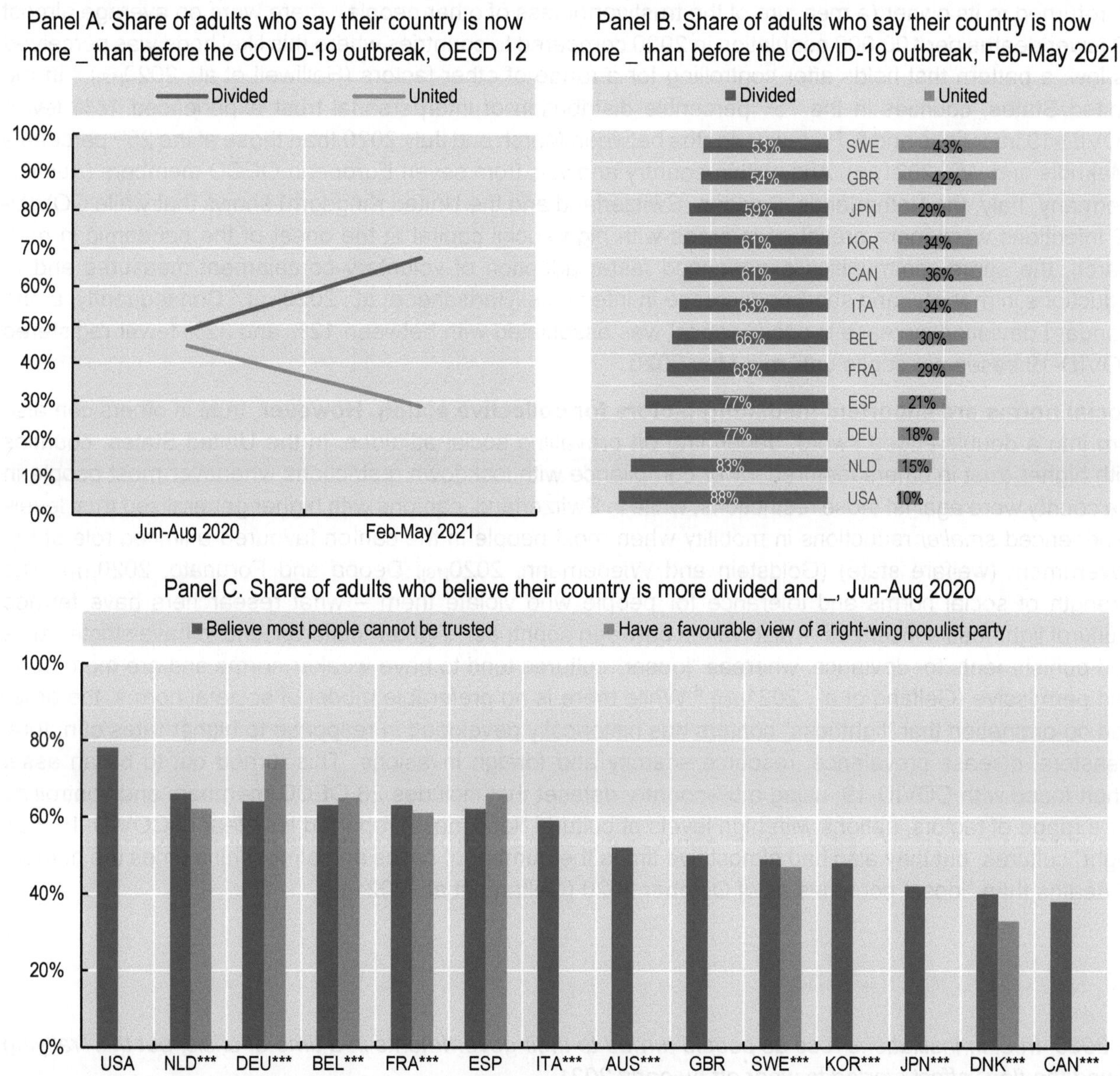

Note: Sample size is around 1 000 people per country. Those who did not answer are not shown. In Panel A, the OECD average incudes only those 12 countries shown in Panel B. In Panel C, countries followed by *** saw statistically significant (at the 5% level) differences between the share of people believing that most people can be trusted and those who believe most people cannot be trusted. For perceptions of right-wing populist parties, only countries with significant differences between those with favourable and unfavourable views are shown. Right-wing populist parties refer to the Flemish Interest in Belgium, Danish People's Party in Denmark, AfD in Germany, National Front in France, Party for Freedom in the Netherlands, Vox in Spain and Sweden Democrats in Sweden.

Source: Pew Research Center (2020[10]), *Most Approve of National Response to COVID-19 in 14 Advanced Economies*, https://www.pewresearch.org/global/2020/08/27/most-approve-of-national-response-to-covid-19-in-14-advanced-economies/; and Pew Research Center (2021[11]), *People in Advanced Economies Say Their Society Is More Divided Than Before Pandemic*, https://www.pewresearch.org/global/2021/06/23/people-in-advanced-economies-say-their-society-is-more-divided-than-before-pandemic/.

StatLink https://stat.link/8fi6wn

Interpersonal trust was an important resilience factor in 2020

More trusting communities were better protected from pandemic effects in the medium-term.[5] Higher interpersonal trust has been associated with better hygienic practices, greater compliance with social distancing, and lower mortality rates. In Germany, for instance, high interpersonal trust was linked to adherence to more hygienic practices as well as to greater willingness to be vaccinated (DIW, 2021[12]). In countries where a comparatively high share of people (in 2019) felt it likely that a dropped wallet would be returned to its owner (a measure of the trustworthiness of other people), there were on average almost 50 fewer deaths per 100 000 population in 2020 compared to countries where this likelihood was perceived as low, a pattern that holds after controlling for a range of other factors (Helliwell et al., 2020[13]).[6] In the United States, counties in the 75th percentile distribution of interpersonal trust experienced 18% fewer COVID-19 infections and 5.7% fewer deaths between March and July 2020 than those at the 25th percentile (Makridis and Wu, 2021[14]). And, within-country analysis from seven European OECD members (Austria, Germany, Italy, the Netherlands, Sweden, Switzerland and the United Kingdom) shows that while COVID-19 infections were more prevalent in areas with high social capital at the onset of the pandemic in mid-March, the same communities experienced faster adoption of voluntary containment measures and of reductions in mobility, and sharper decrease in infections (Bartscher et al., 2020[15]).[7] Consequently, a one standard deviation increase in social capital was associated with between 12% and 32% fewer registered COVID-19 cases per capita until mid-May 2020.

Social norms are important mediating factors for collective action. However, trust in others can also turn into a double-edged sword, depending on prevailing social attitudes. In the United States, counties with higher trust in others featured *lower* compliance with lockdown restrictions whenever most people in the county were against those restrictions; while in Switzerland, cantons with higher generalised trust levels experienced *smaller* reductions in mobility when most people in the canton favoured a limited role of the government (welfare state) (Goldstein and Wiedemann, 2020[16]; Deopa and Forunato, 2020[17]). The strength of social norms and tolerance for people who violate them – what researchers have termed "cultural tightness–looseness" – also varies between countries. "Tighter" cultures tend to have stricter rules and punishments for deviance, whereas "looser" cultures tend to have weaker norms and are more open and permissive (Gelfand et al., 2021[18]).[8] While there is no preferable model of societal norms, the order and co-ordination that "tightness" confers has historically developed in response to higher rates of natural disasters, disease prevalence, resource scarcity and foreign invasions. This turned out to be an asset when faced with COVID-19: using a 57-country dataset that includes 28 OECD members and controlling for a range of factors, nations with high levels of cultural "looseness" reported less fear of COVID-19 than "tight" cultures, but they also had almost five times the number of cases and almost nine times the number of deaths than "loose" countries as of October 2020 (Gelfand et al., 2021[18]).

10.3. Trust in institutions

In 2020, trust in institutions rose as people turned to their governments in a time of crisis, but this "rallying round the flag" effect started to wear off by early 2021

Like trust in others, trust in institutions has been a key factor for successful pandemic management. As has been shown by past pandemics such as the Ebola outbreak in West Africa in 2014-16, greater trust in government is associated with higher compliance with health policies (Blair, Morse and Tsai, 2017[19]). Across European regions, trust in policy makers pre-outbreak was associated with stronger decreases in mobility around the time of lockdown announcements in mid-March 2000, while the efficiency of policy stringency in terms of mobility reduction significantly increased with trust (Bargain and Aminjonov, 2020[20]). Results from a nationally representative survey in Denmark at the end of February 2020 showed that trust in governments was positively correlated with people's willingness to practice physical distancing

(Olsen and Hjorth, 2020[21]). In Finland, respondents to a Citizens' Pulse Survey (carried out in co-operation with the OECD) who said that they were unwilling to comply with COVID-19 restrictions in November 2020 also reported statistically significant lower levels of trust in public institutions (Figure 10.4).

Figure 10.4. In Finland, people willing to comply with COVID-19 restrictions had higher trust in institutions

Average institutional trust levels of people in Finland willing and unwilling to comply with COVID-19 restrictions, on a scale of 1 (no trust at all) to 10 (complete trust), Nov-2020

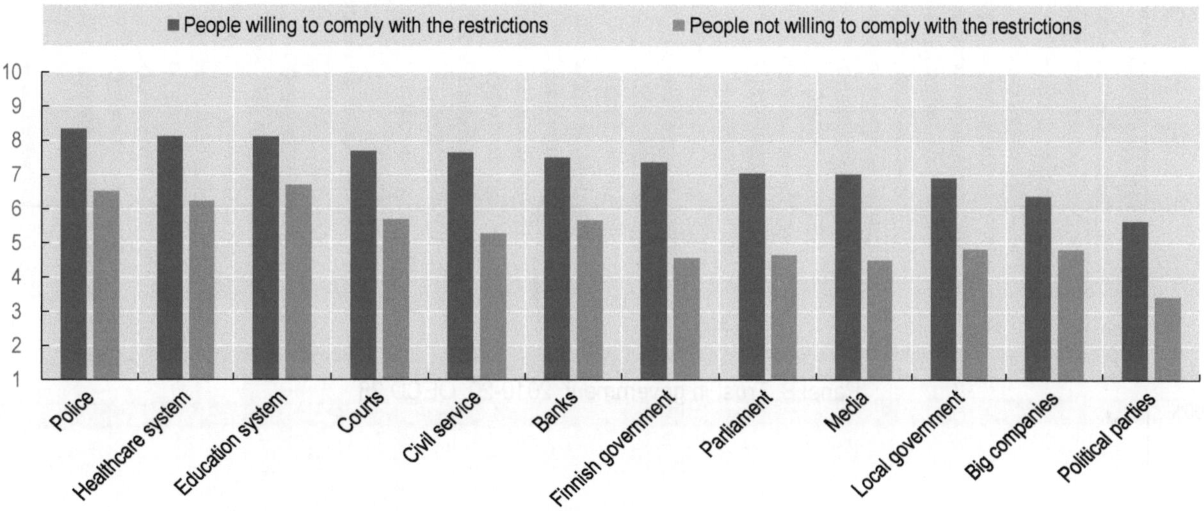

Note: Willingness to comply with COVID-19 restrictions refers to the share of respondents answering "well" and "quite well" to the question: "How well have other people followed the instructions given by the authorities during the coronavirus crisis?".
Source: OECD (2021[22]), *Drivers of Trust in Public Institutions in Finland*, https://doi.org/10.1787/52600c9e-en.

StatLink https://stat.link/w643me

In most OECD countries, institutional trust in 2020 was at its highest since records began in 2006, and it continued to rise until the end of the year. Trust in national governments rose markedly in the majority of OECD countries (with the exception of Eastern Europe) as COVID-19 unfolded: although "only" 50% of people in OECD countries reported confidence in national governments throughout 2020, this is a 5 percentage point increase relative to the previous year (Figure 10.5, Panel A). Historically, OECD average trust in government fell consistently in the five-year period following the Global Financial Crisis (GFC) in 2008, beginning an unsteady climb-back from 2014. In 2019, it exceeded pre-GFC levels, and it continued to rise in 2020, reaching its highest point since data collection started in 2006 (Figure 10.5, Panel B).

Figure 10.5. Trust in institutions was at an all-time high in 2020 in most OECD countries

Share of people answering "yes" to a question about confidence in the national government

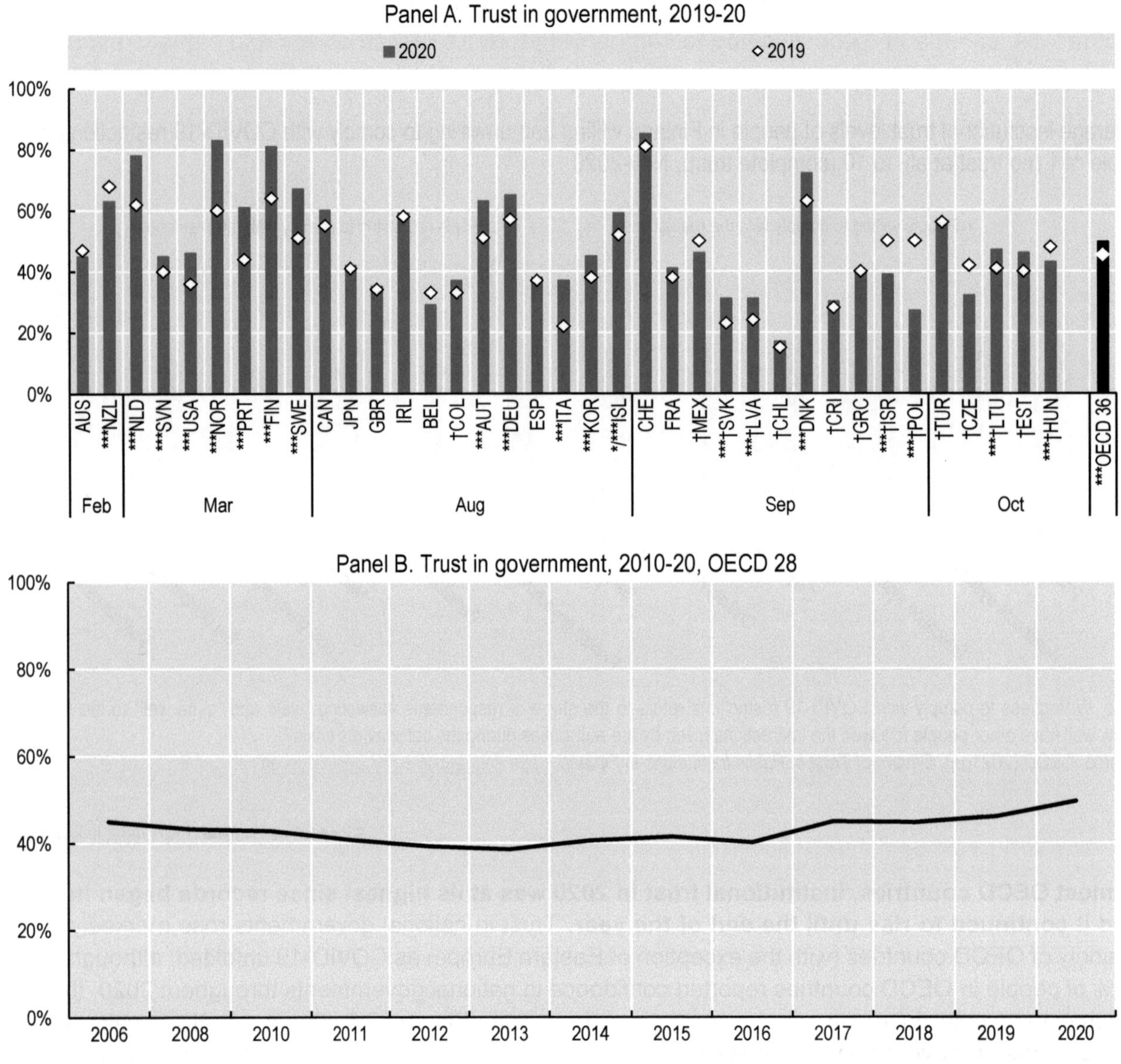

Note: In Panel A, † denotes countries in which the mode of data collection changed between 2019 and 2020 (generally, moving from face-to-face interviews to phone-based interviews). * denotes countries with between 301 and 500 observations. More than 500 observations are available for all other countries. Countries preceded by *** saw statistically significant (at the 5% level) changes from 2019-2020. The OECD average excludes Luxembourg (no data in 2020) and the Czech Republic (no data in 2019). The 2019 value for the Czech Republic refers to 2018. Countries are ranked by fieldwork start date (earliest to latest) in 2020. Refer to the Reader's Guide for a complete list of Gallup World Poll data collection dates in 2020, and to Box 3.4 for additional information about the data collection methodology. In Panel B, the OECD average excludes Chile, the Czech Republic, Estonia, Greece, Iceland, Latvia, Luxembourg, Norway, Slovenia and the Slovak Republic due to missing data for at least one of the years. 2010 has been selected as the starting year (vs. 2006 when the Gallup World Poll was launched) to maximise country coverage.

Source: OECD calculations based on the *Gallup World Poll* (n.d.[4]) (database), https://www.gallup.com/178667/gallup-world-poll-work.aspx.

StatLink https://stat.link/fvl3qn

The increase of trust in institutions carries many elements of a "rallying round the flag" effect. This phenomenon refers to national unity in the face of common threats, and is characterised by temporary surges in public approval for governments or political leaders during periods of crisis or war (such as in the aftermath of 9/11), as well as less attention to other policy issues (Mueller, 1970[23]; Chatagnier, 2012[24]; OECD, 2021[25]). In the context of COVID-19, lockdown measures in European countries between March-April 2020 were associated with stronger support for the party of the incumbent prime minister/president, as well as with higher trust in government and satisfaction with democracy, without affecting traditional left-right attitudes (Bol et al., 2021[26]). In Spain, demand for strong leadership, willingness to give up individual freedoms and support for technocratic governance all increased in March 2020 (Amat et al., 2020[27]). Panel data from the Netherlands in March 2020 also show that some of the traditional drivers of institutional trust, such as people's evaluations of economic performance, lost their explanatory power and were superseded by collective distress as infections rose (Schraff, 2020[28]).

The "rallying round the flag" phenomenon also contributed to the narrowing of inequalities in institutional trust throughout 2020. As the pandemic unfolded, the share of people with confidence in the national government rose for all age and income groups, including for those at the bottom of the income distribution who traditionally trust institutions less, and for young people, even though they were affected most by school and university closures and employment losses (Figure 10.6).[9] Trust in government increased the most for those aged 65 or over, who are most at risk from (and likely have the greatest fear of) the virus.

Figure 10.6. Trust in institutions rose across all ages and income groups in 2020

Share of people answering "yes" to a question about confidence in the national government, OECD 28, 2010-20

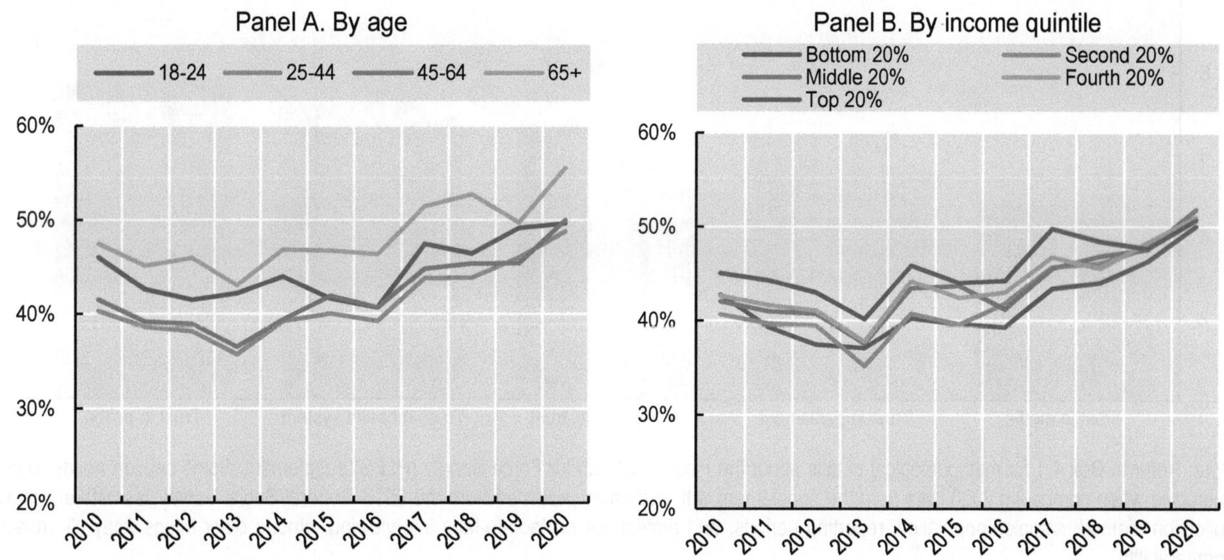

Note: The OECD average excludes Switzerland, the Czech Republic, Estonia, Greece, Iceland, Latvia, Luxembourg, Norway, Slovenia and the Slovak Republic due to missing data for at least one of the years. 2010 has been selected as the starting year (vs. 2006 when the Gallup World Poll launched) to maximise country coverage.

Source: OECD calculations based on the *Gallup World Poll* (n.d.[4]) (database), https://www.gallup.com/178667/gallup-world-poll-work.aspx.

StatLink https://stat.link/jfvbwp

These gains in institutional trust are likely to be temporary and by early 2021 they showed signs of wearing off. In New Zealand, where the initial impacts of the pandemic have been limited by rapid shutdowns and strict border controls, trust in various public institutions was slightly higher in June 2020 compared to 2018 but, except for parliament and the health system, returned to baseline levels by September and remained there until March 2021 (Figure 10.7).[10] In Finland, trust in various institutions (the government, parliament, civil service and political parties) in April 2021 was lower than in May 2020, despite a temporary rebound in January 2021, which might be attributed partially to the relatively good handling of the second wave of the pandemic (OECD, 2021[22]). Overall in Europe, trust in the government, the police and the media started to edge down slowly between April-May 2020 and January-February 2021, while across the OECD there are signs that people were more critically evaluating their leaders in the first months of vaccine rollout (Figure 10.8, Figure 10.9).[11] According to the Edelman Trust Barometer survey covering 14 OECD members, trust in government in January 2021 was still higher than a year prior (before COVID-19 hit) in all countries except Japan and Korea, but had started to fall compared to May 2020 (Edelman, 2021[29]).[12] If the "rally round the flag" effect wears off, and the traditional drivers of institutional trust such as job and financial security regain importance, then limiting the impact of phasing out government support programmes is likely to play an important role in institutional trust in the future (see Chapter 1).[13]

Figure 10.7. In New Zealand, mid-2020 gains in people's trust in institution were mostly short-lived

Average trust ratings in New Zealand on a 0 (lowest possible trust) to 10 (highest possible trust) scale

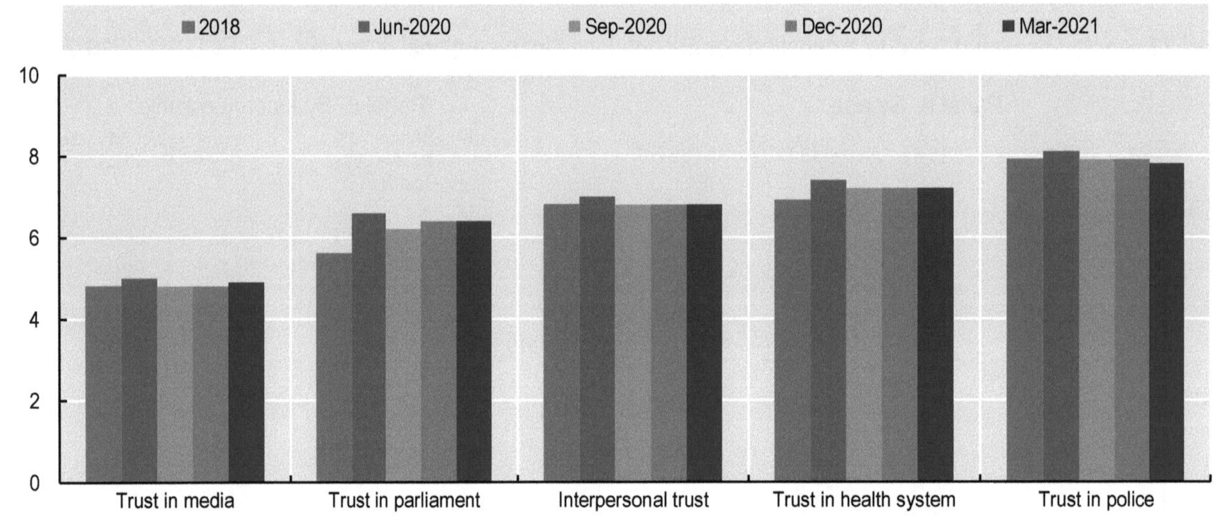

Note: Refer to Box 4.1 for methodological details about the Household Labour Force Survey (HLFS) supplement. Some caution needs to be exercised when comparing 2020 data from the supplement with estimates produced from the 2018 General Social Survey, as differences in collection method, sampled population, reporting periods, and restrictions on face-to-face interviewing, among other things, may all impact comparability.

Source: StatsNZ (2021[30]), *Wellbeing statistics: A year in review (June 2020 to March 2021 quarter)*, https://www.stats.govt.nz/reports/wellbeing-statistics-a-year-in-review-june-2020-to-march-2021-quarter#worse.

StatLink https://stat.link/ra9ox1

Figure 10.8. A year after the COVID-19 outbreak, trust in institutions is showing signs of decline in Europe

Trust in institutions on a scale from 1 (do not trust at all) to 10 (trust completely), OECD 22, 2016, Apr-May 2020, Jun-Jul 2020, Feb-Mar 2021

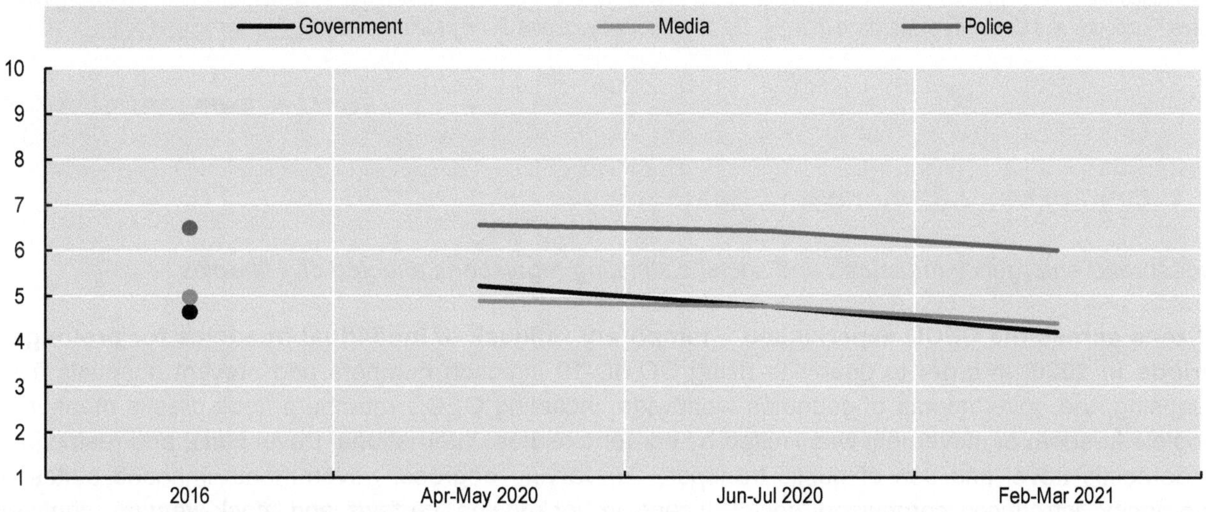

Note: The OECD average includes Austria, Belgium, the Czech Republic, Denmark, Estonia, France, Finland, Germany, Greece, Hungary, Ireland, Italy, Lithuania, Latvia, Luxembourg, the Netherlands, Poland, Portugal, Slovenia, the Slovak Republic, Spain and Sweden. Refer to Box 2.1 for methodological details on the Living, working and COVID-19 e-survey. The 2020-2021 and 2016 data, from the Eurofound Living, working and Covid-19 e-survey and the European Quality of Life Survey are not directly comparable due to different sampling designs.

Source: Eurofound (2018[31]), *European Quality of Life Survey 2016*, https://www.eurofound.europa.eu/publications/report/2017/fourth-european-quality-of-life-survey-overview-report; and Eurofound (n.d.[32]), *Living, working and COVID-19 e-survey* (database), http://eurofound.link/covid19data.

StatLink https://stat.link/q5jut7

Figure 10.9. Government health officials enjoy higher trust than friends and family members when it comes to recommendations on vaccines, but trust in politicians declined in early 2021

Share of people reporting being more likely to get vaccinations if recommended by family and friends, government health officials or politicians, OECD 25, 27 Dec 2020 - 30 Apr 2021

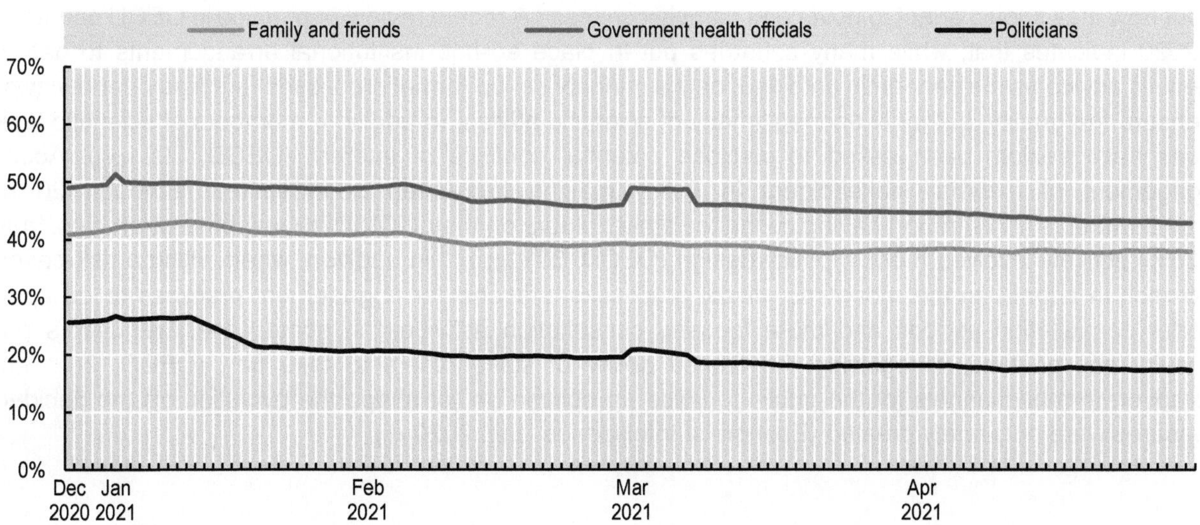

Note: The COVID-19 World Symptoms Survey is a partnership between Facebook and academic institutions. A sample of Facebook users in 115 countries is invited on a daily basis (over half a million responses are collected daily) to report on topics including COVID-19 symptoms, social distancing behaviour, vaccine acceptance, mental health issues and financial constraints. Aggregate statistics here are weighted by Facebook to reduce non-response and coverage bias. Observations with less than 500 responses per day have been dropped. The OECD average includes Australia, Austria, Belgium, Canada, Chile, Colombia, Costa Rica, the Czech Republic, Denmark, Finland, France, Germany, Greece, Ireland, Italy, Japan, Mexico, the Netherlands, New Zealand, Poland, Portugal, the Slovak Republic, Switzerland, Sweden and the United Kingdom.
Source: Facebook and University of Maryland (n.d.[33]), *Covid-19 World Symptoms Survey* (database), https://covidmap.umd.edu/.

StatLink https://stat.link/35u4t6

10.4. Quality of institutions and democracy

Widespread emergency measures and social distancing regulations affected civil liberties…

Citizens across the OECD experienced a temporary rollback of individual freedoms for prolonged periods in 2020. In order to deal with rising COVID-19 infection numbers and prevent hospitals from collapsing, the governments of countries worldwide, including OECD members, took drastic measures: people's freedom of movement was limited by border closures, international travel bans, and restrictions on domestic travel and use of public transport. To varying degrees, governments imposed states of emergency; introduced compulsory social distancing, lockdowns, curfews and mask-wearing; confined people to their homes, except for limited activities; prevented public gatherings other than for small crowds; closed educational and cultural establishments; postponed elections; enacted surveillance on citizens' movements via mobile phone applications; and used the force of the law, including the military, for enforcement (IDEA, 2021[34]; ICNL, n.d.[35]; CIVICUS, 2021[36]; Carnegie Europe, 2020[37]; Open Government Partnership, n.d.[38]; OECD, 2020[39]). Consequently, 2020 scores for the "private civil liberties" component on the V-DEM Varieties of Democracy Project, an expert-based dataset trying to capture nations' state of democracy, fell by 80% across OECD countries year-on-year (V-Dem Institute, n.d.[40]).[14] Other expert-based measures such as the Economist Intelligence Unit Civil Liberties Index come to similar conclusions (Economist Intelligence Unit, 2020[41]).

…and the COVID-19 response has posed certain risks for government transparency

The speed and scale with which governments implemented their response to the unprecedented nature of COVID-19 have posed risks for transparency, openness and stakeholder consultation. At the outset of the pandemic, few OECD governments had structured capacity to gather scientific advice about how they should adapt to novel and complex crises.[15] A recent review of practice in OECD countries in 2020 indicates that, while many countries put in place ad-hoc institutional arrangements to gather scientific advice as the pandemic unfolded, only a minority set up formal processes (such as peer reviews) to ensure the quality, authority and legitimacy of scientific advice. In addition, members of scientific task forces have seldom been asked to disclose potential conflicts of interest (OECD, 2021[25]). Active engagement of external stakeholders in policy making has often been limited: although 20 of 26 governments (77%) report having consulted stakeholders on their COVID-19 response strategies, only 9 (35%) actively involved them in policy design (OECD, 2021[25]).[16] In addition, when taking a risk-based approach in prioritising the most time-critical processes, stakeholder engagement practices relied upon shorter consultation periods and more focused consultation activities; in some cases, regulators put consultations on hold, recognising the limited ability of stakeholders to take part (OECD, 2021[25]). Moreover, formal channels for the public to voice an opinion on (or shape the evolution of) the decided measures were only rarely created (Economist Intelligence Unit, 2020[41]).[17]

Governments also had to fast-track many new regulations and cut back on impact assessments and the usual system of checks and balances. Prior to the crisis, only around one-third of OECD countries had established some form of exception to the requirement to carry out regulatory impact assessments (RIAs) in emergency responses (OECD, 2018[42]). Various flexible approaches were therefore employed towards RIA during COVID-19. These ranged from exemptions (e.g. Australia, Belgium) to ensuring that policy documents at least discussed qualitative impacts (e.g. the United Kingdom).The usual procedures to scrutinise the quality of RIAs for emergency regulations were often not followed or were shortened, although some oversight bodies have required follow-up once evidence becomes available, and in many cases the use of temporary regulations and sunset clauses has offset the risks to democratic oversight (OECD, 2020[43]). In addition, while most parliaments adopted fast-track legislative acts initiated by the government or converted into law the decrees adopted in response to the pandemic, the executive branch played a more dominant role in most OECD countries – particularly in those where legislative oversight of government was already comparably low pre-COVID-19 (Griglio, 2020[44]; European Parliament Think Tank, 2020[45]; V-Dem Institute, n.d.[40]; World Justice Project, n.d.[46]). In some OECD countries, requests by citizens to access information were either delayed or the timeline for answering them was officially extended or suspended (e.g. in Canada, Colombia, France, Hungary, Italy, Mexico, Poland, Slovenia, Spain, the United Kingdom and the United States) (ICNL, n.d.[35]).[18]

Although restrictions might be necessary in light of the extraordinary public health threat that citizens faced, democratic engagement and oversight should be quickly restored to avoid long-term damage to both policy quality and trust in institutions. Recent OECD research pointed to the risk of "mission creep", i.e. once new powers are introduced they are difficult to reverse, even when a crisis has passed (OECD, 2020[39]; OECD, 2020[47]). The importance of procedural utility (i.e. the importance of *how* outcomes are achieved, beyond the outcomes themselves) for trust in institutions and life satisfaction is well established (Benz, Frey and Stutzer, 2002[48]), pointing to the importance of quickly restoring good government practices in the aftermath of the crisis. Already prior to COVID-19, in 2018, only 35% of people in 22 European OECD countries reported feeling confident participating in politics, and 40% of people in 26 European OECD countries believed the political system in their countries allowed people like them to have a say in what the government does (OECD, 2021[25]). In addition, in line with institutional trust, citizens' satisfaction with democracy rose in the initial months of the pandemic but peaked by early 2021: for example, in Germany, the mean score for satisfaction with democracy on a 0-10 scale was 6.2 in January-February 2021 – considerably higher than the 2016 level of 5.8, but below the April-June heights of 6.5 (SOEP-CoV, n.d.[49]). Similar patterns are emerging for other European countries (Eurofound, n.d.[32]). The OECD has identified three areas as crucial for boosting trust and transparency, and for safeguarding democracy: tackling misinformation; ensuring that public decision-making and services are more transparent, fair and representative of the diverse nature of societies; and strengthening foresight and governance mechanisms, including data-sharing across agencies, to be more prepared for future crises (OECD, 2021[25]).

10.5. Gender parity and diversity in politics

Gender parity in politics slowly progressed in 2020, but remains far from parity, including in COVID-19 task forces

Progress towards gender parity and diversity in politics continued in 2020, although most countries remain far from equality. The share of women in politics is an important indicator of the inclusiveness of decision-making, and of gender equality more generally (Beaman et al., 2012[50]; OECD, 2020[51]). The share of female members of parliament increased in 10 out of 14 legislative elections that took place between January 2020 and June 2021 (Figure 10.10). In Ireland, women gained six additional seats in the indirectly elected Seanad Éireann (upper chamber), bringing the average to 40%, 10 percentage points higher than the share since 2011. However, compared to 2016, the share of women in the Dáil Éireann (lower chamber) remained stable at 22.5%, despite a record number of female candidates (IPU, 2021[52]). The United States experienced historically high levels of women's representation in Congress (26.9% combined for both chambers), and elected its first female and Black vice president, as well as the first person in this position of South Asian descent. After the October 2020 elections, New Zealand now has the most diverse government in the world, with almost half of MPs being women, 11% identifying as LGBTQ+, and both Māori and people with Pacific Island heritage represented at a slightly higher rate than in the general population. In addition, for the first time both major party candidates for prime minister were women (CNN, 2020[53]). Nevertheless, in only four of the legislative bodies that were re-elected in 2020 (the New Zealand Parliament, the Netherland's House of Representatives and the French and Irish upper houses) the share of women exceeded one-third, while the share of women in parliament declined in the Czech Republic and in the 2021 Israeli elections. On average across OECD countries, 31.6% of the seats in the lower/single houses of their parliaments were held by women in 2021, compared to 26% almost a decade ago (OECD, 2021[25]).[19]

Figure 10.10. The share of women in parliament increased in 10 out of 14 legislative elections that took place in 2020 and mid-2021

Share of women in national parliament in OECD countries with 2020 or 2021 elections

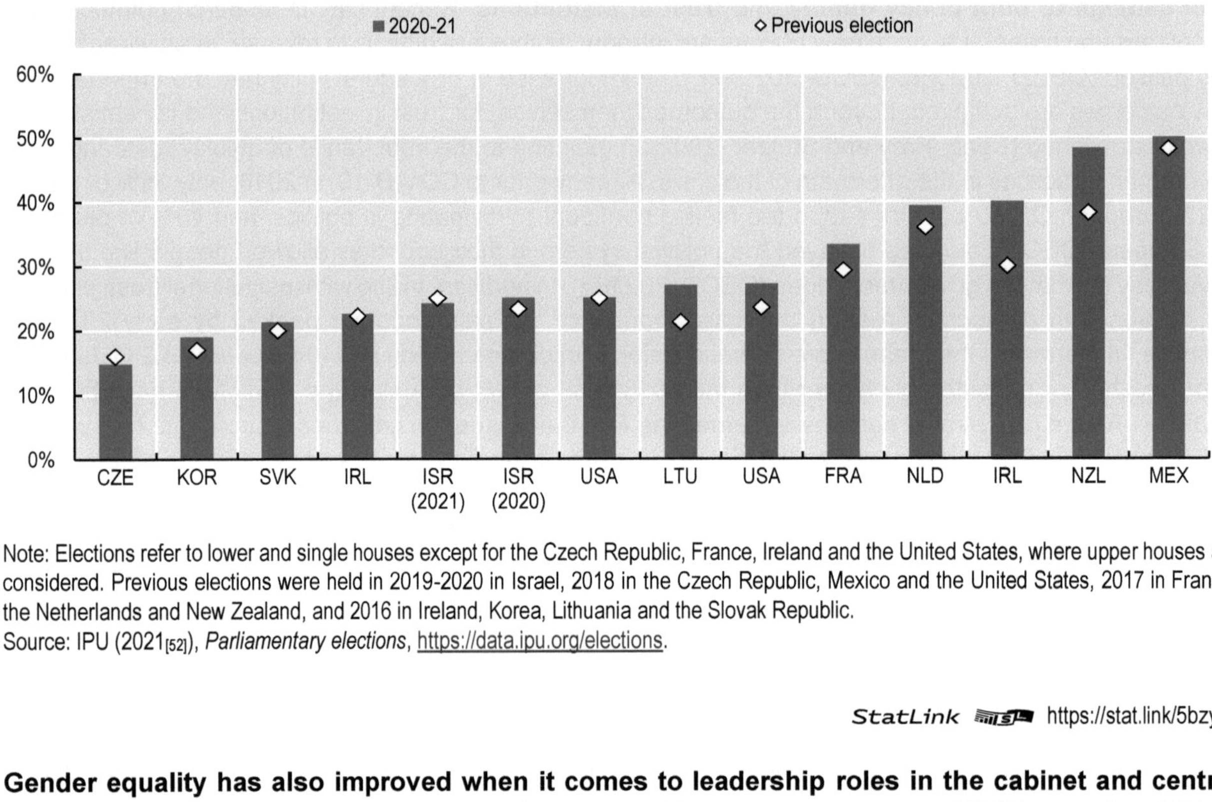

Note: Elections refer to lower and single houses except for the Czech Republic, France, Ireland and the United States, where upper houses are considered. Previous elections were held in 2019-2020 in Israel, 2018 in the Czech Republic, Mexico and the United States, 2017 in France, the Netherlands and New Zealand, and 2016 in Ireland, Korea, Lithuania and the Slovak Republic.
Source: IPU (2021[52]), *Parliamentary elections*, https://data.ipu.org/elections.

StatLink https://stat.link/5bzyc9

Gender equality has also improved when it comes to leadership roles in the cabinet and central government as well as in COVID-19 task forces. In 2021, on average across OECD countries, 34% of federal/central government ministerial positions were held by women, an increase of 6 percentage points since 2017 (OECD, 2021[25]). But, while the share of women in senior positions in central government increased in most OECD countries since 2015, on average, only 37% of senior roles in central government were held by women in 2020 (OECD, 2021[25]). In almost all OECD countries, the share of women in middle and senior management is lower than for other central government positions, suggesting obstacles in climbing the leadership ladder (OECD, 2021[25]). Moreover, women represented only 35% of the members of COVID-19 task forces by March 2021 (Figure 10.11).

Figure 10.11. Women are under-represented in COVID-19 task forces in 22 out 27 OECD countries with available data

Share of women in COVID-19 task forces by Mar-2021

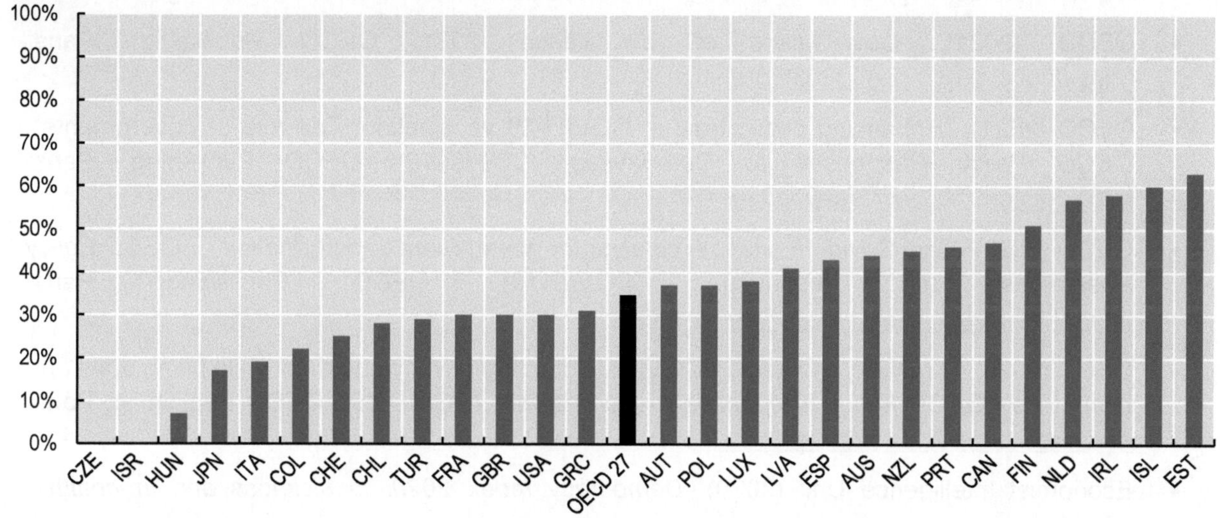

Note: The OECD average includes only those 27 countries shown. Only task forces with sex-disaggregated composition data are considered.
Source: UNDP, UN WOMEN and University of Pittsburgh (n.d.[54]), *COVID-19 Global Gender Response Tracker*, https://www.undp.org/content/dam/undp/library/km-qap/UNDP-UNWomen-UPitt-COVID19-Task-Force-Participation.pdf/.

StatLink https://stat.link/6cm3ro

The move towards remote and digital parliamentary practices has both positive and negative implications for female participation in politics

The pandemic changed the way parliaments operated in 2020, with some of these changes being beneficial for women and others introducing new obstacles to female representation. The shift to remote, technology-based parliamentary practices might have a positive long-term impact for women: the use of new technology for debates resulted in new forms of personal interaction, breaking up "old boy" practices that had previously excluded the full participation of women (IPU, 2021[52]; IPU, 2020[55]). Virtual voting and sittings helped participation by members for whom travel is more difficult, including those with disabilities or with young children. Going forward, if legislatures retain these flexible workplace practices, more women might be able to combine caregiving with political careers. However, the pandemic-related disruption of formal political processes towards ad-hoc, informal practices might have also favoured dominant (male) groups. In addition, the increased digital nature of policy making might have increased the exposure of women in politics to online harassment, which is on the rise worldwide (IPU, 2021[52]; Carnegie Endowment for International Peace, 2020[56]). Lastly, as omen across OECD countries were more likely than men to drop out of the labour force during the pandemic, often to return to traditional roles as primary caregivers, it remains to be seen whether the future supply of female candidacies for political office will be interrupted.

Youth remain under-represented in politics

While democracy does not necessarily require institutions to mirror demographics, youth's under-representation in parliament indicates the existence of norms, rules and regulations that hamper their participation to democratic processes. In 2020, on average across OECD countries, 22% of members of parliaments were under 40, ranging from 36% in Norway to 8% in France. In comparison, 20-39 year-olds represent 34% of the voting-age population across OECD countries, a gap in representation exceeding 12 percentage points (OECD, 2021[25]).[20]

Box 10.1. Further reading

- OECD, (forthcoming), *Building a new Paradigm for Public Trust*, OECD Publishing, Paris
- OECD (2021), *Government at a Glance 2021*, OECD Publishing, Paris, https://doi.org/10.1787/1c258f55-en
- OECD (2021), "Enhancing public trust in COVID-19 vaccination: The role of governments", *OECD Policy Responses to Coronavirus (COVID-19)*, OECD Publishing, Paris, https://doi.org/10.1787/eae0ec5a-en
- OECD (2020), "The Covid-19 crisis: A catalyst for government transformation?", *OECD Policy Responses to Coronavirus (COVID-19)*, OECD Publishing, Paris, https://doi.org/10.1787/1d0c0788-en
- OECD (2020), "Tracking and tracing COVID: Protecting privacy and data while using apps and biometrics", *OECD Policy Responses to Coronavirus (COVID-19),* OECD Publishing, Paris, https://doi.org/10.1787/8f394636-en
- Economist Intelligence Unit (2020), *Democracy Index 2020: In sickness and in health?,* https://www.eiu.com/n/campaigns/democracy-index-2020
- Inter-Parliamentary Union (2021), *Women in Parliament in 2020,* https://www.ipu.org/women-in-parliament-2020

References

Aassve, A. et al. (2020), *Pandemics and social capital: From the Spanish flu of 1918-19 to COVID-19*, VOX Cepr Policy Journal, https://voxeu.org/article/pandemics-and-social-capital. [8]

ABS (2021), *Household Impacts of COVID-19 Survey*, https://www.abs.gov.au/statistics/people/people-and-communities/household-impacts-covid-19-survey/latest-release#voluntary-work-and-unpaid-help. [1]

Aldrich, A. and N. Lotito (2020), "Pandemic Performance: Women Leaders in the COVID-19 Crisis", *Politics & Gender*, Vol. 16/4, http://dx.doi.org/10.1017/S1743923X20000549. [58]

Amat, F. et al. (2020), "Pandemics meet democracy. Experimental evidence from the COVID-19 crisis in Spain", https://osf.io/preprints/socarxiv/dkusw/. [27]

Ananyev, M. and S. Guriev (2019), "Effect of Income on Trust: Evidence from the 2009 Economic Crisis in Russia", *The Economic Journal*, Vol. 129/619, http://dx.doi.org/10.1111/ecoj.12612. [9]

Bargain, O. and U. Aminjonov (2020), "Trust and Compliance to Public Health Policies in Times of COVID-19", http://bordeauxeconomicswp.u-bordeaux.fr/2020/2020-06.pdf. [20]

Bartscher, A. et al. (2020), "Social Capital and the Spread of COVID-19: Insights from European Countries", *IZA DP*, No. 13310, https://www.iza.org/publications/dp/13310/social-capital-and-the-spread-of-covid-19-insights-from-european-countries. [15]

Beaman, L. et al. (2012), "Female Leadership Raises Aspirations and Educational Attainment for Girls: A Policy Experiment in India", *Science*, Vol. 335/6068, pp. 582-586, https://dx.doi.org/10.1126%2Fscience.1212382. [50]

Benz, M., B. Frey and A. Stutzer (2002), "Introducing Procedural Utility: Not Only What, But Also How Matters", *SSRN Electronic Journal*, http://dx.doi.org/10.2139/ssrn.338568. [48]

Biddle, N. and M. Gray (2020), "The experience of volunteers during the early stages of the COVID-19 pandemic", https://csrm.cass.anu.edu.au/sites/default/files/docs/2020/6/The_experience_of_volunteers_during_the_early_stages_of_the_COVID-19_pandemic_0.pdf. [3]

Blair, R., B. Morse and L. Tsai (2017), "Public health and public trust: Survey evidence from the Ebola Virus Disease epidemic in Liberia", *Social Science & Medicine*, Vol. 172, http://dx.doi.org/10.1016/j.socscimed.2016.11.016. [19]

Bol, D. et al. (2021), "The effect of COVID-19 lockdowns on political support: Some good news for democracy?", *European Journal of Political Research*, Vol. 60/2, http://dx.doi.org/10.1111/1475-6765.12401. [26]

Carnegie Endowment for International Peace (2020), *Tackling Online Abuse and Disinformation Targeting Women in Politics*, https://carnegieendowment.org/2020/11/30/tackling-online-abuse-and-disinformation-targeting-women-in-politics-pub-83331. [56]

Carnegie Europe (2020), *Does the Coronavirus Endanger Democracy in Europe?*, https://carnegieeurope.eu/2020/06/23/does-coronavirus-endanger-democracy-in-europe-pub-82110. [37]

Chatagnier, J. (2012), "The effect of trust in government on rallies 'round the flag", *Journal of Peace Research*, Vol. 49/5, http://dx.doi.org/10.1177/0022343312440808. [24]

CIVICUS (2021), *Civic Freedoms and the COVID19 Pandemic: A snapshot of restrictions*, https://www.civicus.org/index.php/media-resources/reports-publications/4396-civic-freedoms-and-the-covid19-pandemic-a-snapshot-of-restrictions (accessed on 21 June 2021). [36]

CNN (2020), *New Zealand has just elected one of the most diverse parliaments in the world. Here's how it stacks up*, https://edition.cnn.com/2020/11/16/asia/new-zealand-parliament-diverse-intl-hnk-dst/index.html. [53]

Deopa, N. and P. Forunato (2020), "Coronagraben. Culture and Social Distancing in Times of COVID-19", *SSRN Electronic Journal*, http://dx.doi.org/10.2139/ssrn.3635287. [17]

DIE ZEIT (2020), "Deutsche haben in der Krise mehr Vertrauen in Politik und Zusammenhalt", https://www.zeit.de/gesellschaft/zeitgeschehen/2020-07/coronavirus-deutschland-vertrauen-demokratie-zusammenhalt-soep-nrw/seite-2. [6]

Dietz, N. and R. Grimm (2019), "A Less Charitable Nation: The Decline of Volunteering and Giving in the United States", *Explaining Declines in Volunteering and Giving*, https://cppp.usc.edu/wp-content/uploads/2019/03/Grimm-Robert-Dietz-and-Grimm_A-Less-Charitable-Nation_March-2019-USC-Conference-Paper.pdf. [62]

DIW (2021), *Corona-Pandemie: Vertrauensvolle Menschen sind eher zur Impfung bereit und halten sich eher an AHA-Regeln*, https://www.diw.de/de/diw_01.c.820366.de/publikationen/diw_aktuell/2021_0066/corona-pandemie__vertrauensvolle_menschen_sind_eher_zur_impfung_bereit_und_halten_sich_eher_an_aha-regeln.html. [12]

Economist Intelligence Unit (2020), *Democracy Index 2020: In sickness and in health?*, https://www.eiu.com/n/campaigns/democracy-index-2020/. [41]

Edelman (2021), *Edelman Trust Barometer*, https://www.edelman.com/sites/g/files/aatuss191/files/2021-03/2021%20Edelman%20Trust%20Barometer.pdf. [29]

Eurofound (2018), *European Quality of Life Survey 2016*, Publications Office of the European Union, Luxembourg, https://www.eurofound.europa.eu/publications/report/2017/fourth-european-quality-of-life-survey-overview-report. [31]

Eurofound (n.d.), *Living, working and COVID-19 dataset*, https://www.eurofound.europa.eu/data/covid-19 (accessed on 21 August 2021). [32]

European Parliament Think Tank (2020), "States of emergency in response to the coronavirus crisis: Normative response and parliamentary oversight in EU Member States during the first wave of the pandemic", https://www.europarl.europa.eu/thinktank/en/document.html?reference=EPRS_STU(2020)659385. [45]

Facebook and University of Maryland (n.d.), *COVID-19 World Symptoms Survey*, https://covidmap.umd.edu/ (accessed on 21 June 2021). [33]

Gallup (n.d.), *Gallup World Poll (database)*, https://www.gallup.com/178667/gallup-world-poll-work.aspx (accessed on 18 June 2021). [4]

Gelfand, M. et al. (2021), "The relationship between cultural tightness–looseness and COVID-19 cases and deaths: a global analysis", *The Lancet Planetary Health*, Vol. 5/3, http://dx.doi.org/10.1016/S2542-5196(20)30301-6. [18]

Goldstein, D. and J. Wiedemann (2020), "Who Do You Trust? The Consequences of Partisanship and Trust in Government for Public Responsiveness to COVID-19", *SSRN Electronic Journal*, http://dx.doi.org/10.2139/ssrn.3580547. [16]

Griglio, E. (2020), "Parliamentary oversight under the Covid-19 emergency: striving against executive dominance", *The Theory and Practice of Legislation*, Vol. 8/1-2, http://dx.doi.org/10.1080/20508840.2020.1789935. [44]

Helliwell, J. et al. (2020), "Happiness, trust, and deaths under COVID-19", in *World Happiness Report*, https://worldhappiness.report/ed/2021/happiness-trust-and-deaths-under-covid-19/#fn13. [13]

ICNL (n.d.), *COVID-19 Civic Freedom Tracker*, https://www.icnl.org/covid19tracker/?location=6,7,11,17,23,25,26,27,31,34,38,41,42,46,48,54,55,59,60,61,63,71,75,203,80,217,89,93,100,147,105,112,113,115,116,144,121,246,128,133,134&issue=&date=&type= (accessed on 21 June 2021). [35]

IDEA (2021), *Global overview of COVID-19: Impact on elections*, https://www.idea.int/news-media/multimedia-reports/global-overview-covid-19-impact-elections. [34]

Imperial College London YouGov (2020), *Covid 19 Behaviour Tracker Data Hub*, https://github.com/YouGov-Data/covid-19-tracker. [5]

IPU (2021), *Women in Parliament in 2020*, https://www.ipu.org/women-in-parliament-2020. [52]

IPU (2020), *Country compilation of parliamentary responses to the pandemic*, https://www.ipu.org/country-compilation-parliamentary-responses-pandemic. [55]

Kühne, S. et al. (2020), "The need for household panel surveys in times of crisis: The case of SOEP-CoV", *Survey Research Methods*, Vol. 14/2, pp. 195-203, https://doi.org/10.18148/srm/2020.v14i2.7748. [7]

Makridis, C. and C. Wu (2021), "How social capital helps communities weather the COVID-19 pandemic", *PLOS ONE*, Vol. 16/1, http://dx.doi.org/10.1371/journal.pone.0245135. [14]

Mueller, J. (1970), "Presidential Popularity from Truman to Johnson", *American Political Science Review*, Vol. 64/1, http://dx.doi.org/10.2307/1955610. [23]

Murtin, F. et al. (2018), "Trust and its determinants: Evidence from the Trustlab experiment", *OECD Statistics Working Papers*, No. 2018/2, OECD Publishing, Paris, https://dx.doi.org/10.1787/869ef2ec-en. [64]

OECD (2021), *Drivers of Trust in Public Institutions in Finland*, OECD Publishing, Paris, https://dx.doi.org/10.1787/52600c9e-en. [22]

OECD (2021), *Government at a Glance 2021*, OECD Publishing, Paris, https://doi.org/10.1787/1c258f55-en. [25]

OECD (2020), *How's Life? 2020 - Measuring Well-being*, OECD Publishing, Paris, https://doi.org/10.1787/9870c393-en. [51]

OECD (2020), "Regulatory quality and COVID-19: Managing the risks and supporting the recovery", *OECD Policy Responses to Coronavirus (COVID-19)*, OECD Publishing, Paris, https://dx.doi.org/10.1787/3f752e60-en. [43]

OECD (2020), "The Covid-19 crisis: A catalyst for government transformation?", *OECD Policy Responses to Coronavirus (COVID-19)*, OECD Publishing, Paris, https://dx.doi.org/10.1787/1d0c0788-en. [39]

OECD (2020), "Tracking and tracing COVID: Protecting privacy and data while using apps and biometrics", *OECD Policy Responses to Coronavirus (COVID-19)*, OECD Publishing, Paris, https://dx.doi.org/10.1787/8f394636-en. [47]

OECD (2020), "Youth and COVID-19: Response, recovery and resilience", *OECD Policy Responses to Coronavirus (COVID-19)*, OECD Publishing, Paris, https://dx.doi.org/10.1787/c40e61c6-en. [65]

OECD (2018), *OECD Regulatory Policy Outlook 2018*, OECD Publishing, Paris, https://dx.doi.org/10.1787/9789264303072-en. [42]

OECD (2018), *Scientific Advice During Crises: Facilitating Transnational Co-operation and Exchange of Information*, OECD Publishing, Paris, https://dx.doi.org/10.1787/9789264304413-en. [60]

OECD (2017), *Trust and Public Policy: How Better Governance Can Help Rebuild Public Trust*, OECD Public Governance Reviews, OECD Publishing, Paris, https://dx.doi.org/10.1787/9789264268920-en. [61]

OECD (2016), *Trends in Risk Communication Policies and Practices*, OECD Reviews of Risk Management Policies, OECD Publishing, Paris, https://dx.doi.org/10.1787/9789264260467-en. [59]

Olsen, A. and F. Hjorth (2020), "Willingness to Distance in the COVID-19 Pandemic", https://osf.io/xpwg2/. [21]

Open Government Partnership (n.d.), *State of Open Government During COVID-19*, https://www.opengovpartnership.org/state-of-open-government-during-covid-19/ (accessed on 21 June 2021). [38]

Pew Research Center (2020), *Most Approve of National Response to COVID-19 in 14 Advanced Economies*, https://www.pewresearch.org/global/2020/08/27/most-approve-of-national-response-to-covid-19-in-14-advanced-economies/. [10]

Pew Research Centre (2021), *People in Advanced Economies Say Their Society Is More Divided Than Before Pandemic*, https://www.pewresearch.org/global/2021/06/23/people-in-advanced-economies-say-their-society-is-more-divided-than-before-pandemic/?utm_source=Pew+Research+Center&utm_campaign=eb70cab40f-Weekly_2021_06_26&utm_medium=email&utm_term=0_3e953b9b70-eb70cab40f-401039990. [11]

Piscopo, J. (2020), "Women Leaders and Pandemic Performance: A Spurious Correlation", *Politics & Gender*, Vol. 16/4, http://dx.doi.org/10.1017/S1743923X20000525. [57]

Schraff, D. (2020), "Political trust during the Covid-19 pandemic: Rally around the flag or lockdown effects?", *European Journal of Political Research*, http://dx.doi.org/10.1111/1475-6765.12425. [28]

SOEP-CoV (n.d.), *SOEP-CoV The Spread of the Coronavirus in Germany: Socio-Economic Factors and Consequences*, https://www.soep-cov.de/Startseite/ (accessed on 21 May 2021). [49]

StatsNZ (2021), *Wellbeing statistics: A year in review (June 2020 to March 2021 quarter)*, https://www.stats.govt.nz/reports/wellbeing-statistics-a-year-in-review-june-2020-to-march-2021-quarter#worse. [30]

Toshkov, D., K. Yesilkagit and B. Carroll (2020), "Government Capacity, Societal Trust or Party Preferences? What Accounts for the Variety of National Policy Responses to the COVID-19 Pandemic in Europe?", https://osf.io/7chpu/. [63]

UNDP, UN WOMEN and University of Pittsburgh (n.d.), *Covid-19 Global Gender Response Tracker*, https://www.undp.org/content/dam/undp/library/km-qap/UNDP-UNWomen-UPitt-COVID19-Task-Force-Participation.pdf (accessed on 26 July 2021). [54]

V-Dem Institute (n.d.), *Varieties of Democracy*, https://www.v-dem.net/en/ (accessed on 21 June 2021). [40]

What Works Wellbeing (2020), *Volunteering in the time of COVID-19 – five things the evidence shows us*, https://whatworkswellbeing.org/blog/volunteering-covid-evidence/. [2]

World Justice Project (n.d.), *World Justice Project Rule of Law Index*, https://worldjusticeproject.org/rule-of-law-index/ (accessed on 23 July 2021). [46]

Notes

1 Reasons for the decline in volunteering via established organisations are complex, but include consolidations of churches and schools especially in rural areas and declining rates of home ownership (which are likely to make a person more interested in giving back to a specific community) (Dietz and Grimm, 2019[62]).

2 The most common reasons for people not volunteering for an organisation or group in the last four weeks were that they could not fit volunteering in around paid work (31%) and they could not fit it around family or caring commitments (22%).

3 Evidence from a Citizens' Pulse Survey carried out in co-operation with the OECD in Finland between May and November 2020 indicates that while respondents initially considered others to be complying with COVID-19-related restrictions, this share progressively fell starting in June (OECD, 2021[22]).

4 Some caution needs to be exercised when comparing 2020 data from the Household Labour Force Survey (HLFS) supplement (see Box 4.1) with estimates produced from the General Social Survey, as

differences in collection method, sampled population, reporting periods, and restrictions on face-to-face interviewing, among other things, may all impact on comparability.

5 There is some evidence that in the early stages of the pandemic, before April 2020, European countries with higher levels of interpersonal trust, government effectiveness, and freedom were generally slower in implementing containment measures such as school closures, national lockdowns and states of emergency. Factors associated with a faster initial response include decentralisation, separate ministries of health and health ministers with a medical background (Toshkov, Yesilkagit and Carroll, 2020[63]).

6 This study included 142 countries worldwide, including all OECD members.

7 The authors repeat their analysis with different measures of social capital that are all related to interpersonal trust: voter turnout in the 2019 European elections, blood donations and historical literacy rates.

8 To assess cultural tightness–looseness, the level of agreement with a battery of survey items is used, including items such as, "There are many social norms that people are supposed to abide by in this country", "There are very clear expectations for how people should act in most situations", "In this country, if someone acts in an inappropriate way, others will strongly disapprove", and, "People in this country almost always comply with social norms".

9 Snapshot data from an OECD survey of youth organisations in April 2020 also shows that, on aggregate, trust in government had increased for 43% of the youth organisations surveyed across 48 countries since the outbreak of COVID-19 (OECD, 2020[65]).

10 Over the four quarters, Māori consistently gave lower mean ratings for trust in the health system than people with European, Pacific peoples or Asian ethnicity, and the national average. The mean ratings given by Māori were 7.1 in the June 2020 quarter (national average:7.4), 6.8 in the September 2020 quarter (national average: 7.2), 6.7 in the December 2020 quarter (national average: 7.2) and 6.8 in the March 2021 quarter (national average: 7.2) (StatsNZ, 2021[30]).

11 Recent OECD work has addressed the role of governments in promoting confidence in the effectiveness and safety of vaccines through effective communication, as well as trust in their ability to procure and distribute the vaccines efficiently and equitably (OECD, 2021[25]).

12 OECD members covered by the Edelman Trust Barometer are Australia, Canada, Colombia, France, Italy, Ireland, Japan, Germany, Mexico, the Netherlands, Spain, South Korea, the United Kingdom and the United States.

13 In addition, government competencies and values have been identified as important drivers of trust pre-COVID (Murtin et al., 2018[64]; OECD, 2017[61]; OECD, 2021[22]).

14 This measure takes into account whether citizens enjoy freedom of foreign and domestic movement, freedom of religion and organisation, property rights as well as freedom from forced labour, with the freedom of movement components constituting about one-fourth of the overall score.

15 In 2018, only half of OECD countries had a specific government department or institution whose purpose was to identify novel, unforeseen or complex crises (OECD, 2018[60]).

16 Although 73% of centres of government increased the number of stakeholders joining co-ordination meetings, there are no data on the extent to which groups other than scientific experts were involved (OECD, 2021[25]).

[17] Traditional crisis communication has often been implemented in a top-down manner, with messages delivered from governments to citizens (OECD, 2016[59]). During COVID-19, some countries have innovated by developing two-way crisis communication to foster dialogue and help governments understand citizens' questions and concerns. For example, Slovenia established a call centre for citizens to engage with public health professionals. This allowed citizens to receive immediate responses to health and safety issues and gave government a more thorough and immediate knowledge of citizens' concerns (OECD, 2021[25]).

[18] There were also practical reasons that limited the governments' ability to respond to requests for access to information, with public officials working from home and difficulties to access government records, and some countries introduced legal changes for filing requests to allow electronic means and prioritised requests relating to the pandemic.

[19] While media attention in 2020 focused on the claim that women were more effective political leaders throughout the pandemic, this is a spurious correlation: both female and male leaders were better able to respond to the pandemic in wealthy, liberal democracies with high state capacity and good governance (Piscopo, 2020[57]). In addition, data from 132 countries up until mid-June 2020 shows that the gender of executive leaders and legislators was not a factor in determining the timing of adapting information campaigns and containment policies such as stay-at home orders and school closures, nor their duration. However, the likelihood of school closures being *delayed* increased with the share of women in legislatures (Aldrich and Lotito, 2020[58]).

[20] Representation gaps are even more pronounced within countries' political leadership. In 2018, the average age of cabinet members ranged from 45 years in Iceland to 62 years in Japan, with an OECD average of 53 years. The five youngest cabinets across OECD countries were in Iceland (45 years), Norway (46.2), Estonia (47.1), Denmark (47.4) and Finland (47.4). In 2018, across the OECD, only 51 of the then-incumbent cabinet members were under 40 (8%) and only 20 were aged 35 or below (3%) (OECD, 2021[25]).

11 Natural capital and COVID-19

Natural capital underpins human health and well-being, both directly and by supporting economic activity. Few data currently exist to assess the impacts of COVID-19 on natural capital, and this chapter therefore covers only selected aspects of biodiversity and climate. The suspension of economic and social activity during the pandemic has done little to ease the overall pressures on natural systems, which have been mounting over many decades. Biodiversity loss creates a wide variety of risks for well-being, including contributing to climate change and increasing the risk of disease transmission between humans and animals. A brief reprieve in energy-related CO_2 emissions (-5.8%, globally) will have little bearing on atmospheric concentrations of greenhouse gases without concerted policy action to accelerate emissions reductions. Analysis of COVID-19 stimulus measures across OECD and partner countries indicates that the volume of environmentally negative or mixed spending will at least match that spent on environmentally positive measures.

The essential link between natural resources and human health and well-being has been reinforced by the pandemic. For example, land-use change and wildlife exploitation are known to influence the emergence, incidence and distribution of infectious diseases (IPBES, 2020[1]; OECD, 2020[2]). At the same time, some studies indicate that air pollution may contribute to more severe COVID-19 outcomes, while access to green space has been a valuable resource during lockdowns (as discussed in Chapters 3 and 6). Better management of natural capital[1] lies at the heart of multiple, interlinked crises that governments currently face: biodiversity loss, climate change, novel infectious diseases, and the fundamental threats these pose to both healthy economies and healthy lives (OECD, 2021[3]). Yet natural capital is often side-lined in economic decision-making and has faced chronic underinvestment. It has been estimated that between 1992 and 2014, produced capital per person doubled globally, human capital per person increased by about 13%, but the stock of natural capital per person declined by nearly 40% (Dasgupta, 2021[4]).

The focus of this report is on changes in well-being in the first 15 months of the pandemic, considering both current well-being outcomes and the resources (capitals) that will support them in the future. However, capturing the evolution of natural capital during this period is challenging and should be complemented with a longer-term perspective. 2020 data are lacking for the large majority of the natural capital indicators (covering stocks and flows, risks and resilience factors) typically included in the OECD's *How's Life?* and *Environment at a Glance* dashboards. While frequent monitoring is important (and abrupt changes can signal important shifts in the state of natural capital, particularly those related to human actions), long-run trends in natural capital are typically the main focus of policy analysis – as described in other OECD work (OECD, 2021[5]; OECD, 2020[6]). Alongside this, monitoring of policy responses such as the OECD Green Recovery Database (OECD, 2021[7]) and the International Programme for Action on Climate (IPAC) initiative (OECD, 2021[8]) provides timely feedback to policy makers. A key concern for the pandemic recovery is ensuring that major threats to future well-being, in the form of climate change and biodiversity loss in particular, remain at the top of the policy agenda, and that they are fully integrated in recovery packages (see also Chapter 1 of this report). The evidence that follows is therefore focused on these two areas, which represent only a subsection of the natural capital considerations addressed in the *How's Life?* report.[2]

11.1. Biodiversity

Biodiversity[3] and ecosystem services underpin human health and well-being via critical life support functions such as clean air provisioning. Biodiversity also underpins economic activity, both directly and indirectly (Dasgupta, 2021[4]). The goods and services provided by biodiversity range from raw materials, fuel and food to clean air and water, space for recreation, protection against erosion and flooding, and processes such as pollination, nutrient cycling and carbon sequestration (OECD, 2021[3]). Biodiversity loss also increases the risk of infectious diseases being transferred across wildlife, livestock and people (United Nations, 2020[9]; Gottdenker et al., 2014[10]). For example, wildlife exploitation and land-use change (such as agricultural expansion close to wilderness areas) can bring people and domestic animals into closer proximity to pathogen-carrying wildlife. Human activities can also disrupt the ecological processes and high levels of species diversity that help to regulate and contain disease transmission in natural areas (OECD, 2020[2]).

Pressure on biodiversity has been increasing globally due to land and sea-use change, pollution, natural resource over-exploitation, climate change and invasive alien species (IPBES, 2019[11]). Biodiversity is declining faster than at any time in human history (Dasgupta, 2021[4]). Twenty-five percent of the world's remaining species are now threatened with extinction, and populations of mammals, birds, reptiles, amphibians and fish have shrunk on average by 68% since 1970 (OECD, 2021[3]). Since 1992, 2.9% of natural or semi-natural vegetated land (i.e. tree-covered areas, grassland, wetland, shrubland and sparse vegetation) worldwide have been lost to other types of land cover. This represents an area four times the size of Spain, with OECD and G20 countries accounting for over half of this loss (OECD, 2021[5]). Urban areas have doubled in size since 1990 (OECD, 2021[3]). Biodiversity loss and climate change are intrinsically linked. On the one hand, land use change (such as deforestation) contributes to climate change; on the other hand, the changing climate is a significant, and growing, driver of biodiversity loss (OECD, 2021[3]).

Available evidence suggests that the pandemic has not slowed the pace of land use change in some of the most at-risk biodiverse regions. For example, pandemic restrictions have not stopped deforestation in Latin America (UNDP Latin America and the Caribbean, 2020[12]). External threats to these forests from mining, oil, agricultural and forestry companies, cattle ranchers, farmers, illegal groups and land speculators have increased markedly over the last decade (Walker et al., 2020[13]; Ellis et al., 2017[14]). With the arrival of the pandemic, governments had to limit their monitoring and enforcement efforts, for both health and budgetary reasons, thereby exacerbating the vulnerability of forests, water and other natural resources, including those in Indigenous territories (ECLAC, 2020[15]).

It will be some time before the full impact of COVID-19 on biodiversity is known. 2020 data are not yet available for most of the indicators currently used by the OECD to assess these aspects of natural capital (OECD, 2021[5]; OECD, 2020[6]), and even when data are available, long-term implications are difficult to determine. For the Red List Index of threatened species and the share of marine and terrestrial protected areas, there has been little or no change in the values reported between 2019 and 2021 for OECD countries. The main pattern of note for the Red List Index is the further worsening since 2000, particularly in those OECD countries already facing significant pressures on threatened species (Figure 11.1). Protected areas, which reflect policy efforts to conserve biodiversity, have increased nearly eight-fold since 2000 for marine areas across OECD countries on average, while terrestrial areas have increased by 6 percentage points (Figure 11.2). Nevertheless, progress has been weak since 2019, as several OECD countries approach or even exceed levels embodied in Aichi Biodiversity Target 11.[4] Many protected areas still lack effective management and, worldwide, their coverage is not yet representative of the diversity of ecosystems on the planet (OECD, 2021[3]).

Figure 11.1. Threats to species have increased since 2000, particularly in countries that already face significant biodiversity pressures

Red List Index of threatened species, from 1.0 = all species qualifying as "Least Concern" to 0 = all species having gone extinct

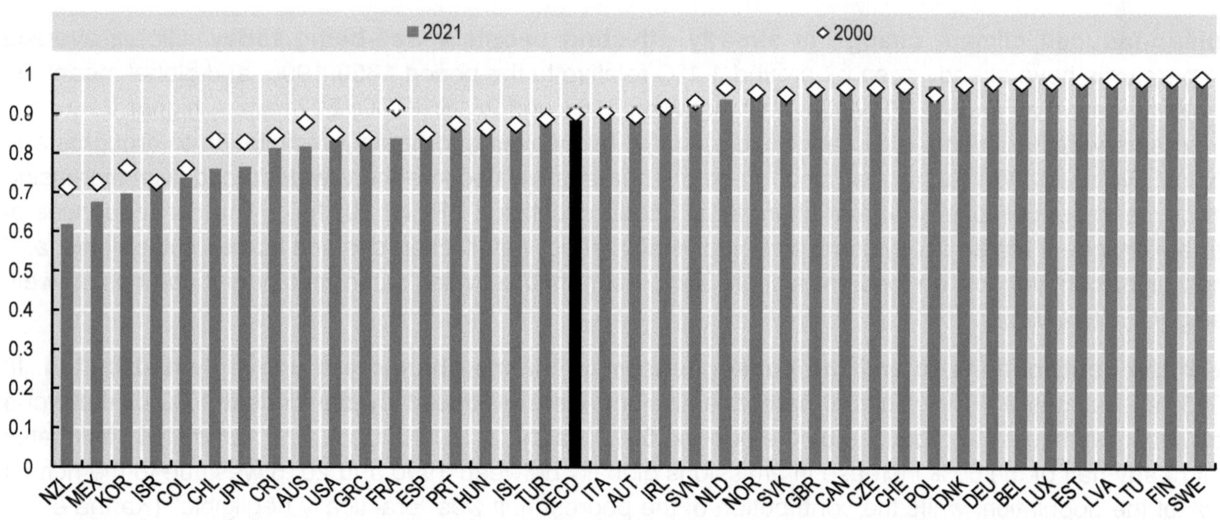

Note: The Red List Index is a combined indicator of extinction risk for birds, mammals, amphibians, cycads and corals.
Source: UN DESA (n.d.[16]), *Global SDG Indicator Database, indicator 15.5.1*, https://unstats.un.org/sdgs/indicators/database/.

StatLink https://stat.link/kgytfv

Figure 11.2. The share of territory designated as protected areas has increased substantially since 2000 in OECD countries on average, but there have been few changes in recent years

Marine protected areas, as a share of each country's exclusive economic zone, and terrestrial protected areas, as a share of total land area, OECD Total

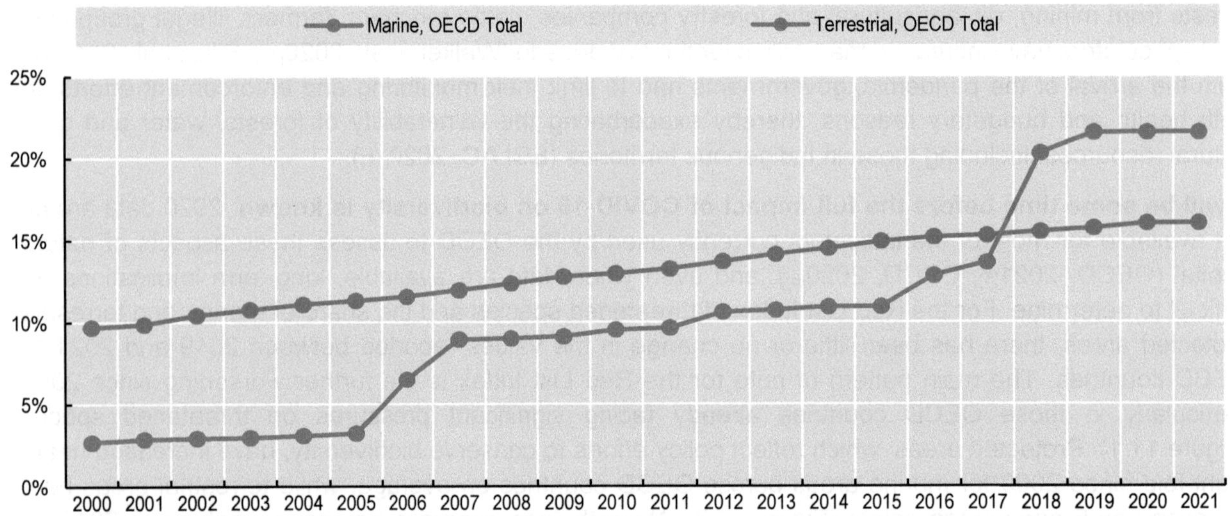

Note: The OECD Total for terrestrial areas excludes Turkey, as no data are available. The OECD Total for marine areas excludes Turkey, as no data are available, and Austria, the Czech Republic, Hungary, Luxembourg, the Slovak Republic and Switzerland due to a lack of marine areas.
Source: OECD (n.d.[17]), *Environment Statistics Database: Biodiversity*, https://stats.oecd.org/Index.aspx?DataSetCode=PROTECTED_AREAS.

StatLink https://stat.link/3m5lnr

11.2. Climate change

Human-induced climate change is already affecting people's well-being today. Global average temperatures have already risen by around 1.1°C relative to the period 1850-1900, and global mean sea levels increased by around 20 centimetres between 1901 and 2018 (IPCC, 2021[18]). A higher frequency of extreme weather events is already visible – from heatwaves and heavy precipitation to droughts and tropical cyclones. With further warming, these phenomena will become more widespread, with increasing risk of ice sheet collapse or abrupt changes in ocean circulation (IPCC, 2021[18]). The consequences of climate change threaten ecosystems and biodiversity, affect water resources and human settlements, and imply significant impacts on food production, socio-economic activities, economic output and human well-being (OECD, 2021[5]).

Both the contributions to and the consequences of climate change are unevenly distributed. In 2015, an estimated 49% of global carbon emissions were produced by the richest 10% of the world population, with just 7% produced by the poorest 50% (Kartha et al., 2020[19]). The same study estimates that nearly half of the 60% increase in emissions globally between 1990 and 2015 was due to the richest 10% of the population, while the contribution of the poorest half was "practically negligible" (Kartha et al., 2020[19]). Meanwhile, the impacts of environmental degradation are concentrated among vulnerable groups and households (OECD, 2021[20]). For example, climate change is projected to have significant impacts on rural and coastal communities dependent on farming or fisheries, while extreme heat and weather events will particularly affect outdoor workers, who are often low-earners (OECD, 2021[20]). At the same time, heat stress in urban areas is more likely to affect impoverished communities. In the United States, evidence suggests that communities of colour are particularly exposed, due to neighbourhood characteristics such as a lack of tree cover and wide expanses of heat-absorbing concrete (Witze, 2021[21]).

The collapse in economic and social activity caused by the pandemic has led to some temporary reductions in global emissions. While official national estimates of greenhouse gas emissions are not yet available for 2020,[5] global emissions of anthropogenic fossil CO_2 are thought to have reduced by around 7% (with estimates ranging from 5.8% to 13%) (IPCC, 2021[18]). The International Energy Agency (IEA) estimates that total energy-related CO_2 emissions (which account for around two-thirds of all greenhouse gas emissions) fell by 5.8% globally in 2020, the largest annual percentage fall since the Second World War (IEA, 2021[22]). Reductions in energy-related CO_2 emissions were estimated to be largest in advanced economies (almost 10% on average), while emissions from emerging market and developing economies fell by 4% relative to 2019 (IEA, 2021[22]).

Reductions in transport contributed the largest falls in global energy-related CO_2 emissions. Over 50% of the total fall is accounted for by lower oil use in the transport sector (IEA, 2021[22]). For example, emissions from international aviation fell by almost 45% in 2020, and road transport's demand for oil fell 10% relative to 2019. Only one sector was estimated to have increased energy-related CO_2 emissions in 2020: sport utility vehicles (SUVs), whose emissions went up by an estimated 0.5% (IEA, 2021[23]).[6] Energy-related CO_2 emissions in the power sector fell by 3.3% globally, due to the combined impact of reduced electricity demand and increased power generation from renewables, which increased their share of global electricity generation from 27% in 2019 to 29% in 2020 (IEA, 2021[22]).

Figure 11.3. In December 2020, global energy-related CO2 emissions were estimated to be 2.1% higher than in December 2019

Monthly evolution of global energy-related CO_2 emissions, percentage change, 2020 relative to 2019

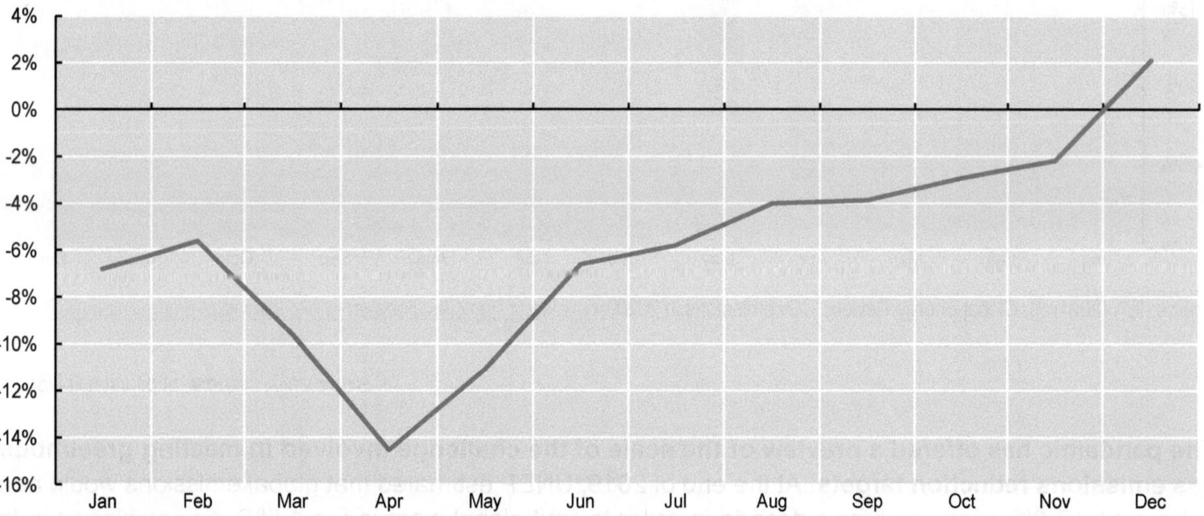

Note: January 2020 energy-related CO2 emissions were lower than in January 2019 due to milder-than-usual weather, which reduced heating needs in major economies (such as the United States, Germany, the United Kingdom and the Russian Federation) by 15-20%.
Source: IEA (2021[22]), Global Energy Review: CO_2 emissions in 2020, www.iea.org/articles/global-energy-review-co2-emissions-in-2020.

StatLink https://stat.link/deuv10

This temporary fall in CO_2 emissions, however, will have little bearing on climate change unless followed up with strong policy action in the recovery (OECD, 2020[24]). 2020 emissions reductions have not prevented an overall rise in atmospheric concentrations of CO_2 in 2020 (IPCC, 2021[18]; NOAA Global Monitoring Laboratory, 2021[25]), and evidence from past crises suggests that a strong rebound in emissions is likely as economic activity picks up (United Nations Environment Programme, 2020[26]; OECD, 2020[24]). Indeed, monthly energy-related CO_2 emissions estimates for 2020 suggest a gradual return to business as usual, with global emissions in December 2020 2.1% higher than in the previous year (Figure 11.3). In the final months of 2020, many advanced economies were entering their second wave of the pandemic and applying new restrictions, yet the impact on energy demand of these second-wave lockdowns was lower than in the first, meaning that many advanced economies were close to reverting to 2019 emissions levels by the end of the year (IEA, 2021[22]). For example, in the European Union, a 10% net reduction in energy-related CO_2 emissions over the course of 2020 was mostly concentrated in the first eight months of the year (Figure 11.4).

Figure 11.4. In the European Union, a 10% net reduction in energy-related CO2 emissions over the course of 2020 was concentrated in the first eight months of the year

Energy-related CO_2 emissions in the European Union, monthly percentage change, 2020 relative to 2019

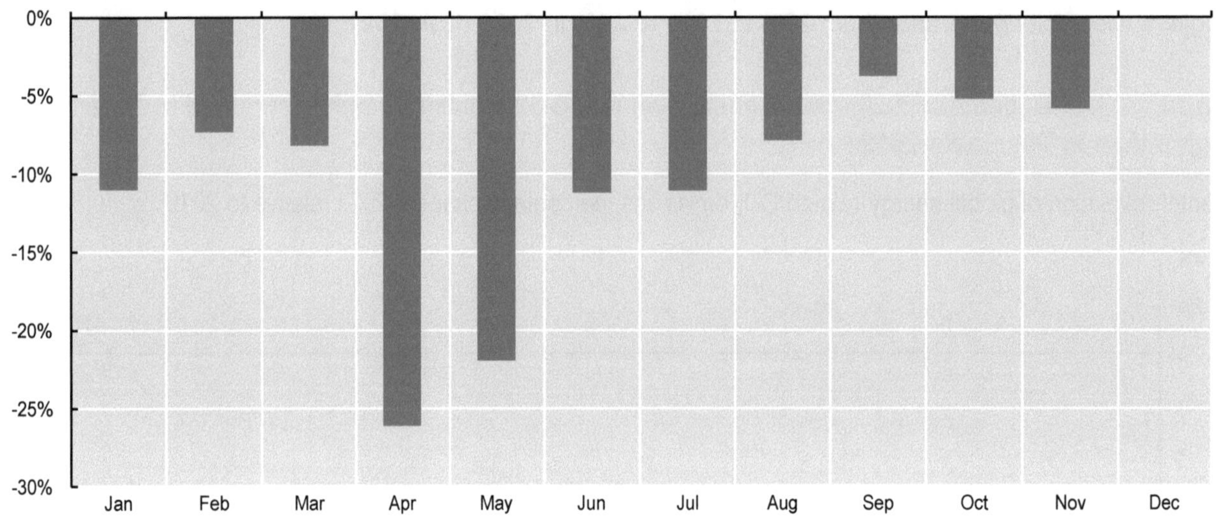

Source: IEA (2021[22]), Global Energy Review: CO_2 emissions in 2020, www.iea.org/articles/global-energy-review-co2-emissions-in-2020.

StatLink https://stat.link/64a0q9

The pandemic has offered a preview of the scale of the challenge involved in meeting greenhouse gas emissions reduction targets. At the end of 2019, UNEP estimated that global emissions would need to be cut by 7.6% every year for a decade in order to limit global warming to 1.5°C, as envisioned in the 2015 Paris agreement (United Nations Environment Programme, 2019[27]). This implies that global emissions reductions of a scale similar to those achieved during the first year of the pandemic would need to be repeated, year-on-year, for a further nine years.

Policy choices made in COVID-19 recovery packages will shape future developments, at a time when both biodiversity loss and climate change are at critical junctures. OECD and key partner governments have so far announced very substantial stimulus and recovery packages, to respond to the consequences of COVID-19 and to reignite economic activity (see Chapter 1). This spending will set the direction for future economic development in OECD countries for years to come, and could do so in a way that will either help or harm biodiversity loss and climate change. Preliminary OECD analysis (from

February 2021) concluded that, across 43 countries,[7] green measures make up a small proportion (17%) of overall stimulus packages – and, within that amount, only 7% of green stimulus supports biodiversity (OECD, 2021[7]). In addition, there is a lack of coherence across this spending – with the volume of stimulus that is deemed to have negative or mixed consequences for the environment set to be at least as large as that which is environmentally-positive (OECD, 2021[7]).

Box 11.1. Further reading

- OECD (2021), *Environment at a Glance Indicators*, OECD Publishing, Paris, https://dx.doi.org/10.1787/ac4b8b89-en
- OECD (2021), "Biodiversity, natural capital and the economy: A policy guide for finance, economic and environment ministers", *OECD Environment Policy Papers*, No. 26, OECD Publishing, Paris, https://doi.org/10.1787/1a1ae114-en
- OECD (2021), *International Programme for Action on Climate*, OECD, Paris, https://www.oecd.org/climate-change/ipac/
- OECD (2021), "The inequalities-environment nexus: Towards a people-centred green transition", *OECD Green Growth Papers*, No. 2021/01, OECD Publishing, Paris, https://doi.org/10.1787/ca9d8479-en
- OECD (2020), "Biodiversity and the economic response to COVID-19: Ensuring a green and resilient recovery", *OECD Policy Responses to Coronavirus (COVID-19)*, OECD Publishing, Paris, https://doi.org/10.1787/d98b5a09-enhttps://www.oecd.org/coronavirus/policy-responses/biodiversity-and-the-economic-response-to-covid-19-ensuring-a-green-and-resilient-recovery-d98b5a09/
- OECD (2019), *Accelerating Climate Action: Refocusing Policies through a Well-being Lens*, OECD Publishing, Paris, https://doi.org/10.1787/2f4c8c9a-en

References

Brondizio, E. et al. (eds.) (2019), *Global assessment report on biodiversity and ecosystem services of the Intergovernmental Science-Policy Platform on Biodiversity and Ecosystem Services*, https://doi.org/10.5281/zenodo.3831673. [11]

Dasgupta, P. (2021), *The Economics of Biodiversity: The Dasgupta Review*, HM Treasury, London, https://www.gov.uk/government/publications/final-report-the-economics-of-biodiversity-the-dasgupta-review. [4]

Daszak, P. et al. (eds.) (2020), *Workshop Report on Biodiversity and Pandemics of the Intergovernmental Platform on Biodiversity and Ecosystem Services*, IPBES Secretariat, Bonn, http://dx.doi.org/10.5281/zenodo.4147317. [1]

ECLAC (2020), *The part played by natural resources in addressing the COVID-19 pandemic in Latin America and the Caribbean | Insights | Economic Commission for Latin America and the Caribbean*, https://www.cepal.org/en/insights/part-played-natural-resources-addressing-covid-19-pandemic-latin-america-and-caribbean?utm_source=CiviCRM&utm_medium=email&utm_campaign=20200914_natural_resources_bulletin_1. [15]

Ellis, E. et al. (2017), "Private property and Mennonites are major drivers of forest cover loss in central Yucatan Peninsula, Mexico", *Land Use Policy*, Vol. 69, pp. 474-484, http://dx.doi.org/10.1016/j.landusepol.2017.09.048. [14]

Gottdenker, N. et al. (2014), "Anthropogenic Land Use Change and Infectious Diseases: A Review of the Evidence", http://dx.doi.org/10.1007/s10393-014-0941-z. [10]

IEA (2021), *Carbon emissions fell across all sectors in 2020 except for one – SUVs*, IEA, Paris, https://www.iea.org/commentaries/carbon-emissions-fell-across-all-sectors-in-2020-except-for-one-suvs. [23]

IEA (2021), *Global Energy Review: CO2 Emissions in 2020*, IEA, Paris, https://www.iea.org/articles/global-energy-review-co2-emissions-in-2020. [22]

IPCC (2021), *Climate Change 2021: The Physical Science Basis. Contribution of Working Group I to the Sixth Assessment Report of the Intergovernmental Panel on Climate Change*, Cambridge University Press, Cambridge, https://www.ipcc.ch/report/ar6/wg1/#FullReport. [18]

Kartha, S. et al. (2020), *The Carbon Inequality Era: An assessment of the global distribution of consumption emissions among individuals from 1990 to 2015 and beyond*, Stockholm Environment Institute and Oxfam International, Oxford, http://dx.doi.org/10.21201/2020.6492. [19]

NOAA Global Monitoring Laboratory (2021), *Can we see a change in the CO2 record because of COVID-19?*, https://gml.noaa.gov/ccgg/covid2.html (accessed on 9 August 2021). [25]

OECD (2021), "Biodiversity, natural capital and the economy: A policy guide for finance, economic and environment ministers", *OECD Environment Policy Papers*, No. 26, OECD Publishing, Paris, https://doi.org/10.1787/1a1ae114-en. [3]

OECD (2021), *Environment at a Glance Indicators*, OECD Publishing, Paris, https://dx.doi.org/10.1787/ac4b8b89-en. [5]

OECD (2021), *International Programme for Action on Climate*, https://www.oecd.org/climate-change/ipac/ (accessed on 10 August 2021). [8]

OECD (2021), "The inequalities-environment nexus: Towards a people-centred green transition", *OECD Green Growth Papers*, No. 2021/1, OECD Publishing, Paris, https://doi.org/10.1787/ca9d8479-en. [20]

OECD (2021), "The OECD Green Recovery Database: Examining the environmental implications of COVID-19 recovery policies", *OECD Policy Responses to Coronavirus (COVID-19)*, OECD Publishing, Paris, https://dx.doi.org/10.1787/47ae0f0d-en. [7]

OECD (2020), "Biodiversity and the economic response to COVID-19: Ensuring a green and resilient recovery", *OECD Policy Responses to Coronavirus (COVID-19)*, OECD Publishing, Paris, https://dx.doi.org/10.1787/d98b5a09-en. [2]

OECD (2020), "COVID-19 and the low-carbon transition: Impacts and possible policy responses", *OECD Policy Responses to Coronavirus (COVID-19)*, OECD Publishing, Paris, https://dx.doi.org/10.1787/749738fc-en. [24]

OECD (2020), *How's Life? 2020: Measuring Well-being*, OECD Publishing, Paris, https://dx.doi.org/10.1787/9870c393-en. [6]

OECD (n.d.), *Environment Statistics Database: Biodiversity*, https://stats.oecd.org/Index.aspx?DataSetCode=PROTECTED_AREAS (accessed on 22 September 2021). [17]

UN DESA (n.d.), *Global SDG Indicator Database, indicator 15.5.1*, https://unstats.un.org/sdgs/indicators/database/ (accessed on 20 September 2021). [16]

UNDP Latin America and the Caribbean (2020), *Lessons from COVID-19 for a Sustainability Agenda in Latin America and the Caribbean*, https://www.latinamerica.undp.org/content/rblac/en/home/library/crisis_prevention_and_recovery/lecciones-del-covid-19-para-una-agenda-de-sostenibilidad-en-amer.html. [12]

United Nations (2020), *The Sustainable Development Goals Report*, https://unstats.un.org/sdgs/report/2020/The-Sustainable-Development-Goals-Report-2020.pdf. [9]

United Nations Environment Programme (2020), *Emissions Gap Report 2020*, UNEP, Nairobi, https://www.unep.org/emissions-gap-report-2020. [26]

United Nations Environment Programme (2019), *Emissions Gap Report 2019. UNEP, Nairobi.*, UNEP, Nairobi, https://www.unep.org/resources/emissions-gap-report-2019. [27]

Walker, W. et al. (2020), "The role of forest conversion, degradation, and disturbance in the carbon dynamics of Amazon indigenous territories and protected areas", *Proceedings of the National Academy of Sciences of the United States of America*, Vol. 117/6, pp. 3015-3025, http://dx.doi.org/10.1073/pnas.1913321117. [13]

Witze, A. (2021), "Racism is magnifying the deadly impact of rising city heat", *Nature*, Vol. 595/7867, http://dx.doi.org/10.1038/d41586-021-01881-4. [21]

Notes

[1] Natural capital concerns both natural assets (e.g. natural land cover, biodiversity) and ecosystems and their services (e.g. oceans, forests, soil and the atmosphere). Alternative terms used to denote natural capital include *nature, the natural environment, the biosphere,* and *the natural world.* In the context of the OECD Well-Being Framework, indicators of natural capital include stocks and flows into and out of these natural systems, as well as risk and resilience factors affecting them. Four elements are examined in different issues of the OECD report *How's Life?*: biological resources and biodiversity, climate change, soil quality and freshwater resources, and waste and materials.

[2] For example, topics such as water and soil quality, and waste and materials – pressures on all of which also interact with biodiversity and climate change.

[3] According to Article 2 of the Convention on Biological Diversity, biodiversity or "biological diversity" means the variability among living organisms from all sources including, inter alia, terrestrial, marine and other aquatic ecosystems and the ecological complexes of which they are part; this includes diversity within species, between species and of ecosystems (https://www.cbd.int/convention/text/).

[4] Aichi Biodiversity Target 11 states: "By 2020, at least 17 per cent of terrestrial and inland water areas and 10 per cent of coastal and marine areas, especially areas of particular importance for biodiversity and ecosystem services, are conserved through effectively and equitably managed, ecologically representative and well-connected systems of protected areas and other effective area-based conservation measures, and integrated into the wider landscape and seascape" (https://www.cbd.int/sp/).

[5] National Inventory Submissions 2020 to the *United Nations Framework Convention on Climate Change* (UNFCCC), combined with replies to the OECD State of the Environment Questionnaire, provide greenhouse gas emissions data up to 2018; 2021 submissions will address the situation up to 2019.

[6] This continues a trend that has seen carbon emissions from SUVs triple globally over the past decade, to a level that is now equivalent to the entire maritime industry, including international shipping (IEA, 2021[23]). By contrast, in advanced economies, all other sectors (including electricity generation, heating of buildings, manufacturing and heavy industry, and other forms of transport) have either stabilised or reduced energy-related CO_2 emissions over the 2010-2020 period.

[7] In addition to the 38 OECD members, 5 OECD key partner countries are included: Brazil, China, India, Indonesia and South Africa.

Printed by Libri Plureos GmbH in Hamburg,
Germany

9 789264 871830